BSAVA Manual of Canine and Feline Infectious Diseases

Editors:

Ian K. Ramsey
BVSc PhD DSAM DipECVIM MRCVS
Department of Veterinary Clinical Studies
University of Glasgow
Bearsden Road
Glasgow G61 1QH

and

Bryn J. Tennant
BVSc PhD CertVR MRCVS
Capital Diagnostics
SAC Veterinary Science Division
Bush Estate
Penicuik
Midlothian EH26 0QE

Published by:

British Small Animal Veterinary Association
Woodrow House, 1 Telford Way,
Waterwells Business Park, Quedgeley,
Gloucester GL2 4AB

A Company Limited by Guarantee in England.
Registered Company No. 2837793.
Registered as a Charity.

Copyright © 2001 BSAVA

All rights reserved. No part of this publication may be reproduced, stored in a retrieval system, or transmitted, in form or by any means, electronic, mechanical, photocopying, recording or otherwise without prior written permission of the copyright holder.

A catalogue record for this book is available from the British Library.

ISBN 0 905214 53 6

The publishers and contributors cannot take responsibility for information provided on dosages and methods of application of drugs mentioned in this publication. Details of this kind must be verified by individual users from the appropriate literature.

Typeset by: Fusion Design, Fordingbridge, Hampshire, UK

Printed by: Lookers, Upton, Poole, Dorset, UK

Other titles in the BSAVA Manuals series:

Manual of Advanced Veterinary Nursing
Manual of Canine and Feline Emergency and Critical Care
Manual of Canine and Feline Gastroenterology
Manual of Canine and Feline Haematology and Transfusion Medicine
Manual of Canine and Feline Nephrology and Urology
Manual of Companion Animal Nutrition and Feeding
Manual of Canine Behaviour
Manual of Exotic Pets
Manual of Feline Behaviour
Manual of Ornamental Fish
Manual of Psittacine Birds
Manual of Rabbit Medicine and Surgery
Manual of Raptors, Pigeons and Waterfowl
Manual of Reptiles
Manual of Small Animal Anaesthesia and Analgesia
Manual of Small Animal Arthrology
Manual of Small Animal Clinical Pathology
Manual of Small Animal Dentistry, 2nd edition
Manual of Small Animal Dermatology
Manual of Small Animal Diagnostic Imaging
Manual of Small Animal Endocrinology, 2nd edition
Manual of Small Animal Fracture Repair and Management
Manual of Small Animal Neurology, 2nd edition
Manual of Small Animal Oncology
Manual of Small Animal Ophthalmology
Manual of Small Animal Reproduction and Neonatology
Manual of Veterinary Care
Manual of Veterinary Nursing

For information on these and all BSAVA publications please visit our website: www.bsava.com

Contents

List of contributors		v
Foreword		vii
Preface		viii
1	**The laboratory diagnosis of infectious diseases** *Diane Addie and Ian Ramsey*	1
2	**Antimicrobial and antiparasitic chemotherapy** *Jonathan Elliott*	19
3	**Vaccination** *Oswald Jarrett and Ian Ramsey*	41
4	**Control of infectious diseases in multi-animal environments** *Danièlle Gunn-Moore*	51
5	**The haemopoietic and lymphoreticular systems** *Ian Ramsey, Danièlle Gunn-Moore and Susan Shaw*	65
6	**The respiratory tract** *Kim Willoughby and Susan Dawson*	89
7	**The cardiovascular system** *Clive Elwood*	117
8	**The alimentary tract** *Bryn Tennant*	129
9	**The peritoneal cavity** *Danièlle Gunn-Moore and Diane Addie*	151
10	**The urinary system** *Bryn Tennant*	167
11	**The liver, pancreas and spleen** *Bryn Tennant*	175
12	**The reproductive tract and neonate** *Gary England*	185
13	**The skin** *Ian Mason, Ross Bond, Danièlle Gunn-Moore and Andrew Sparkes*	197
14	**The musculoskeletal system** *Chris May*	219
15	**The nervous system** *Clare Rusbridge*	231
16	**The eye** *David Gould*	251
Appendices		
	1 *Sending samples by post*	266
	2 *Pet travel outside the UK and Eire*	268
	3 *Drug dosages*	271
Index		279

Contributors

Diane Addie BVMS PhD MRCVS
Department of Veterinary Pathology, University of Glasgow Veterinary School, Bearsden Road, Bearsden, Glasgow G61 1QH

Ross Bond BVMS PhD DVD DipECVD MRCVS
Royal Veterinary College, University of London, Hawkshead Lane, North Mymms, Hatfield, Herts AL9 7TA

Susan Dawson BVMS PhD MRCVS
Department of Veterinary Clinical Science and Animal Husbandry, University of Liverpool, Small Animal Hospital, Crown Street, Liverpool L7 7EX

Jonathan Elliott MA VetMB PhD CertSAC DipECVPT MRCVS
Department of Veterinary Basic Sciences, Royal Veterinary College, University of London, Royal College Street, London NW1 0TU

Clive M. Elwood MA VetMB MSc PhD CertSAC DipACVIM DECVIM MRCVS
Davies White, Unit 5, Manor Farm Business Park, Higham Road, Higham Gobion, Herts SG5 3HR

Professor Gary C.W. England BVetMed PhD DVetMed CertVA DVR DVRep DipECAR DipACT FRCVS
Professor of Veterinary Reproduction, Royal Veterinary College, University of London, Hawkshead Lane, North Mymms, Hatfield, Herts AL9 7TA

David Gould BSc BVM&S PhD DVOphthal MRCVS
University of Bristol, Department of Veterinary Medicine, Langford House, Langford, Bristol BS40 5DU

Danièlle Gunn-Moore BSc BVM&S PhD MACVSc MRCVS
The R(D)SVS Hospital for Small Animals, The University of Edinburgh, Easter Bush Veterinary Centre, Roslin, Midlothian EH25 9RG

Professor Oswald Jarrett BVMS PhD MRCVS FRSE
Department of Veterinary Pathology, University of Glasgow Veterinary School, Bearsden Road, Bearsden, Glasgow G61 1QH

Ian S. Mason BVetMed PhD CertSAD DECVD MRCVS
Veterinary Dermatology Consultants, 2 Kempton Court, Kempton Avenue, Sunbury on Thames, Middx TW16 5PA

Chris May MA VetMB PhD CertSAO MRCVS
Willows Referral Service, 78 Tanworth Lane, Shirley, Solihull B90 4DF

Ian K. Ramsey BVSc PhD DSAM DipECVIM MRCVS
Department of Veterinary Clinical Studies, University of Glasgow Veterinary School, Bearsden Road, Bearsden, Glasgow G61 1QH

Clare Rusbridge BVMS DipECVN MRCVS
Stone Lion Veterinary Centre, 41 High Street, Wimbledon, London SW19 5AU

Susan Shaw BVSc(Hons) MSc DipACVIM FACVSc MRCVS
Department of Veterinary Medicine, University of Bristol, Langford House, Langford, Bristol BS40 5DU

Andrew H. Sparkes BVetMed PhD DipECVIM MRCVS
Department of Clinical Studies, Animal Health Trust, Lanwades Park, Newmarket, Suffolk CB8 7DW

Bryn J. Tennant BVSc PhD CertVR MRCVS
Capital Diagnostics, SAC Veterinary Science Division, Bush Estate, Penicuik, Midlothian EH26 0QE

Kim Willoughby BVMS PhD MRCVS
University of Liverpool, Small Animal Hospital, Crown Street, Liverpool L69 7ZJ

Foreword

Every veterinary surgeon working in small animal practice has to diagnose and treat infectious disease in dogs and cats on a daily basis.

In this new manual the infections described are grouped according to the body system affected, making it much easier for the practitioner to access information quickly when faced with a diagnostic problem. Viral, bacterial, parasitic, fungal and protozoal diseases are all covered and where there are zoonotic implications these are highlighted.

There is information not only on common diseases in the UK but also on exotic diseases. Obviously rabies is described, but most importantly the diagnosis, treatment, prevention and control of diseases that may be imported into the UK following the introduction of the Pet Travel Scheme are also covered.

In-depth microbiological details are not given but modern diagnostic techniques essential in the accurate diagnosis of many conditions are and these will become more significant as expansion of current knowledge occurs.

The Editors and the BSAVA Publishing Manager are to be congratulated on the production of this manual for its clinical and scientific content and for its presentation and layout. They have combined the expertise of all the authors to make this a very fine text.

This excellent new manual in the BSAVA manual series is destined to be a great success as it provides a quick and yet detailed reference for the busy practitioner and is a welcome addition to all practice libraries.

Lynn Turner MA VetMB MRCVS
BSAVA President 2000–2001

Preface

Infectious diseases are amongst the commonest conditions seen in small animal practice. This completely new manual describes diseases of dogs and cats caused by bacteria, fungi, viruses, protozoans and other parasites. The book concentrates on conditions common in the UK such as cat 'flu, infectious diarrhoea and pyoderma, although numerous exotic diseases are also presented. Detailed information is provided on a number of important diseases that may be seen in animals imported into the UK under the Pet Travel Scheme. Other infectious diseases that might be seen in quarantined animals are covered in less depth. Important non-infectious differential diagnoses are noted in the text where appropriate.

A problem-oriented rather than a 'pattern recognition' approach has been adopted. Infections are grouped by the affected body systems rather than by taxonomic classification. Thus, all gastrointestinal viruses, bacteria and parasites are considered in one chapter. When an infectious agent has more than one presentation (e.g. canine distemper virus), the main details of clinical signs, diagnosis, treatment and control and to be found in one chapter. Other chapters contain relevant details for the particular system and the reader is cross-referred to the main chapter. This allows infectious agents from different taxonomic groups but which are associated with similar clinical signs to be grouped together. It is hoped that this approach is more relevant to the busy practitioner.

The Manual does not provide details of microbial structure, replication, molecular biology and post-mortem findings that are not directly important to the practitioner. Modern diagnostic techniques, including molecular biology, are described. In a rapidly advancing field such as molecular biology it is inevitable that techniques will become available which allow new infectious agents to be identified and well known agents to be diagnosed with greater accuracy. These techniques must be carefully scrutinized against accepted standards before they are used on a large scale. There is much still to be learned about the application of these techniques in clinical practice. It is hoped that this book will assist veterinary surgeons in the selection and interpretation of such tests.

We have done our best to ensure that the book is free of errors and omissions, but we would be grateful for any suggestions that readers may have for improvements.

The Editors would like to thank all the authors who gave their time and experience to this project. They would also like to thank Marion Jowett and the staff of BSAVA for their help and hard work. The book is dedicated to the Editors' families in recognition of their love and support.

Ian Ramsey BVSc PhD DSAM DipECVIM MRCVS
Bryn Tennant BVSc PhD CertVR MRCVS

February 2001

CHAPTER ONE

The Laboratory Diagnosis of Infectious Diseases

Diane Addie and Ian Ramsey

CHAPTER PLAN

Introduction
   Choosing a laboratory test
   Sending samples to the laboratory
Virological techniques
   Virus isolation
   Electron microscopy
   Haemagglutination
   Histopathology
Bacteriological techniques
   Direct identification
   Bacterial culture
Mycological techniques
   Direct identification
   Mycological culture
Parasitological techniques
   Ectoparasites: coat brushings, follicular smears, ear swabs, skin scrapes, histopathology, faecal examination
   Endoparasites: faecal smears, flotation techniques, bronchial lavage, blood smears, microfilarial concentration techniques
Serological techniques
   Virus neutralizing antibody testing
   Agar gel immunodiffusion
   Haemagglutination inhibition
   Latex agglutination
   Immunofluorescence
   Immunoblotting
   Enzyme-linked immunosorbent assay
   Rapid immunomigration assay
References and further reading

INTRODUCTION

Choosing a laboratory test

Laboratory tests are the cornerstone of the diagnosis of most infectious diseases. Specific recommendations on which test to use for a particular infection are covered in relevant chapters.

There are no regulatory authorities that govern the provision of veterinary diagnostic services in the UK. To obtain valid results it is essential to use tests validated by the scientific veterinary community. It is the veterinary surgeon's responsibility to ensure that a test is reputable, regardless of whether they are using it directly in a practice laboratory or indirectly through a commercial laboratory. Good commercial laboratories will supply validation data that have been published in peer-reviewed journals such as the *Journal of Small Animal Practice* or in appropriate textbooks. When assessing the value of a test, consideration must be given to its sensitivity, specificity and predictive values. These terms are defined in Figure 1.1.

The decision about whether to send samples to a commercial laboratory or to perform in-house tests depends on several factors, including cost, technical experience and facilities. Many tests must be performed by experienced laboratory staff using specialized equipment. Commercial laboratories offer the advantage that trained technicians are employed with extensive experience in specific assays. Some tests are, however, best performed in the practice, and a well equipped practice laboratory is highly desirable. In-house laboratory tests may provide rapid confirmation of some infectious diseases. All practice laboratories must adhere to strict safety standards (for advice contact the Health and Safety Executive). In-house virus testing kits offer the advantages of both convenience and speed but they should only be used with an awareness of their limitations; no test is either 100% sensitive or 100% specific.

Sending samples to the laboratory

Veterinary practices wishing to submit samples to diagnostic laboratories for bacterial culture should stock both plain swabs and those containing charcoal medium. The latter are required for Gram-negative and anaerobic infections as the organisms die rapidly on a dry swab. Faeces are always preferred to rectal swabs. Bacterial transport media can be stored at room temperature. Viral and chlamydial transport media are kept in the refrigerator and may last up to 6 months. Some viral media can be frozen and will then last for years.

	Test results	
	+	**−**
+	a	b
−	c	d

Definitive assay

$$\text{Sensitivity} = \frac{a}{a+b}$$

$$\text{Specificity} = \frac{d}{c+d}$$

$$\text{Positive predictive value} = \frac{a}{a+c}$$

$$\text{Negative predictive value} = \frac{d}{b+d}$$

Sensitivity
This is a measure of the test's ability to identify diseased animals correctly. The proportion of negative test results that are obtained from sick animals (the 'false negative rate') is inversely related to the sensitivity. The better the sensitivity, the lower the number of false negative results that are encountered. The 'false positive rate' cannot be determined from this measure.

Specificity
This is a measure of the test's ability to identify healthy animals correctly. The proportion of positive results that are obtained from healthy animals (i.e. the 'false positive rate') is inversely related to the specificity. The better the specificity, the lower the number of false positive results. The 'false negative rate' cannot be determined from this measure.

Positive predictive value
This is a measure of the value of a positive test result. Although it is related to the sensitivity, it is also influenced by disease prevalence (which the sensitivity of the test is not) and is therefore a more meaningful measure of the value of a positive test result to a clinician.

Negative predictive value
This is a measure of the value of a negative test result. Although it is related to the specificity, it is also influenced by disease prevalence (which the sensitivity of the test is not) and is therefore a more meaningful measure of the value of a negative test result to a clinician.

Figure 1.1: Terms used in the comparison of laboratory tests. The sensitivity, specificity, and positive and negative predictive values can be calculated for any laboratory test that can be compared against a definitive method such as histopathology. The selection of appropriate control populations is important, as this will affect the values of the predictive values. The letters a, b, c and d refer to the numbers of results in each category. For example, b is the number of negative test results when the definitive assay is positive, i.e. false negative results.

Serum or plasma should be separated from red cells prior to posting in order to eliminate haemolysis as a cause of artefactual biochemical or serological results. Serum is preferred for practically all routine biochemical and serological assays.

Packaging of samples for diagnostic laboratories has come under some scrutiny in recent years. Current Post Office guidelines are presented in Appendix 1.

VIROLOGICAL TECHNIQUES

Virus isolation
Virus isolation is one of the definitive methods of demonstrating the presence of a particular virus. It is widely used for the diagnosis of feline leukaemia virus (FeLV) (Figure 1.2), feline calicivirus (FCV), feline herpesvirus (FHV) and feline poxvirus. It is also used for suspected canine adenovirus (CAV) and canine herpesvirus (CHV) infections; however, other techniques are more commonly used. Virus isolation is a time-consuming expensive technique and is restricted to specialized laboratories. Different viruses require different cell types in which to grow and repeated subcultures may be necessary. Virus isolation should not be attempted by non-specialists. Virus isolation is the technique of choice for detection and culture of unknown viruses or novel strains of known viruses.

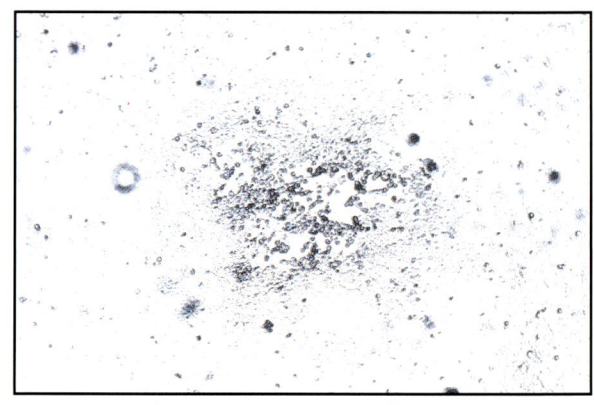

Figure 1.2: Laboratory cells (QN10S) that have been infected with feline leukaemia virus (FeLV). The virus has transformed the cells, resulting in a change in morphology and loss of cells from the plastic on which they are growing. The resulting focus of infection confirms the presence of infectious FeLV in the sample. Other viruses, e.g. feline immunodeficiency virus, do not transform QN10S cells. (Photograph courtesy of Professor Oswald Jarrett.)

Some viruses, such as canine distemper virus and feline coronavirus, are notoriously difficult to isolate in cell culture, and serological tests are more commonly used in these infections. Viruses may not be present in secretions, blood or tissues by the time clinical signs appear or they may not survive outside the host even in transport media.

Electron microscopy

Electron microscopy is a rapid method of identifying families, although not usually individual viruses from their characteristic structures. The availability of equipment is restricted by cost and considerable expertise is required. Another problem is the relative ease with which some viruses can change their morphology. For example, coronaviruses may lose their characteristic club-like projections.

The technique is relatively insensitive as natural infections only sometimes produce the high levels of viral particles needed. One exception to this is poxvirus infection in cats, which produces high concentrations of viral particles that are incorporated into crusts of exudates. Poxvirus infections also produce high concentrations of viral particles in cell cultures, which can also be detected by electron microscopy (Figure 1.3).

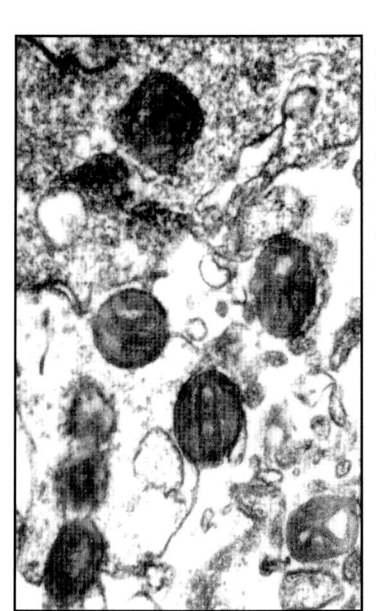

Figure 1.3: Electron micrograph of feline poxvirus from an exudative crust. This is one of the few viruses that replicates in sufficient numbers to allow this technique to be used for routine diagnosis.

Haemagglutination

Some viruses (particularly parvoviruses) cause red blood cells of certain species to agglutinate. The most common example of this phenomenon is the agglutination of porcine red blood cells by canine and feline parvoviruses (CPV and FPV). The haemagglutination (HA) test for these viruses requires considerable experience and a source of fresh pig blood. It is not suitable for in-practice use. This test is relatively insensitive as it requires high concentrations of viral particles. The test is non-specific, but CPV (which causes agglutination at pH 7.2) can be differentiated from FPV (pH 6.4). Haemagglutination inhibition (HI) is a development of haemagglutination and is more specific (see below). The test can be used to confirm the identity of a virus but is more usually used to quantify antiviral antibodies.

Polymerase chain reaction

The polymerase chain reaction (PCR) technique repeatedly amplifies tiny quantities of DNA using a heat-resistant DNA polymerase enzyme to copy from a template DNA/RNA sequence (Figure 1.4). The starting point for this amplification is a short sequence of DNA, called a primer, that binds to a specific region on the DNA of the organism. After each polymerization phase, the reaction mixture is heated to split the DNA strands, thereby providing more templates for further cycles of polymerization. The amplified DNA is then separated from the reaction mixture of nucleotides using a gel matrix and can be detected by a variety of techniques (the most common is a stain that is fluorescent under ultraviolet light). The technique can be adapted for RNA-containing viruses by the prior addition of an enzyme, reverse transcriptase (RT), which results in the making of a DNA 'copy' of the RNA. The principle of RT-PCR is shown in Figure 1.5. The main advantage of this technique is its high sensitivity. In theory, it can detect a single organism, although in practice several hundred are often required. The PCR technique is very specific (providing the primers have been carefully chosen).

The main drawback of PCR is that its sensitivity makes it prone to producing false positive results as a result of sample, primer, enzyme or nucleotide contamination. Whilst laboratories should prevent contamination of their reagents and run appropriate controls to ensure that any contamination is detected, sample contamination may occur within the practice. The high sensitivity leads to problems relating to the interpretation of positive results. Most PCR assays are qualitative although some may be semi-quantitative. Qualitative assays only provide information regarding the presence or absence of an organism. For some infections low numbers of an organism may not be clinically significant and therefore it is easy to overdiagnose an infectious disorder using PCR technology. Another, albeit lesser, problem with the technology is the very high specificity of the technique. Inappropriate choice of primers can result in 'false' negative results. False negative results may also occur in RT-PCRs due to RNA degradation by ubiquitous enzymes. Primers should be generated from known DNA sequences that have been shown to be conserved between different strains of virus isolated from geographically distinct areas over several years.

PCR-based diagnostic tests are now available for a wide variety of infectious organisms including FeLV, FIV, FHV, FCV, FCoV, CPV, *Chlamydophila felis* (formerly *Chlamydia psittaci* var. *felis*) and

4   Manual of Canine and Feline Infectious Diseases

1 Double-stranded DNA is separated by heating

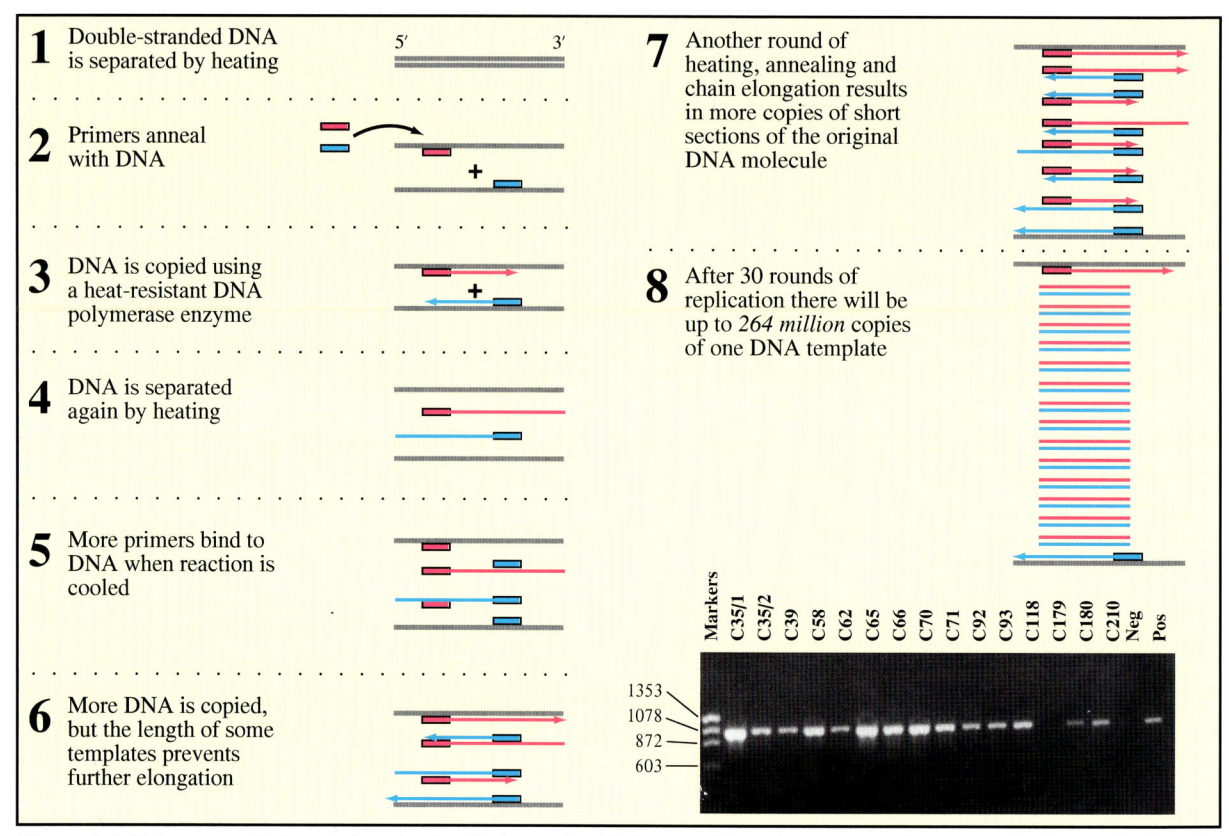

2 Primers anneal with DNA

3 DNA is copied using a heat-resistant DNA polymerase enzyme

4 DNA is separated again by heating

5 More primers bind to DNA when reaction is cooled

6 More DNA is copied, but the length of some templates prevents further elongation

7 Another round of heating, annealing and chain elongation results in more copies of short sections of the original DNA molecule

8 After 30 rounds of replication there will be up to *264 million* copies of one DNA template

Figure 1.4: Polymerase chain reaction. A pair of primers that bind to specific regions on complementary single strands of DNA (produced by heating duplex DNA) are used as the starting point for polymerization. Repeated rounds (20 to 30 times) of separating, binding and polymerization result in an amplification of a specific section of DNA. The resulting reaction mixture is then separated by gel electrophoresis and the DNA in the gels stained (often using a fluorescent compound called ethidium bromide). In the photograph, C35/1 to C210 are test samples, the left hand column contains markers of specified sizes; the far right columns are negative ('Neg') and positive ('Pos') controls. (Photograph courtesy of Mr Michael McDonald.)

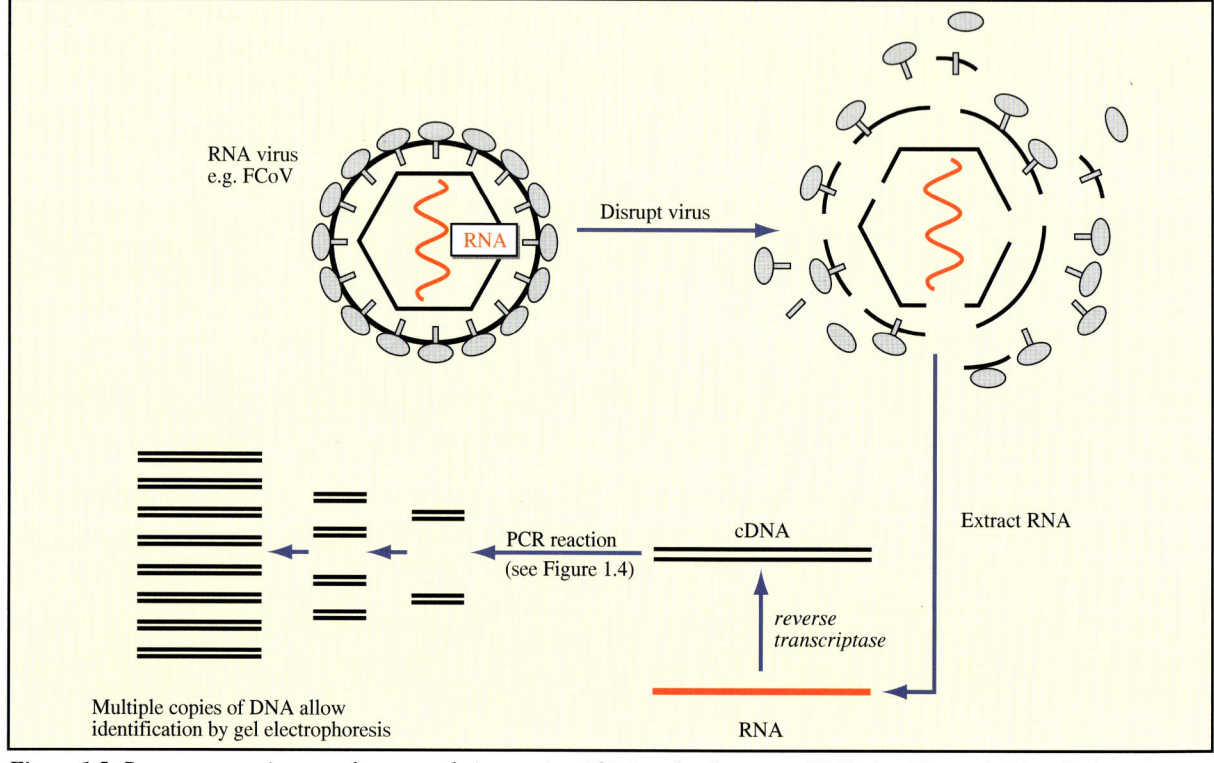

Figure 1.5: Reverse transcriptase polymerase chain reaction. This is a development of PCR (see Figure 1.4) in which an enzyme (reverse transcriptase) converts an RNA template into a single-stranded DNA template. Complementary DNA is then made by a single round of polymerization.

Haemobartonella felis. It is likely that more will become available in the future. The interpretation of results obtained using this technology must always be considered in the light of the clinical information, and a diagnosis should not be made purely on a PCR result.

Histopathology, immunohistochemistry and *in situ* techniques

The value of routine histopathology in the diagnosis of viral diseases should not be overlooked. Many viruses produce characteristic pathological changes and viral inclusion bodies. The main disadvantages of this technique are that suitable biopsies need to be obtained, and interpretation of such material requires time and experienced personnel.

Immunohistochemistry may be used with routine histopathology to detect an infectious organism. The principle of immunohistochemistry is similar to that of immunofluorescence (see below) but it uses fixed tissues rather than cell cultures. Different conjugates and development techniques are also required.

In situ hybridization is used to demonstrate the presence of specific DNA sequences (e.g. viral regulatory genes) within fixed tissues. Such techniques may require special fixatives, and formalin-fixed tissue may not be suitable. There are no examples of such technology being used commercially in the diagnosis of infectious diseases. *In situ* PCR reactions may become more useful in the future, but again their application is currently limited to experimental situations.

Serological methods

There are several serological methods for detecting viruses. These techniques are described later in this chapter.

BACTERIOLOGICAL TECHNIQUES

It is often possible to demonstrate bacteria in stained smears. In most cases, however, a definitive diagnosis cannot be made because the agent cannot be specifically identified on morphological or staining characteristics alone. Culture is necessary for the identification of most bacterial species. Bacterial culture may be performed in a practice laboratory or the sample can be sent to a commercial laboratory. In general, a commercial laboratory is preferred for the following reasons:

- There are many health and safety regulations with regard to the work of the staff performing the test and to the safe disposal of cultured material. In the UK a Category 2 laboratory is required for handling routine samples and a Category 3 laboratory (including a Class 1 safety cabinet) for organisms such as *Mycobacterium* spp. and *Chlamydophila felis* (see McCandlish and Taylor, 1998)

- For many bacteria, an incubator set above room temperature will be necessary. Using incubators of different temperatures may be helpful in differentiating between strains of some species of bacteria (e.g. *Pseudomonas* spp., *Campylobacter* spp.)
- A variety of selective media is required to favour the growth of specific bacteria (e.g. *Streptococcus* spp., *Campylobacter* spp.) by selectively inhibiting the growth of other organisms. Selective media may also allow the rapid identification of specific bacteria (e.g. *Salmonella* spp., *Bordetella* spp., *Streptococcus* spp.). Enrichment media that promote the growth of more fastidious bacteria are also required
- Considerable expertise is required to identify cultured bacteria and to perfom sensitivity testing correctly.

It is important to take samples for bacteriology from areas that are representative of the lesions and to inform the laboratory of the exact sampling site. Such information is essential for the choice of appropriate culture media and for sensitivity testing against antibacterial agents. It is useful to make an impression smear on a glass slide, either directly from a lesion or with a swab. This can then be examined using Gram staining to allow the appropriate culture medium to be chosen. Some organisms, such as *Campylobacter* spp., *Brachyspira* spp., *Helicobacter* spp. and yeasts, can be identified on a Gram-stained smear but cannot be subsequently isolated, either because of their fastidious growth requirements or because other bacteria (e.g. *Proteus* spp.) overgrow the plates.

Direct identification

Dark field microscopy

Most bacteria cannot be identified by direct microscopy; however, it is possible to demonstrate spirochaetes such as *Leptospira* spp. in urine by dark field microscopy. Unfortunately this is only possible within 30 minutes of voiding because changes in urine pH rapidly destroy the organism. Identification of *Leptospira* spp. by this method also requires some experience and the ready availability of a suitable microscope.

Haematological and cytological stains

All haematological and cytological stains will stain bacteria. The most commonly used stains in commercial and practice laboratories are of the Romanowsky type (e.g. modified Wright's, May-Grünwald-Giemsa stain and Leishman's). These stain bacteria a dark blue colour and are particularly useful for the identification of intracellular bacteria and epi-erythrocytic organisms such as *Haemobartonella felis* (see Figure 5.8).

Some practices prefer to use rapid stains such as Diff-Quik®. However, as these tend to stain eukaryotic cells a darker blue colour, it is important to look more carefully for intracellular or epi-erythrocytic bacteria than with conventional cytological stains. Stain precipitate is more of a problem with rapid stains, and such precipitates can easily be mistaken for bacteria by inexperienced individuals.

Gram stain

This is the most important stain used in bacteriology. It relies on a basic para-rosaniline dye (such as crystal violet, methyl violet or a mixture of the two, called gentian violet) reacting with iodine to form an insoluble dark purple compound in the bacterial cell wall. This compound is removed with a decolorizing solvent (such as acetone or alcohol). The rate of decolorizing depends on the character and thickness of the bacterial cell wall. A lighter coloured counterstain is used to demonstrate those organisms that have been decolorized. Gram-positive bacteria resist the decolorizing process and stain dark purple. This resistance is not absolute, and prolonged decolorization will remove the stain. Gram-negative organisms stain pink, together with all other material in a cytological preparation. Cultures and samples containing Gram-positive organisms may contain a proportion of Gram-negative cells, especially if the samples are old.

There are several different protocols published for Gram staining. Only the order of the reagents, the length of decolorization and adequate removal of each reagent are critical (Figure 1.6). Commercial kits for Gram staining are available and the manufacturer's instructions should be followed.

Ziehl–Neelsen stain

The Ziehl–Neelsen (ZN) stain is used to detect acid-fast bacteria. The stain relies on the ability of the cell walls of a few species of bacteria to resist decolorization with strong acids once stained with an aniline dye (such as fuchsin). Such bacterial cell walls are hard to stain in the first instance and so a combination of heat and phenol is used to allow the dye to penetrate the cell wall. The preparation is counterstained with methylene blue to provide contrast with the red stained acid-fast bacilli (Figure 1.7).

The ZN stain is an important stain as the organisms it detects, *Mycobacterium* spp. and some *Nocardia* isolates, are difficult to culture and are also potentially zoonotic. The detection of acid-fast organisms in a cytological smear is always significant.

Method
1. Heat fix the slide by passing it a couple of times over a blue Bunsen flame
2. Flood the slide with 0.5% methyl violet or 1% crystal violet for 1 minute
3. Wash with tap water
4. Flood the slide with 1% Lugol's iodine solution for 1 minute
5. Wash with tap water
6. Flood the slide with 95% alcohol and tilt it gently until no more colour comes out of the smear. This will take 30 seconds or longer. If the smear is very thick, fresh alcohol may be used to hasten the decolorization
7. Wash the slide once with tap water
8. Counterstain with 0.5% basic fuchsin for 30 seconds, 0.1% neutral red for 2 minutes or 0.5% safranine for 10 seconds.

Notes
- Acetone may be used as a decolorizer. It is more rapid than alcohol (about 2 seconds is sufficient) but is more likely to result in excessive decolorization
- Acetone is more harmful than alcohol if splashed on skin or clothes.

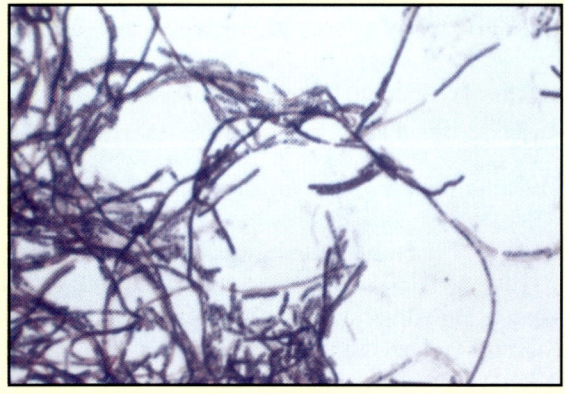

Gram-positive bacilli	Gram-negative cocci

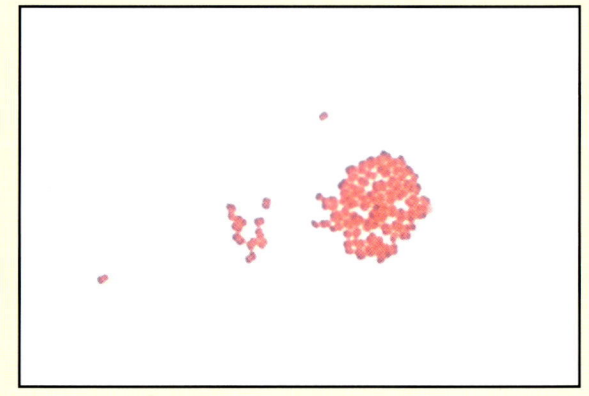

Figure 1.6: Gram staining. (Photographs courtesy of Dr David Taylor.)

Method
1. Flood the slide with 1% carbol fuchsin
2. Heat the slide over a Bunsen flame until steam rises from the solution
3. Keep the slide hot for 5 minutes by periodic reheating
4. Do not allow the solution to dry out. Add more carbol fuschin if required
5. Wash the slide with tap water
6. Flood the slide with 20% sulphuric acid for 5 minutes
7. Wash the slide with tap water
8. Repeat the acid treatment until no more colour comes out of the slide (this will require at least 10 minutes)
9. Flood the slide with 95% alcohol for 2 minutes
10. Wash with tap water
11. Counterstain with Loeffler's methylene blue or 0.1% malachite green for 20 seconds

Notes
- Some of the solutions used in this technique are very corrosive. Safety goggles should always be worn. Use laboratory safety precautions
- Modified ZN staining requires the acid in step 6 to be replaced with 5% sulphuric acid.

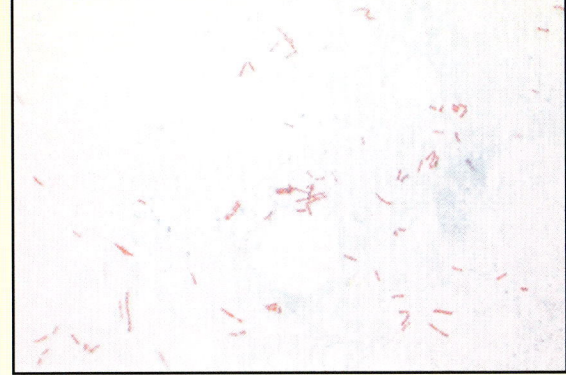

ZN-positive bacilli

Figure 1.7: Ziehl–Neelsen staining. Photograph of Mycobacterium tuberculosis *from a cat is courtesy of Dr David Taylor.*

If *Mycobacterium* spp. infection is suspected on the basis of a ZN stain, then samples should be submitted to an appropriate laboratory with a **clearly visible warning**. It would be prudent to telephone the laboratory prior to dispatching the sample.

Weak acid-fast organisms resist decolorization with 5% sulphuric acid (the modified ZN technique) but not 20% sulphuric acid. Such organisms include *Brucella* spp. and *Nocardia* spp.

Histopathology
Bacterial organisms may be identified on routine histopathology although this only usually provides morphological information (e.g. rods, cocci). Occasionally more precise identification is possible; for example, leptospires in renal biopsy samples, *Helicobacter* spp. in gastric biopsy samples, or *Campylobacter* spp. in colonic biopsy samples.

Bacterial culture
Bacterial isolation is the definitive method of confirming the presence of most species of bacteria. Suitable samples include swabs, fluids, tissues or faeces. Many anticoagulants, including EDTA, heparin and citrate, are bacteriostatic or bactericidal for some bacteria and should be avoided for submitting fluids or blood for culture. A comprehensive list of preferred media, temperature requirements and culture characteristics of various bacteria that infect dogs and cats has been presented by McCandlish and Taylor (1998). The accurate identification of bacteria is best left to specialist bacteriologists.

Bacterial culture is usually accompanied by tests of sensitivity to antibacterial agents. Using a Petri dish, discs impregnated with various antibacterials are placed on top of the inoculated medium. Bacteria are said to be 'sensitive' or 'resistant' depending on the degree of growth around the discs. The limitations of this information and the use of minimum inhibitory concentrations (MICs) as an alternative assessment of a bacterium's sensitivity are discussed in Chapter 2. It is difficult to assess the drug sensitivity of slow-growing bacteria, such as *Campylobacter,* and of many anaerobes using the disc method as the drug contained within the disc diffuses out too quickly compared to the bacterial growth rate. Once one antibacterial agent has diffused into the region of another the test becomes meaningless.

An in-house test system for bacterial culture and sensitivity is available. The value of such kits lies in the speed with which they produce results. The main drawback is the limited culture media that such kits use, resulting in growth of only some bacterial species.

In-house culture is preferable for urease-positive bacteria from gastric biopsy samples.

Blood culture
The culture of organisms directly from blood is a useful technique, but it requires special liquid media and meticulous sampling procedures. Most anticoagulants are bacteriostatic or bactericidal to at least some bacteria, and clotted blood is unsuitable for culture. It is important to note that incubation of the blood must be started as soon as possible after collection. For this reason samples must be inoculated into the liquid

media before they are dispatched to a commercial laboratory. The organisms most likely to be isolated from blood are unlikely to die at room temperature once they are in the media. The presence of antibodies, complement and antibacterial agents in the blood may produce false negative results. Contamination with skin bacteria during the sampling process may give rise to false positive results.

Culture of urease-positive bacteria from gastric biopsy samples

Some bacteria, including *Helicobacter* spp., produce ureases that split urea into ammonia and carbon dioxide. This reaction can be demonstrated by a change in colour of a pH indicator included in the culture medium. If such a reaction is obtained on culture of a gastric biopsy sample obtained endoscopically, it suggests the presence of *Helicobacter* spp. The colour change normally occurs within 2 hours.

Polymerase chain reaction

PCR technology is described earlier in the chapter (see Figure 1.4). Several pathogenic bacteria that are hard to culture have been identified using PCR. One of the best known examples is *Bartonella henselae*, the causative agent of bacillary angiomatosis ('cat scratch' disease) in humans. *Bartonella* can be identified by PCR in blood from cats but takes several weeks to culture. The technique is also routinely used to identify *Chlamydophila felis*, and methods have been described for the demonstration of *Salmonella* spp. and *Campylobacter* spp.

Serological techniques

Serological techniques for detecting bacteria are described later in the chapter. The number of applications is limited. One example of such a technique is the Rose Bengal test for *Brucella canis* that is performed in countries where this infection is endemic.

MYCOLOGICAL TECHNIQUES

Direct identification

Ultraviolet fluorescence

Some dermatophytes fluoresce with an apple-green colour under certain wavelengths of ultraviolet light. Of the fungi commonly seen in dogs and cats, only 50-60% of *Microsporum canis* strains fluoresce; other species do not. The precise nature of the fluorescent material is unknown but it may be an excreted fungal metabolite or an altered substance present in the hair shaft.

Many practices possess a Wood's lamp to examine animals for these fungi; however, it is important that this test is performed properly, in particular:

- The test must be performed in a darkened room
- The Wood's lamp must be allowed to achieve the correct wavelength (i.e. to 'warm up')
- The light should not be shone into animal or human eyes as UV light damages the retina.

Care should also be taken to distinguish true fluorescence associated with dermatophyte infections from the bluish autofluorescence seen with scales and crusts. Positive results from Wood's lamp examination should be confirmed by microscopy and fungal culture. Negative Wood's lamp results do not exclude a diagnosis of dermatophytosis.

Microscopic examination of plucked hairs

Microscopic examination of plucked hairs is useful in the diagnosis of dermatophytosis. Hairs obtained from areas that have fluoresced under Wood's lamp examination are particularly suitable. The hairs are placed on a slide with a drop of 10% potassium hydroxide. A cover slip is then added and the slide left for 30 minutes. Fungal hyphae or spores will be visible microscopically on infected hair shafts. Although specific and rapid, this technique is not very sensitive, and fungal culture should still be used in all cases of suspected dermatophytosis.

Microscopic examination of stained adhesive tape preparations or material obtained by a skin scrape from skin lesions is used in the diagnosis of *Malassezia* infection. The yeast has a characteristic 'peanut'-shaped morphology (see Chapter 13).

Mycological culture

Mycological cultures are used to confirm the presence of various fungi, including dermatophytes, *Malassezia* spp., *Candida albicans* and *Aspergillus fumigatus*. Mycological culture may be performed in a practice laboratory. The following are required:

- Dedicated incubators: fungal cultures that are not incubated correctly produce anomalous results due to temperature variations
- Specialist culture media: unfortunately these do not have long shelf lives
- Experienced personnel: correct identification of fungal cultures can be difficult and examination of macroconidia etc. may be required.

Before a sample of hair for dermatophyte culture is sent to a commercial laboratory it should be ascertained that the laboratory has suitable facilities and personnel to handle the material. Hairs should be plucked from a representative area at the edge of a lesion and submitted inside a labelled paper envelope. The paper envelope should in turn be sealed within a plastic container. Hairs should not be placed directly into plastic as the resulting static electricity will make it difficult to examine the hair.

Some fungi, including dermatophytes, *Candida* spp. and *Aspergillus fumigatus*, are potentially zoonotic, and cultures of these should only be handled by experienced laboratory staff.

Dermatophyte test media

Commercial kits containing media with a pH indicator may be used to culture dermatophytes (Figure 1.8). A small sample of scale and hair should be taken from the suspected area, placed on the medium and covered with the plastic lid. Most kits are stored and cultured at room temperature. It is important to examine the plate daily for change in medium colour and fungal growth.

Dermatophytic colonies are white, whereas saprophytic colonies are brown, greyish or green. Dermatophytes cause the medium to change from yellow to red before or at the same time as fungal growth is visible (usually 2–12 days). Saprophytes cause the colour of the medium to change after the appearance of fungal growth (usually after 12 days). Some dermatophytes are slow growing, and cultures should be maintained for 21 days before they can be considered negative. In addition, *Microsporum* spp. may be differentiated from *Trichophyton* spp. by colony morphology:

- *Microsporum* colonies are white, large and fluffy, similar to cotton wool. The undersurface of the colony is pale yellowish to brownish
- *Trichophyton* colonies are smaller, white to cream in colour and more powdery in appearance. The undersurface of the colony is light brown to brown.

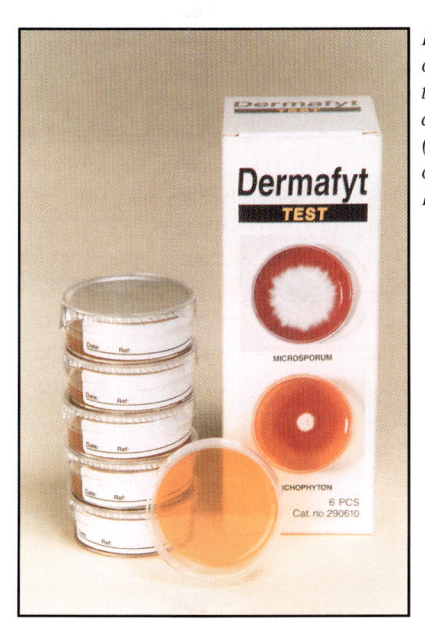

Figure 1.8: A commercial kit for the culture of dermatophytes. (Photograph courtesy of Kruuse UK.)

It is important to confirm that a fungal colony is a dermatophyte even if the colour of the colony and morphology is indicative of a pathogenic species. It is usual to submit such positive culture results to experienced mycologists for identification of the conidia. To examine a colony by microscopy, clear tape should be pressed against the colony, mounted on a slide, stained with lactophenol blue and then examined for macroconidia. If the macroconidia cannot be seen clearly, the first culture should be inoculated on to Sabouraud's agar and recultured before retesting.

- *Microsporum canis* macroconidia are numerous, spindle-shaped and have an uneven, thick wall. The microconidia are fewer in number, club-shaped and smooth
- *Microsporum gypseum* macroconidia are found in large numbers and are cigar-shaped with rounded ends. The microconidia are thin-walled and club-shaped
- *Trichophyton mentagrophytes* macroconidia are only occasionally found. If present, they are cigar-shaped and thin-walled. The microconidia are very round and clustered on branched conidiophores.

PARASITOLOGICAL TECHNIQUES

Ectoparasites

Direct identification

Lice (*Trichodectes canis, Linognathus setosus, Felicola subrostratus*), harvest mites (*Neotrombicula autumnalis*) and fleas (*Ctenocephalides* spp.) can all be directly observed in the coat. The sensitivity of direct examination depends on the colour and density of the coat, the visual acuity of the veterinary surgeon, and the time spent examining the animal. A hand lens is often useful.

Adult lice are easily seen but their eggs are more common. *Trichodectes* (a biting louse) is yellow, whereas *Linognathus* (a sucking louse) is bluish. *Felicola* (a biting louse) is the only louse found on cats. *N. autumnalis* mites are bright orange, usually found in a cluster, and about the size of a pinhead.

Adhesive tape impressions may be used as an aid to direct identification of smaller parasites such as *Cheyletiella*. As fleas spend much of their time off the animal, examination for flea faeces is a more sensitive test than looking for adults.

Coat brushings

A coat brushing is useful for the identification of flea faeces and *Cheyletiella* spp. The technique is described in Chapter 13. Brushing the coat with a new or sterilized toothbrush may be used to gather samples for dermatophyte culture. The toothbrush is placed in direct contact with the dermatophyte culture medium.

Follicular/pustule smears

Follicular/pustule smears are useful for demonstrating *Demodex* spp., which reside in the hair follicle. The technique is described in Chapter 13. Potassium hydroxide can be used to clear the slide but may damage *Demodex* mites and so is not generally recommended.

Ear swabs

Ear swabs are useful for identifying the ear mite *Otodectes cynotis*. Ear wax should be gently removed using a cotton bud, mixed with an equal volume of 5-10% potassium hydroxide on a glass slide and examined immediately. If the first examination is negative, the wax should be re-examined after 20-30 minutes' clearance. The mites are large, with long legs.

Skin scrapes

The technique for performing a skin scrape is described in Chapter 13. Skin scrapes should always be examined within a few hours, and it is highly desirable that the practice laboratory is equipped to allow such examinations. If samples have to be sent away, they should be preserved either in mineral oil or with a small drop of water. Samples should not be stored in potassium hydroxide as the mites will become desiccated.

Histopathology

Demodex spp. and, very occasionally, *Sarcoptes* spp. and *Notoedres* spp. can be identified during examination of skin biopsy samples, although in general this is a poor method of attempting to diagnose these infestations.

Faecal examination

Mites may be ingested and may be found in the faeces of animals with heavy burdens.

Serology

Serological techniques are described later in this chapter. Their main application to ectoparasites has been the development of flea saliva antigen assays.

Endoparasites

Faecal smears

Faecal smears are useful for identifying motile parasites. Smears are commonly made from diarrhoeic or mucoid faecal samples. Faeces that are as fresh as possible should be used. The method is described in Figure 1.9.

Method
1. Place a drop of saline solution on a clean glass slide
2. Collect a rectal sample of faeces using a gloved finger (or touch a gloved finger or swab to a fresh sample already collected)
3. Smear very thinly on a clean slide and cover with a cover slip
4. Use less light than normal on microscopic examination because of the clear colour of most unstained parasites.

Notes
Dried smears may be stained with Ziehl-Neelsen, carbol-fuchsin, or Diff-Quik® stains.

Figure 1.9: Faecal smears.

Unfortunately negative results are inconclusive and it is necessary to perform a concentration technique, such as zinc sulphate flotation or centrifugation, on all samples that show nothing on direct smear examination. Identification of parasitic eggs can be straightforward with appropriate guides (see Chapter 8). Identification of parasitic larvae is more difficult, and an experienced parasitologist or authoritative textbook should be consulted.

Cryptosporidium parvum can be identified using a modified ZN stain (see above); however, a fluorescent technique is also available (Figure 1.10).

Method
1. Fix air-dried faecal smears in ethanol
2. Incubate smears in formalin for 20 minutes at room temperature
3. Stain with phenol/auramine (auramine O 0.03 g, phenol 3.0 g, distilled water 100 ml) for 10 minutes
4. Wash in tap water
5. Decolorize with 1% hydrochloric acid in 70% methylated spirit for 5 minutes
6. Counterstain for 30 seconds with 0.01% Evans blue
7. Examine microscopically under ultraviolet light for fluorescing cryptosporidia.

Figure 1.10: Fluorescent staining of faecal smears for Cryptosporidium parvum.

Flotation techniques

Zinc sulphate: Many intestinal parasites are best diagnosed by the presence of their oocysts and eggs in faeces. Examples include *Giardia* spp., *Ancylostoma* spp., *Toxocara* spp., *Toxascaris leonina*, *Toxoplasma gondii* and *Trichuris vulpis*. In addition some parasites of the respiratory tract produce larvae that are coughed up and swallowed, and are therefore present in faeces, e.g. *Aelurostrongylus abstrusus*, *Angiostrongylus vasorum*.

Flotation methods rely on using a liquid with a specific gravity higher than that of the eggs and larvae. Old solutions that have begun to form crystals are therefore useless and should be discarded.

To perform this test a fresh sample of faeces is mixed well with an equal volume of zinc sulphate solution (33 g $ZnSO_4.7H_2O$ (about 6 or 7 rounded teaspoons) in 100 ml water) and left to stand for 15 minutes. The specific gravity should be between 1.20 and 1.25. Eggs and larvae will rise to the surface, where they can be gently collected on a cover slip which is placed on the surface of the liquid and then removed vertically and placed on a glass slide (Figure 1.11).

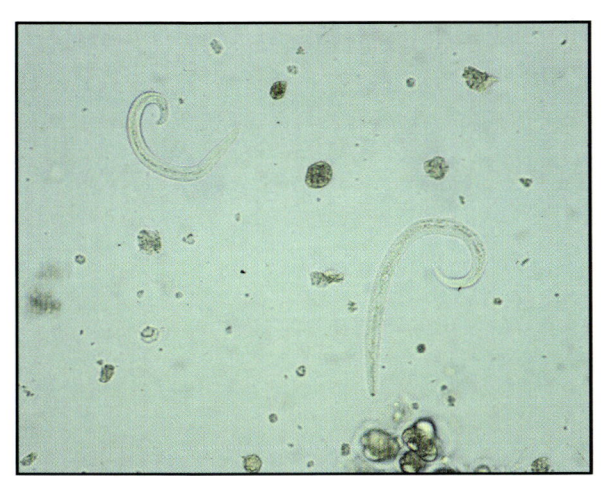

Figure 1.11: Angiostrongylus vasorum *larvae in a zinc sulphate flotation preparation. (Courtesy of Mr Alasdair Hotston-Moore.)*

Sugar: This is easier to obtain than zinc sulphate, but sugar solutions distort *Giardia* cysts and some roundworm eggs. The procedure is as described above. A sucrose solution of specific gravity 1.20–1.25 is made by dissolving 45 g of sucrose in 35 ml of water (gentle heating may be required). Formalin (1 ml) or phenol (0.1 g) can be added as a preservative.

Centrifugation
Centrifugation can be used to concentrate intestinal helminth eggs, larvae, protozoan cysts and coccidian oocysts. These techniques involve mixing faeces with formalin (5–10% solution) and ethyl acetate before centrifugation at 500 *g* for 10 minutes. The parasites will collect at the bottom of the centrifugation tube. Faecal debris and fat will collect at the boundary between the formalin and ethyl acetate. These solutions are harmful and should only be centrifuged in sealed containers. Fixed angle centrifuges cannot be used for these techniques.

Sedimentation of lungworm larvae (Baermann method)
Most lungworm larvae are detected using a sedimentation rather than a flotation technique. Faeces are placed in a sieve with 0.25 mm apertures that is laid on a funnel with a clamped rubber tube attached to the bottom. Water is added until the faeces are immersed. The apparatus is left overnight at room temperature. The clamp is removed the next morning and the first few drops of water examined under a microscope at low power. This technique does not require special solutions but does require appropriate laboratory equipment.

A simple adaptation of this technique is to suspend 10 g of faeces enclosed in gauze in a large beaker filled with lukewarm (tepid) water and leave for at least 6 hours. Any larvae will leave the cold faeces, migrate through the gauze and settle at the bottom of the glass once the water has cooled. After siphoning off most of the supernatant, the sediment is examined under low power.

Endoscopy and bronchial lavage
As the eggs, larvae and adult forms of several of the parasites mentioned below can sometimes be identified in faeces, it is worth submitting a sample prior to performing endoscopy. Faecal analysis is cheaper and less invasive than endoscopy and does not require specialist equipment (see above).

The grey-white nodules produced by *Oslerus osleri* are occasionally seen during endoscopic investigation. Identification of most parasites of the respiratory tree such as *Aelurostrongylus abstrusus*, *Angiostrongylus vasorum* and *O. osleri* is achieved by bronchial lavage. This technique is described in Chapter 6.

Some parasites of the gastrointestinal tract, e.g. *Toxocara canis*, may be seen during routine endoscopy. *Spirocerca lupi* produces nodules in the oesophagus, but this parasite is not endemic in the UK and so infections are confined to imported dogs.

Blood smears
Blood smears may be examined for several blood-borne parasites. It is important that the blood smear is prepared properly and that staining is of a high standard (Figure 1.12). Blood smears should always be prepared immediately after withdrawal of the blood from the animal. Anticoagulants tend to cause artefacts in the interpretation of such smears, and in particular epi-erythrocytic parasites, such as *Haemobartonella felis*, can be dislodged from the surface of red blood cells. Any of several Romanowsky-type stains (e.g. Giemsa, Leishman's) are suitable. Organisms that can be demonstrated by this technique include *Haemobartonella felis*, *H. canis*, *Babesia canis*, *Leishmania infantum*, *Ehrlichia canis* and *Dirofilaria immitis*. Several of these organisms are not endemic in the UK but are occasionally diagnosed in imported dogs.

Haemobartonella felis can also be detected using several nuclear stains. The most widely used of these is acridine orange (Figure 1.13).

Microfilarial concentration techniques
There are several methods available for concentrating blood-borne parasites. The most widely used of these is the modified Knott's test (Figure 1.14).

There are also filter concentration methods, which are available as commercial kits. A negative test result using either method is not reliable as about 25% of dogs infected with heartworm do not have microfilariae in their blood at any given time.

Equipment: 2 ml syringe, 23 gauge needle, several glass slides, one spreader glass slide (made by cutting a small corner off a normal glass slide with a tile or glass cutter), Romanowsky-type stain

Preparing stains:

May–Grünwald
Add 0.3 g of powdered dye to a 200–250 ml flask. Add 100 ml methanol and warm to 50°C. Allow to cool to room temperature and shake several times during the day. After standing 24 hours, filter the solution.

Giemsa
Weigh 1 g of powdered dye and put into a flask. Add 100 ml methanol and warm to 50°C, keep at this temperature for 15 mins with occasional shaking, then filter. It will improve on standing.

Sorensen's buffered water
A 9.1 g/l KH_2PO_4
B 9.5 g/l NA_2HPO_4 or 11.9 g/l $Na_2HPO_4.2H_2O$

To obtain pH 6.8, add 50.8 ml of solution A to 49.2 ml of solution B.

Method
1. Take 1 ml of blood using a 23 gauge needle
2. Put a small drop of blood at the end of each of two glass slides
3. Take a third glass slide and place it end on to the blood drop at an angle of about 45 degrees
4. Draw the slide rapidly but smoothly along the length of the lower slide. Repeat for the second slide
5. Air dry the smears
6. Fix in methanol for 10–20 minutes
7. Transfer to a slide jar containing May-Grünwald's stain freshly diluted with an equal volume of buffered water
8. After 15 minutes, transfer without washing to a jar of Giemsa's stain freshly diluted with 9 volumes of buffered water
9. After 10–15 minutes, transfer slide to a jar of buffered water and rapidly wash in 3 or 4 changes of water
10. Stand undisturbed in water for 2–5 minutes
11. Stand slides upright to dry
12. Rapid staining solutions, such as Diff-Quik®, may be used (according to the manufacturer's instructions) but the results are usually less successful.

Notes
- It is important that the drop is small; thin smears are better than thick smears
- The smaller bore needle helps to control the size of the drop, and damage to the red cells is minimized by a gentle blood sampling technique
- Precipitate from the stain is easy to mistake for epi-erythrocytic parasites such as *Haemobartonella felis* or *H. canis*.

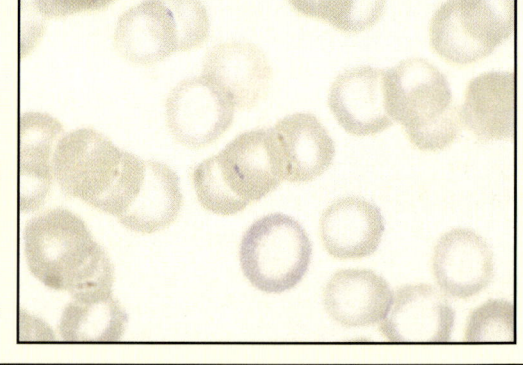

Figure 1.12: Preparing a blood smear. The photograph shows Haemobartonella canis *in a blood smear.*

Method
1. Mix 100 μl of whole blood with 100 ml of freshly diluted 1:20 000 acridine orange in Sorenson's borate buffer, pH 9.0
2. Place a drop of the mixture on a slide that has been cleaned with alcohol and protect with a cover slip
3. Leave in a moist chamber for 5 minutes before examining microscopically under ultraviolet light. Keep the slides away from light until they are examined

OR
1. Flood the air-dried slide with acridine orange solution for 5 minutes
2. Examine microscopically under ultraviolet light.

Small fluorescing inclusions on the surface of red blood cells are positive for *Haemobartonella*.

Figure 1.13: Acridine orange staining for Haemobartonella felis. *An example of the results is shown in Figure 5.8a.*

Method
1. Mix 1 ml of whole blood with 10 ml of 2% formalin for 15 minutes
2. Centrifuge the mixture for 5 minutes at 1500 rpm
3. Discard the supernatant and resuspend the deposit in a drop of 1:1000 methylene blue
4. Place a small drop of the stained mixture on a slide and add a cover slip.

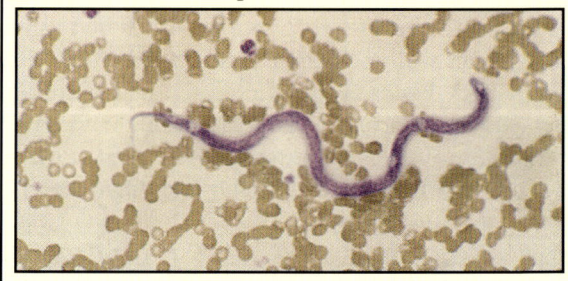

Figure 1.14: The modified Knott's test. The photograph shows the microfilarial form of Dirofilaria immitis. *It can be difficult to distinguish this parasite from the harmless microfilariae of* Dipetalonema reconditum, *and expert advice may be needed. (Photograph courtesy of Dr Susan Shaw.)*

SEROLOGICAL TECHNIQUES

It has become commonplace to attempt to diagnose infectious diseases by demonstrating specific antibody responses to organisms – usually those that are difficult or expensive to identify by other methods. Serology is widely used in population studies, in some screening programmes and in the testing of vaccines.

There are several problems with the use of serology:

- The presence of antibodies may not indicate an active infection but may reflect previous infections
- Antibodies may reflect exposure to a closely related non-pathogenic organism
- Antibody responses take time to develop and so serological tests are less useful in acute infectious diseases
- If using paired samples for serology tests, antibody concentrations may be maximal by the time clinical signs are seen
- Antibody titres may not increase in animals that are immunocompromised.

Most of these factors tend to ensure that the prevalence of seroconversion exceeds the prevalence of clinical disease. **Clinicians should never confuse seroconversion with the demonstration of a pathogenic organism.**

It is important that serological tests use target proteins that are relevant to the disease in question. For example, tests that employ farm animal or human strains of infectious agents that also cause disease in small animals are likely to produce false negative results. Equally, the presence of maternal antibodies can lead to false positive results. In addition to the above caveats, it should be remembered that alterations in test conditions may lead to false negative and false positive results despite the presence (or absence) of appropriate antibody. These can occur either as a result of antibodies being unable to bind to their target proteins or as a result of non-specific antibodies binding to the target proteins.

Paired samples

Classically a 4-fold rise in antibody titre has been taken to indicate active infection with an organism. Unfortunately an appropriate sample taken during the initial period of illness is often not available. Even if an appropriate sample is taken, in some diseases, e.g. parvovirus infections, the rise in antibody level is so rapid that even at the initial presentation the titre is already maximal. Furthermore, animals infected with immunosuppressive viruses, e.g. canine distemper virus, may never show a rise in titre. Testing for specific IgM antibodies may replace paired samples in the future.

Antibody classes

Several tests are now available that detect only the IgM antibodies that are directed against a particular pathogen, e.g. *Toxoplasma gondii*. IgM antibody responses do not usually persist after infection, and therefore a high IgM titre is suggestive of recent infection. The length of time that an IgM response lasts varies between individual animals and the target antigen. For example, anti-*T. gondii* IgM antibodies may persist for 6 weeks in most cats but for 6 months in some. Measuring IgM responses can be difficult, and cross reactions with IgG are a problem.

Virus neutralizing antibody testing

Virus neutralizing antibody (VNA) tests are performed by incubating a serum sample with the virus for a short time then introducing susceptible cells and allowing them to grow. If the virus has been neutralized then no viral plaques will develop. The demonstration of a virus neutralizing capability in serum is one of the most direct ways of confirming the presence of antibodies to the virus. Those antibodies that are detected by VNA testing are an important group because they suggest that the animal is immune to the virus (although this is not the case for some viruses, e.g. FCoV and FIV). The major disadvantage of VNA testing is the handling of live virus and cell cultures. The procedures are usually technically demanding, and the tests may take several days to perform. In many viral infections, antibody titres assessed by other means (e.g. ELISA) have been found to correlate with VNA tests, rendering the latter of academic interest only. For example, anti-parvovirus antibody titres measured by haemagglutination correlate with VNA tests. One exception to this is VNA testing for anti-FeLV antibodies, which does not correlate with other tests.

Agar gel immunodiffusion

Agar gel immunodiffusion is one of the simplest serological techniques. It relies on the passive diffusion of antigen and antibody towards each other. The site of immune complex formation is seen as a white line in the gel. Very high concentrations of antibody and antigen are required for this technique to succeed, and there are few diagnostic tests that rely on this technique. One example is serology for *Aspergillus fumigatus*.

Haemagglutination inhibition

Haemagglutination inhibition (HI) is a development of haemagglutination (see earlier) and is particularly used for the assessment of anti-parvoviral antibody titres. The test is conducted in a similar fashion to the HA test. The serum sample under test is mixed with a known amount of virus and the reduction in haemagglutinating ability of the virus assessed. A titre can be obtained by diluting the serum sample. The principle of HI is illustrated in Figure 1.15.

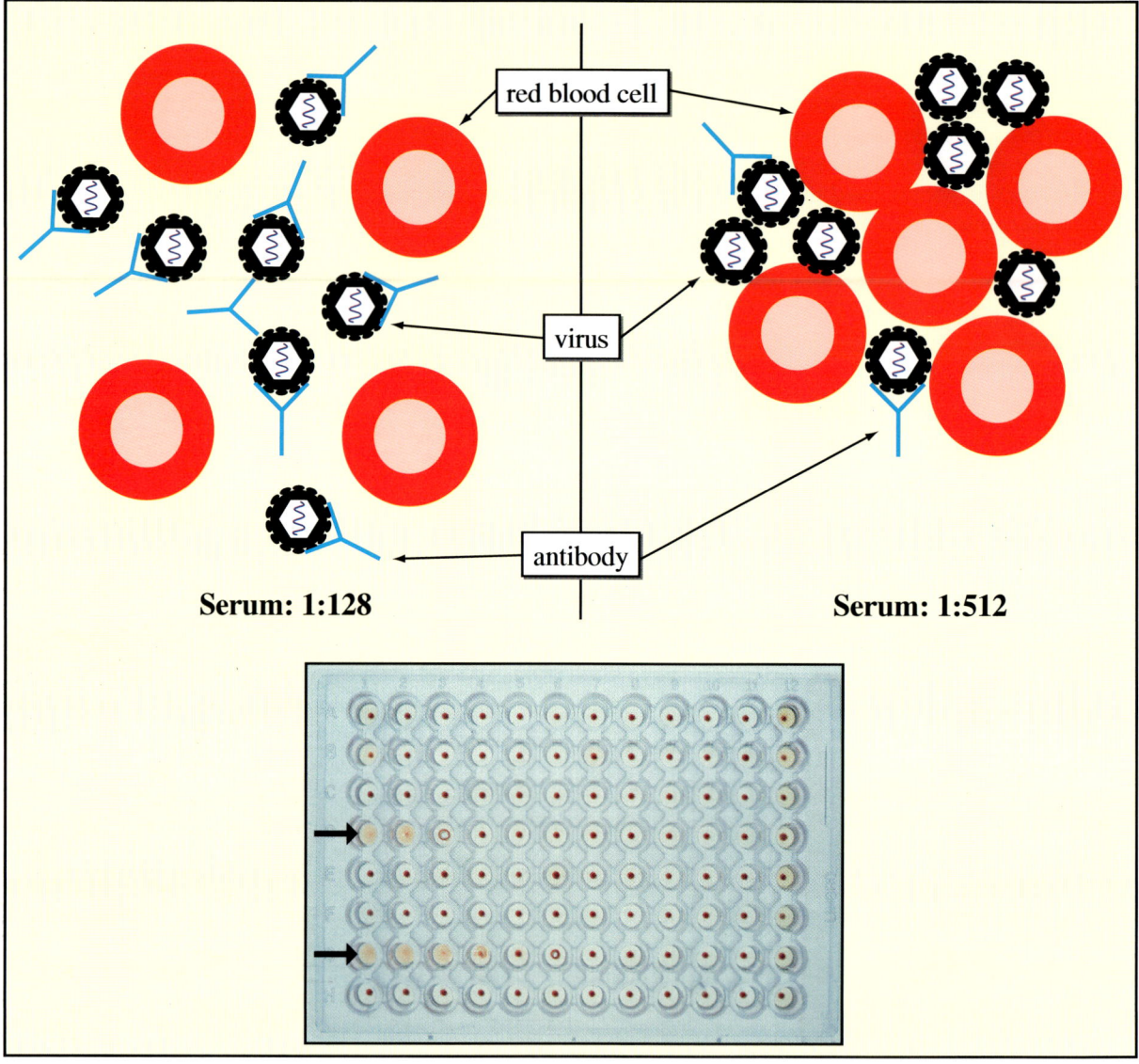

Figure 1.15: *Haemagglutination inhibition test. Virus will normally cause the erythrocytes to agglutinate. The presence of sufficient antibody to the virus interferes with the process. Samples in arrowed rows are positive for antibodies. As the serum is diluted, the concentration of antibody becomes too low to inhibit haemagglutination. The recorded titre is that at which haemagglutination again occurs. The photograph is reproduced from the* Manual of Small Animal Clinical Pathology, *edited by Davidson, Else and Lumsden (1998) and published by BSAVA.*

Latex agglutination

Latex agglutination is analogous to haemagglutination except that the red blood cells are replaced by antigen-coated latex beads. The test is relatively insensitive, and only high concentrations of antibody can be detected. Antibodies against *Toxoplasma gondii* and *Aspergillus fumigatus* are often demonstrated using this technique.

Immunofluorescent antibody assays

Direct immunofluorescent antibody (IFA) testing uses a fluorescein-labelled antibody that binds to target proteins on the surface of a cell and fluoresces under ultraviolet light. Unattached antibodies are washed off before the test is examined. The technique is invaluable for demonstrating infected cells within a tissue.

Indirect IFA may be used to demonstrate the presence of antibodies in a serum sample by using fluorescein-labelled anti-immunoglobulin. Cells infected in the laboratory are used as a target for the serum antibodies. The principle of this test is illustrated in Figure 1.16.

Adequately darkened rooms, microscopes with an ultraviolet light source and cell culture facilities are required for both these tests.

A positive test result is shown by fluorescence of infected but not uninfected cells. Non-specific fluorescence is a common problem with IFA tests, and a mixture of infected and uninfected cells is usually used to reduce the effect of this problem. If all the cells are seen to fluoresce, despite some being uninfected, then clearly a non-specific reaction is occurring that cannot be interpreted. The fluorescence fades with time and in

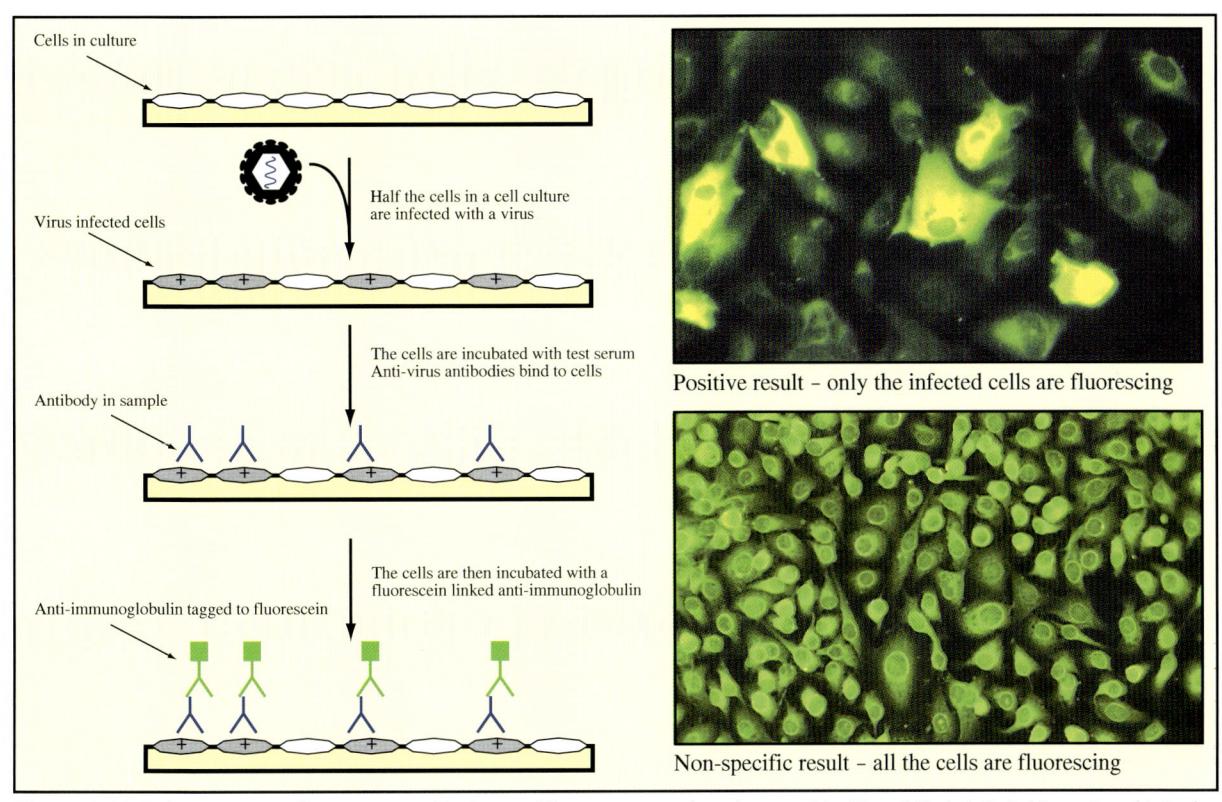

Figure 1.16: Indirect immunofluorescent antibody test. The serum sample to be tested is diluted (1:4, 1:8, 1:16, etc.) and it is the last dilution that still shows fluorescence which is the animal's antibody titre. The uninfected cells provide an internal negative control for every dilution of serum. If all the cells fluoresce then the reaction is non-specific and another test, such as immunoblotting, is necessary. The photograph of non-specific fluorescence is courtesy of Mr Matt Golder.

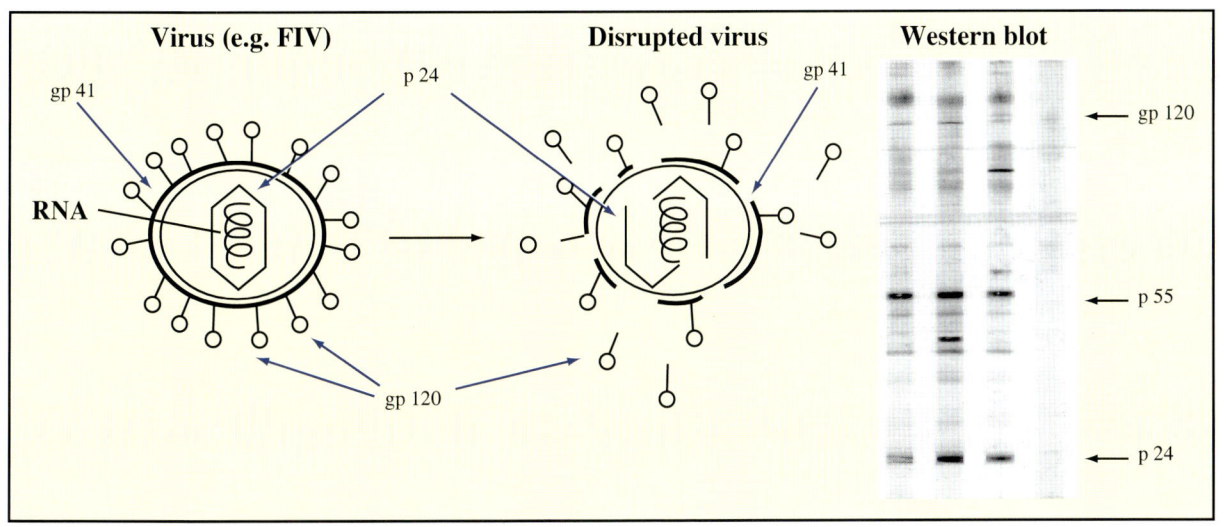

Figure 1.17: Western blotting. To make a Western blot, virus is purified, disrupted, and run down a polyacrylamide gel. In this example, feline immunodeficiency virus is used. The viral proteins are then transferred onto a nitrocellulose membrane and the membrane reacted with antibody. The antibody bands can then be visualized with a special stain. The photograph of the results for FIV is courtesy of Dr Margaret Hosie.

ultraviolet light. Thus, the test cannot be re-examined at a later date but must be repeated. Experienced technicians are required to distinguish true fluorescence from non-specific fluorescence.

Immunoblotting

Immunoblotting (also known as Western blotting) is used to identify not just the binding of antibody to a virus, but also which particular proteins are recognized by the antibodies. The principle of the test is shown in Figure 1.17.

The virus or bacterial proteins are usually denatured with strong detergent to produce long chains of amino acids without higher orders of structure. These chains of amino acids are separated by electrophoresis through a polyacrylamide gel. Once separated the

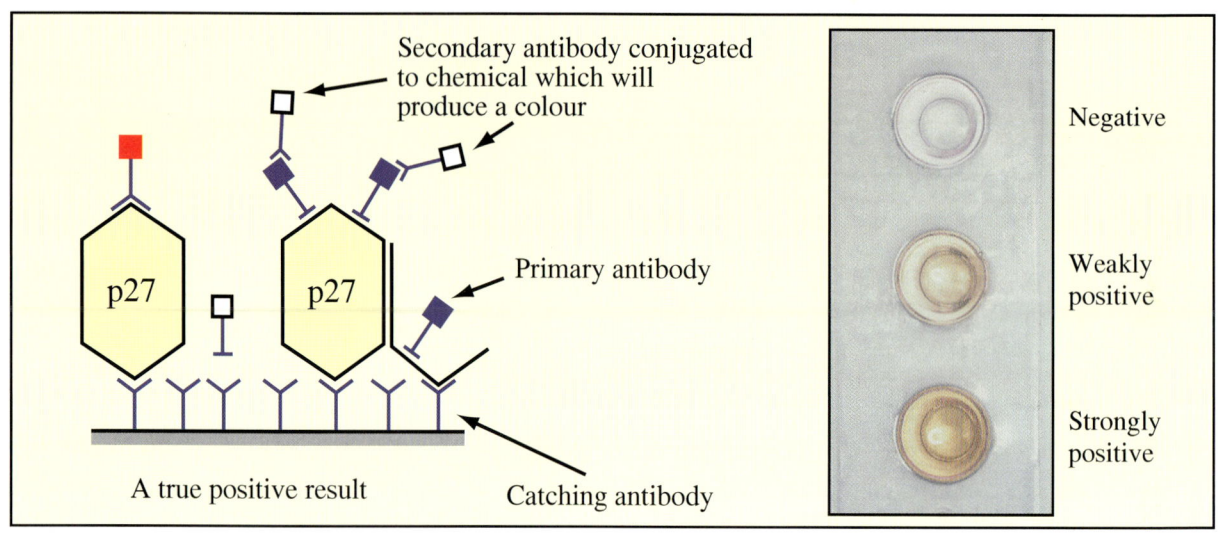

16 Manual of Canine and Feline Infectious Diseases

Figure 1.18: Enzyme-linked immunosorbent assay. In this example, the ELISA is detecting protein p27 of FeLV. The photograph of results is courtesy of Professor Oswald Jarrett.

proteins are transferred on to a nitrocellulose or nylon membrane, which is then immersed in a bath of diluted antibody. The binding of the antibody to the viral proteins is detected by a second enzyme-linked anti-immunoglobulin.

Immunoblotting is time-consuming and expensive. It is rarely necessary for diagnostic purposes unless equivocal results have been obtained with other immunological tests. It is, however, considered to be the definitive test for some infections, the best example of which is FIV.

Enzyme-linked immunosorbent assay

Enzyme-linked immunosorbent assays (ELISAs) are one of the most versatile serological techniques for the diagnosis of infectious diseases and can be adapted equally well to antigen (e.g. FeLV) or antibody (e.g. FIV) detection. The principle of the ELISA is shown in Figure 1.18. It relies on the immobilization of an antigen in a plastic antibody-lined well, which is then detected with a second antibody. An anti-immunoglobulin linked to an enzyme is used to detect the antibody-antigen-antibody complex. There are numerous variations on this theme.

The major advantage of the ELISA is the amplification that is achieved by each enzyme-linked antibody being able to react with many molecules of substrate to produce a coloured product. The technology is generally cheap and reliable and can be adapted for large scale testing. The major disadvantage of the ELISA is that, because reactions happen in the liquid phase, several solutions are required and accurate pipetting is essential. Cross contamination between the wells can have disastrous consequences. For these reasons ELISAs are used mostly in commercial laboratories by experienced technicians. Some ELISAs have been developed for use in practice (e.g. CITE tests). In most cases the solid well has been replaced by a special membrane. As the reactions still occur in the liquid phase it is important not to let the membrane dry out once the test has started.

Rapid immunomigration assay

The rapid immunomigration assay (Figure 1.19) has much in common with the ELISA and CITE. It has proven to be adaptable to the practice situation and is now a popular method for diagnosing many viral diseases or demonstrating seroconversion to causative agents. The assay relies on the binding of antibody-coated colloidal gold or latex particles to viral proteins or serum antibodies (Figure 1.20). The complexes diffuse along a membrane until they cross a line of specific antibodies against the protein under test. The colloid-protein-antibody complexes aggregate along this line and produce a colour change. A control strip is included to ensure that the device has worked and the colloid-protein-antibody complexes have diffused far enough (Figure 1.19). If this control line does not develop, the test is invalid. If this occurs, the sample should be sent to a reference laboratory for further investigation.

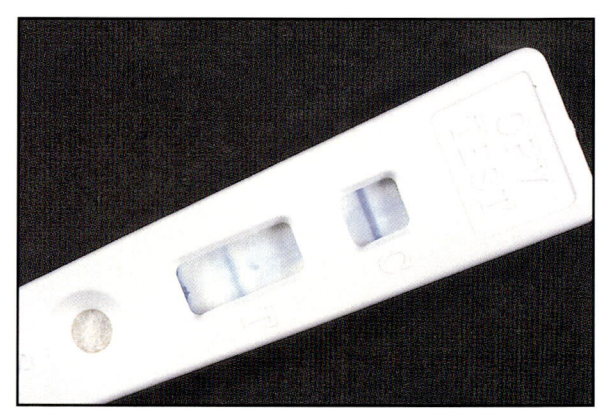

Figure 1.19: An example of a rapid immunomigration test.

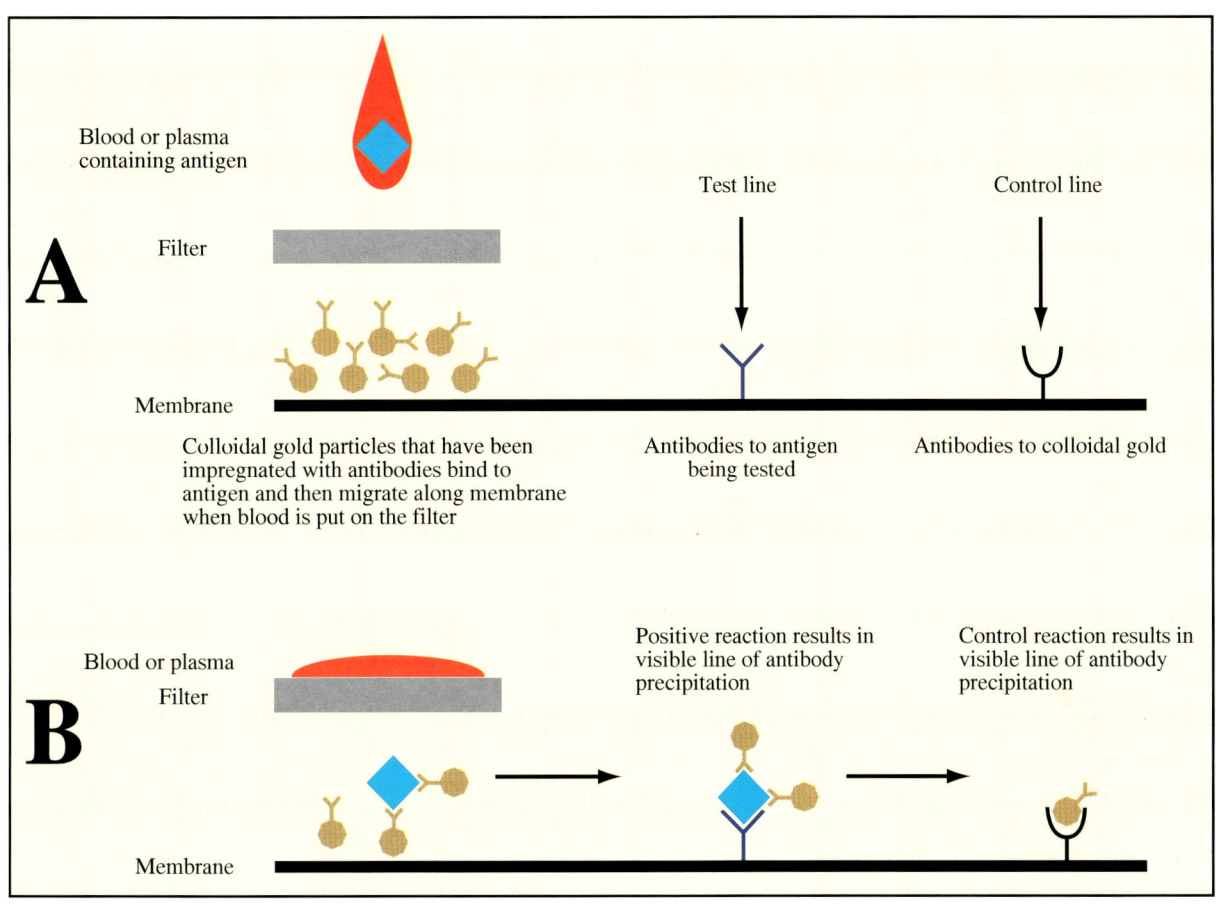

Figure 1.20: The principle of the rapid immunomigration test.

REFERENCES AND FURTHER READING

Lappin MR and Calpin JP (1998) Laboratory diagnosis of protozoal infections. In: *Infectious Diseases of the Dog and Cat, 2nd edn*, ed. CG Greene, pp. 437-441. WB Saunders, Philadelphia

McCandlish IAP and Taylor DJ (1998) Microbiological testing. In: *BSAVA Manual of Small Animal Clinical Pathology*, ed. M Davidson et al., pp. 87-108. BSAVA, Cheltenham

McDonald M, Willett BJ, Jarrett O and Addie DD (1998) A comparison of DNA amplification, isolation and serology for the detection of *Chlamydia psittaci* infection in cats. *Veterinary Record* **143,** 97-101

Meyer DJ, Coles EH and Rich LJ (1992) *Veterinary Laboratory Medicine, Interpretation and Diagnosis*. WB Saunders, Philadelphia

Wade WF and Gaafar SM (1991) Common laboratory procedures for diagnosing parasitism. In: *Diagnostic Parasitology for Veterinary Technicians*, ed. J Colville, pp. 7-50. American Veterinary Publications, California

Waner T, Naveh A, Wudovsky I and Carmichael LE (1996) Assessment of maternal antibody decay and response to canine parvovirus vaccination using a clinic-based enzyme-linked immunosorbent assay. *Journal of Veterinary Diagnostic Investigation* **8,** 427-432

Willard MD, Tvedten H and Turnwald GH (1989) *Small Animal Clinical Diagnosis by Laboratory Methods*. WB Saunders, Philadelphia

Woodward MJ, Swallow C, Kitching A, Dalley C and Sayers AR (1997) Leptospira hardjo serodiagnosis: a comparison of MAT, ELISA and Immunocomb. *Veterinary Record* **141,** 603-604

CHAPTER TWO

Antimicrobial and Antiparasitic Chemotherapy

Jonathan Elliott

CHAPTER PLAN

Introduction
    Mode of action
    Selective toxicity
    Microbial killing and microbial growth inhibition
    Synergistic and antagonistic reactions
    Resistance
Antibacterial drugs
    Spectrum of activity
    Bacterial sensitivity testing
    Combinations
    Pharmacokinetics
        Route of administration and rate of absorption
        Distribution to the site of infection
        Excretion of antibacterial drugs
        Dosing regimens
        Inhibitors of antibacterial drug action
    Adverse effects
        Avoiding adverse reactions: pharmacodynamic considerations
    Selection of resistance in populations of bacteria
Antiviral drugs
    Antiherpes drugs
        Aciclovir (acyclovir)
        Trifluridine
    Antiretroviral drugs
        Zidovudine
        Other antiretroviral drugs
Antifungal drugs
    Therapeutic classification of antifungal drugs
    Antifungal drugs given systemically
Antiparasitic drugs
    Endoparasiticides
        Spectrum of activity and pharmacokinetics
        Toxicity
    Ectoparasiticides
        Spectrum of activity and pharmacokinetics
        Adverse effects
Antiprotozoal drugs
References and further reading

INTRODUCTION

Antimicrobial and antiparasitic drugs are so widely used in small animal practice that it is possible to take these important drugs for granted and become indiscriminate in their use. The logical selection and use of such drugs are important for two reasons:

- The large range of antimicrobial and antiparasitic drugs available in small animal practice creates difficulties in making appropriate choices
- The prescribing practices of veterinary surgeons are under close scrutiny as there are concerns about the emergence of antimicrobial resistance in human pathogens.

Appropriate drug selection can be made by considering three groups of questions:

- **The pathogen**
  - Is the clinical problem caused by a microbial pathogen?
  - What pathogens are likely to be involved?
  - What is the antimicrobial sensitivity of the pathogen?

- **The host**
  - What are the host's natural defences against the pathogen?
  - What barriers within the host may prevent the drug from reaching the pathogen?
  - How will the host in its diseased state handle the drug?

- **The drug**
  - What effect does the drug have on the pathogen?
  - What dose is required, and for how long should the drug be given?
  - What are the side effects of the drug on the host?

The relationships between the host, the pathogen and the drug are summarized by the 'therapeutic triangle' (Figure 2.1).

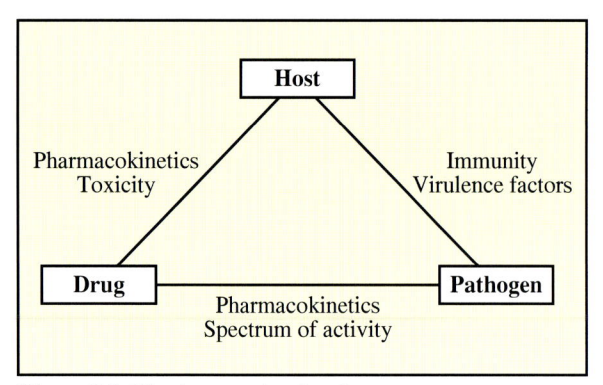

Figure 2.1: The therapeutic triangle.

Mode of action

Understanding the mode of action of an antimicrobial or antiparasitic drug is useful as it provides an explanation for important clinical properties of the drug. The modes of action of the major groups of these drugs are presented in Figures 2.2 to 2.4. The mode of action of a drug predicts:

- The degree of selective toxicity it will achieve
- The effect it will have on the pathogen ('-cidal' versus '-static')
- Whether the drug will interact with another in a synergistic, additive or antagonistic way
- The ease with which resistance occurs.

Selective toxicity

Selective toxicity is the aim of antimicrobial and antiparasitic chemotherapy and relies on the exploitation of a difference between the organism and the mammalian host under treatment. A drug shows complete selective toxicity when, at the concentration of drug achieved in the tissues of the host, the pathogen is damaged but the mammalian host cells remain unaffected. The closer the physiology of the infecting organism resembles that of its host, the more difficult it is to achieve complete selective toxicity. Viruses, for example, use many mammalian enzymes to replicate, and therefore it is difficult to devise strategies that stop them replicating without damaging the host cell they parasitize.

Microbial killing and microbial growth inhibition

The mode of action predicts whether a drug will kill the microbe or parasite ('-cidal') or merely inhibit its growth ('-static'). For example, β-lactam antibacterials cause breakdown of bacterial cell walls and are therefore bactericidal. In contrast, many antibacterial drugs that slow down bacterial protein synthesis are bacteriostatic, stopping cell growth rather than killing the organisms. An exception to this latter group are the aminoglycosides, which cause misreading of the mRNA code, leading to the synthesis of nonsense proteins that cause bacterial cell death.

Drug group	Examples	Mode of action	Effect on bacteria
Penicillins Cephalosporins Glycopeptides	Ampicillin Cephalexin Vancomycin	Inhibition of cell wall synthesis or activation of enzymes disrupting cell walls	Bactericidal
Polymyxins	Polymixin B	Action on cell membrane to alter its permeability leading to loss of intracellular compounds	Bactericidal (fungicidal)
Acetamides Macrolides Lincosamides Fusidic acid	Chloramphenicol Tylosin Clindamycin	Binding to 50S ribosomal subunit causing reversible inhibition of protein synthesis	Bacteriostatic[a]
Aminoglycosides Aminocyclitols Tetracyclines	Streptomycin Spectinomycin Doxycycline	Binding to the 30S subunit causing misreading of the mRNA code or inhibitors of the initiation step of protein synthesis	Bactericidal (aminoglycosides) or bacteriostatic
Fluoroquinolones Rifamycins Nitroimidazoles	Enrofloxacin Rifampicin Metronidazole	Inhibition of enzymes involved in DNA metabolism: e.g. DNA gyrase and DNA-dependent RNA polymerase, or disruption of the DNA template	Bactericidal (all groups)
Sulphonamides Diaminopyrimidines (DHR inhibitors)	Sulphadiazine Trimethoprim	Inhibition of nucleic acid synthesis	Separately bacteriostatic; in combination - bactericidal

Figure 2.2: Modes of action of antibacterial drugs.
DHR = dihydrofolate reductase inhibitors.
[a] *Clindamycin is probably bactericidal to obligate anaerobes.*

Drug group	Examples	Mode of action	Fungicidal or fungistatic
Polyenes	Amphotericin B Nantamycin Nystatin	Bind to ergosterol and disrupt the plasma membrane making it leaky	Fungicidal
Azoles	Clotrimazole Miconazole Enilconazole Ketoconazole Fluconazole Itraconazole	Inhibit cytochrome P_{450} enzymes involved in ergosterol synthesis	Fungistatic
Griseofulvin	–	Binds to the microtubule of fungal cells and disrupts the mitotic spindle apparatus	Fungistatic
Flucytosine	–	Deaminated to 5′-fluorouracil, which is then incorporated into mRNA	Fungicidal at high concentrations (5 × minimum inhibitory concentration)
Allylamines	Terbinafine	Interferes with ergosterol synthesis by inhibiting the fungal enzyme squalene epoxidase. Squalene then accumulates and is toxic to the fungal cell	Fungicidal

Figure 2.3: Modes of action of antifungal drugs.

Drug group	Examples	Mode of action	Consequences
Avermectins/ milbemycins	Selamectin	Opens glycine-operated chloride channels	Causes paralysis of parasite, which leads to its expulsion
Benzimidazoles	Fenbendazole Mebendazole Febental (prodrug)	Binds to tubulin, part of the cellular cytoskeleton Inhibits fumarate reductase	Disrupts the parasite energy metabolism – starves the worms, which are expelled in 2 to 3 days
Dichlorophen		Uncouples oxidative phosphorylation	Kills worms by preventing energy formation
Imidathiazoles	Levamisole	Ganglionic stimulant (cholinometic)	Causes sustained muscle contraction (spastic paralysis) leading to rapid expulsion of the worms
Niclosamide		Inhibits glucose uptake and uncouples oxidative phosphorylation	Kills cestodes by causing accumulation of lactic acid
Nitroscanate		Mechanism of action not well characterized	–
Piperazine		Anticholinergic drug Inhibits succinic acid production	Flaccid paralysis of adult worms leading to their expulsion
Praziquantel		Causes disruption of the parasite's integument	Makes the parasite more permeable to glucose and more susceptible to proteolysis
Tetrahydropyrimidines	Pyrantel	Ganglionic stimulant (cholinomimetic)	Causes spastic paralysis of the worms

*Figure 2.4: Modes of action of antiparasitic drugs. (a) Endoparasites. **(continues overleaf)***

Drug group	Examples	Mode of action	Consequences
Amidines	Amitraz	Stimulates insect octopamine receptors	Increased nervous activity leading to spastic paralysis
Avermectins/ milbemycins	Selamectin[a] Ivermectin	Open glycine-operated chloride channels	Cause paralysis of parasite
Carbamates	Carbaril Propoxur	Reversible cholinesterase inhibitors	Causes spastic paralysis of insects
Chloronicotinyl nitroguanide	Imidacloprid	Binds to and blocks nicotinic receptors in the insect's central nervous system	Causes paralysis and death of the parasite
Insect growth regulators[b] a) juvenile hormone analogues	Methoprene Pyriproxyfen	Mimics the action of juvenile hormone of insects	Disrupts development of larvae so halting life cycle
b) chitin synthesis inhibitors	Lufenuron Cyromazine	Blocks chitin formation	Inhibits development of larvae so disrupting life cycle
Organophosphates	Cythioate Dichlorvos Dimpylate Fenitrothion Phosmet	Irreversible cholinesterase inhibitors	Causes spastic paralysis of insects
Phenylpyrazoles	Fipronil	Blocks the action of the inhibitory transmitter γ-amino butyric acid	Causes rapid death of the invertebrate
Pipronyl butoxide		Inhibits the insect microsomal system	
Pyrethrins and synthetic pyrethroids	Fenvalerate Permethrin Pyrethrin	Sodium channel activators	Cause initial excitement and then paralysis of the parasite

Figure 2.4 continued: Modes of action of antiparasitic drugs. (b) Ectoparasites.
[a] *Selamectin is preferred. Ivermectin is not licensed for use in dogs and cats in the UK and should not be used.*
[b] *These products are a form of environmental control. They should be used with an adulticide initially to control heavy infestations in pets. Methoprene is a component of products that are applied to the environment rather than on the animal.*

Synergistic and antagonistic reactions

Two drugs with differing modes of action may interact synergistically or antagonize each other's effects. Many drug combinations are additive (i.e. the final response is the sum of the two individual responses) but some are synergistic (i.e. the final response exceeds the sum of the individual responses). One example of synergy is the increased penetration of aminoglycosides into Gram-negative organisms when β-lactam antibacterial drugs are also present. In contrast, since aminoglycoside activity depends on the synthesis of nonsense proteins, if another drug that inhibits protein synthesis (e.g. tetracycline) is given as well, then the production of the nonsense proteins will slow down. This will antagonize the effect of the aminoglycoside.

Resistance

Resistance of pathogenic organisms results most readily when an existing protein, essential for the drug's action, can be altered slightly. For example, tetracyclines require a transport protein to enter bacterial cells. Changes in the structure of this protein can prevent it from binding tetracyclines and concentrating them inside the bacterial cell. By contrast, the glycopeptide vancomycin binds to part of the peptidoglycan molecule outside the bacterial cytoplasm. To alter the structure of this macromolecule and prevent vancomycin binding would involve a major change in the bacterial cell's physiology.

ANTIBACTERIAL DRUGS

Antibacterial drugs are one of the most widely used groups of drugs in small animal practice. They are of fundamental importance in the treatment and control of infectious diseases. As such, it is hardly surprising that there is a bewildering range of antibacterial drugs from which to choose for a particular patient. When choosing a drug to treat an infection it is necessary to consider its

- Spectrum of activity
- Pharmacokinetics
- Adverse effects
- Tendency to develop resistance.

Spectrum of activity

The best method of determining the effects of various drugs is to culture bacteria and determine their susceptibility profile in vitro. This approach is not practical for all cases in veterinary practice in which the use of antibacterial drugs is being considered. Appropriate samples may not be accessible, and the organisms may not be easy to culture. In some instances, recognition of the disease suggests the species of bacterium involved and allows the predictability of its susceptibility profile to antibacterial drugs. For example, most cases of superficial pyoderma in the dog are caused by *Staphylococcus intermedius*, which often produces β-lactamase. Simple and inexpensive tests (e.g. Gram-stained smears of exudate) can be undertaken that provide further information where one cannot be certain on clinical grounds. This information may help to determine whether susceptibility testing would be advisable.

It is helpful, for practical drug therapy purposes, to divide antibacterial drugs into categories based on their activity against different groups (Gram-negative aerobes, Gram-positive aerobes and obligate anaerobes). Figure 2.5 provides a summary of information on the spectrum of activity of antibacterial drugs. This figure provides a starting point when deciding which drug might be appropriate for a particular infection. However, it is important to recognize that such a figure is always going to be an oversimplification. Sensitivity testing will be necessary in the clinical situation, particularly for coagulase-positive staphylococci, many Gram-negative Enterobacteriaceae and *Pseudomonas aeruginosa*, whose sensitivities are unpredictable and change due to plasmid-mediated resistance.

The choice of antibacterial drug depends on the site of infection and how well the drug penetrates into that body compartment. For example, tetracyclines are not particularly effective against difficult Gram-negative organisms, such as *P. aeruginosa*, but in cases of urinary tract infection in dogs caused by this organism, members of the tetracycline family are the drugs of choice because such high concentrations are excreted in urine.

In general, drugs that have activity against difficult Gram-negative organisms (e.g. gentamicin, amikacin, tobramycin and the fluoroquinolones) should be reserved for these infections, even though they are active against many species of bacteria.

Figure 2.5 does not reflect the relative efficacy of drugs that act on a particular group. For example, both the aminoglycosides and fluoroquinolones, despite being relatively broad spectrum, are much less effective against streptococcal organisms than are penicillins and cephalosporins.

It should be remembered that although some families of antibacterial drugs share the same antibacterial spectrum of activity (e.g. tetracyclines, sulphonamides, macrolides and lincosamides), members of other families have undergone specific development to increase or change their spectrum of activity (e.g. penicillins, cephalosporins, quinolones and aminoglycosides).

It is important to recognize which organisms are particularly unpredictable in their antibacterial sensitivities. These are summarized in Figure 2.6. If unpredictable organisms could be present then culture and sensitivity testing will be required to determine the most appropriate antibacterial drug. Culture and sensitivity testing are required if an animal has received antibacterial drugs recently (within the past 2 to 3 months) and/or the problem is recurrent.

Bacterial sensitivity testing

There may be wide variation in the sensitivity of organisms to particular antibacterial drugs. Two tests are used for assessing sensitivity in vitro.

Disc sensitivity

This is the traditional method of demonstrating in vitro sensitivity. Discs containing antibacterial drugs are placed on the surface of culture plates that have been previously inoculated with a bacterial strain. The amount of antibacterial drug included in the disc is such that the concentration produced by diffusion in the agar is similar to that which is achieved in plasma following therapeutic doses of the drug. The zone of inhibition of bacterial growth around the disc gives an indication of the sensitivity of the bacterium to the antibacterial drug contained in the disc. The test only provides qualitative information and can be inaccurate. In particular, it is not a suitable method for determining the sensitivity of microaerophilic and slow-growing bacteria.

Dilution test

This method determines the concentration of an antibacterial drug that is required to inhibit the growth of a particular bacterial strain in liquid broth (the minimum inhibitory concentration, MIC). It can also be used to determine the concentration that is required to kill 99.9% of bacteria (minimum bactericidal concentration, MBC). The value of the latter has not been established in clinical practice but the former provides quantitative data on the in vitro susceptibility of a particular bacterial isolate.

Combinations of antibacterial drugs

In some instances it may be necessary to use a combination of antibacterial drugs to treat a particular infection. The reasons for doing this include:

- The combination is more effective than either drug alone
- A very broad spectrum of activity is required (mixed infections; life-threatening infections where the causative organism is not known)
- Combined therapy may decrease toxicity (as lower doses of each drug are required).

24 Manual of Canine and Feline Infectious Diseases

AEROBES AND FACULTATIVE ANAEROBES				SPECIAL ORGANISMS	
Narrow spectrum		Broad spectrum			
Mainly Gram-positive	*Gram-positive plus the fastidious Gram-negative organisms (e.g. Haemophilus, Bordetella etc.)*	*Mainly Gram-negative*	*Many Gram-positive and Gram-negative bacteria*	*Many Gram-positive and Gram-negative bacteria and protozoans (P), rickettsias (R) and Chlamydia (C)*	*Obligate anaerobic bacteria*	*Mycobacteria and mycoplasmas*
Lincosamides[a] Glycopeptides	Natural penicillins[b] **Active versus β-lactamase-producing staphylococci** Isoxazoyl penicillins (e.g. cloxacillin, flucloxacillin) Macrolides[d] Rifampicin[e]	Aminoglycosides (kanamycin, neomycin[c], streptomycin) Nalidixic acid Polymyxins[e]	Aminoglycosides (amikacin[c], gentamicin[c], tobramycin[c]) Aminopenicillins (ampicillin, amoxycillin) Carboxypenicillins[e] (carbenicillin, ticarcillin) (clavulanate potentiation increases spectrum) Cephalosporins (third generation[e]) Trimethoprim Baquiloprim	Chloramphenicol (R, C) Fluoroquinolones[e] (R) Sulphonamides (P, C) Tetracyclines (R, P, C)	Cephalosporins (all) (Cefoxitin) Clindamycin Chloramphenicol Metronidazole Penicillins (all) (Piperacillin) (*Bacteroides fragilis* is resistant to all penicillins except piperacillin and many cephalosporins except cefoxitin)	**Mycobacteria** Rifampicin Streptomycin **Mycoplasmas** Fluoroquinolones[e] Lincosamides Macrolides Tetracyclines

Figure 2.5: Summary of spectrum of activity of antibacterial drugs.
[a] Also very active against obligate anaerobes.
[b] Penicillin G and penicillin V: poor activity against β-lactamase-producing staphylococci.
[c] Antibacterial agents with activity against Pseudomonas aerginosa, which should usually be reserved for treatment of infections by particularly resistant Gram-negative organisms.
[d] Also effective against chlamydial organisms, and some atypical mycobacteria are susceptible to clarithromycin and azithromycin.
[e] Rifampicin also has activity against chlamydias, some protozoans, poxviruses and fungi (not used clinically against the last two).

Predictable	Unpredictable
Obligate anaerobes[a]	Enteric organisms
Actinobacillus spp.	(particularly
Pasteurella spp.	Enterobacteriaceae)
Corynebacterium spp.	*Pseudomonas* spp.
Actinomyces spp.	*Bordetella*
β-haemolytic	*bronchiseptica*
streptococci	Coagulase-positive
Haemophilus spp.	staphylococci[b]

Figure 2.6: Predictability of antibacterial susceptibility of clinically important bacteria.
[a] *Except Bacteroides fragilis.*
[b] *Methicillin-resistant strains can also be seen; these may be resistant to many antibacterials.*

Examples of synergistic combinations include:

- β-lactams and β-lactamase inhibitors that prevent the breakdown of β-lactams by enzymes produced by resistant organisms
- Aminoglycosides and β-lactams, where penetration of the aminoglycosides to their site of action in Gram-negative organisms is enhanced
- Diaminopyrimidines and sulphonamides, where blocking the synthesis of tetrahydrofolate at two different sites in the same pathway produces more than an additive effect. Even if organisms to be treated are resistant to sulphonamides alone, including sulphonamides with trimethoprim or baquiloprim still has a synergistic effect.

In mixed infections, particularly where the causative organisms are not known and the animal to be treated is seriously ill, combinations of drugs are used to enhance the spectrum of activity. There are no drugs currently used in veterinary practice that will provide reliable activity against three major categories of bacteria, namely the Gram-positive aerobes (such as *Staphylococcus*), the Gram-negative aerobes (including *Pseudomonas* and *Klebsiella* spp.) and the obligate anaerobes. Animals with peritonitis secondary to gastrointestinal spillage or febrile neutropenic animals that have received cancer chemotherapy are examples of cases in which extremely broad-spectrum treatment regimens may be necessary. Combinations of two or three different bactericidal drugs would be used in these situations, including:

- Ticarcillin plus clavulanate and a fluoroquinolone or an aminoglycoside
- Amoxycillin plus clavulanate or a second generation cephalosporin and a fluoroquinolone or an aminoglycoside and metronidazole or clindamycin.

It should be remembered that some antibacterial drugs can be antagonistic and so would not be logical to use in combination. For example,

- β-lactams require bacterial cells to be actively dividing if they are to produce a bactericidal effect. If β-lactams were combined with bacteriostatic drugs, they would be ineffective
- Aminoglycosides require nonsense proteins to be synthesized, which then results in the bacterial cell's demise. If combined with another drug that inhibits protein synthesis (e.g. chloramphenicol), this second drug would prevent the bactericidal action of the aminoglycosides.

The toxicity of antibacterial drugs can, in some instances, be reduced by using them in combination. For example, streptomycin and dihydrostreptomycin are used together. Streptomycin is most toxic to the vestibular nerve while dihydrostreptomycin is most toxic to the cochlear nerve. Using the two drugs together at doses below their toxicity thresholds gives additive antibacterial effects but less than additive toxic effects.

Pharmacokinetics

The pharmacokinetic profile of an antibacterial drug is determined by:

- route of administration
- tissue distribution
- metabolism
- excretion.

Knowledge of the pharmacokinetics of antibacterial drugs is important in choosing a drug with the appropriate spectrum of activity that will penetrate to the site of infection. Ideally, having selected the drug based on the sensitivity of the organism and knowing its MIC in vitro, it would be possible to decide from pharmacokinetic studies if the drug would reach sufficient concentration at the site of infection for an adequate proportion of the interdosing interval. Most published pharmacokinetic studies, however, involve measurement of drug concentrations in plasma rather than tissue concentrations. Plasma concentrations depend on the route of administration, the rate of absorption and the rate of clearance. Tissue concentrations also depend on the ability of the drug to cross cell membranes and the fate of the drug in the tissue compartment.

Route of administration and rate of absorption

The route of administration influences the peak plasma concentration achieved following administration of a particular dose. For ease of administration many antibacterial drugs are formulated for oral use. Figure 2.7 details the effect of feeding on oral bioavailability of antibacterial drugs that are absorbed from the gastrointestinal tract.

Recommendation	Drugs or drug groups
Better given on an empty stomach Drug absorption may be impaired by the presence of food Withdraw food for at least 1–2 hours before and 1–2 hours after dosing	Cephalosporins Erythromycin (free base) Erythromycin stearate Lincomycin Most penicillins Most sulphonamides Most tetracyclines[a]
Better given with food Drug availability is improved or gastrointestinal upsets are reduced by dosing with food or after a meal	Doxycycline[b] Erythromycin estolate Erythromycin ethylsuccinate Metronidazole Minocycline Nitrofurantoin
No restriction necessary Can be given before or after feeding	Chloramphenicol Enteric-coated erythromycin formulations Fluoroquinolones[c]

Figure 2.7. Recommendations for timing oral dosing of antibacterial drugs in relation to feeding. Reproduced from Gorman (1999) Canine Medicine and Therapeutics, 4th edn, with the permission of Blackwell Science.
Data from human studies except penicillins and chloramphenicol (see Watson, 1994).
[a] Avoid milk and calcium-rich foods in particular. Antacids will also reduce absorption.
[b] Food may reduce gut irritation without hindering absorption importantly.
[c] Antacids such as magnesium or aluminium hydroxide will reduce absorption; avoid these combinations.

Oral preparations: The oral bioavailability of some drugs is poor, yet they are produced in oral formulations because they are used to treat intestinal infections and are not intended to be used for infections elsewhere. Examples include aminoglycosides and some forms of sulphonamides. Oral bioavailability is affected by food, but quite marked differences exist even between members of the same family of drugs. For example, the bioavailability of ampicillin is markedly reduced by the presence of food whereas the closely related drug amoxycillin is less affected, such that amoxycillin can be given with food.

Injectable preparations: Many antibacterial and some antiparasitic drugs are formulated as slow-release depot preparations for intramuscular or subcutaneous injection. With this type of formulation, although a long duration of effect will be produced by delayed absorption of the drug from the site of administration, the peak plasma concentration (and therefore concentration in the tissues) achieved will be lower than if a different, more rapidly absorbed, formulation were used. There are a number of examples of β-lactam drugs that have been formulated in an oil base to give a depot effect at the site of injection, thereby allowing an increased dosing interval. However, as these drugs are often excreted very rapidly from the body, peak plasma concentrations are lower than for non-depot formulations. Depot preparations are only effective against highly susceptible organisms.

There are relatively few intravenous preparations of antibacterial drugs that are authorized for use in small animals; several human preparations are available for use when indicated. Peak plasma concentrations are relatively high when compared with other formulations. Dosing intervals need to be reduced when compared with oral and depot injectable preparations.

Distribution to the site of infection
The tissue distribution of a drug depends on its physico-chemical properties (Figure 2.8).

Extracellular fluid: Treating infections that are present in extracellular fluid (ECF) only requires the drug to pass from the bloodstream into the fluid. As most antibacterial drugs are relatively small molecules this does not represent a major problem. Even drugs that are highly plasma protein-bound pass into ECF by binding to tissue proteins and inflammatory exudate, thereby maintaining the concentration gradient of the free drug. The major limiting factor is the blood supply to the area of infection. Ancillary measures, such as surgical debridement, are essential to ensure successful management of infections that have a poor blood supply.

There are some drugs that bind to particular tissues where it may be claimed that they are selectively concentrated within that tissue. Examples include tetracyclines, which bind to bone, and aminoglycosides, which bind to kidney tissues. The firm binding of these drugs to tissue components, however, does not provide more free drug molecules needed to interact with

Polar (hydrophilic) drugs of low lipophilicity		Drugs of moderate to high lipophilicity			Highly lipophilic molecules with low ionization
Acids	Bases	Weak acids	Weak bases	Amphoteric	
β-lactams Penicillins Ampicillin Amoxycillin Carbenicillin Isoxazolypenicillins[a] Penicillin G and V Piperacillin Ticarcillin Cephalosporins (all groups) β-lactamase inhibitors Clavulanate	Polymyxins Polymyxin B Polymyxin E (colistin) Aminoglycosides Amikacin Dihydrostreptomycin Gentamicin Kanamycin Neomycin Streptomycin Tobramycin Spectinomycin	Sulphonamides Sulphadiazine Sulphadimethoxine Sulphadoxine Sulphafurazole Sulphamethazine Sulphamethoxazole Sulphathiazole	Diaminopyrimidines Baquiloprim Ormetoprim Trimethoprim Lincosamides Clindamycin Lincomycin Macrolides Clarithromycin Azithromycin Erythromycin Spiramycin Tylosin	Tetracyclines Chlortetracycline Oxytetracycline Tetracycline	Fluoroquinolones Danofloxacin Difloxacin Enrofloxacin Marbofloxacin Lipophilic tetracyclines Minocycline Doxycycline Miscellaneous drugs Chloramphenicol Florphenicol Metronidazole Rifampicin
Do not readily penetrate 'natural body barriers' so that effective concentrations in cerebrospinal fluid, milk and other transcellular fluids will not always be achieved. Adequate concentrations may be achieved in joints and pleural and peritoneal fluids where the barrier to penetration is lower (Penetration may be assisted by acute inflammation)		Cross cellular barriers more readily than polar molecules so enter transcellular fluids to a greater extent Weak bases will be ion trapped (concentrated) in fluids that are more acidic than plasma, e.g. prostatic fluid, milk, intracellular fluid if lipophilic enough to penetrate (e.g.erythromycin) Penetration into cerebrospinal fluid and ocular fluids is affected by plasma-protein binding as well as lipophilicity; sulphonamides and diaminopyrimidines penetrate effectively whereas macrolides, lincosamides and tetracyclines do not			Cross cellular barriers very readily Penetrate into difficult transcellular fluids such as prostatic fluid and bronchial secretions All penetrate into intracellular fluids All penetrate into cerebrospinal fluid except tetracyclines and rifampicin

Figure 2.8: Physicochemical properties and effects on tissue distribution of antibacterial drugs. Reproduced from Gorman (1999) Canine Medicine and Therapeutics, 4th edn, with the permission of Blackwell Science.
[a] *Cloxacillin, oxacillin and flucloxacillin are highly plasma-protein bound (>95%) in the dog; higher dose rates are required than in humans.*

bacteria at these sites and, therefore, such properties are of dubious advantage. Some drugs do seem to have an ability to concentrate inside macrophages and so are delivered to the sites of infection when the inflammatory cells are recruited into infected tissue. Examples of such drugs include the macrolides and the fluoroquinolones, where intracellular concentrations can reach 20 to 30 times those found in ECF.

Transcellular fluids: Some sites of infection in the body are not simply in ECF but are in so-called transcellular fluids of the body. In these circumstances, the drug has to cross another epithelial or mesothelial cell layer to reach the site of infection. Penetration into transcellular fluids depends on lipid solubility of the drug and the barrier caused by the epithelial/mesothelial layer lining the compartment. The presence of inflammation alters the permeability of epithelial/mesothelial barriers. Transcellular fluids include (in approximate order of increasing difficulty of penetration of the barrier by drugs):

- Urine
- Peritoneal, pleural and joint fluids
- Bile and gastrointestinal secretions
- Bronchial secretions
- Prostatic fluid; milk
- Cerebrospinal fluid; ocular fluids.

Only the most lipophilic drugs cross the normal blood–brain barrier and enter ocular fluids following systemic administration. Distribution to urine and bile are considered in Excretion of antibacterial drugs, below.

Milk and prostatic fluid tend to be more acidic than plasma, and drugs that are weak bases will be concentrated within these fluids via a process called ion trapping. The uncharged lipophilic molecule diffuses across the secretory epithelial membrane and, on exposure to the lower pH of the transcellular fluid, becomes protonated and therefore charged, so preventing back diffusion of the molecule out of the transcellular fluid and favouring the concentration gradient for further diffusion of uncharged molecules into that compartment.

It is relatively easy for drugs to penetrate pleural, peritoneal and joint fluids as the mesothelial cells lining these body cavities do not have tight junctions between them. Many antibacterial drugs, unless extensively bound to plasma proteins, penetrate into these fluids.

Excretion of antibacterial drugs

Figure 2.9 summarizes the routes of metabolism and excretion of the commonly used antibacterial drugs. Drugs that are eliminated unchanged into urine or bile would be logical choices for treatment of urinary tract or biliary tract infections.

URINARY EXCRETION[a]			BILIARY EXCRETION OF UNCHANGED DRUG
Hepatic metabolism important for elimination of drug	Urinary excretion of the unchanged drug is the important route of elimination		
Filtration plus good/fair reabsorption	*Filtration plus little/ no reabsorption*	*Filtration plus active secretion in proximal convoluted tubule*	*Secreted in bile and generally undergo enterohepatic circulation*
Chloramphenicol Florphenicol Diaminopyrimidines (especially in alkaline urine) e.g. baquiloprim, ormetoprim, trimethoprim Lincosamides Macrolides (especially in alkaline urine) Metronidazole Sulphonamides (especially in acidic urine) e.g. sulphadimethoxine, sulphadoxine Tetracyclines e.g. doxycycline, minocycline	Aminoglycosides Polymyxins Tetracyclines e.g. oxytetracycline, tetracycline	Cephalosporins (most) Fluoroquinolones Penicillins (all groups) Sulphonamides (short-acting drugs) e.g. sulphadiazine, sulphadimidine, sulphafurazole, sulphamethoxazole, sulphathiazole	Cefoperazone Chloramphenicol[b] Fluoroquinolones Lincosamides Macrolides Rifampicin Tetracyclines (except minocycline)

Figure 2.9: Important routes of excretion of antibacterial drugs. Reproduced from Gorman (1999) Canine Medicine and Therapeutics, 4th edn, with the permission of Blackwell Science.
[a] *Even drugs that are reabsorbed following filtration may still reach urinary concentrations adequate to treat urinary tract infections (e.g. trimethoprim and baquiloprim).*
[b] *Glucuronides of chloramphenicol can be hydrolysed in the gut and the active drug absorbed from the intestine.*

Urine: Urine is a special example of a transcellular fluid. Urinary excretion is a major route of drug elimination from the body. Many hydrophilic drugs are excreted unchanged in urine and so are active against uropathogens. As the kidney reabsorbs most of the water from the glomerular filtrate, if a drug is filtered but not reabsorbed to any great extent, the urine to plasma concentration ratio for that drug will be 100 to 1 (e.g. aminoglycosides and water-soluble tetracyclines). Even lipophilic drugs, which are reabsorbed to a greater extent, will achieve higher concentrations in urine than in plasma, depending on the pH of the urine formed (e.g. baquiloprim, sulphadoxine and macrolides). In some cases, this is sufficient to make these drugs very effective against urinary tract infections (e.g. potentiated sulphonamides). Other drugs are actively secreted into urine and, if they are hydrophilic and not reabsorbed to any extent, can achieve urine to plasma concentration ratios as high as 300 to 1 (e.g. all penicillins, many cephalosporins and short-acting sulphonamides such as sulphadiazine). This makes these drugs extremely effective against urinary tract infections. Fluoroquinolones occupy an intermediate position, being actively secreted, undergoing re-absorption to a certain extent, but still reaching highly effective concentrations in urine.

Bile: Certain drugs are actively secreted into bile as a means of eliminating them from the body. In some cases these drugs are altered metabolically (conjugated) to make them more water soluble, but these conjugates can be broken down within the intestine, releasing the active drug, which can then be absorbed again into the portal circulation. This process is called enterohepatic recycling and can occur with chloramphenicol, macrolides, lincosamides and the water-soluble tetracyclines. Other drugs that are secreted in bile include the fluoroquinolones, aminopenicillins and some cephalosporins (cefoperazone in particular).

Dosing regimens

Bacteriostatic drugs: It seems sensible to devise dosing regimens for bacteriostatic drugs such that the drug concentration at the site of infection remains above the MIC throughout the interdosing interval. This would prevent bacteria from multiplying before the next dose was given; however, this is probably an oversimplification of the situation in vivo because antibacterial drugs do have some effects below MIC concentrations, which can help the host to eliminate the infection. Nevertheless, this concept is one that is applied in determining dosing regimens to be used clinically.

Bactericidal drugs: Determining dosing regimens for bactericidal drugs is more complex as there seem to be two groups that are distinguished by their killing mechanisms:

- Time-dependent killers: these behave very much like the bacteriostatic drugs. They kill the bacteria provided a threshold concentration is achieved and maintained throughout the interdosing interval. The longer the bacteria are exposed to this threshold concentration, the more effective the drug proves. Increasing the concentration much above the threshold has little therapeutic advantage. Drugs that operate time-dependent killing include the β-lactam group (penicillins and ccphalosporins)
- Concentration-dependent killers: the higher the concentration of these drugs that the bacterium is exposed to, the more effective the drug is at killing the organism. Much can be gained by achieving very high concentrations for short periods of time rather than attempting to maintain the drug concentration above a certain threshold for the entire interdosing interval. These drugs are said to produce a marked 'post-antibacterial effect'. Examples of drugs that operate in this way are the aminoglycosides and, to a certain extent, the fluoroquinolones. Pulse dosing regimens of these drugs can be used successfully in the clinical situation.

Inhibitors of antibacterial drug action

The ideal way of determining which antibacterial drug to use is to look at MIC data from in vitro tests and to marry this with pharmacokinetic data where the drug concentration at the site of infection can be predicted. However, there are several factors that influence the action of certain antibacterial drugs at the site of infection and therefore the outcome of the treatment. Examples of these include:

- Purulent material binds and inactivates certain drugs, such as sulphonamides and aminoglycosides. Drainage of purulent material will be essential to aid bacterial therapy in many situations
- Lowered pH and oxygen tension can inhibit the activity of several antibacterial drugs. The lethal action of β-lactams depends on the autolytic enzyme activity in bacteria, which is impaired under acidic conditions. A low pH also substantially reduces the activity of aminoglycosides, erythromycin and fluoroquinolones
- A foreign body at an infected site reduces the likelihood of effective antibacterial drug therapy.

All of these factors show that antibacterial drug therapy is only one element of the management of bacterial infections. Consideration of drainage and debridement of an infected site to improve antibacterial drug penetration and action is also of great importance.

Adverse effects

The final factor to consider when choosing which drug to use is whether the drug treatment will harm the patient under treatment or the person giving the treatment. A summary of the direct toxic effects of antibacterial drugs is presented in Figure 2.10. Many of these effects depend on the physiological state and concomitant drug therapy that the animal is receiving, and some species or breeds within a species may be more susceptible. The significance of the potential toxicity can, therefore, only be assessed on an individual basis. The severity of the infection and the efficacy of alternative, perhaps less toxic, treatment options are important factors to consider. There are several drugs that, because of their direct organ toxicity and/or because of their route of elimination from the body, should be avoided in animals with kidney or liver failure. Recommendations of which drugs to avoid in animals with renal and liver disease and which can be safely given are presented in Figure 2.11 and 2.12. Although these figures provide a useful summary they will not be applicable in all circumstances.

Drug	Adverse reaction	Comment
Acetamides e.g. chloramphenicol, florphenicol	Bone marrow suppression Many drug interactions Cardiotoxic	Anaemia is reversible in cat (compare with humans) Depresses hepatic metabolism of other drugs Depresses cardiac muscle plus vasodilatory effect
Aminoglycosides e.g. gentamicin, amikacin	Neurotoxic Nephrotoxic Cardiotoxic Neuromuscular block	Vestibular and cochlear nerve affected to varying degrees Concentrated in proximal tubular cells producing direct toxicity Depresses cardiac muscle plus vasodilatory effect, see note 3 below See note 2 below
Cephalosporins	Nephrotoxic Bleeding disorders Irritation at site of injection Profound effects on gut flora	Especially cephaloridine and cephalothin Especially those excreted in bile, e.g. cefoperazone e.g. cephalothin See note 1 below
Fluoroquinolones	Damage to articular cartilage Neurotoxic	Seen in young animals Care in epileptics
Lincosamides	Neuromuscular block Cardiodepressive Profound effects on gut flora	See note 2 below
Macrolides e.g. erythromycin	Altered gut flora Irritation at site of injection Many drug interactions	See note 1 below. Erythromycin also has effect on gut motility Depresses hepatic metabolism of other drugs (particularly erythromycin)
Nitroimidazoles	Neurotoxic Teratogenic	Reported in humans and suspected in dogs
Penicillins	Immunoallergenic Profound effects on gut flora	Cross-sensitivity between all penicillins See note 1 below
Polymyxins	Irritation at site of injection Neuromuscular block Nephrotoxic	Seen with sulphates but not sulphonates See note 2 below
Rifamycins	Teratogenic	
Potentiated sulphonamides e.g. trimethoprim, baquiloprim combined with sulphadimidine, sulphamethoxazole	Immunoallergenic Folic acid deficiency Depress thyroxine synthesis Crystalluria Cardiotoxic Irritation at site of injection	Manifests as keratoconjunctivitis sicca, immune-mediated blood dyscrasias, immune-mediated polyarthritis, cutaneous drug reactions, etc. Seen in cats after several weeks of therapy Low thyroxine concentration after only 4 weeks of therapy Acidic urine favours crystal formation. May worsen pre-existing renal disease See note 3 below Specifically sodium salts
Tetracyclines e.g. oxytetracycline, doxycycline	Cardiotoxic Hepatotoxic Nephrotoxic Neuromuscular block Teratogenic Irritation at site of injection Alter gut flora	Depresses cardiac muscle plus vasodilatory effect, see note 3 below Hepatotoxicity only occurs at high doses Nephrotoxicity may relate to impurities in older preparations Due to ability to bind calcium, see note 2 below Stains teeth (only reported in humans)

Figure 2.10: Summary of potential adverse reactions to antibacterial drugs.
Notes:
1. Most antibacterials alter gut flora and can cause diarrhoea. Only those that have marked gastrointestinal effects are shown. Those that have the least detrimental effects on the protective normal gut flora are fluoroquinolones and the potentiated sulphonamides.
2. Those antibacterials that have neuromuscular blocking properties are most likely to cause adverse reactions following parenteral administration or if combined with anaesthetics and other neuromuscular junction blockers.
3. The cardiotoxic effects of antibacterials are most likely to be seen following intravenous administration.

Recommendation	Drugs or group of drugs
Probably safe No dose adjustment necessary either because renal excretion is not a major route of clearance or the drugs have wide therapeutic indices	Chloramphenicol Clindamycin Doxycycline Macrolides Penicillins (including clavulanate)[a]
Consider dosage adjustment In moderate or severe failure based on the plasma creatinine concentration (see Trepanier and Elliott 1998 for further discussion)	Cephalosporins (most) Fluoroquinolones Lincomycin Sulphonamides Sulphonamide-trimethoprim
Hazardous, avoid if possible Accumulation of drug or its metabolites can increase side effects or non-renal toxicity	Nitrofurantoin Tetracycline[b] (except doxycycline)
Nephrotoxic, avoid Drugs will exacerbate renal damage	Aminoglycosides

Figure 2.11: Recommendation for systemic use of antibacterials in dogs and cats with renal failure. Reproduced from Gorman (1999) Canine Medicine and Therapeutics, 4th edn, with the permission of Blackwell Science.
See Watson (1994) for further discussion.
[a] *Sodium or potassium salts of these agents may cause electrolyte abnormalities.*
[b] *There are some reports of nephrotoxicity of tetracyclines that are probably due to impurities in out-dated or improperly stored products.*

Recommendation	Drugs or group of drugs
Probably safe Drugs not known to be hepatotoxic and their clearance is via renal excretion so they do not accumulate	Aminoglycosides Cephalosporins Penicillins
Caution advised Drugs metabolized by the liver that *might* accumulate to toxic levels in hepatopathy	Chloramphenicol[a,b] Lincosamides Macrolides Metronidazole Sulphonamides Tetracyclines
Potentially toxic Drugs that may cause hepatic injury	Chlortetracycline Erythromycin estolate[a] Rifampicin[a] Sulphonamide-trimethoprim

Figure 2.12: Recommendations for systemic administration of antibacterials in dogs and cats with liver failure. Reproduced from Gorman (1999) Canine Medicine and Therapeutics, 4th edn, with the permission of Blackwell Science.
See Watson (1994) for further details. There have been few studies of the effects of liver failure on antibacterial drug kinetics and adverse effects. These warnings are extrapolated from what is known in human medicine.
[a] *These can affect metabolism of other drugs by the liver (chloramphenicol and erythromycin are enzyme inhibitors and rifampicin is an enzyme inducer).*
[b] *Should be avoided in cats with liver disease because of its bone marrow toxicity in this species.*

Avoiding adverse reactions

A number of the toxicities, particularly those affecting the cardiovascular system and neuromuscular function, are acute toxicities that are concentration related and are only seen when rapid intravenous bolus injections of the drugs are given. These can, therefore, be avoided by giving the drugs slowly or by choosing a different route of administration.

Combination drug therapy can increase the risk of toxicity due to pharmacodynamic interactions and should be avoided if possible. If it is not possible to avoid combinations of drugs then care should be taken to ascertain likely interactions between the drugs. There are many examples of such interactions, and readers should consult appropriate sources such as the *BSAVA Small Animal Formulary*. The following are examples of such interactions with antibacterial drugs:

- Neuromuscular junction blockade will be potentiated if some antibacterials are given to animals that are about to be anaesthetized or that are just recovering from an anaesthetic

- Frusemide is ototoxic and, if combined with aminoglycoside drugs, will enhance the risk of ototoxicity
- Frusemide tends to cause dehydration, which enhances the nephrotoxicity of drugs such as the aminoglycosides
- Sulphonamides and their metabolites precipitate in urine which is acidic and so should not be used in animals on acidifying diets or that are taking urinary acidifying drugs.

Pharmacodynamic considerations: Some adverse effects of antibacterial drugs occur because of pharmacokinetic interactions between combinations of drugs. For example, chloramphenicol is an irreversible inhibitor of the hepatic cytochrome P_{450} system responsible for metabolism of barbiturates, phenytoin, anticoagulants (warfarin) and hypoglycaemic drugs. Use of chloramphenicol in patients receiving these drugs of narrow therapeutic index should be avoided. The inhibitory effects of chloramphenicol on clearance of barbiturates can be detected for up to 3 weeks after a single dose, due to the irreversible mechanism of action. Erythromycin is also a potent inhibitor of the cytochrome P_{450} enzyme, and fatal drug interactions have been documented in human medicine in patients taking terfenadine (an antihistamine). In general, well characterized examples of pharmacokinetic drug interactions are lacking in veterinary medicine and extrapolation from the data available from human medicine is often relied upon, findings that may or may not be relevant to veterinary species.

Selection of resistance in populations of bacteria

Whenever antibacterial drugs are used to treat infections, pressure is placed on the exposed population of bacteria that selects for those bacteria with an ability to survive in the presence of the antibacterial drug. The genes that confer resistance are often present within the bacterial population in question already, but at very low levels. Usually, once exposure to the antibacterial drug ceases, the bacteria possessing these genes are diluted as the sensitive bacteria are able to multiply again. If antibacterial drugs are used continuously in an environment where there are large numbers of diseased animals or people in close proximity, drug resistance may transfer more rapidly both within and between species of bacteria. Intensive care units in human hospitals are good examples where this process of selection for resistance occurs.

Hospitalized small animals could represent a similar population of animals, although the duration of stay and intensity and duration of treatment tend to be less in veterinary practice. However, the close proximity between people and their pets, and the tendency for the bacteria to cross over between them, should be recognized. This means that with bacteria of zoonotic potential in particular, careful selection of antibacterial drugs should be made to avoid resistance being transferred into the human bacterial population.

ANTIVIRAL DRUGS

Of all the microorganisms that cause disease in the dog and cat, viruses are the most challenging to treat without causing harm to the patient. The reasons for this are:

- Viruses are obligate intracellular parasites and their replication depends primarily on synthetic processes in the host cell
- In many viral infections, replication of the virus peaks before the onset of clinical signs.

Most antiviral drugs currently available are drugs with very low therapeutic indices, and these should be used with great care. Human medicine is actively searching for chemicals that inhibit virus-specific functions. The main area in which antiviral drugs have been used in veterinary practice is in ophthalmology for the treatment of feline herpesvirus (FHV) infections.

There are several steps in viral replication that are potential sites for drug action. These are listed in Figure 2.13 with some examples.

Step in viral replication	Examples
1. Adsorption to and penetration into susceptible cells	Gamma globulins (by stearic hinderance)
2. Uncoating of viral nucleic acid	Amatadine inhibits uncoating viral RNA of the influenza A virus
3. Synthesis of early regulatory proteins	No drugs have been developed that act at this stage
4. Nucleic acid synthesis	Purine and pyrimidine analogues, e.g. dideoxyinosine, dideoxycytidine Reverse transcriptase inhibitors, e.g. azidothymidine
5. Synthesis of late structural proteins	No drugs have been developed that act at this stage
6. Assembly (maturation) of viral particles	Rifampicin
7. Release of virus particles from the cell	No drugs have been developed that act at this stage

Figure 2.13: Steps in viral replication that are potential sites for drug action, with examples.

Antiherpes drugs

All antiherpes drugs currently available for human use are analogues of nucleotides that inhibit viral DNA polymerase activity. Two have been used in veterinary medicine.

Aciclovir (acyclovir)

Aciclovir is an acyclic guanosine derivative, which is activated following phosphorylation by the herpesvirus-specific thymidine kinase. The active drug only accumulates inside infected cells. Phosphorylated aciclovir inhibits viral DNA replication by competitively binding to viral DNA polymerase. If this fails and the drug is incorporated into viral DNA then chain termination occurs. This drug is available in intravenous, oral and topical formulations, the last of which is used in veterinary practice to treat conjunctivitis and keratitis caused by FHV. There is some in vitro evidence that suggests that aciclovir is not very effective against FHV. Adverse effects are reported in human medicine following systemic administration of this drug but are relatively uncommon.

Trifluridine

Trifluridine is a fluorinated pyrimidine nucleoside. It is phosphorylated intracellularly by host cell enzymes to produce the active form that competes with thymidine triphosphate for incorporation into viral DNA. Because it is activated by host cell enzymes, this drug lacks specificity for infected cells and is too toxic to use by routes other than topical administration to the site of infection. Eye drops can be obtained (only through pharmacists) containing 1% trifluridine.

Antiretroviral drugs

Over the past few years several antiretroviral drugs have entered the human market to treat HIV infection. Veterinary medicine is in the early stages of examining the efficacy of these drugs in the management of cats infected with FIV.

Zidovudine

Zidovudine (previously known as azidothymidine, AZT) is the main antiretroviral drug that has been used to treat FIV-infected cats showing signs of immunodeficiency. The active form of the drug is a competitive inhibitor of reverse transcriptase. In humans the major route of clearance of the drug from the body is hepatic metabolism to form the inactive glucuronide derivative. The relative inability of cats to glucuronidate drugs influences the pharmacokinetics of the drug. Interactions with other drugs that require hepatic metabolism or that alter liver enzyme activity are also likely to occur. These factors may influence the efficacy and safety of the drug in cats. Reported adverse effects in cats include bone marrow suppression, leading to neutropenia and anaemia, and hepatotoxicity. Zidovudine should be regarded as having a very narrow therapeutic index and should be used with similar caution to cancer chemotherapy drugs. It does not eliminate the infection but may ameliorate its effects in the short to medium term.

Other antiretroviral drugs

Zalcitabine (also known as dideoxycytidine, ddC) and didanosine (also known as dideoxyinosine, ddI) are nucleoside analogues that function in a similar manner to zidovudine. Non-nucleoside reverse transcriptase inhibitors include lamuvidine and stavudine. None of these has been tested in clinical practice and their empirical use is not encouraged.

ANTIFUNGAL DRUGS

Compared with antibacterial drugs, antifungal drugs tend to be more toxic to the animals under treatment because fungal cells are eukaryotes and share many of the biological characteristics of mammalian cells. Fortunately, many of the fungal infections found in the UK are amenable to topical therapy, and exposure of the major organ systems of animals to many of these drugs is not necessary. The recent introduction of the relatively non-toxic orally active antifungal azoles has revolutionized the management of serious systemic fungal infections. The modes of action of the antifungal drugs currently available are summarized in Figure 2.3.

Therapeutic classification of antifungal drugs

The major fungal infections facing practitioners in veterinary practice in the UK include dermatophytosis, nasal aspergillosis and yeast infections (candidiasis, cryptococcosis and *Malassezia pachydermatis* infection). The specific management of these infections is covered elsewhere in this manual. Figure 2.14 summarizes the spectrum of activity, route of administration and clinical indications for the antifungal drugs currently available. The antifungal drugs can be divided into those that are only used topically to treat local infections in various superficial areas of the body, because they are too toxic to use systemically, and those drugs that are safe enough to use systemically to treat more generalized infections, albeit with caution in many cases.

Antifungal drugs given systemically

It is important to select a drug that, when given by the proposed route of administration and dose rate, will reach the site of infection at an effective concentration but without adversely harming the patient. Figure 2.15 summarizes the important points relating to the pharmacokinetics and toxicity of these drugs. It should be noted that the newer triazoles, in particular itraconazole and fluconazole, are broad-spectrum antifungal drugs that are active following oral administration and are relatively non-toxic.

Drug group	Examples	Route of administration	Spectrum of action and main clinical use
Polyenes	Amphotericin B	Parenteral or oral (for GIT infections); can be used topically	Very broad spectrum; used for life-threatening systemic mycoses
	Nystatin	Topical only	Broad spectrum; used in ear preparations
Azoles	Clotrimazole Enilconazole	Topical only	Broad spectrum; used in treatment of dermatophytosis, candidiasis, *Malassezia* infections and aspergillosis
	Fluconazole Itraconazole Ketoconazole	Oral (all) or i.v. (fluconazole) Can be used topically	Broad spectrum; itraconazole and fluconazole are preferred to ketoconazole. Itraconazole is used for refractory dermatophytosis; fluconazole is used to treat cryptococcal meningitis in humans
Griseofulvin	-	Oral only (inactive if applied topically)	Dermatophytes (all species) only
Flucytosine	-	Parenteral (oral preparation is available but only on a named patient basis from Bell and Croydon)	Narrow spectrum (yeasts; cryptococcosis and candidiasis). Synergisitic with amphotericin
Allylamines	Terbinafine	Oral	Narrow spectrum; dermatophytosis, particularly for onychomycosis in human medicine

Figure 2.14: Routes of administration, spectrum of action and clinical uses of antifungal drugs.

ANTIPARASITIC DRUGS

Endoparasiticides

In addition to the principles described above for antibacterial drugs, the life cycle of the parasite needs to be considered when treating a parasitic infection. Different stages of a parasite's life cycle may vary in susceptibility to a drug. The mechanism of actions of the antiparasitic drugs used in canine and feline practice are summarized in Figure 2.4.

Spectrum of activity and pharmacokinetics

Figure 2.16 summarizes the spectrum of activity of the commonly used endoparasiticides. In some cases, efficacy against non-intestinal forms of the parasites (arrested larvae, migrating larvae, lung and heart worms) require different dosing regimens, often more prolonged, than standard treatments for intestinal parasites. Dichlorophen, niclosamide and nitroscanate are poorly absorbed from the intestinal tract following oral dosing. Absorption of pyrantel depends on the exact formulation used. Ivermectin, levamisole, piperazine and praziquantel are readily absorbed from the intestine. The benzimidazoles are slowly absorbed to a limited extent due to their low water solubility, although the rate of absorption in dogs and cats is higher than in ruminants, pigs and horses. As the benzimidazoles kill helminths by depriving them of glucose, prolonged exposure is necessary, and repeated dosing over several days may be required depending on the metabolic rate of the target parasite.

Among the drugs that are effective against round worms, the benzimidazoles are effective against all stages of the life cycle (i.e. eggs, larvae and adults).

Levamisole and ivermectin have activity against adults and many of the larval stages of nematodes. Pyrantel is active against larval and adult forms of nematodes but is not active against migrating or arrested larvae. Mature parasites are much more susceptible to the actions of piperazine than are the younger stages; the lumen-dwelling larvae are only partially eliminated following a single dose of this drug. Hence, repeated and frequent dosing regimens are important for effective use of products containing piperazine.

Toxicity

Most of the anthelmintic drugs used in dogs and cats have broad safety margins. In some cases this is because they are poorly absorbed from the gastrointestinal tract, so the chances of systemic toxicity following oral administration are slight (e.g. dichlorophen and niclosamide). The benzimidazoles have very wide therapeutic indices. The early members of this group showed some teratogenic effects, but mebendazole and fenbendazole have been extensively tested in pregnant animals, including dogs, and shown to be without ill effects even at dose rates that greatly exceed those recommended in the data sheet. Likewise, praziquantel is safe at 20 to 40 times the recommended dose rate, even when given to pregnant animals. Care should be taken when calculating doses for puppies and kittens as significant overdoses can cause signs of toxicity.

The only contraindication with piperazine is the treatment of extremely heavy infestations of ascarids. Because this drug causes rapid death of the adult worms, intestinal blockage or even rupture can occur as large masses of worms are expelled from the intestine simultaneously. In such situations, benzimidazoles

Antimicrobial and Antiparasitic Chemotherapy 35

Drug	Oral bioavailability	Distribution and route of elimination	Drug interactions	Adverse effects
Amphotericin B	Poor; used orally to treat infections of the gastrointestinal tract	Heavily plasma-protein bound so does not get into cerebrospinal fluid	Other nephrotoxic drugs Aminoglycosides Cyclosporine	Renal toxicity often occurs during treatment but is reversible if recognized. Renal tubular acidosis and potassium and magnesium wasting occur. Sodium loading may reduce toxicity Acute toxicity related to drug infusion includes hypotension, fever, vomiting, malaise and depression. Cardiac arrhythmias can develop during infusions, and thrombophlebitis can occur
Fluconazole	Excellent; not affected by antacids	Most of the administered dose is metabolized by the liver but a small amount is excreted unchanged in the urine	Hypokalaemia[a] that results may increase digoxin toxicity Diuretic use concomitantly may increase risks of hypokalaemia	Least toxic of all the azoles
		Most effective of all the azoles at penetrating into cerebrospinal fluid; can be given by intravenous infusion to facilitate this Cleared by renal excretion	Inhibits hepatic cytochrome P$_{450}$-dependent microsomal enzymes (least effective of all azoles). Avoid concomitant use of drugs mentioned under ketoconazole and itraconazole	Hepatotoxicity and teratogenicity are potential problems
Itraconazole and ketoconazole	Variable; antacids, adsorbents and ulcer healing drugs inhibit absorption (an acid environment is necessary for optimal dissolution of these poorly water-soluble drugs)	Poor penetration into cerebrospinal fluid Cleared by hepatic metabolism	Inhibit hepatic cyt P$_{450}$-dependent microsomal enzymes (ketoconazole more than itraconazole). Data in dogs and cats are lacking, but avoid antihistamines, cyclosporine, cisapride, warfarin	Hepatotoxicity and teratogenicity Inhibit adrenal and gonadal steroid synthesis (ketoconazole only at therapeutic doses), leading to infertility and other endocrine abnormalities
Griseofulvin	Variable; absorption is improved if given with fatty foods	Deposited on newly forming skin, where it binds to keratin Cleared by hepatic metabolism	Antiepileptic drugs increase the rate of hepatic metabolism of griseofulvin and *vice versa*. Griseofulvin also increases rate of metabolism of anticoagulants	Teratogenic Bone marrow suppression (cats positive for feline immunodeficiency virus) Hepatotoxicity Pure bred cats may be more susceptible to toxic effects
Flucytosine	Well absorbed	Low plasma-protein binding; penetrates well into all fluid compartments, including cerebrospinal fluid Rate of excretion depends on glomerular filtration rate	None reported	Some of the oral dose is converted by gastrointestinal flora to 5-fluorouracil (cytotoxic) leading to bone marrow toxicity Use with caution in face of renal impairment

Figure 2.15: Pharmacokinetics and adverse effects of systemic antifungal drugs.
[a] Less common side effect in dogs and cats than in humans.

Drug	Tapeworms			Round worms					
	Echinococcus	*Taenia*	*Dipylidium*	*Toxocara/ Toxascaris*	*Toxocara* arrested larvae[a]	Hook worms *Uncinaria*	Whip worms *Trichuris*	Lung worms *Filaroides* and *Aelurostronglyus*	Heart worm[b] *Angiostrongylus*
Dichlorophen	–	+	+	–	–	–	–	–	–
Febental	–	+	–	+	–	+	+	–	–
Fenbendazole	–	+	–	+	+	+	+	+	+[c]
Levamisole[d]	–	–	–	+	–	+	–	+	+
Mebendazole	+[e]	+	–	+	–	+	+	–	–
Niclosamide[d]	+/–	+	+	–	–	–	–	–	–
Nitroscanate[f]	+/–	+	+	+	–	+	–	–	–
Piperazine	–	–	–	+	–	+	–	–	–
Praziquantel	+[g]	+	+	–	–	–	–	–	–
Pyrantel	–	–	–	+	–	+	–	–	–
Selamectin	–	–	–	+	+[h,c]	+	+	–	+

Figure 2.16: *Spectrum of activity of endoparasiticides for use in dogs and cats.*
+ *Data sheet claims of efficacy or, if drug not licensed for dogs and cats, data from the literature suggest efficacy.*
– *No data sheet claims for efficacy or data in the literature suggesting efficacy.*
+/– *Limited efficacy.*
[a] *Used to prevent transmission from dam to offspring.*
[b] *Treatment and prevention of* Dirofilaria immitis *involves drugs that are mostly not licensed for the dog in the UK. See Chapter 7 for further information on treatment.*
[c] *Not a data sheet recommendation but data in the literature suggest efficacy.*
[d] *Not licensed for use in dogs and cats in the UK.*
[e] *Only active against* Echinococcus granulosus granulosus.
[f] *Not suitable for cats.*
[g] *Effective against* Echinococcus granulosus granulosus *and* E. multilocularis.
[h] *Treatment of the dam during pregnancy (last dose 10 days before whelping) and lactation (first dose 10 days after whelping) is effective in preventing perinatal and lactogenic* Toxocara canis *infestation.*

would be preferred because their mode of killing is more prolonged, and the expulsion of dead worms occurs over an extended period.

Levamisole should be considered as a drug with a relatively narrow therapeutic index, particularly when compared with other anthelmintic drugs like the benzimidazoles. This drug is a cholinomimetic. The signs of levamisole toxicity are a mixture of overstimulation of the parasympathetic and sympathetic systems and include salivation, defecation, respiratory distress and cardiac arrhythmias. Dogs and cats tolerate levamisole much better if it is given by the oral rather than intravenous route. Combinations of organophosphates or pyrantel with levamisole are not advisable because these drugs, theoretically, might have additive or even synergistic toxic effects.

Ivermectin is not licensed for dogs or cats in the UK. In the USA, this drug is used routinely as a preventive measure against heart worm, and a dose of 0.006 to 0.012 mg/kg is given once a month. There is no evidence that at this low dose the drug has any toxic effects. Signs of toxicity can be seen at the higher doses (0.1 to 0.2 mg/kg) that are needed to affect other nematode parasites. Collies are particularly susceptible, but cases of ivermectin toxicity have occurred in other breeds. Clinical signs of toxicity include depression, ataxia, tremors, recumbency and mydriasis. Death can occur, and this drug should be used with extreme caution. Formulations for large animal species may behave quite differently in dogs and cats in terms of their bioavailability, efficacy and potential toxicity. Selamectin is a newly licensed avermectin and is much safer to use in dogs and cats. Its safety has been extensively evaluated, and it produces no adverse effects at therapeutic dose rates in avermectin-sensitive collies (Novotny *et al.*, 2000).

Ectoparasiticides

Spectrum of activity and pharmacokinetics

The major ectoparasitic drugs used in dogs and cats are listed in Figure 2.17 with an indication of their spectrum of activity. The drugs listed can be divided into two main groups: those that kill ectoparasites following direct contact and those that kill following ingestion of the animal's blood. The latter group can be given orally or as spot-on formulations designed for absorption across the skin into the bloodstream. The group includes ivermectin, cythioate, fenthion and phosmet.

For some ectoparasites, environmental control is important in the overall treatment strategy. This is certainly the case for fleas where much of the life cycle occurs in the animal's home rather than on the animal itself. Organophosphates and synthetic pyrethroids can be used in this way, and licensed products exist that give a persistent effect within the home to prevent

Drug	Fleas (adults)	Ticks	Lice	Mites						
				Otodectes	Sarcoptes	Notoedres	Demodex	Trombicula	Cheyletiella
Amitraz[a]					+		+		
Carbamates Carbaril[b] Propoxur	+								
Fipronil	+	+	+		(+)[c]			(+)[c]	(+)[c]
Imidacloprid	+								
Monosulphiram				+					
Organophosphate Cythioate[b,d] Diazinon[b] Dichlorvos plus fenitrothion Fenthion[d] Phosmet[b,d]	+ + + + +	+ + 			 (+)[c]		(+)[c]		(+)[c]	(+)[c]
Pyrethrins[e] Pyrethroids Fenvalerate Permethrin	+ + +	 + +	(+)[c] (+)[c]		 + 				
Selamectin	+	(+)[f]		+	+				
Selenium sulphide									(+)[c]
Thiabendazole				+					

Figure 2.17: Spectrum of activity of ectoparasiticides for use in dogs and cats.
+ Data sheet recommendation for the use of this drug against this parasite or data in the literature supports efficacy (if product not licensed).
[a] Not recommended for use in cats. Do not use in Chihuahuas.
[b] Not licensed for use in the UK in dogs or cats.
[c] Data sheets do not claim activity against these parasites, but fipronil, cythioate, phosmet, permethrin or selenium sulphide may aid in their control.
[d] Systemically acting ectoparasiticides; fenthion and phosmet are applied topically as spot-ons, which are absorbed systemically. All other drugs are applied and act topically.
[e] Natural extracts of pyrethrum flowers; often coformulated with pipronyl butoxide, which acts synergistically. The combination may be active against some mites.
[f] Data sheet does not claim efficacy but data in the literature suggest good activity in experimental infestations of dogs with Rhipicephalus sanguineus and Dermacentor variabilis.

reinfestation of the environment. The insect growth regulator methoprene is formulated with pyrethrins to prevent larval development. Sodium polyborate (borax) is a chemical that is larvicidal and can be used very successfully in environmental flea control. Lufenuron is a drug that achieves environmental flea control despite being given to the animal rather than being sprayed in the environment. This drug, which inhibits chitin formation, is ingested by adult fleas as they feed and is incorporated into their eggs, preventing viable larvae from hatching. The drug becomes incorporated into the fat stores of the host, which act as a slow-release depot. A single injectable dose can be effective for 6 months in cats. The highly lipid-soluble nature of this drug means that if the oral route of administration is chosen the drug must be given with food to stimulate sufficient biliary secretion to allow effective absorption of the drug.

Flea adulticides that have a persistent action once given to an animal are preferred because they allow long intervals between treatments, during which time the food supply necessary for the adult fleas to continue to reproduce is unavailable. For example, fipronil persists for between 1 and 3 months and during this time will kill any adult flea before they have a chance to lay eggs. Fleas that do not feed for this period will not die but will not lay eggs, thereby reducing environmental contamination. The persistence of the drug on or in the host's system depends not only on the nature of the active ingredient but also on the formulation of the product used, and the data sheet recommendations of each formulation should be consulted.

Adverse effects
The adverse effects of several groups of ectoparasiticides have been well documented in the literature.

These are summarized in Figure 2.18. The drugs that have been developed in the past 5 to 10 years seem to have very few acute adverse effects. Imidacloprid, a drug that binds to cholinoceptors in insects, has a much higher affinity for these receptors when compared with their mammalian counterparts, explaining its very low toxic potential. Fipronil also has a very good safety profile and is one of the few insecticides which, in the spray formulation, can be recommended for use in puppies and kittens from 2 days of age. The use of ivermectin to treat ectoparasite infestations in dogs and cats is not recommended. Selamectin has a much better safety profile and is effective against a wide range of ectoparasites.

Drug or drug group	Clinical signs	Mechanism of toxicity/ predisposing factors	Recommended treatment
Amitraz	Transient sedation, lethargy, central nervous system depression, bradycardia, shallow breathing	Amitraz has agonist activity at mammalian α_2-adrenoceptors. Sedation with α_2-agonists is not recommended. Do not use in Chihuahuas. Take care in other small breeds	The signs usually subside in 24 hours or less. Wash in soapy water (not detergent) to remove drug from skin and provide supportive therapy. If signs persist, give atipamezole (0.2 mg/kg)
Carbamates (carbaril; propoxur)	Vomiting, diarrhoea, bradycardia, salivation, lacrimation and miosis. Muscle fasciculations leading to weakness and paralysis. Anxiety and restlessness, progressing to central nervous system depression	Inhibition of the breakdown of acetylcholine at synapses in the periphery and in the central nervous system. Organophosphates used concomitantly with carbamates will produce additive effects	Wash animal to remove source of carbamate. Atropine should be used to control the parasympathetic overstimulation; dose to effect. Toxic effects of carbamates are much shorter lasting than those of the organophosphates. Use of pralidoxime is contraindicated
Ivermectin[a]	Central nervous system depression, listlessness mydriasis, ataxia, recumbency and death	In the mammalian central nervous system, ivermectin enhances γ-amino butyric acid (inhibitory neurotransmitter) binding to its receptor. Benzodiazepines enhance toxicity. Collies and collie cross breeds seem to be more susceptible to the toxic effects and may show signs at dose rates required to treat ectoparasites; possibly because the drug traverses their blood-brain barrier more easily than it does in other breeds	Supportive therapy
Organophosphates	Same signs as for carbamates	Same mechanism as for carbamates but organophosphates have longer lasting effects because of irreversible action. Other drugs that are substrates for plasma cholinesterase can potentiate the action, e.g. phenothiazines and procaine. Organophosphates enhance and prolong the action of suxamethonium	As for carbamates except pralidoxime (20-50 mg/kg i.v. slowly) is recommended to regenerate the phosphorylated enzyme (if given before the enzyme-drug complex has aged)
Pyrethroids and pyrethrins	Vomiting, diarrhoea, hyperexcitability and hyperaesthesia	Activation of sodium channels in central and peripheral nerve fibres	Diazepam to reduce central nervous system excitability. Supportive care

Figure 2.18: Adverse effects of ectoparasiticides.
[a] *In contrast, no adverse effects have been seen with selamectin in avermectin-sensitive collies at dose rates recommended for the management of ectoparasites.*

ANTIPROTOZOAL DRUGS

Fortunately, only a few protozoal infections are endemic to the UK. These include giardiasis, toxoplasmosis and neosporosis. As pet travel increases, however, more cases of leishmaniasis and other protozoal infections are likely to be seen in the UK. As with antifungal drugs, antiprotozoal drugs tend to be more toxic to the host animals than are antibacterial drugs because protozoans are eukaryotes and share many of the biological characteristics of mammalian cells. Figure 2.19 lists drugs that are available for the treatment of protozoal infections.

It should be noted that several widely available antibacterial and endoparasiticide drugs also have useful antiprotozoal activity. The preceding sections on these drugs should be consulted. The choices of antiprotozoal drugs to treat leishmaniasis, ehrlichiosis and babesiosis are covered in Chapter 5. The treatment of giardiasis is covered in Chapter 8 and that of toxoplasmosis and neosporosis in Chapter 15.

Group	Antiprotozoal drug	Spectrum of activity	Comments
Aminoglycosides	Paromomycin	*Leishmania*	Binds to small ribosomal subunit causing failure of protein synthesis Poor oral absorption; systemic use is associated with nephrotoxicity. Used topically for cutaneous leishmaniasis
Antimonials	Meglumine antimonate Sodium stibogluconate	*Leishmania*	Inhibitors of glycolysis and fatty acid metabolism. Variety of toxic side effects. Given parenterally Often combined with allopurinol
Benzimidazoles	Fenbendazole Albendazole	*Giardia*	Binds to tubulin Poorly absorbed from gastrointestinal tract
Diamidines	Pentamidine Imidocarb Diminazine aceturate	*Pneumocystis* *Babesia* Trypanosomes	Mechanism of action unknown Nephrotoxic (pentamidine) and neurotoxic (imidocarb, diminazine). Sensitivity varies between protozoans
Diaminopyrimidine	Pyrimethamine[a] Trimethoprim	*Toxoplasma* *Neospora* *Pneumocystis* Coccidia	Dihydrofolate reductase inhibitors (usually combined with sulphonamides, which may cause a variety of toxic effects; see Figure 2.10)
Macrolides/lincosamides	Clindamycin Spiramycin	*Toxoplasma* *Neospora*	Binds to large ribosomal subunit causing reversible inhibition of protein synthesis
Nitrofurans	Furazolidone	*Giardia* Coccidia	Mechanism of action unknown but depends on metabolism of drug by nitroreductase enzymes of the microbe Poorly absorbed from gastrointestinal tract Can cause central nervous system and haemostatic problems Potentially carcinogenic
Nitroimidazoles	Metronidazole	*Giardia*	Inhibition of DNA metabolism Benzimidazoles are more effective
Pyrazolopyrimidines	Allopurinol	*Leishmania*	Disrupts DNA synthesis by the production of altered nucleotides Used in conjunction with antimonials Well absorbed from gastrointestinal tract
Sulphonamides	Sulphadimidine	*Toxoplasma* *Neospora* *Pneumocystis* Coccidia	Inhibition of folic acid synthesis (usually combined with diaminopyrimidine) Variety of toxic effects (often immune-mediated) (see Figure 2.10)
Tetracyclines	Doxycycline	*Ehrlichia*	Binds to small ribosomal subunit causing failure of protein synthesis
Thiamine inhibitors	Amprolium	Coccidia	Inhibits parasite's thiamine usage

Figure 2.19: Antiprotozoal drugs for use in dogs and cats.
[a] *Pyrimethamine is more effective than trimethoprim against protozoans.*

REFERENCES AND FURTHER READING

Bishop Y (2000) *The Veterinary Formulary, 5th edn*. Pharmaceutical Press, London

Fisher MA (1998) Fleas and flea control. In: *Canine Medicine and Therapeutics, 4th edn*, ed. NT Gorman, pp. 903-913. Blackwell Science, Oxford

Green CE and Watson ADJ (1998) Antiprotozoal chemotherapy. In: *Infectious Diseases of the Dog and Cat, 2nd edn*, ed. CG Greene, pp. 441-444. WB Saunders, Philadelphia

Krautmann MJ, Novotny MJ, DeKeulenaer K, Godin CS, Evans EI, McCall JW, Wang C, Rowan TG and Jernigan AD (2000) Safety of selamectin in cats. *Veterinary Parasitology* **9**, 393-403

Novotny MJ, Krautmann MJ, Ehrhart JC, Godin CS, Evans EI, McCall JW, Sun F, Rowan TG and Jernigan AD (2000) Safety of selamectin in dogs. *Veterinary Parasitology* **9**, 377-391

Prescott JF and Baggot JD (2000) *Antimicrobial Therapy in Veterinary Medicine, 3rd edn*. Iowa State University Press, Ames, Iowa

Safrin S and Chambers HF (1998) Antiviral agents. In: *Basic and Clinical Pharmacology, 7th edn*, ed. BG Katzung, pp. 788-802. Appleton and Lange, Connecticut

Sheppard D and Lampiris HW (1998) Antifungal agents. In: *Basic and Clinical Pharmacology, 7th edn*, ed. BG Katzung, pp. 780-787. Appleton and Lange, Connecticut

Tennant B (1999) *Small Animal Formulary, 3rd edn*. BSAVA Publications, Cheltenham

Trepanier L and Elliott J (1998) Good prescribing practice. In: *Canine Medicine and Therapeutics, 4th edn*, ed. NT Gorman, pp. 3-23. Blackwell Science, Oxford

Vaden SL and Papich MG (1995) Empiric antibiotic therapy. In: *Kirk's Current Veterinary Therapy XII*, ed. JD Bonagura, pp. 276-279. WB Saunders, Philadelphia

Watson ADJ (1994) Appropriate use of antimicrobial drugs in dogs and cats. In: *Antimicrobial Prescribing Guidelines for Veterinarians*, ed. BS Copper, pp. 55-81. Postgraduate Foundation, University of Sydney

Watson ADJ, Elliott J and Maddison JE (1998) Rational use of antibacterial drugs. In: *Canine Medicine and Therapeutics, 4th edn*, ed. NT Gorman, pp. 53-72. Blackwell Science, Oxford

Wilcke JR ed. (1990) Clinical pharmacology: problems in antimicrobial therapy. *Problems in Veterinary Medicine* **2**

Wolfe AM (1994) Antifungal agents. In: *Consultations in Feline Medicine 2, 2nd edn*, ed. JR August pp. 53-56. WB Saunders, Philadelphia

CHAPTER THREE

Vaccination

Oswald Jarrett and Ian Ramsey

CHAPTER PLAN

The need for vaccination
Types of vaccine
　Modified live vaccines
　Non-living vaccines
　Adjuvants
　Routes of adminstration
Factors influencing vaccine efficacy
　Vaccine factors
　　Annual revaccination
　Host factors
　　Maternal antibodies
　　Pre-existing infections
　　Immune system function
　Human factors
　Environmental factors
Risks of vaccination
　Adverse reactions
　Lack of efficacy
Investigation of suspected vaccine breakdowns
Alternatives to vaccination
　Isolation
　Control of vectors and reservoir hosts
　Treatment
　Serological testing
References and further reading

THE NEED FOR VACCINATION

Vaccination is an effective way of controlling infectious diseases and has achieved spectacular success in promoting human and animal welfare. Dogs and cats are susceptible to several common and potentially fatal infections that can be avoided by vaccination. The impact of infectious disease on a fully susceptible population was seen dramatically in the late 1970s and early 1980s when canine parvovirus (CPV) emerged as a lethal infection of young and old dogs. The success of effective vaccination in controlling that infection was equally dramatic. The sources of infectious diseases for pet cats and dogs are varied. Animals may be exposed to infectious agents from diseased animals, healthy carrier animals and contaminated environments. Vaccination provides a convenient solution to the prevention of diseases that may be acquired from known or unsuspected sources.

The aim of vaccination is to make susceptible animals immune and thereby resistant to infectious disease. It is doubtful whether any vaccine provides a level of immunity that totally prevents infection following natural exposure. The growth of an infectious agent in the vaccinated animal following exposure provides a boost to vaccination-induced immunity, resulting in a more effective containment of infection. Although an infection may not be totally prevented, the quantity of infectious agent in vaccinated animals may be much reduced after exposure. This reduction results in protection from clinical disease and a large reduction in the amount of the agent excreted by the animal. Vaccination of companion animals is primarily concerned with the prevention of disease in individual animals. However, when most of the susceptible individuals in a population are protected from infection and subclinical infection is rare, the agent may be eradicated as it cannot spread in the community. For example, this result may have been achieved for canine distemper virus (CDV) in many populations of dogs.

Although vaccination is a convenient option for controlling infectious disease, there are many factors that have to be considered if a vaccination programme is to be successful. These include:

- The infectious agent involved
- The inherent efficacy of the vaccine
- The storage and administration of the vaccine
- The effects of maternally derived antibodies
- The duration of immunity
- The short- and long-term adverse reactions of vaccination.

An understanding of these elements helps to ensure that animals are properly protected from many potentially fatal viral and bacterial infections.

TYPES OF VACCINE

Vaccines are of two general types: modified live or non-living. Modified live vaccines may be attenuated by cultivation in vitro or by genetic modification. Non-living vaccines may be inactivated organisms, components of organisms or genetically engineered subunits. The variety of vaccine types is illustrated in Figure 3.1, and a selection of such vaccines available for cats and dogs in the UK is given in Figure 3.2.

Live attenuated organisms
- Serially passaged organisms that have developed disabling mutations
- Potential advantages
    - Rapid protection
    - Cell mediated immunity stimulated
    - Lower antigenic mass
- Potential disadvantages
    - Reversion to virulence
    - Disease even without reversion
    - Adventitious agents

Inactivated organisms
- Killed organisms whose antigenic structure is often altered
- Advantages
    - No reversion to virulence
    - Stable
- Disadvantages
    - Inappropriate responses
    - Lower titres of antibody
    - Adjuvant required

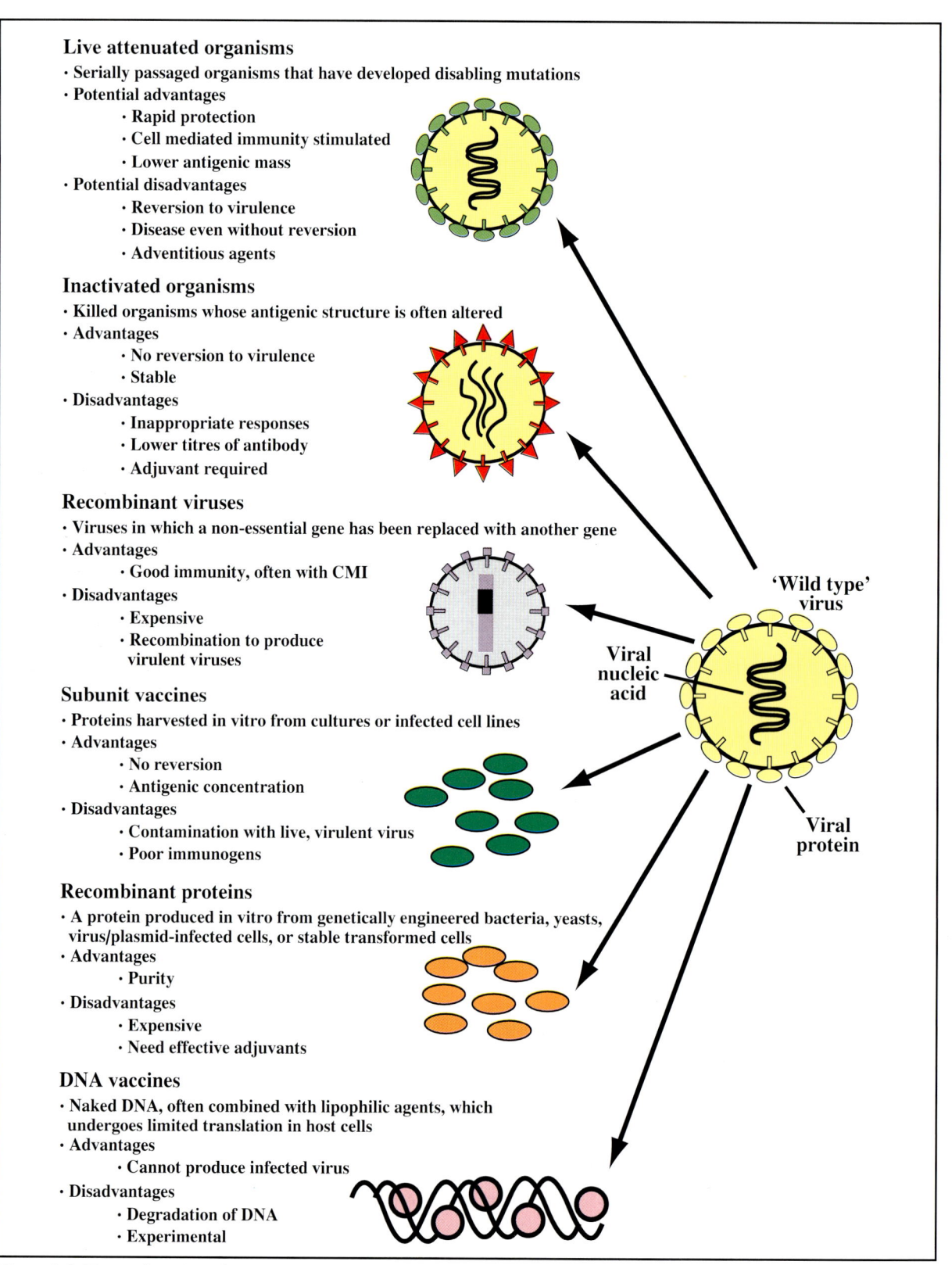

Recombinant viruses
- Viruses in which a non-essential gene has been replaced with another gene
- Advantages
    - Good immunity, often with CMI
- Disadvantages
    - Expensive
    - Recombination to produce virulent viruses

Subunit vaccines
- Proteins harvested in vitro from cultures or infected cell lines
- Advantages
    - No reversion
    - Antigenic concentration
- Disadvantages
    - Contamination with live, virulent virus
    - Poor immunogens

Recombinant proteins
- A protein produced in vitro from genetically engineered bacteria, yeasts, virus/plasmid-infected cells, or stable transformed cells
- Advantages
    - Purity
- Disadvantages
    - Expensive
    - Need effective adjuvants

DNA vaccines
- Naked DNA, often combined with lipophilic agents, which undergoes limited translation in host cells
- Advantages
    - Cannot produce infected virus
- Disadvantages
    - Degradation of DNA
    - Experimental

Figure 3.1: Types of vaccines that are, or probably soon will be, available in small animal practice, with their advantages and disadvantages.

Type of vaccine	Source	Applicable small animal infections	
		Cat	Dog
Live	Attenuated	Feline calicivirus Feline herpesvirus Feline parvovirus *Chlamydophila felis* (formerly *Chlamydia psittaci* var. *felis*)	Canine distemper virus Canine parvovirus Canine adenovirus Canine parainfluenza virus *Bordetella bronchiseptica*
	Genetically modified recombinants	Canarypox-feline leukaemia virus	Vaccinia-rabies (red fox)
Non-living	Chemically inactivated	Feline parvovirus Feline leukaemia virus Rabies	Canine parvovirus Rabies
	Disrupted virus	Feline calicivirus Feline herpesvirus	
	Recombinant protein	Feline leukaemia virus	

Figure 3.2: Examples of vaccines available for small animals.

Modified live vaccines

Most vaccines for dogs and cats contain living organisms. The aim of vaccination with live agents is to achieve a quality of response that simulates naturally acquired immunity. Clearly, live vaccines must contain non-pathogenic organisms. Traditionally this attenuation was achieved by cultivating wild-type infectious agents in conditions that selected for mutants that were apathogenic but retained the antigenic properties of the wild-type organism. These mutants were then used to induce a protective immune response when given to animals.

It is generally considered that live vaccines provide a better quality of immune response than non-living vaccines because they replicate in the animal. Three main features that contribute to this greater efficacy are:

- Exposure of the host's immune system to all of the antigens of the organism. During their period of growth in the host, live organisms express all of their proteins and consequently expose the animal to a range of antigenic determinants that may induce a protective immune response. For example, following administration of a live viral vaccine, the host is presented with not only the surface structural proteins of the virus that are the major components of most non-living virus vaccines, but also with internal proteins of the virus particle, and in addition non-structural viral proteins. All or any of these antigens may contribute to the induction of protective immunity
- Induction of cell-mediated immunity through appropriate presentation of antigens. By replicating within the cells of a vaccinated animal, antigens are presented to the immune system in such a way as to stimulate cell-mediated immunity (CMI) through cytotoxic T lymphocytes (CTLs), which subsequently recognize and kill infected cells. In this process, a proportion of the viral or bacterial proteins that are synthesized within the infected cell is digested into peptides of around nine amino acids. These peptides are then transported through the endoplasmic reticulum where they are bound to, and subsequently presented on, the surface of the cell by major histocompatibility complex (MHC) class I molecules. This pathway of antigen presentation is called the 'endogenous' pathway. The peptide–MHC molecule complex is recognized by the T-cell receptor of an antigen-specific precursor CTL, which is consequently activated to provide a large population of effector CTLs within a few days. These cells then recognize infected cells through the same surface peptide–MHC molecule combination on the cell surface and kill them by lysing their plasma membranes. In this way virus-infected cells may be killed even before progeny virus is assembled in the cell and spreads to other cells
- Generation of mucosal immunity (if given orally or intranasally). This is best achieved by administration of live vaccines to mucosal surfaces, for example by intranasal instillation. Parenteral administration of live vaccines has been shown to generate significant mucosal immunity in some models, but research in small animals in this area is somewhat limited.

Live vaccines do not require as many infectious agents as non-living vaccines and consequently are less expensive to manufacture. However, there are also potential disadvantages of live vaccines:

- Incomplete attenuation. In large measure, the extent of attenuation of a vaccine is inversely proportional to the quality of the immune

response that it induces. In attempting to improve the immunity generated by a vaccine, the degree of attenuation may be reduced. Although great care is taken by vaccine manufacturers, on rare occasions a vaccine that is safe in laboratory trials is found to be virulent in the field and has to be withdrawn. An example of this problem was the occurrence of post-vaccinal encephalitis in dogs given a particular batch of combined CDV/canine adenovirus vaccine in which the CDV component was shown to be poorly attenuated (Ek-Kommonen *et al.*, 1997)
- Reversion of the attenuated organism to virulence – although this is very rare for small animal vaccines
- Inactivation of the organism through environmental factors, e.g. heat
- Neutralization of infectivity of the organism by maternally derived antibody (see below).

Genetically modified live vaccines

Techniques for genetic modification have been employed to produce vaccines of a defined non-pathogenic phenotype (see Figure 3.2). The simplest genetically modified vaccine is one in which genes that encode proteins known to be associated with virulence have been inactivated. There are no examples of this kind of vaccine currently available for use in dogs or cats.

A second type of genetically modified live vaccine consists of a virus vector into which has been inserted a gene encoding a foreign protein that induces a protective immune response. The best known example is a vaccine of recombinant vaccinia virus containing the gene for the G glycoprotein of rabies virus. This glycoprotein is recognized as the prime antigen in inducing protective immunity against rabies virus infection. When the live recombinant virus grows in vaccinated animals, the proteins encoded by both the vector and the foreign gene are expressed and immunize the host against rabies. This vaccine has been used with remarkable success in immunizing red foxes of continental western Europe. The programme has been so successful that it is expected that the infection will soon be eradicated in that area. Although not yet licensed for use in domestic animals (for which excellent inactivated rabies virus vaccines are available), the recombinant virus has been shown to be effective in dogs and cats. An analogous vaccine is a canarypox–feline leukaemia virus recombinant that produces excellent protection against challenge with FeLV in cats.

Other viral and bacterial vectors that have been used experimentally include herpesviruses, adenoviruses and *Salmonella*, but none of these has yet been developed as a platform technology for commercial use.

A recent interesting development in vaccine technology is DNA vaccination. In this process, the gene encoding the relevant immunogens is inserted into a bacterial plasmid. This construct is grown to large quantities in bacteria, purified and used as a vaccine. When inoculated into an animal, the construct is taken up by cells of the host where the gene is expressed. The expressed proteins are then processed by the immune system to produce a protective response. DNA vaccines have been shown to induce immunity to many infectious diseases but have yet to be developed for use in the field.

Non-living vaccines

There are three main types of non-living vaccines.

Chemically inactivated vaccines

Most non-living vaccines are made from living and potentially virulent organisms treated with a chemical agent that renders them non-infectious but does not affect their immunogenicity. Antibody responses are often directed at native conformational determinants on antigens, so it is important that these structures are retained in the vaccine. This can be a problem with chemically inactivated organisms and with recombinant proteins which may have different conformations. The latter group may have to be solubilized by denaturing agents such as urea to extract them from the bacteria in which they have been expressed.

Common inactivating agents for viral vaccines are β-propiolactone and aziridine compounds. These agents interact with viral nucleic acid preventing it from replicating, while having little effect on proteins. Formaldehyde, which was widely used previously, is now rarely employed because it is difficult to achieve the high levels of inactivation required for vaccine safety without compromising immunogenicity.

Subunit vaccines

These are made by disrupting the whole organism, for example with detergents, to release immunogenic subunits. This is an uncommon and relatively expensive method of production, and the only small animal examples of this type are vaccines against feline calicivirus (FCV) and feline herpesvirus (FHV).

Genetically engineered subunit vaccines

These are made by expressing components of the agent that are known to be immunogenic in bacteria, yeasts, insect or mammalian cells. The major attraction of this type of approach to vaccine production is that the immunogen can be produced on a very large scale, relatively inexpensively. However, success of the process depends on maintenance of immunogenicity during expression and purification of the antigen.

The only current example of this type is a vaccine for FeLV. Because the surface envelope glycoprotein of FeLV was known to be responsible for inducing a protective immune response in cats, the gene encoding the protein was cloned, inserted into an appropriate plasmid and expressed in *Escherichia coli* (Figure 3.3). However, the viral protein purified from the bacteria is rather different from the native glycoprotein in the viral particle. It is not glycosylated and is in a denatured form. Both features might be expected to impair the immunogenicity of the vaccine. Nonetheless, the protein does elicit an effective immune response against FeLV infection, probably through the induction of CMI.

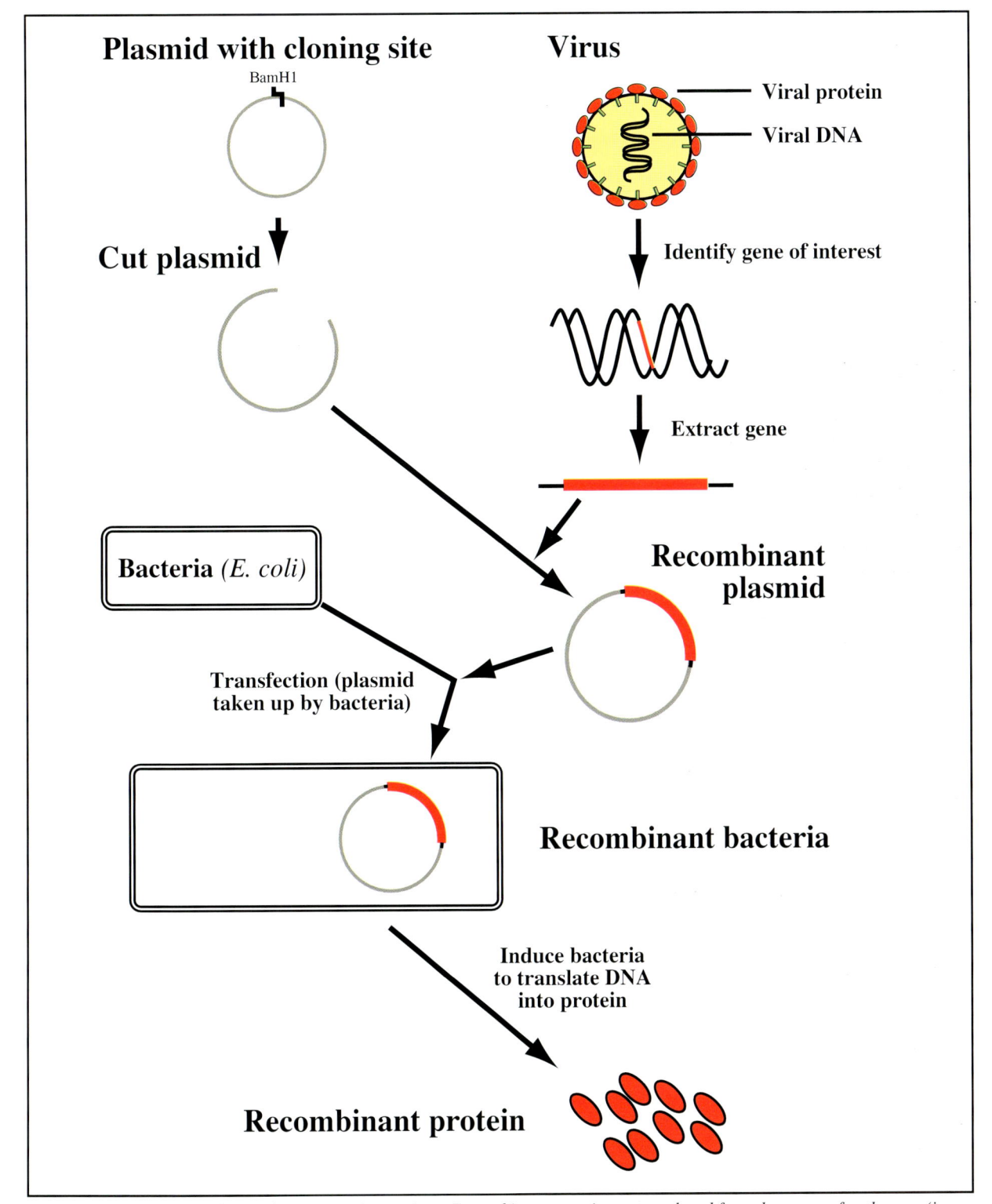

Figure 3.3: Production of recombinant protein vaccines. Recombinant proteins are produced from the genes of pathogens (in this case a virus) that have been inserted into bacteria, yeasts or other cells. The expression of these genes is controlled by an inducible promotor (not shown). The samples of recombinant proteins are very pure and do not contain any infectious organisms.

Adjuvants

All non-living vaccines require an adjuvant to provide an adequate immune response. A wide range of adjuvants is used in small animal vaccines including aluminium salts and derivatives of the glycoside saponin. Adjuvants are believed to have two main modes of action:

- Slow release of antigen by forming a depot of vaccine at the site of inoculation, which promotes the generation of an immune response of high affinity
- Attraction of antigen-presenting cells, such as macrophages and dendritic cells, to the inoculation site. These cells process the antigen for presentation to the lymphocytes, which need to be activated to assist the development of immune responses.

Previously it was generally considered that non-living viral vaccines were poor inducers of CMI responses, including CTLs. However, the nature of the response can be modified by the type of adjuvant incorporated into the vaccine. Recent studies indicate that non-living vaccines can indeed induce CMI, although perhaps not at the levels achieved by live vaccines.

The major theoretical advantage of non-living vaccines over live vaccines is that they are safer because they are incapable of replication. Their main disadvantages are that higher doses of the organism have to be given, and they do not present such a wide range of potential immunogens to the immune system. The adjuvant contained in non-living vaccines may cause adverse reactions in the host.

Routes of administration

Most vaccines for small animals are given by subcutaneous or intramuscular inoculation to induce a systemic immune response. However, some are designed for direct application to mucosal surfaces and are given intranasally or orally, for example the vaccine against *Bordetella bronchiseptica* in dogs. There are many advantages to the mucosal route of administration for agents that infect the respiratory or enteric tracts, not least of which is the induction of a very powerful mucosal immune response. Such vaccines may also induce a systemic response. Intranasal administration of some vaccines may be effective even in the face of maternally derived antibody in young animals.

FACTORS INFLUENCING VACCINE EFFICACY

The efficacy of a vaccine depends on an interaction between vaccine, host, human and environmental factors (Figure 3.4).

Vaccine factors
Correct strain/immunogen
Degree of attenuation
Adjuvant
Host factors
Maternal antibodies
Pre-existing infections
Immune system function
Human factors
Storage and mixing
Timing of vaccination
Route of administration
Environmental factors
Challenge

Figure 3.4: *Factors influencing vaccine efficacy.*

Vaccine factors

Extensive research is undertaken before a vaccine is released for general use. This ensures that the vaccine, if used properly, induces protection from challenge in a high percentage of vaccinated animals. This is achieved by presenting the correct antigen in a safe manner to the host's immune system; however, wild-type organisms change with time and place. Vaccines that were effective may become ineffective due to antigenic drift.

Annual revaccination

Vaccine manufacturers often recommend that booster doses of vaccine should be given following a primary course. In most cases this advice is based on their own duration of immunity studies showing that animals given a primary course of vaccination are protected when challenged 12, or sometimes 24, months later. From observations on the persistence of antibody levels following vaccination, particularly to the canine viruses, it has been suggested that dogs do not require to be vaccinated annually, and a period of 3 years between vaccinations has been suggested. Apart from studies on some rabies virus vaccines, there is very little experimental evidence on protective immunity following challenge on which to base a recommendation that vaccinated cats or dogs should be given booster vaccinations at longer intervals than 1 year. There would be serious welfare and financial implications of carrying out such laboratory trials of efficacy.

Host factors

All animals do not respond equally well to vaccination, and some may not mount an effective immune response to a vaccine. Fortunately, non-responders to the common vaccines are few. The host factor most affecting vaccine efficacy is the presence of maternally derived antibodies (MDA).

Maternal antibodies
Many newborn animals acquire immunoglobulins from their mother in the immediate perinatal period by one of two passive routes of transfer:

- In utero: this route is responsible for 2-18% of the total immunoglobulins transferred
- Colostrum: this is responsible for the remainder of transfer.

Passive transfer of antibodies is so successful that many neonates have titres almost equal to that of their dam after the first few days of suckling. Neonatal antibody titres are lower in larger litters or if suckling is impaired. Initial titres are important in determining the time for which a neonate will be protected (Figure 3.5).

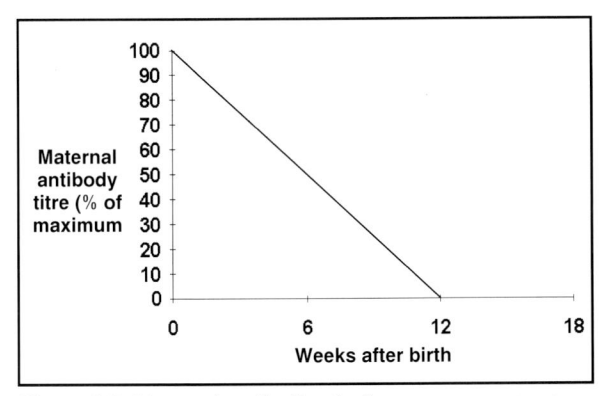

Figure 3.5: Maternal antibodies decline at a constant rate. The rate is determined to a large extent by the antibody type. As different viruses produce different proportions of antibody types so their rates of decline vary. For example, maternal antibodies against canine distemper virus have a half life of 8.4 days whereas those against feline leukaemia virus have a half life of 15 days.

Maternal antibodies can interfere with the ability of vaccines to induce immunity. This is particularly true for live virus vaccines that contain relatively small amounts of infectious virus and may be readily neutralized by MDA. For example, the early CPV vaccines when given at the conventional times (i.e. 9 and 12 weeks old) left many puppies unprotected as their levels of MDA were sufficient to neutralize the virus used in the vaccine. This sort of problem can be overcome by:

- Giving a third dose of vaccine when the animal is over 12 weeks old, by which time MDA will have gone in the vast majority of animals
- Increasing the virus titre in the vaccine
- Establishing the serum antibody level to the virus to ensure freedom from MDA before vaccination (see below).

Colostrum-deprived individuals should be vaccinated earlier than normal animals. There are only limited data on the timing of such vaccinations, and no vaccine is licensed for use in these circumstances. The authors suggest giving half the standard dose to animals 2-3 weeks old and repeating every 3 weeks until they are 9 weeks old.

Pre-existing infections
Infectious organisms require an incubation period before clinical signs of disease become apparent. This incubation period may be as short as a few hours or as long as a few years but in general is a few days. If an animal is incubating an infectious disease at the time of vaccination then it may well develop clinical signs. The host's immune response may be impaired, thereby reducing the response to vaccination. The vaccination may be more likely to induce unwanted side effects, although this has not been documented in small animals.

Young animals from large multi-animal environments will be particularly likely to be incubating diseases at the time of first or second vaccination. Diseases may be acquired from the veterinary surgery by direct contact or fomite transmission. It is particularly important that veterinary surgeons' examination tables and hands are thoroughly cleaned before an unvaccinated animal is examined. It is sensible to encourage owners to wait 1 week after acquiring a new puppy or kitten before requesting vaccination. In that time the animal should be isolated from other animals in the household.

Immune system function
An animal must have an effective immune system if it is to respond appropriately to a vaccine. Animals that are very old, very young, pregnant, sick or receiving drugs (particularly glucocorticoids and cytotoxic agents) may have a reduced ability to respond appropriately to vaccination. The effect of these factors on the ability to respond to vaccination has not been extensively investigated, and those studies that have been performed have produced variable results. For example, it is likely that low doses of glucocorticoids do not significantly reduce the response to vaccination. In contrast, hyperthermic puppies (>39.8°C, 103.6°F) are unable to mount an effective immune response to CDV vaccination and will succumb to disease if subsequently challenged. Anaesthetics have not been shown to influence vaccine efficacy on their own, but the stress of surgical procedures may affect the ability of the immune system to respond effectively.

Human factors
There are several factors within the control of the veterinary surgeon that may affect vaccine efficacy. First, vaccines should be stored at the appropriate temperature recommended by the manufacturer, usually 4°C. This is especially true for live vaccines, which might be inactivated at higher temperatures. Each vaccine has an expiry date printed on the vial which

should be strictly adhered to. Vaccines should be reconstituted with the diluent with which they are supplied. Once reconstituted they should be used immediately (or at least within a couple of hours provided they are stored at 4°C).

There are also several factors within the control of the owner that may affect vaccine efficacy. Owners should not allow animals to leave isolation until 1 week after the second (or in some cases third) dose. The secondary (anamnestic) response takes a short time to develop and, until it has, the animal will not be fully protected (Figure 3.6). It is also important that owners adhere to the vaccination schedule advised by their veterinary surgeon. Excessive or decreased delays between the first and second doses reduces the secondary antibody response and therefore both the length and quality of the immunity produced.

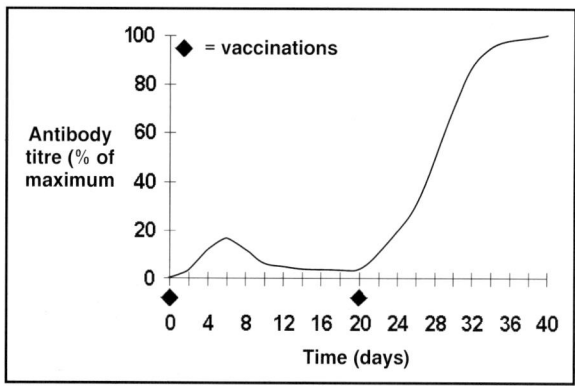

Figure 3.6: Primary and secondary immune response. Vaccination achieves immunity by induction of a secondary (anamnestic) response. This response requires that a primary response has been elicited in the days preceding the second dose. If the interval is too short then the primary response renders the second dose of vaccine ineffective. If the interval is too long then the secondary response does not occur. Some vaccines that undergo limited replication within the host can provoke both a primary and a secondary response as they are still present as the primary response abates.

Environmental factors

Although vaccination programmes may be adequate to control infectious disease under 'normal' conditions of exposure, it should be remembered that they may not protect under severe conditions of challenge. This situation has been observed in kittens infected with feline parvovirus (FPV). In many cases FPV was not suspected initially as a cause of death because vaccination was performed in the households in which disease occurred. The infection was diagnosed only by the application of specific diagnostic tests for FPV. Disease was thought to develop as a result of an accumulation of virus in an environment that either overcame vaccinal immunity in the affected kittens or infected the kittens in the period between the waning of maternal antibodies and the administration of the vaccine.

RISKS OF VACCINATION

To be granted a product licence, a vaccine must be shown to be of adequate quality, safety and efficacy. Studies on these criteria are often conducted in the target species in laboratory settings. There is always a possibility that when vaccines that have proved to be effective in these studies are then applied on a large scale in field conditions, they do not meet these exacting standards. There are two main problems that have been encountered following release of vaccines for general use:

- Adverse reactions
- Lack of efficacy.

Measures are in place to detect adverse reactions in the UK through reporting by veterinary surgeons to the Veterinary Medicines Directorate so that vaccines suspected of giving trouble should be identified and investigated. Lack of efficacy may not, however, be immediately evident.

Adverse reactions

The case of postvaccinal encephalitis in dogs given a live CDV vaccine has been described above. There are two other exmples of adverse reactions that have caused concern. One example was the appearance in kittens of polyarthritis and lameness shortly after the administration of a live FCV vaccine. That particular problem was resolved, but transient lameness may still occur in cats vaccinated with similar vaccines. The occurrence of this reaction is so rare that it is considered that the benefit outweighs the cost.

Another example of an adverse reaction has been the development of fibrosarcomas at injection sites in cats, particularly in North America. The cause is unknown. It may involve adjuvants or live virus or may result from multiple injections of any sort. Although some authorities recommend that vaccines should be inoculated at different sites on each occasion, there is no evidence that dividing injection sites reduces the risk of sarcoma development. Indeed, increasing the number of injection sites may actually increase the risk of tumour formation.

Many other types of adverse reactions have been reported following vaccination, ranging from relatively trivial (e.g. reactions at the injection site, pain, transient pyrexia, anorexia and depression) to more serious side effects. These include anaphylaxis and some autoimmune diseases such as immune-mediated haemolytic anaemia (Duval and Giger, 1996). It is these serious, but rare, reactions that have led to the controversial advocacy of alternatives to vaccination, including homeopathic products and serological screening to establish the immune state of an animal.

Care must be taken to ensure that vaccines are not given by an inappropriate route, either directly or indirectly. Accidental intranasal administration of feline respiratory virus vaccines intended to be inoculated subcutaneously may result in the replication of virus in the oropharynx and clinical disease. Accidental infection of susceptible non-target hosts with vaccinal virus may cause serious problems. An example is the occurrence of encephalitis in young puppies caused by CDV given to their dam in a booster vaccine when the puppies were 3 days old.

Lack of efficacy

Lack of efficacy may be identified when a vaccinated animal is not protected following natural exposure to an agent. This failure is likely to be relatively easy to detect when the infection is acute, such as CPV or FHV infection. It is much less likely to be suspected when the infection is more chronic, such as FeLV, or when the agent is absent from the community.

A dramatic example of the latter was the epizootic of canine distemper that occurred in Finland in 1996. It seems that the low efficacy of the vaccine used in that country for several years had not been recognized because the prevalence of CDV infection in Finland was low or zero (no case of distemper had occurred there for 16 years). However, when CDV was reintroduced to Finland from Russia, the consequences of the poor quality of the vaccine became immediately evident when at least 5000 cases of distemper were recorded. This situation might have been avoided if dogs had been screened to determine whether they had levels of virus neutralizing antibodies indicative of protection.

INVESTIGATION OF SUSPECTED VACCINE BREAKDOWNS

Vaccination failures are uncommon but when they occur owners often seek to blame the veterinary surgeon and/or manufacturer. Vaccines may fail to provide adequate protection for many reasons, some of which are beyond the control of either the veterinary surgeon or the vaccine company. The term 'vaccination' should not be confused with 'immunization' in literature given to owners. No vaccine produces 100% immunity. A variety of host factors, vaccine factors and veterinary factors may also be involved (Figure 3.7). The commonest reasons are pre-existent infections and high titres of maternal antibodies. The investigation of a suspected vaccine breakdown should proceed in a stepwise pattern. All suspected vaccine breakdowns, whether confirmed or not, should be reported to the Veterinary Medicines Directorate:

1. **Obtain a definitive diagnosis.** This may be achieved by isolation of the organism, histopathology or serology. Clinical signs alone are not sufficient evidence to confirm a vaccine breakdown as other diseases may produce similar clinical signs to the disease being vaccinated against.

Pre-existing infections
High titres of maternal antibodies
Pyrexia, hyperthermia, hypothermia
Immunosuppression
Age: very young or very old
Concurrent disease
Pregnancy
Malnutrition
'Stress'
Concomitant drug therapy, e.g. glucocorticoids
Wrong strain/immunogen in vaccine
Excessive attenuation of vaccine
Poor adjuvant
Overwhelming exposure
Poor storage
Poor mixing
Wrong timing of vaccination, e.g. delay between initial and second doses
Exposing animal to infection at the time of vaccination
Wrong route of administration
Disinfectant on syringe

Figure 3.7: Causes of vaccine breakdowns.

---

2. **Eliminate the possibility of pre-existing disease.** It may be possible with some infections to determine whether the virus or bacteria is antigenically related to the strain of virus in the vaccine. In other cases, knowledge of the incubation period is used to distinguish between true vaccine failure and the development of pre-existing disease. Pre-existing infections tend to produce clinical signs soon after vaccination. For example, a puppy that develops signs of parvoviral enteritis 24 hours after vaccination will have been incubating the disease at the time of vaccination as the incubation period is known to be at least 5 days.

3. **Obtain an accurate history of the vaccination.** It is essential that the vaccine batch should be checked to ensure it is 'in date'. It is also pertinent to review the storage facilities of the vaccine and that it is being given in an appropriate way. The timing of the first and second vaccinations should be checked against the manufacturer's recommendations. Check that no other drugs have been given around the time of vaccination.

4. **Obtain more information about the vaccinated animal.** In particular, re-evaluate the health status of the animal at the time of vaccination (e.g. rectal temperature, signs of systemic illness). It may also be useful to enquire about the environment in which the animal is living. Excessive challenges can overcome vaccine-induced immunity in some instances.

5. **Check the effectiveness of the vaccine in other animals.** This may be done by measuring antibody titres before and after vaccination. It may be useful to contact the manufacturer for help with this.

ALTERNATIVES TO VACCINATION

Owners of animals that have shown signs that may be due an adverse reaction to a vaccine are often unwilling to revaccinate their pet but many owners will still want to try to provide some form of protection. In addition there are a small number of owners who, for ethical or economical reasons, do not wish to vaccinate their pets. In the latter case encouragement at least to complete a primary course of vaccinations should be contemplated. There are four alternatives to vaccination: isolation; control of vectors and reservoir hosts; treatment; and serological testing.

Isolation

Isolating animals from other animals that are sources of infection prevents those animals from acquiring the infection. As long as such isolation is performed in an effective and humane manner, then it is the optimum method of control of infectious disease. The most widely used example of this is the 'test and remove' scheme that has kept a large number of catteries free of FeLV for some years.

Control of vectors and reservoir hosts

Tick-borne diseases and those that are spread by biting insects can be prevented by reducing the exposure to the vectors. Reservoir hosts (usually wild animals) allow a disease to be maintained in a population in which it would otherwise disappear. This method of control can be effective on the medium to large scale. It is rarely effective at the level of the individual household. Few of the diseases that are currently vaccinated against are spread by vectors. *Leptospira icterohaemorrhagica* is maintained in a reservoir host (rats and other rodents), and effective control of these can reduce the contamination of water sources from which the infection is contracted by companion animals.

Treatment

Some infectious diseases may be controlled by treatment of outbreaks rather than vaccination. This may be a cost-effective alternative for the control of *Bordetella bronchiseptica* and *Chlamydophila felis*. This approach is not appropriate for pathogens such as canine parvovirus that induce life-threatening diseases.

Serological testing

For those pet owners who are concerned about possible adverse reactions or who do not wish their pets to be 'over-vaccinated,' a pragmatic solution to their problem is to measure serum antibody titres. This will establish whether the animal is likely to be immune and therefore does not require to be vaccinated. Asessment of serum antibody titres to several canine and feline pathogens allows the state of protective immunity to be predicted accurately (provided an appropriate serological test is performed). This is not the case for agents such as *Leptospira* spp., canine parainfluenza virus or *B. bronchiseptica* in the dog, or FeLV in the cat.

A special case of the measurement of antibody levels induced by vaccination is rabies virus. To enter the UK from a specified rabies-free area, dogs or cats must be vaccinated with a licensed rabies virus vaccine and be shown to have responded by having a titre of at least 0.5 IU/ml of rabies virus neutralizing antibodies in their serum. In this case the quality of the serological tests is controlled by an international authority, and the tests are carried out only in licensed laboratories.

REFERENCES AND FURTHER READING

Anon (1999) Vaccine-associated feline sarcoma task force guidelines. Diagnosis and treatment of suspected sarcomas. *Journal of the American Veterinary Medical Association* **214**, 1745

Brochier B, Kieny MP, Costy F *et al.* (1991) Large scale eradication of rabies using recombinant vaccinia-rabies vaccine. *Nature* **354**, 520–522

Duval D and Giger U (1996) Vaccine associated immune mediated hemolytic anemia in the dog. *Journal of Veterinary Internal Medicine* **10**, 290–295

Ek-Kommonen C, Sihvonen L, Pekkanen K, Rikula U and Nuotio L (1997) Outbreak of canine distemper in vaccinated dogs in Finland. *Veterinary Record* **141**, 380–383

Greene CE (1998) Immunoprophylaxis and immunotherapy. In: *Infectious Diseases of the Dog and Cat*, 3rd edn, ed. CE Greene, pp. 717–750. WB Saunders, Philadelphia

Kruth SA and Ellis JA (1998) Vaccination of dogs and cats: general principles and duration of immunity. *Canadian Veterinary Journal* **39**, 423–426

McCandlish IA, Cornwell HJ, Thompson H, Nash AS and Lowe CM (1992) Distemper encephalitis in pups after vaccination of the dam. *Veterinary Record* **130**, 27–30

Marciani DJ, Kensil CR, Beltz GA, Hung CH, Cronier J and Aubert A (1991) Genetically-engineered subunit vaccine against feline leukaemia virus: protective immune response in cats. *Vaccine* **9**, 89–96

Tartaglia J, Jarrett O, Neil JC, Desmettre P and Paoletti E (1993) Protection of cats against feline leukaemia virus by vaccination with a canarypox virus recombinant, ALVAC-FL. *Journal of Virology* **67**, 2370–2375

Rikula U, Nuotio L and Sihvonen L (2000) Canine distemper virus neutralising antibodies in vaccinated dogs. *Veterinary Record* **147**, 598–603

CHAPTER FOUR

Control of Infectious Diseases in Multi-Animal Environments

Danièlle Gunn-Moore

CHAPTER PLAN

Introduction
    Factors determining the extent of disease
    Prevention is better than cure
Common infectious organisms
    The multifactorial nature of disease
    Method of dissemination
Construction of facilities
Disinfection of environments
Management of facilities
    Numbers of animals
    Grouping animals
    Hygiene measures
Breeding establishments
    Special considerations
    Kittening/whelping rooms
Investigating outbreaks of infectious diseases
Veterinary practices
    Nosocomial infections
    Veterinary factors predisposing to spread
      of nosocomial infections
    Preventing nosocomial infections
References and further reading

INTRODUCTION

The dynamics of infectious disease within a group of animals vary with the dynamics of the host population (Figure 4.1). Animals may be kept in groups for a variety of reasons. Populations are generally described as either stable or transient:

- Stable populations are usually found in households containing large numbers of pets, breeding establishments, laboratory colonies and kennelled hounds
- Transient populations occur in veterinary practices, grooming and boarding establishments and animal shelters.

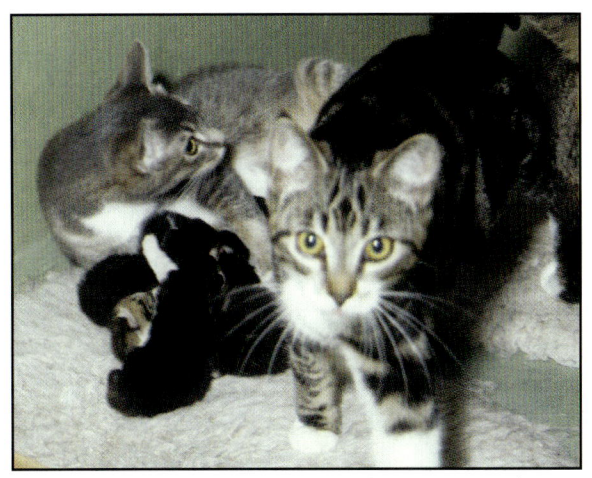

Figure 4.1: Example of a multi-animal environment where infectious diseases will be able to spread rapidly.

Some populations have stable and transient characteristics, such as shelters with a non-euthanasia policy, and feral populations.

Whether a population is stable or transient affects the amount and type of infectious diseases that are present. It may also affect the importance attached to disease control. Control of infectious disease is difficult in transient populations, given the random source of the animals, their short stay within the group, the high levels of stress and the frequent reintroduction of infectious organisms. It is generally easier to control infectious disease in stable populations, usually via a combination of quarantine, vaccination, parasite control and disease surveillance.

Although certain types of establishment require specific considerations, several risk factors for infectious disease can be considered more generally. These are listed below. Control of these factors and discussion of special situations, such as neonates in breeding establishments and the risk of nosocomial infections in veterinary practices, are considered in later sections.

Under the Animal Boarding Establishments Act 1963 licensed premises must conform to the criteria detailed in *Model Licence Conditions and Guidance for Cat Boarding Establishments* and *Model Licence Conditions and Guidance for Dog Boarding Establishments*.

Factors determining the extent of disease

Factors that determine the extent of infectious disease within a multi-animal environment are:

- The presence of infectious organisms
- The dose of organisms to which animals may be exposed; this relates to population density and/or environmental contamination
- The presence of concurrent disease, particularly if immunosuppressive in nature
- The level of stress to which the animals are subjected, e.g. overcrowding, weaning, rehoming
- The age of the animals
- The genetics of the animals.

Infectious diseases are found most commonly in animals with reduced immunocompetence, e.g. young or old animals, those with immunosuppressive or debilitating diseases, or animals that are stressed because of overcrowding. All these factors should be considered when trying to reduce the level of disease within a multi-animal environment.

The motivation towards reducing infectious disease varies with the function of the establishment. In all cases animal welfare should be the prime concern, but professional reputation, the cost of medical treatment or the loss of income from unsold or undersold stock will also be involved. When a veterinary surgeon is called to advise on infectious disease control it is useful to determine which of these factors are important.

Prevention is better than cure

If possible, a veterinary surgeon who is responsible for the care of a particular group of animals should be involved in the design of the facility and the planning of the disease control policy. This will result in fewer disease outbreaks and is considerably more rewarding than providing an emergency service when problems arise (see sections on design and management of multi-animal facilities).

COMMON INFECTIOUS ORGANISMS

The multifactorial nature of disease

Many infectious diseases that are seen in multi-animal environments present with similar clinical signs, such as coughing or diarrhoea. It is advisable to identify which organisms are involved in a disease outbreak. In multi-animal environments, disease may be multifactorial, with several infectious organisms being involved and non-infectious (often environmental) factors complicating the situation (Figure 4.2). For example,

Clinical sign	Infectious causes		Non-infectious causes
	Dogs	**Cats**	
Respiratory, e.g. coughing, sneezing, ocular discharges, nasal discharges (see also Chapter 6)	Canine parainfluenza virus, canine adenovirus type1, canine adenovirus type 2, canine distemper virus, mycoplasmosis, bordetellosis, pasteurellosis	Feline herpesvirus, feline calicivirus, feline coronavirus, chlamydophilosis, mycoplasmosis, bordetellosis, pasteurellosis	Poor ventilation/dusty environment, irritant chemicals/residual disinfectant
Gastrointestinal, e.g. diarrhoea and/or vomiting (see also Chapter 8)	Canine distemper virus, canine parvovirus, canine coronavirus, canine adenovirus type1 (rare), giardiasis, coccidiosis, cryptosporidiosis, campylobacteriosis, salmonellosis	Feline panleucopenia virus, feline coronavirus, giardiasis, coccidiosis, cryptosporidiosis, campylobacteriosis, salmonellosis	Nutritional indiscretions, unsuitable diet, lack of colostrum, stress
Neurological, e.g. collapse, seizures (see also Chapter 15)	Canine distemper virus, canine herpesvirus - neonatal (rare), tetanus - iatrogenic spread (rare), botulism	Feline coronavirus, feline panleucopenia virus, tetanus - iatrogenic spread (rare), botulism	Heat stress, poisoning (e.g. lead, metaldehyde, strychnine, some plants, fungi)
Reproductive, e.g. infertility, abortion, neonatal deaths ('fading kittens/puppies') (see also Chapter 12)	Canine parvovirus, canine distemper virus, canine adenovirus type1, canine herpesvirus (rare), salmonellosis - rare	Feline leukaemia virus, feline panleucopenia virus, feline immunodeficiency virus, feline coronavirus, salmonellosis - rare	Lack of colostrum, inappropriate nutrition/management, congenital disorders
Dermatological, e.g. alopecia/skin irritation (see also Chapter 13)	Fleas, lice, mites, ticks, dermatophytosis, bacterial infections (*Staphylococcus*), whip-worms	Fleas, lice, mites, ticks, dermatophytosis, bacterial infections (*Staphylococcus*), feline cowpox virus - rare	Irritant chemicals/residual disinfectant Poor hygiene
Musculoskeletal, e.g. polyarthritis (see also Chapter 14)		Feline calicivirus, *Streptococcus*	Poor hygiene resulting in bacterial 'joint ill'

Figure 4.2: Presenting signs of infectious diseases in multi-animal establishments and their causes. This table lists those infectious agents that may cause outbreaks of clinical disease in multi-animal environments in the UK. It does not include infectious diseases that only affect an individual within such an environment. The table also includes non-infectious differential diagnoses that need to be considered when large numbers of animals become ill within a multi-animal establishment.

respiratory disease in cats may be caused by feline herpesvirus (FHV), feline calicivirus (FCV), feline coronavirus (FCoV) and a variety of bacteria (including *Bordetella bronchiseptica, Pasteurella* spp. and *Chlamydophila felis* (formerly *Chlamydia psittaci* var. *felis*)). Poor ventilation, high humidity and overcrowding increase their clinical effects and the likelihood of spread. To reduce respiratory disease within an affected facility, it is necessary to address infectious and non-infectious causes. Improving ventilation, reducing overcrowding, treating with antibacterials, instigating a suitable vaccination programme and/or isolation may all be required (see later sections for detailed information).

Method of dissemination

The type of infectious disease found within a multi-animal establishment depends on the function of the facility and the measures taken to limit the dissemination of infectious organisms. Nosocomial infections are more likely to be found in veterinary practices, dermatophytes in grooming parlours, and respiratory and enteric infections in rescue centres. To prevent the spread of infection, it is necessary to understand how easily and by what route organisms are usually transmitted. To do this it is helpful to classify organisms by their infectious potential (Figure 4.3, overleaf):

- **Class 1** organisms have little chance of spreading between individuals, and the zoonotic potential is low
- **Class 2** organisms require close contact or vector transmission; these organisms are not environmentally resistant
- **Class 3** organisms can be transmitted by close or direct contact with infected body secretions; these organisms have moderate environmental resistance or zoonotic potential
- **Class 4** organisms are serious zoonotic pathogens or are easily transmitted (animals with these infections should be dealt with in isolation facilities).

Interspecies spread of disease

Several infections can cross between species, either affecting both cats and dogs or having a zoonotic or reverse zoonotic risk. This is true for many bacterial and protozoal infections, e.g. *Bordetella bronchiseptica* infection may pass between dogs and cats and may also have zoonotic and reverse zoonotic potential. Some viral infections may infect more than one species, e.g. 10-20% of canine parvovirus isolates cause disease indistinguishable from that caused by feline panleucopenia virus (FPV) in cats (Truyen, 1999).

Humans are an often forgotten source of infectious disease; not only may they shed several enteric infections, including *Salmonella, Giardia* and *Campylobacter*, but they can act as a reservoir for pulmonary tuberculosis. Humans can also act as vectors, disseminating infection on hands, clothes or footwear.

CONSTRUCTION OF FACILITIES

Animal accommodation should be comfortable, easy to clean, safe and secure. Because disease control is a major concern in multi-animal establishments, it should be addressed at the design stage of construction. Later alterations are usually difficult and expensive.

- Space is important. Ideally, an average cat should have about 8000 cm^2 of floor space. This is increased proportionately for larger cats and dogs and for animals in long-term housing. Animals in short-term housing or intensive care facilities can have less space
- All animal facilities should be non-hazardous. Wood preserver and paint must be suitable for use around animals, and sharp edges or loose wires must be covered. Concrete-based runs should be properly maintained as broken surfaces are dangerous and difficult to clean
- All areas accessible to animals must be easy to clean (see Figure 4.4). Everything that an animal can contact should be either disinfected or disposed of before the next animal takes up residence. A water supply for cleaning and hand washing should be available in all areas
- Open walkways should be at least 91 cm wide, as cats and dogs can sneeze viral particles to a distance of 61 cm or more. Where animals are housed side by side, then solid partitions are essential. In cat housing, these partitions should reach the ceiling to prevent residents climbing up and sneezing down on neighbours
- Dog runs should be easy to clean. Individual rather than communal runs are recommended. Ideally they should have a solid base (such as concrete). Grass and gravel runs are difficult to clean and maintain
- Facilities should be available for the safe disposal of all waste products, including adequate and appropriate drainage for urine and faeces (see Figure 4.4)
- To reduce air-borne infections, ventilation should allow 6-12 air changes per hour, depending on the number of animals within each air space. Air should be vented directly outside, not from one room to another
- Relative humidity should ideally be less than 55% and temperature between 15 and 24°C (check with a nursery thermometer or, better still, a maximum-minimum mercury thermometer)
- Buildings should be designed to allow movement of staff and visitors from clean to dirty areas, not the reverse
- Rodent access should be prevented.

Organism (classification of infectivity)	Method of spread	Significance of environmental contamination	Control of infection
Class 1			
Canine herpesvirus (CHV) (puppies)	Neonatal infection from dam or littermates	Rare	Improve management of puppies
Class 2			
Most (antibacterial-sensitive) bacteria	Variable	Variable	Improve hygiene, appropriate use of antibacterials
Feline leukaemia virus	Vertical transmission and horizontal transmission via saliva, urine and faeces	Minimal, generally requires prolonged duration of contact for transmission	Vaccination, 'test and remove' policy
Feline immunodeficiency virus	Mainly by biting. Vertical transmission can occur	None	Prevent biting, night curfew, neuter toms
Feline coronavirus	Mainly orofaecal, some via saliva and urine. Fomite transmission can occur	Minor, but virus can exist for days to weeks in organic matter	Improve hygiene, isolation breeding and early weaning
Class 3			
Giardia	Orofaecal	Significant, mainly via contaminated water	Improve hygiene, prevent exposure
Cryptosporidium	Orofaecal, especially in immunosuppressed individuals	Rare but significant when occurs, via contaminated water or food	Improve hygiene, prevent exposure
Coccidia (e.g. *Isospora*)	Orofaecal and eating infected intermediate hosts (e.g. mice)	Significant, via contaminated water and food	Improve hygiene, prevent exposure
Dermatophytes	Direct contact with affected and carrier animals and spores	Significant, via spore contamination	Improve hygiene, prevent exposure, screen for carriers
Leptospira	Mainly urine, also saliva, venereal or placental transfer	Significant, via urine contamination of water, bedding, etc.	Vaccination, prevent exposure
Campylobacter	Orofaecal	Significant, via contaminated water or food	Improve hygiene, prevent exposure
Antibacterial-resistant bacteria (e.g. *Pseudomonas*)	Variable	Variable	Improve hygiene, appropriate use of antibacterials
Enteric helminths (e.g. *Toxocara*)	Orofaecal, some vertically via milk	Significant	Improve hygiene, use of anthelmintics
Ectoparasites (e.g. fleas, lice, mites)	Direct contact, fomites	Highly significant	Use of topical and environmental antiparasitics
Class 4			
Canine parvovirus/feline panleucopenia virus	Orofaecal	Highly significant	Vaccination, quarantine procedures
Canine distemper virus	Orofaecal	Highly significant	Vaccination, quarantine procedures
Canine parainfluenza virus	Oronasal, aerosol	Moderate	Vaccination
Canine adenovirus type 1	Oronasal, urine and faeces	Significant	Vaccination
Canine adenovirus type 2	Oronasal	Significant	Vaccination
Feline calicivirus/feline herpesvirus	Oronasal, aerosol	Significant	Vaccination, quarantine procedures
Chlamydophila felis (formerly *Chlamydia psittaci* var. *felis*)	Direct contact	Minimal	Vaccination, appropriate use of antibacterials
Bordetella	Oronasal, aerosol; a carrier state exists	Moderate	Improve hygiene, vaccination, appropriate use of antibacterials
Salmonella	Orofaecal, food, water, fomites, rarely airborne	Highly significant, ubiquitous in nature	Improve hygiene, quarantine procedures

Figure 4.3: Classification of some infectious organisms found in multi-animal environments, their method of dissemination and control. Agents listed in Figure 4.2 are classified according to their zoonotic potential and ability to spread to other animals (based on Greene, 1998). The higher the classification, the more serious the agent is as a zoonosis or the more able it is to spread to other animals.

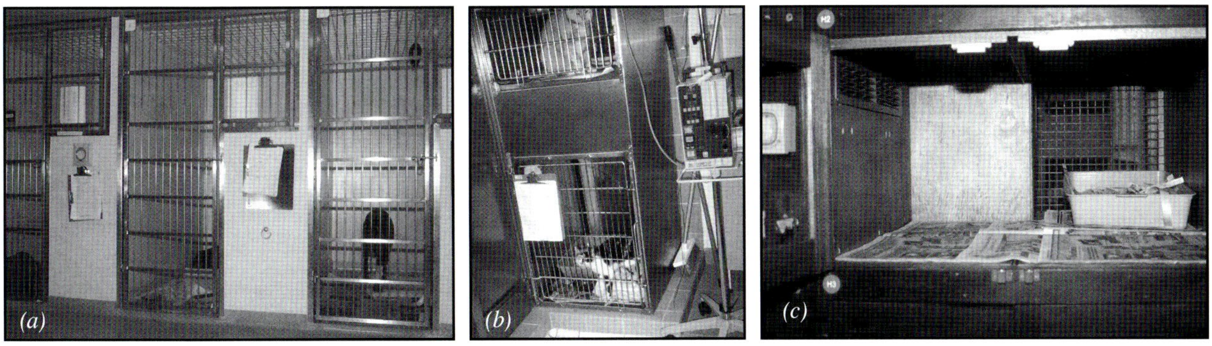

Figure 4.4: Examples of good and poor kennel design. (a) These kennels are large enough for large breed dogs. The floor slopes toward the door. Drip sets can be suspended from the roof such that the patients can still move about the kennel. (Courtesy of Mr Michael Herrtage.) (b) Inadequate guttering means that any spillage of urine or faeces in the upper cage will contaminate the cage below. (c) Poor choice of materials (in this case wood) and poor design mean that effective cleaning is difficult. (Courtesy of Dr Ian Ramsey.)

DISINFECTION OF ENVIRONMENTS

The aim of disinfection is to prevent the spread of infectious organisms between animals and in some cases from animals to humans. Of the organisms that can infect dogs and cats in multi-animal establishments, the cat 'flu' viruses and parvoviruses are of particular importance. Because parvoviruses are highly infectious and somewhat resistant to disinfection, they are often used as the 'gold standard' by which disinfectants are judged. Of the other important pathogens, most bacteria are fairly readily destroyed by disinfectants, but acid-fast bacteria and bacterial and fungal spores are more resistant. Figure 4.5 shows disinfectant activity against the more resistant microbial groups.

Where an area is known to be contaminated with a particular pathogen, disinfection should be tailored to that organism.

Particular care must be taken when choosing a disinfectant for use near cats as they are less able than most mammals to detoxify phenolic compounds. Other disinfectants are generally safe, provided that manufacturer's instructions are strictly followed. Although individual disinfectant compounds can be used, better results are often gained using proprietary mixtures. Homemade mixtures are not recommended as they may be ineffective or unsafe. As with all disinfectants, it is important to check their labels for information on safety and efficacy before use.

Type of disinfectant	Examples	Activity against				
		Acid-fast bacteria	Resistant bacteria	Bacterial spores	Fungi	Non-enveloped viruses
Alcohols	Ethanol	+	+	–	–	+
	Isopropyl	+	+	–	–	–
Phenolic compounds[a,b]	Coal tar derivatives	+	+	–	+	+/–
	Cresol	+	+	–	+	+/–
	Xylenol-rich cresylic acid	+	+	–	+	+/–
Biguanides[c]	Chlorhexidine[d]	–	+	–	–	–
Surface-active agents Cationic[e]	Quaternary ammonium compounds, e.g. cetrimide and benzalkonium chloride	–	–	–	+/–	–
Amphoteric	TEGO compounds	+	+	–	+	–
Aldehydes	Glutaraldehyde	+	+	+	+	+
	Formaldehyde	+	+	+	+	+
Halogens[c]	Chlorine (sodium hypochlorite)	+	+	+	+	+
	Iodine (povidone-iodine)	+	+	+/–	+	+/–
Combination products	Variable mixtures of the above	Check label for established activities				

Figure 4.5: Commonly available disinfectants and their antimicrobial activity.
+, effective; –, not effective; +/–, partially effective. [a] *Retain activity in the presence of organic matter.*
[b] *Not to be used where cats have access (see above).* [c] *Loses activity in heavily soiled situations.*
[d] *Low tissue toxicity and therefore useful for skin preparation.*
[e] *Unusually, Giardia cysts are sensitive to quaternary ammonium disinfectants.*

Before disinfection it is important to ensure that organic matter (e.g. faeces, hair, food) has been removed. Whichever disinfectant is chosen, it should be allowed the recommended contact time. It is necessary to rinse the area, as pools of disinfectant, even when made to the correct concentration, can cause inflammation of paws and respiratory tract. The area should be dried after rinsing, as pools of rinse water permit the rapid growth of bacteria.

MANAGEMENT OF FACILITIES

Although this section considers rescue centres, breeding units and boarding facilities in particular, much of the discussion also relates to other multi-animal establishments. Cleaning protocols, use of isolation facilities, methods to reduce stress and vaccination policies are also directly applicable to veterinary practices. Additional considerations for breeding establishments and veterinary practices are discussed later.

Preventing or reducing infectious disease in animals housed in groups can be difficult, time-consuming and expensive. Figure 4.6 presents a list of methods for reducing the incidence of infectious disease in multi-animal environments.

Reduce overcrowding
Maintain stable groups
Keep animals in single units
Improve hygiene
Have a standard cleaning protocol
Limit the number of times each pen is entered
Have and use an isolation facility
Reduce stress
Have a suitable vaccination policy

Figure 4.6: *Methods of reducing infectious disease within a multi-animal facility.*

Numbers of animals

Infectious disease is found most often when animals are kept in large groups or overcrowded conditions. This is because:

- When animals from different sources are mixed together there is an increased risk that infectious organisms will be introduced
- Infection spreads quickly in overcrowded conditions. Newly introduced animals become infected with organisms already present within the group, and infections from the newly introduced animals spread to the resident population
- In a large group of animals it is highly likely that at least some of the group will be infectious at any given time
- Animals may receive high doses of infectious organisms directly from other animals and indirectly from the environment. This is exacerbated by the difficulty of effective cleaning when large groups of animals are housed together
- Overcrowding causes stress and increases the incidence of concurrent infections
- Group feeding in overcrowded conditions can lead to malnutrition in weaker individuals.

Taken together, these factors increase the dissemination of infectious organisms and act to weaken animals' immune responses, so increasing the risk of disease developing.

Although no 'hard and fast' rules can be made, it is generally inadvisable to keep more than 8-10 cats in a domestic residence, unless purpose-built accommodation is also available. Figures for dogs have not been suggested.

Grouping animals

- With stable populations animals will often be kept in small groups. Individuals should be removed from the group if they show signs that may be due to an infectious disease
- With transient populations the most effective way to control infectious disease is to house animals individually. The only exception to this is animals arriving in an established group, when the group can be considered as a single unit. Whereas individual housing generally occurs in boarding establishments and grooming parlours, only a few rescue centres keep animals in this manner
- Where there is no alternative to group housing, it is advisable to quarantine all new arrivals until they have been examined for clinical signs of common infections. Animals should then be separated by age and disease status (with sick animals being attended to individually). Animals should not be transferred from one group to another. In this way, when disease outbreaks do occur infection can hopefully be confined to a single group
- Screening for some common infections (e.g. feline leukaemia virus) is sometimes performed and is useful for controlling that infection within the population. The value of such testing is limited by the large number of potential infectious agents.

Hygiene measures

Effective hygiene is the most important method of limiting the spread of infection in a multi-animal facility.

- Ideally, each animal should be housed separately. It should have its own set of utensils, which should be cleaned daily (food and water bowls, litter boxes for cats)

Kittening/whelping rooms

A practical way to reduce infectious disease in neonates is to let the dam give birth and rear her offspring in isolation. In some cases it may be advisable to wean the dam from her offspring when they are 5-6 weeks of age (see below). When neonates are orphaned or their mother is unable to care for them, the risk of infectious disease is increased, so even greater care is required.

- To reduce environmental contamination the room should be easy to clean, well ventilated and away from other animals
- The kittening/whelping room/isolation facility should always be cleaned and ideally left empty for a week before introducing the dam. If possible, the dam should be allowed to settle in before the birth
- During their time in isolation the dam and offspring should be kept under quarantine conditions (see previous section). No other animals should be allowed into the room. The room should have a dedicated set of food and water bowls, bedding and cleaning utensils (and litter boxes for cats)
- The youngest animals should be cleaned out first each day, followed by older kittens or puppies, then adults
- The dam will usually pass maternally derived antibodies (MDAs) on to her offspring. If the offspring suckle sufficiently when first born and environmental contamination is not extensive, MDAs are usually sufficient to protect offspring from infections for the first few weeks of life. The exact length of this protection varies with the dam's own immunity but 6 to 8 weeks is typical
- With some infectious diseases (e.g. FCoV infection) a dam known to be carrying the organism should be removed from her offspring once they are 5-6 weeks old. At this time the MDAs begin to wane and the offspring are at risk of being infected by their mother. If such infectious diseases are not present then this practice is not recommended (see below)
- Ideally, kittens and puppies should be kept in isolation until they are old enough to be rehomed. Separate litters should not be mixed as this increases their risk of infectious disease
- All kittens and puppies should be regularly dewormed and treated for fleas.

Problems with early weaning and isolation

Although it is well established that isolation and early weaning reduces the risk of neonates developing infectious disease, the practice is not without its difficulties.

- Isolation facilities can be expensive to build and time consuming to maintain
- If the offspring are small (e.g. kittens weaned at less than 500-550 g body weight), they are at an increased risk of developing problems such as wasting syndromes after separation from their mother
- Unless the facility provides environmental interest (e.g. toys, radios, vacuum cleaners) animals reared in isolation may become poorly socialized. This may be exacerbated if the litter size is small. Poorly socialized animals make poor pets, so it is important to consider this aspect of development when designing the facility.

INVESTIGATING OUTBREAKS OF INFECTIOUS DISEASES

Outbreaks of infectious diseases in multi-animal environments are common. Their impact on the animals and their owners and carers can be considerable. Only by conducting a full investigation and making a definitive diagnosis can the correct management changes be instigated. This will require:

- Examination of all sick animals
- Collection of samples. When collecting samples, whether by mouth swab, faeces or urine collection, coat brushing, skin scraping or at post mortem examination, it is essential to discuss the procedure with the laboratory that will be undertaking the analysis. Incorrect sample handling can produce non-diagnostic or erroneous results
- Post mortem examinations. Although many establishments are reluctant to have post mortem examinations performed, all deaths should be investigated. In many cases it is the only method of achieving a diagnosis, and other information gained during the procedure is often useful
- Examination of records. It is strongly advised that records should be kept of all animals entering and leaving multi-animal establishments. For breeding establishments, details of litter sizes and birth weights should be recorded. In all cases incidents of disease should be noted, particularly when thought to be infectious or when resulting in fatality. It is by noting changes in the morbidity and mortality patterns that problems can be recognized early. Although there is often reluctance to keep these records, they are invaluable in the long-term control of infectious disease
- Identification of recent changes in management policy. This will require a detailed history to be obtained from the owner or carer
- Visiting the premises.

Visiting the facilities

It is advisable to visit the facility in person, ideally taking photographs but at least making detailed notes for later reference. If this is not possible, then detailed building plans, photographs and step-by-step cleaning protocols can be useful alternatives. Since practice and policy are rarely identical, it is important to speak not only to the facility manager but also to the day-to-day cleaning staff.

When visiting a multi-animal facility it is useful to have a checklist of things to assess:

- Structural suitability of the facility (size of rooms, method of construction, ventilation, temperature, drainage, etc.)
- Vaccination policy (prerequisite for current vaccination, whether or not non-vaccinated animals are admitted)
- Source of new animals
- Genetic relationships
- Isolation procedures
- Separation of animals by health status, age, etc.
- Size of groups
- Routine cleaning procedure (type and concentration of disinfectant), movement of people, use of protective clothing, movement and use of equipment, including bedding, brushes, combs, leads, toys, etc.)
- Spacing of food bowls in relation to defecation area
- Use of communal runs.

VETERINARY PRACTICES

Nosocomial infections

Nosocomial infections are infections that are gained in, or whose development is favoured by, a hospital environment. Disease as a result of these infections may be seen while the animal is hospitalized or after it has returned home.

Nosocomial infections can arise endogenously from the opportunistic spread of normal microflora or exogenously from contamination within the veterinary practice. The prevalence of nosocomial infections in veterinary clinics is believed to be 5-10% of hospitalized patients (Greene, 1998). Disease is more likely to be found in immunocompromised patients and those with impaired mucocutaneous defences. Factors predisposing veterinary patients to the development of nosocomial infections are considered in Figure 4.7.

The most common nosocomial infections in human hospitals are urinary tract infections followed by pneumonias, surgical wound infections and bacteraemia (Emori and Gaynes, 1993). Although specific information is sparse the situation is believed to be similar in veterinary hospitals (Johnson and Murtaugh, 1997a,b). Figure 4.8 shows some common nosocomial bacterial infections in veterinary hospitals; all the organisms listed in Figure 4.2 can also be acquired in the hospital environment.

Mechanism	Examples
Impaired mucocutaneous defences	Surgery Intravenous or urinary catheters Skin wounds Endotracheal intubation Endoscopy/bronchoscopy Transtracheal wash, bronchoalveolar lavage Nebulization Respiratory/alimentary/urinary tract disease
Impaired immunity	Immunosuppressive infection Glucocorticoids Antineoplastic drugs Malnutrition Lack of colostrum
Altered microflora	Antibacterial therapy Respiratory or alimentary disease Contaminated equipment

Figure 4.7: Factors predisposing veterinary patients to the development of nosocomial infections.

Organism	Typical sources
Pseudomonas	Multiuse bottles, water sources
Serratia	Intravenous catheters, endotracheal tubes
Staphylococcus	Skin infections, dirty clippers
Escherichia	Faecal contamination of hospital equipment
Klebsiella	Faecal contamination of hospital equipment
Salmonella	Poor cleaning of kennels or runs, food contamination
Campylobacter	Poor cleaning of kennels or runs, food contamination

Figure 4.8: Examples of bacteria that are associated with nosocomial infections in veterinary hospitals and their typical sources.

Veterinary factors predisposing to spread of nosocomial infections

- Poor facility design – air flow, drainage, ease of cleaning
- Poor management policies – lack of segregation of patients by age and vaccine status, poor procedure for cleaning, etc.
- Poor design or use of isolation facilities
- Poor maintenance and cleaning of equipment – endoscopes, endotracheal tubes, oesophageal stethoscopes, laryngoscopes, auroscopes, thermometers, stethoscopes, multi-use drug bottles, multi-use ear preparations, multi-use topical anaesthetic/eye drops, examination tables,

carrying baskets, clippers, nebulizers, etc. may all spread infections between patients
- Poor wound management
- Incorrect vaccination procedure when using live vaccines. Animals can develop clinical disease via inhalation of aerosols generated when drawing-up live vaccines or by licking at vaccine-contaminated fur or skin
- Poorly organized puppy parties
- Use of blood donors without prior health screening.

Preventing nosocomial infections

Many of the factors discussed in the design and management of multi-animal facilities also apply to the design and management of veterinary practices (see relevant sections). In particular, suitable ventilation systems, isolation areas and vaccination policies are required. In addition, the following should be addressed:

- Ensure good cleaning practices, including disinfection of commonly used equipment. Where possible use disinfection protocols recommended by the manufacturers. Surgical equipment should be autoclaved or treated by ethylene oxide. Cold disinfection increases the risk of infection with soil saprophytes *(Clostridium tetani).* Stethoscopes should be cleaned periodically and especially after being used on patients with dermatological disease. Auroscopes should be cleaned between each patient. Endoscopes should be cleaned according to manufacturers' instructions after each patient. Particular attention should be paid to biopsy channels. Using fully immersible endoscopes makes cleaning easier
- Mark all sterilized equipment with the date of sterilization and store in dust-free cupboards
- Wash hands frequently. Dirty hands are the single easiest way to spread disease within a veterinary clinic. Some microbes, e.g. *Pseudomonas*, can live in liquid soap dispensing bottles. These bottles should be regularly emptied, cleaned, disinfected and refilled
- Disinfect hands, wear gloves and have a good surgical technique
- Use antibacterials correctly (see Chapter 2)
- Place and maintain intravenous and urinary catheters in a sterile fashion (see below).

Specific situations

Urinary catheterization

- Perform this procedure only when necessary. Repeated catheterization may be better in the short term than placing an indwelling catheter. In the long term an indwelling catheter is preferred to reduce urethral trauma

- Use a sterile non-traumatic technique
- Unless the catheter is in place for less than 4 days, antimicrobial therapy that is initiated while the catheter is still in place will select for resistant organisms (Johnson and Murtaugh, 1997a; Sedor and Mulholland, 1999)
- Where long-term catheterization is required, antimicrobial therapy should begin only when the catheter is removed, according to culture and sensitivity of the catheter.

Intravenous catheterization

- Clip a reasonable area of fur and prepare the catheter site aseptically
- Because the risk of local infection is increased when a cut-down procedure is performed, this should only be undertaken when necessary. Some makes of catheter require cutdown more often than others
- Secure the catheter firmly with sterile dressing. Note the time and date of placement
- After 24 hours, check and replace the dressing. Replace dressing whenever it becomes soiled or wet
- Unless absolutely essential do not leave a catheter in place for more than 72 hours
- Disconnect catheter circuits as rarely as possible
- For small volumes and slow infusion rates over many days it is better to use multiple small infusion bags or bottles rather than one large one
- When adding drugs via the additive port ensure that the drug is sterile, then add it to the giving set or infusion bag in uncontaminated surroundings in a sterile manner. Swab the additive port with surgical spirit before and after giving the drug. Figure 4.9 shows an example of poor catheter management

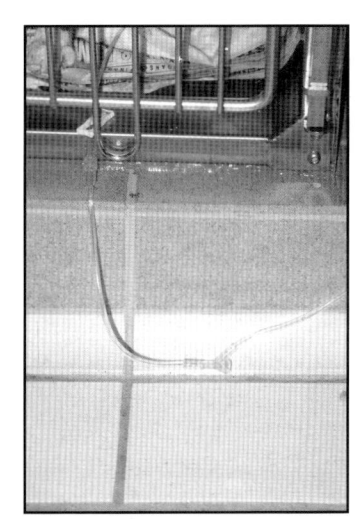

Figure 4.9: An example of poor catheter management. The giving set has been left in the gutter, thereby greatly increasing the risk of intravenous catheter-associated infections.

62 Manual of Canine and Feline Infectious Diseases

- Infection can enter the catheter circuit at the catheter tip, the additive port, hairline cracks in the infusion bags/giving sets, via an influx of room air created when the vacuum is released or at the connection of the infusion set and the hub of the catheter
- Many solutions for intravenous administration support bacterial growth. *Pseudomonas* can grow in distilled water, normal saline and even iodophores. *Serratia marcescens* is an organism that is often incriminated in infections from intravenous catheters in veterinary practice. It has been found growing in alcohol-soaked cottonwool balls. Many organisms can grow in parenteral nutrition solutions, 5% dextrose solutions, blood products and drugs that are packaged in multi-use bottles
- Clinical signs of catheter-associated infections: local – warmth, pain, swelling, redness and venous thrombosis; systemic – fever, hypotension, tachycardia, vomiting, diarrhoea, CNS signs, endotoxic shock, collapse, coma and death
- If intravenous catheter-associated infection is suspected, the catheter should be removed and the catheter tip cultured. Samples of the animal's blood should also be cultured.

Nosocomial pneumonia

- The risk of nosocomial pneumonia is increased by endotracheal intubation, bronchoscopy, transtracheal washing, bronchoalveolar lavage and nebulization. All of these procedures compromise local defence mechanisms. Inadequately sterilized equipment can carry infection from one patient to another
- Nosocomial infection is most common in patients with inherent respiratory compromise; i.e. those with chronic lung disease, impaired pulmonary macrophage function, neuromuscular paralysis or central depression of respiration
- Nosocomial pneumonia is more prevalent in patients that undergo anaesthesia and endotracheal intubation while receiving histamine H_2-receptor antagonists. This is believed to result from bacterial reflux from the stomach resulting in contamination of the oropharynx.

Cutaneous infections

- Nosocomial skin infections commonly result from contamination of surgical wounds, decubital ulcers and burns or secondary contamination of primary skin infections
- Surgical wound contamination may relate to poor surgical technique, compromised blood supply, inappropriately applied or maintained surgical dressings or inadequate postoperative care (Figure 4.10)

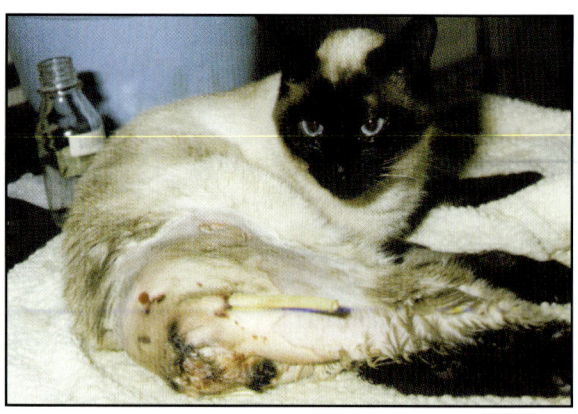

Figure 4.10: Devitalized tissue, such as this tail injury, is at much greater risk of developing nosocomial infection than healthy tissue.

- Decubital ulcers are seen most commonly in immobile or recumbent animals that have inadequate bedding or are moved too infrequently. Pressure results in devitalization of the skin; secondary bacterial infection then follows
- Treatment requires suitable antibacterial therapy and correction of the underlying problem.

Enteric infections

- Outbreaks of disease usually result from poor hygiene, often associated with overcrowding. Infection can be harboured in exercise runs, cages, wards, treatment areas, the waiting room and examination tables or on thermometers (Figure 4.11), feeding and cleaning utensils or protective clothing
- When outbreaks of enteric disease occur, faeces should be cultured to determine the cause and, wherever possible, the source of the infection should be located
- Methods to prevent the spread of enteric infections are discussed in the section on management in multi-animal facilities.

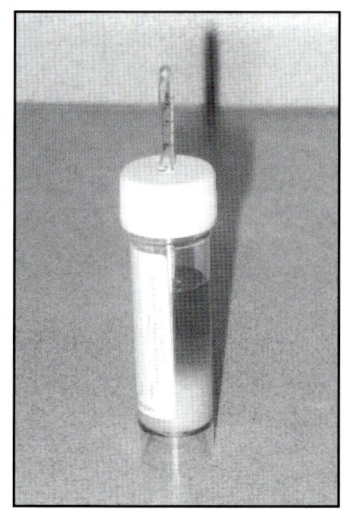

Figure 4.11: Thermometers are an overlooked source of nosocomial enteric infections. Several pathogens are not inactivated by the antiseptic solutions commonly used for storage of thermometers. Some pathogens can even grow in these solutions. Careful cleaning of the thermometer after use and frequent changes of the storage solution reduce the chance of nosocomial infections.

REFERENCES AND FURTHER READING

Chartered Institute of Environmental Health (1995) *Model Licence Conditions and Guidance for Cat Boarding Establishments.* Chartered Institute of Environmental Health, London

Chartered Institute of Environmental Health (1995) *Model Licence Conditions and Guidance for Dog Boarding Establishments.* Chartered Institute of Environmental Health, London

Emori TG and Gaynes RP (1993) An overview of nosocomial infection, including the role of the microbiology laboratory. *Clinical Microbial Review* **6**, 428-442

Feline Advisory Bureau (1993) *Boarding Cattery Construction and Management.* Feline Advisory Bureau, Tisbury, Wiltshire

Feline Advisory Bureau (1998) *FAB Code of Practice for Cat Rescue Facilities.* Feline Advisory Bureau, Tisbury, Wiltshire

Greene CE (1998) Environmental factors in infectious disease. In: *Infectious Diseases of the Dog and Cat, 3rd edn*, ed. CE Greene, pp. 673-682. WB Saunders, Philadelphia

Johnson JA and Murtaugh RJ (1997a) Preventing and treating nosocomial infections: part 1. Urinary tract infections and pneumonia. *Compendium on Continuing Education for the Practicing Veterinarian* **19**, 581-603

Johnson JA and Murtaugh RJ (1997b) Preventing and treating nosocomial infections: part 2. Wound, blood, and gastrointestinal infections. *Compendium on Continuing Education for the Practicing Veterinarian* **19**, 693-703

Lawler DF (1998) Prevention and management of infection in catteries. In: *Infectious Diseases of the Dog and Cat, 3rd edn*, ed. CE Greene, pp. 701-705. WB Saunders, Philadelphia

Lawler DF (1998) Prevention and management of infection in kennels. In: *Infectious Diseases of the Dog and Cat, 3rd edn*, ed. CE Greene, pp. 706-709. WB Saunders, Philadelphia

Sedor J and Mulholland SG (1999) Hospital acquired urinary tract infections associated with the indwelling catheter. *Urology Clinics of North America* **26**, 821-828

Truyen U (1999) Emergence and evolution of canine parvovirus. *Veterinary Microbiology* **69**, 47-50

CHAPTER FIVE

The Haemopoietic and Lymphoreticular Systems

Ian Ramsey, Danièlle Gunn-Moore and Susan Shaw

CHAPTER PLAN

Infections associated with tumours and other masses
  Feline leukaemia virus
  Other viral causes of neoplasia
  Lymphadenopathy
  Other masses
Infections associated with anaemia
  Viral causes of anaemia
  Bacterial causes of anaemia
  Other infectious causes of anaemia
Infections associated with immunosuppression
  History
  Physical examination
  Laboratory investigations
  Feline immunodeficiency virus
  Other infectious causes of immunosuppression
Infections associated with immune-mediated diseases
  History and physical examination
  Laboratory tests
  Leishmaniasis
  Ehrlichiosis
References and further reading

INTRODUCTION

Primary infections of the haemopoietic and lymphoreticular system are relatively common in small animals. In addition, many other infectious agents may cause changes (such as lymphadenopathy) within the haemopoietic and lymphoreticular systems as a secondary effect. Primary infections are often associated with high morbidity and mortality. These infections can be placed into four broad groups according to their association with: tumours and other masses; anaemia; immunosuppression; or immune-mediated disease. Individual infections may, however, be associated with more than one group.

INFECTIONS ASSOCIATED WITH TUMOURS AND OTHER MASSES

Infections may produce neoplasia, lymphadenopathy, abscesses and granulomas. Infections associated with tumours and other masses are listed in Figure 5.1. The clinical signs produced by these infections depend on the location of the mass (or masses). When investigating a mass it is important to try to establish the following information:

- The length of time the mass has been present
- The structures from which the mass originates and those that it invades
- The size, shape and texture of the mass and how it is has changed
- The degree of pain produced by the mass
- The size and texture of the local lymph nodes
- The involvement of distant sites in the disease process.

When investigating a mass, direct palpation and visual inspection may be possible, but in many cases some form of diagnostic imaging will also be required. Diagnostic imaging is essential for the assessment of distant organ involvement in the disease process (especially for lungs, liver and some lymph nodes). If an infectious aetiology is considered to be a differential diagnosis then it is sensible to proceed rapidly to specific tests for the suspected agent. This is particularly true when the suspected agent is zoonotic (e.g. *Mycobacterium* spp.).

Haematology is usually unhelpful in the diagnosis of cases with tumours and other masses, although it can be diagnostic in cases of leukaemia. In particular, neutrophilia may be seen with many tumours and abscesses but is also seen with immune-mediated diseases and glucocorticoid administration. Serum biochemistry is helpful in the general assessment of metabolic status of these cases but is usually of minimal diagnostic value. Hypercalcaemia may occasionally be seen in association with malignancy or granulomatous disease. Urinalysis (including urine cytology) may be helpful if masses involve the urinary tract or when a change in urine colour or urination pattern has been noted by the owner.

	Cats	**Dogs**
Tumours	Feline leukaemia virus (FeLV) (+ feline sarcoma virus) Feline immunodeficiency virus (FIV)	Canine papilloma virus
Lymphadenopathy*	FeLV Feline infectious peritonitis (FIP) FIV *Streptococcus canis* (cervical lymphadenitis) *Bartonella* spp. *Cryptococcus neoformans* *Histoplasma capsulatum* (peripheral or visceral lymph nodes)	*Borrelia* spp. (Lyme disease; see Chapter 14) *Leishmania* spp. *Yersinia pestis* *Pseudomonas mallei* *Brucella canis* (see Chapter 12) *Actinomyces/Nocardia* *Francisella tularensis* *Ehrlichia* spp. *Rickettsia rickettsii* (Rocky Mountain spotted fever) *Blastomyces* spp. (see Chapter 6) *Histoplasma capsulatum* (visceral lymph nodes) *Coccidioides immitis* *Cryptococcus neoformans* *Babesia* spp. *Bartonella* spp.
Abscesses	Many species of bacteria	Many species of bacteria
Granulomas	FIP *Mycobacterium* spp.	*Mycobacterium* spp.

Figure 5.1: Infectious causes of tumours and other masses in dogs and cats.
*Lymphadenopathy is also found in many systemic infections in which other signs predominate and in lymph nodes draining sites of localized infection (e.g. abscesses).

Fine needle aspirates (FNAs) are indispensable for the rapid assessment of most masses. Samples can be obtained cheaply, quickly and with relatively little risk. Cytological interpretation is available through most commercial laboratories. Even if a definitive diagnosis is not possible, it is usually possible to determine the nature of the pathophysiological process occurring within the lesion. Obtaining FNAs of most abdominal organs or intra-abdominal masses requires ultrasound guidance to avoid lacerating organs or puncturing fluid-containing masses such as abscesses or haemorrhagic tumours.

Biopsy is the definitive diagnostic technique for most masses. Representative samples should be placed in an adequate volume of fixative (typically 10 volumes of buffered formalin are required for 1 volume of tissue) and sent to an experienced veterinary pathologist. Smaller tissue samples are fixed more rapidly and, in many instances, core or 'Trucut' biopsies are preferred. These can be obtained from abdominal lesions under ultrasound guidance. Unfixed samples may be submitted for routine and, when indicated, specialist culture.

Feline leukaemia virus

Feline leukaemia virus (FeLV) is an important cause of neoplasia in cats; it also causes anaemia, immunosuppression and immune-mediated diseases. The latter group of presentations is more common than the lymphoproliferative diseases.

Prevalence

The prevalence of FeLV infection in the general healthy cat population is quite high (about 40% of cats show evidence of exposure). However, as most cats recover from infection, the prevalence of viraemia is much less (1-2%). These figures hide a large variation in local prevalence rates that are linked to the number of cats in households and history of exposure to FeLV. In situations where close social contact exists between cats, such as multiple cat households, up to 90% of cats show evidence of FeLV infection and up to 40% may be viraemic. The prevalence of FeLV infection in the general sick cat population is approximately 11-17% (Hosie *et al.*, 1989; Swenson *et al.*, 1990). For certain conditions, such as lymphoblastic leukaemia, the incidence is much higher and can be almost 100%.

Despite vaccination and 'test and remove' schemes, there is little evidence to suggest that the overall prevalence of FeLV has been reduced in the past 20 years. Furthermore, recent work suggests that FeLV may have a role in the development of lymphomas in cats that have recovered from infection. If this is the case then previous estimates of the prevalence of FeLV viraemia may have underestimated the population that is at risk.

Adult cats are less susceptible to FeLV than kittens and therefore most FeLV viraemic cats are under 6 years old. This age-related resistance is not absolute, and it can be overcome by high doses of virus or the use of corticosteroids. There is no breed or sex predilection.

Transmission and pathogenesis

FeLV is present in saliva and infection occurs by the oronasal route, presumably by mutual grooming between cats. After the virus has entered the cat it spreads to systemic lymphoid tissues. At this stage many cats eliminate the infection without developing clinical signs. Alternatively, the virus may disseminate widely throughout the body. Once the stem cells of the bone marrow have become infected (which is marked by the appearance of infected neutrophils in the peripheral blood) then the cat will be persistently viraemic. As a third alternative, the cat may contain the infection within the bone marrow in a latent state for a variable period (Figure 5.2). Occasionally, such latently infected cats may revert to the viraemic state. This may occur spontaneously, when they are given immunosuppressive doses of steroids or after physiological stresses, such as lactation. In most cats, however, the latent infection is eventually eliminated.

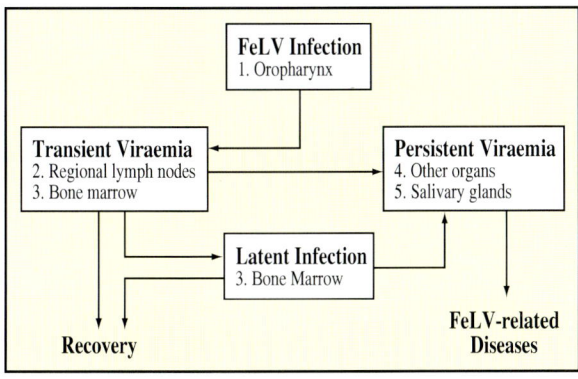

Figure 5.2: Schematic representation of the transmission and pathogenesis of feline leukaemia virus. The numbers refer to the order in which the virus first appears in various tissues.

Malignant diseases	
Lymphomas	Mediastinal
	Multicentric
	Alimentary
	Extranodal – spinal, renal, etc.
Leukaemia	Lymphoid leukaemias
	Myeloid leukaemias
	Erythroleukaemia
	Reticuloendotheliosis
Non-malignant diseases	
Anaemia: Non-regenerative	Pure red cell aplasia
	Myelophthesis
	Myelofibrosis
	Medullary osteosclerosis
	Haemorrhage from tumours
Regenerative	Coinfection with *Haemobartonella felis*
	Immune-mediated thrombocytopenias
	Immune-mediated haemolytic anaemias
Immunosuppression	Various secondary infections
Others	Glomerulonephritis
	Infertility
	Neurological disorders

Figure 5.3: Diseases associated with feline leukaemia virus infection.

FeLV has been shown to exist in three subgroups (A, B and C). FeLV-A can be passed from cat to cat. FeLV-B and FeLV-C arise from FeLV-A. FeLV-C, and maybe FeLV-B, are more pathogenic than FeLV-A. Other, more pathogenic, forms of FeLV-A may also arise within an infected cat with time without changing subgroup.

Diseases associated with FeLV infection

FeLV causes a range of degenerative and proliferative diseases of myeloid, lymphoid and erythroid origin (Figure 5.3). The importance of FeLV as a cause of neoplasia, anaemia and immunosuppression varies with locality (as FeLV prevalence varies).

The most common tumour associated with FeLV infection is lymphoma. Various forms (mediastinal, alimentary, etc.) have been described based on the distribution of the tumour cells within the lymphatic system. In addition, extra-nodal lymphoma can occur anywhere in the body. The incidence of FeLV in each anatomical group varies. In most studies about 90% of cases of mediastinal lymphoma are found to be FeLV positive, whereas for alimentary lymphoma the figure is lower, at about 30%. There may be some local variation in the prevalence of FeLV in a particular anatomical group. In those countries with a low prevalence of FeLV the proportions of various lymphoma types may be different (Court *et al.*, 1997). Many of these tumours present with vague signs of weight loss, lethargy and inappetence but in addition more specific clinical signs may be seen:

- Mediastinal lymphomas may present with dyspnoea or regurgitation and a loss of cranial thoracic compressibility. Horner's syndrome is seen occasionally
- Alimentary lymphomas tend to present with diarrhoea, with or without vomiting, but non-specific weight loss is also common
- Spinal lymphomas tend to produce acute neurological signs after an initial insiduous course
- Renal lymphomas tend to produce bilateral renomegaly (Figure 5.4a) with biochemical evidence of renal failure.

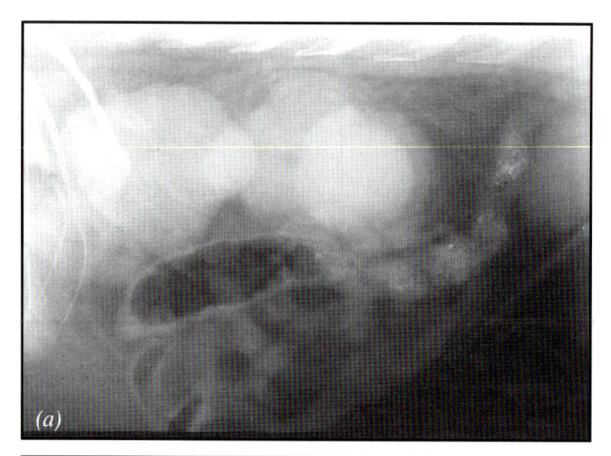

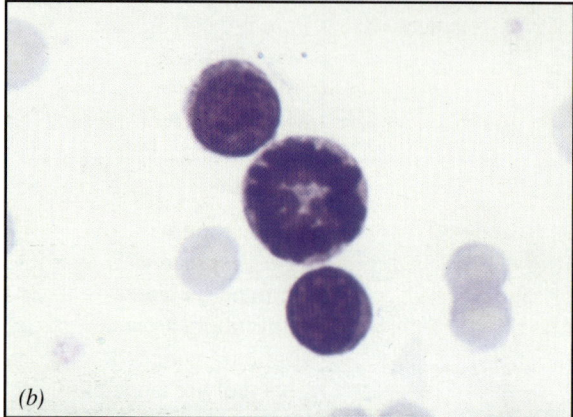

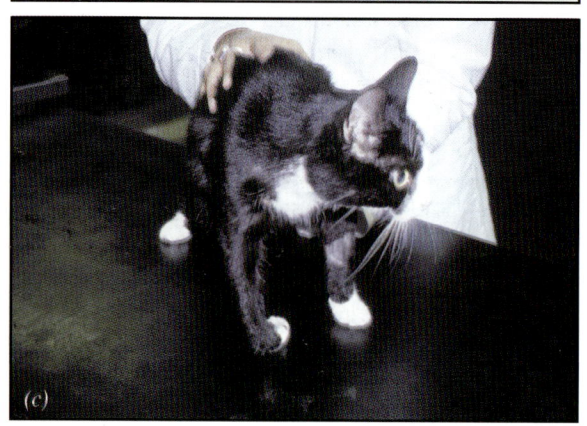

68 Manual of Canine and Feline Infectious Diseases

Figure 5.4: Three manifestations of feline leukaemia virus infection. (a) Bilateral renomegaly is evident in this radiograph. Renal lymphoma was confirmed by cytological examination of fine needle aspirates. (b) A mitotic figure in a peripheral blood smear from a cat with acute lymphoblastic leukaemia. (Reproduced from Ramsey and Gould (1999) In Practice, with permission). (c) A peripheral neuropathy (note the position of the right paw). A peripheral nerve root tumour would be a differential diagnosis of this presentation.

Many of these tumours are solitary at the time of diagnosis – for example, in one study 22 of 23 spinal lymphomas were solitary tumours (Lane *et al.*, 1994). Despite the name of the virus, few infected cats develop leukaemia (Figure 5.4b). A few cats may develop multicentric fibrosarcomas as a result of a recombination event between FeLV and a cellular oncogene that results in the production of a replication-defective feline sarcoma virus (FeSV).

There are many mechanisms by which FeLV causes anaemia (see Figure 5.3). The clinical signs produced are similar to other causes of anaemia (see below). The best studied cause of FeLV-induced anaemia is pure red cell aplasia (PRCA). This is one of the most acute degenerative retrovirus diseases known and is uniquely associated with FeLV-C. PRCA results in a severe non-regenerative anaemia without a significant leucopenia or thrombocytopenia. In addition, about one third of FeLV-induced lymphoproliferative diseases are associated with anaemia. Although a physical 'crowding out' of the bone marrow is partly responsible for the development of the anaemia in leukaemic animals, an altered cytokine environment may be a more important factor in the pathogenesis.

Immunosuppression is common in FeLV-infected cats. Persistent lymphopenia is thought to be due to virus-induced apoptosis. Clinical signs associated with immunosuppression are similar to those seen with feline immunodeficiency virus (FIV; see below). Unlike FIV, there have been few specific associations made with other infections but the role of FeLV in an individual immunosuppressed cat should not be underestimated. Various other diseases, such as glomerulonephritis, severe gastroenteritis and reproductive disorders, are also associated with FeLV. These presentations are uncommon or rare.

The prognosis for a persistently infected cat in a multiple cat household is poor, as approximately 85% die within 3 years of diagnosis. Persistently viraemic cats in single cat households may have a slightly improved prognosis as the number of opportunistic infections to which they are exposed may be less. More infected cats die from myeloid and erythroid aplasias that lead to immunosuppression and anaemia, respectively, than from neoplasia.

Diagnosis
On physical examination pale mucous membranes are common and haematology should be used to check for anaemia. It can be difficult to decide if anaemia in an FeLV-positive cat is regenerative or not. FeLV-positive cats may have an increased mean cell volume (MCV) due to erythrocytic macrocytosis even when they have a non-regenerative anaemia, and for this reason interpretation of MCV values is especially problematical in FeLV-positive cats. Evaluation of a blood smear can be helpful, as in erythrocytic macrocytosis the macrocytes are normochromic whereas in regenerative anaemias they tend to be polychromic. Normoblasts are often present in peripheral blood smears of FeLV-positive cats, reflecting bone marrow disease.

Diagnostic imaging is often useful in assessing cats with FeLV-related tumours. It is less valuable in assessing cases with anaemia, immunosuppression or other diseases.

A variety of tests are available to demonstrate FeLV (Figure 5.5). The most widely used tests in

Type of test	What is detected	Advantages/disadvantages
ELISA	Feline leukaemia virus (FeLV) p27 antigen in blood or serum	Rapid and easy to use Possibility of false positives – should confirm positives by virus isolation
Rapid immunomigratory (RIM) assays	FeLV p27 antigen in blood or serum	Rapid and easy to use Possibility of false positives – should confirm positives by virus isolation
Virus isolation (VI)	Infectious FeLV in serum	Gold standard test if performed by experienced laboratory Takes 7–10 days. Blood should reach laboratory within 2 days because virus is quite labile
Immunofluorescence (IFA)	FeLV antigen in neutrophils and platelets	Gold standard if performed by experienced laboratory Quality of blood smear affects results Anticoagulant affects results, so air-dried smears are recommended
Virus neutralizing antibody (VNA) test	VNAs are an indicator of natural immunity to FeLV	Useful if need to know whether safe to leave FeLV-negative cat in-contact with FeLV-positive cat

Figure 5.5: Tests for feline leukaemia virus.

practice are based on enzyme-linked immunosorbent assay (ELISA) and rapid immunomigratory (RIM) assay technologies (see Chapter 1). These tests are not equally efficient at detecting FeLV and some manufacturers' kits produce more invalid results than others (Hartmann *et al.*, 2001).

Several points should be remembered when interpreting the results of these tests:

- Positive in-house tests should always be confirmed by virus isolation or immunofluorescence. This is particularly important when a healthy cat is found to be positive, as the implications for this cat and others with which it interacts are considerable. The positive predictive value of even the best in-practice tests is only 80–90% (Hartmann *et al.*, 2001)
- FeLV vaccines do not produce false positive results on these tests as there is insufficient circulating antigen after inoculation
- Healthy cats should be tested about 12 weeks after exposure to a known FeLV-positive cat; testing before this may detect a transient viraemia
- False negatives are rare with most in-practice tests as the negative predictive value is typically 95–99% (Hartmann *et al.*, 2001). This is most often suspected when a cat has a problem that strongly suggests FeLV infection, such as a tumour of the haemolymphoreticular system, a severe non-regenerative anaemia or immunosuppression, but is apparently negative. An alternative test method (e.g. virus isolation or immunofluorescence) should be used to confirm the cat's FeLV status
- A few cats consistently produce discordant results when tested with ELISA (or RIM) and virus isolation (or immunofluorescence). This suggests that they have viral antigen in their blood but not infectious virus. On repeated monthly tests about 50% of these discordant cats become negative on both tests, some remain discordant and some become positive by both ELISA or RIM and virus isolation. The reason some cats produce these discordant results is not known
- The diagnostic efficiency of testing by polymerase chain reaction (PCR) is comparable to serological methods, but there have been few large scale studies.

Some specialist laboratories can test for antibodies against feline oncornavirus-associated cell membrane antigen (FOCMA). FOCMA is a heterogeneous group of proteins that may be products of endogenous FeLV (enFeLV) but which are only expressed when exogenous FeLV infects the cell. All cats that recover from FeLV develop anti-FOCMA antibodies. Testing for anti-FOCMA antibodies can be used as a method of assessing prior exposure to FeLV. Some persistently viraemic cats may also possess anti-FOCMA antibodies, which indicates that such antibodies do not protect against the development of persistent viraemia; however, such cats may be at less risk of developing FeLV-induced neoplastic disease.

Treatment

Healthy FeLV-infected cats: Cats are sometimes found to be FeLV positive when they are screened before vaccination or breeding. They should be isolated from other cats and retested 12 weeks later. Most will be negative on the second test, indicating that they were transiently infected and are now likely to be immune from further infection. Several experimental treatments (similar to those listed below for FIV) have been tried for persistently viraemic cats that are otherwise healthy. One (a combination of zidovudine, interferon-α and adoptive transfer of activated T lymphocytes) proved to be successful in 4 of 9 cats (Zeidner *et al.*, 1995). However, no treatment has proved to be practical and successful.

Sick cats: As persistent infection with FeLV is associated with a range of usually fatal conditions, it is debatable whether treatment other than euthanasia is indicated for any of them. Cats with a regenerative anaemia carry a slightly better prognosis as some of the causes are manageable, even though the cat's viral status remains unchanged. Some conditions may respond to appropriate therapy, although the long term prognosis remains poor:

- Recurrent infections associated with immunosuppression can be managed with long courses of antibacterial agents (see also FIV below)
- Anaemia associated with coinfection with *Haemobartonella felis* can be managed with tetracyclines and glucocorticoids. Cats may live for considerable periods after appropriate therapy
- Immune-mediated haemolytic anaemia can be treated with glucocorticoids, and some cats have subsequently become virus negative, suggesting that in these cases the virus had not yet become established in the bone marrow
- Severe non-regenerative anaemia associated with erythroid aplasia can be managed temporarily with blood transfusions, which may last up to 2 months
- FeLV-induced lymphomas can be managed with chemotherapy. The tumours are as chemosensitive as non-FeLV-associated lymphomas. The response rate is high, and similar periods of remission can be achieved in both groups of cats. However, the FeLV-positive cats remain infectious to other cats and susceptible to other FeLV-related diseases.

Control

In-contact cats: The best method of preventing spread of infection is to isolate infected individuals. Vaccination is essential, but see notes below on relative efficacy of FeLV vaccination. No prophylactic treatment is suitable for cats that are currently in-contact with an FeLV-positive cat, as antiretroviral drugs are too toxic for healthy cats. No prophylactic treatment is required for cats that have been introduced into a household that previously contained an FeLV-infected cat, as the virus does not persist in the environment.

'Test and remove' schemes: Until vaccination became widespread, 'test and remove' schemes were the only effective way of controlling FeLV in an infected household. The principle of such a scheme is to identify all cats that are infected and separate them from non-infected individuals (Figure 5.6). As many cats infected with FeLV subsequently recover, it is important that positive test results are checked more than 12 weeks later. During this period positive cats should be isolated. As FeLV is a delicate virus and fomite transmission is very unlikely, isolation of FeLV-positive cats only requires physical separation (e.g. in a separate room). Changes in footwear or clothing are not necessary.

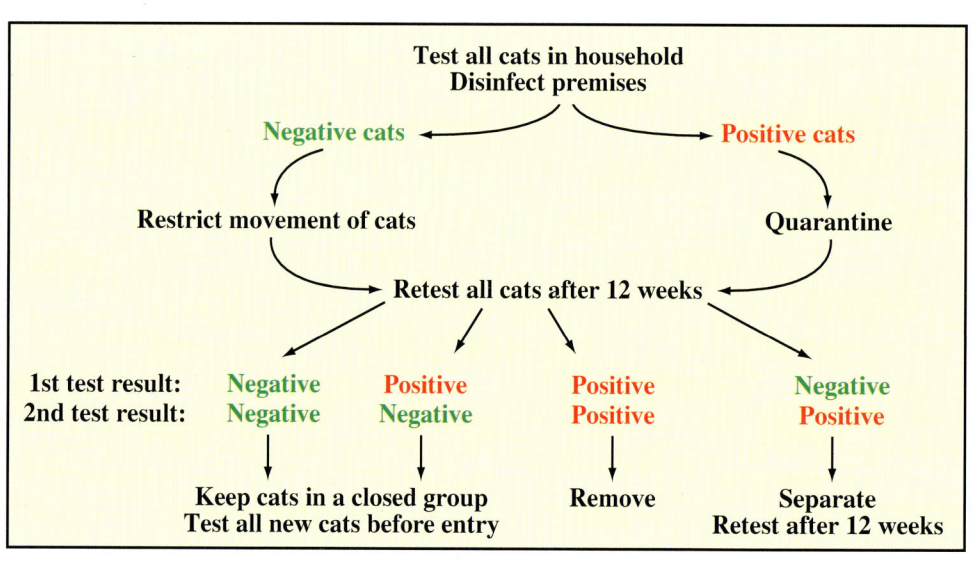

Figure 5.6: Test and remove scheme for feline leukaemia virus.

The test and remove scheme illustrated in Figure 5.6 is a cheap and effective method of controlling FeLV. It is particularly useful for cats in households that do not allow access to the outside or living in areas with a low density of cat-owning households. In these households a single FeLV test of all the cats often establishes that the household is clear of infection. Provided no untested cats are introduced, the household will remain free of FeLV, and vaccination will be unnecessary.

Vaccination: Several different types of FeLV vaccine have been licensed for use in the UK; a 'traditional' inactivated virus vaccine, a recombinant protein vaccine, and a subunit vaccine. Likely developments in the future include the introduction of a recombinant canarypox vaccine. All of these vaccines provide some protection against the development of persistent viraemia; however, as there has been no consensus between the protocols used in various vaccine trials for FeLV, it is not known which vaccine offers the best chance of protection. It is known from the few comparative studies that have been performed that the degree of protection conferred varies (Jarrett and Ganiere, 1996). The ideal FeLV vaccine should induce virus neutralizing antibodies against FeLV-A. No currently available vaccine achieves this.

Except for those animals kept in closed catteries and those that are already infected, all cats are at risk from FeLV infection and therefore will benefit from FeLV vaccination. However, as not all cats are at the same risk of becoming infected with FeLV, more effort should be made to convince those owners whose cats are likely to be exposed to FeLV of the value of vaccination. If a cat is highly unlikely to be exposed to FeLV in the future then the value of vaccination is less. Owners may prefer to test such cats with the intention of setting up an FeLV-negative household. A good example of this situation would be a kitten that is being housed as a single cat in a flat, without access to other cats.

Cats are most susceptible to the development of persistent viraemia after FeLV challenge between 6 and 16 weeks. This is when maternal antibody has waned but age-related resistance has not developed. The most appropriate time to vaccinate a cat is early in life, but vaccination may be considered at any age.

It is probable that vaccination of latently infected or persistently viraemic cats will do no harm to an individual cat, although it is unlikely to provide any beneficial effects. However, the vaccination of a persistently viraemic cat is detrimental to the control of FeLV. This is because a vaccinated persistently viraemic cat still remains a source of infection to other cats. It follows that prevaccination testing for FeLV is highly desirable. Realistically, even when the value of such testing is carefully explained to owners, the costs of testing are sometimes prohibitive. It is therefore of paramount importance that those cats at increased risk of having been in contact with FeLV are identified and particular effort made to convince their owners of the value of prevaccination testing.

Cats that are at an increased risk include:

- Those from rescue centres
- Those from multicat households that do not practice any form of FeLV control
- Those from uncertain backgrounds.

If an owner declines FeLV testing of a cat then they should be made aware that vaccination will not be effective in preventing the spread of, or the diseases that result from, a pre-existent FeLV infection. This is of particular importance when a cat is being introduced into a multicat household. An untested vaccinated cat is no safer to other cats in that household than an untested unvaccinated cat.

Any cat that is positive on a prevaccination screen should be isolated for 3 months and then retested. Most will be found to be FeLV negative on the second test and can be vaccinated (although they are likely to be immune).

Other viral causes of neoplasia

Feline immunodeficiency virus
See the section on FIV for more information.

Canine papillomavirus
See Chapter 8 for further information.

Lymphadenopathy

Cervical lymphadenitis
This condition is seen in 3- to 7-month-old kittens and is caused by streptococci of Lancefield group G, which are usually classified as *Streptococcus canis.* Whereas most streptococcal infections in cats and dogs are opportunistic, this condition does not seem to have any predisposing factors. Several kittens may be infected in a litter. The condition may be unilateral or bilateral and results in lymphadenopathy, which may progress to abscessation. Systemic spread is possible. Group G streptococci are very susceptible to penicillins. The condition has not been reported in the dog for many years.

A sterile lymphadenopathy predominantly affecting the head and neck lymph nodes of juvenile dogs is seen occasionally and is colloquially known as 'puppy strangles.' This condition may be confused with cervical lymphadenitis; however, it has not been shown to have an infectious aetiology. A mineral-associated lymphadenopathy of mature dogs might also be confused with cervical lymphadenitis. Biopsies should be submitted for culture and histopathology to distinguish these conditions, preferably before antibacterials are administered.

Bartonellosis

Bartonella spp. are a group of fastidious Gram-negative bacteria that are found in cats and, to a lesser extent, dogs. The number and names of members of this genus are still changing, and more research is required. Organisms previously placed in the genera of *Rochalimaea* and *Grahamella* are now included in the *Bartonella* genus. *Bartonella* spp. are found throughout the world in 10–80% of cats (depending on the populations sampled). The organisms can be detected by PCR, serology and prolonged blood culture. Lymphadenopathy, vague systemic signs and uveitis have been associated with infections in cats. The pathogenic potential of *Bartonella* spp. in dogs has not yet been fully investigated, although case reports have associated *Bartonella henselae* infection with the vasculoproliferative disease peliosis hepatis and *Bartonella vinsonii* subsp. *berkhoffi* infection with granulomatous lymphadenitis, endocarditis and granulomatous rhinitis.

The major importance of this genus is its zoonotic potential. The genus contains the causal agents of cat-scratch disease (*B. henselae* and *B. clarridgeiae*). Cat-scratch disease is seen in humans in association with animal contact (often, but not always, cats). The disease may be transmitted by bites, scratches and ectoparasites. The disease has a wide variety of manifestations, but localized persistent lymphadenopathy is the most common finding. In immunocompromised individuals (particularly those with AIDS), a more widespread vascular proliferative disease called bacillary angiomatosis may develop (and may be fatal). Some medical practitioners recommend that such patients do not share their house with a cat, although the risk of pet ownership to immunocompromised individuals is unknown. Until more is known, it would seem prudent to provide adequate ectoparasite control and to avoid play patterns that might result in scratches. Thorough cleaning of any bite or scratch wounds is recommended. Treatment of *Bartonella* infections in cats is often ineffective.

Others

Tularaemia: *Francisella tularensis,* a Gram-negative bacillus, is a rare cause of disease in cats and dogs. It is zoonotic, and the disease in humans is often fatal. It has been reported in Europe, USA and elsewhere. It has not been reported in the UK. The bacterium is transmitted by ticks and may be acquired by ingestion of wild animals, especially rabbits and hares. Infected animals may show vague clinical signs such as pyrexia, lymphadenopathy (with abscessation), oral ulceration and panleucopenia. If clinical signs develop, most affected animals die. Diagnosis is by culture on specialized media. Serological tests are used in humans, but the titres in clinically affected animals are quite low. There is no information on treatment, but fluoroquinolones may be effective.

Q fever: *Coxiella burnetti*, the causative agent of Q fever, is found in a wide range of domestic animals and humans in Europe and elsewhere. It has not been identified in dogs and cats in the UK. It is very rarely associated with clinical disease in small animals but, like *Bartonella* spp., it does cause significant disease in humans. The disease may be spread directly or by vectors such as ticks. In humans Q fever is associated with pyrexia, headaches and myalgia, but other manifestations are also reported. The mortality is low. Veterinary surgeons and people in other animal-oriented occupations are particularly at risk. Clinical signs in small animals are vague (pyrexia, anorexia, depression), and the diagnosis is by serology.

Actinomycosis/Nocardiosis: *Actinomyces* spp. may cause cervicofacial infections that are characterized by soft tissue swellings with discharging sinuses and lymphadenopathy. The organisms are facultive anaerobes and are hard to culture. Diagnosis often relies on histopathology. *Actinomyces* is Gram positive and is not acid-fast.

In contrast, *Nocardia* spp. are aerobic, weakly acid-fast and relatively easy to culture. They are normally associated with pleural infections, but they may occasionally be isolated from non-pulmonary sites such as lymph nodes (see Chapter 6).

Plague: Infection with *Yersinia pestis* may present solely with lymphadenopathy. The infection has not been reported in Europe for many years but is present in the USA (see Chapter 6).

Glanders: Dogs and cats are susceptible to infection with *Pseudomonas mallei* but require exposure to infected horses or horse meat. A suppurative lymphadenitis is seen and may be confused with tuberculosis. Potentiated sulphonamides and tetracyclines are said to be effective. The disease has not been recorded in small animals in the UK.

Anthrax: Dogs and cats are relatively resistant to infection with *Bacillus anthracis*. When it does occur it is usually acquired through ingestion of contaminated carcasses or animal by-products. Local inflammation of the upper gastrointestinal tract is followed by local and mesenteric lymphadenopathy. Examination of Gram-stained blood films or FNAs is the safest method of making the diagnosis. The organism is a Gram-positive bacillus. This is a notifiable disease in the UK and other countries. Suspected cases should not be handled without consulting the local veterinary authorities (in the UK this is the Divisional Veterinary Officer).

Systemic fungal infections: Most systemic fungal diseases can present with lymphadenopathy, but this is rarely the only clinical sign. Many of these diseases are not present in the UK (e.g. blastomycosis and histoplasmosis). Those that are include candidiasis, aspergillosis, penicillinosis and cryptococcosis. These diseases are more often confined to one area of the body (e.g. nasal cavity) and only become disseminated in immunosuppressed patients. FNAs, biopsies and, in some cases, serological testing are useful in confirming the diagnosis (see Chapters 6, 8 and 15 for advice on diagnosis and treatment).

Other masses

Abscesses

An abscess is a focal accumulation of pus resulting from liquefactive necrosis which, when fully developed, is contained within a capsule. Abscesses are common conditions in small animal practice and occur in many organs. Their specific diagnosis and treatment are covered in the relevant chapters in this book. The organisms involved vary depending on the site and cause of the abscess. Bacteria gain entry into soft tissues to form abscesses by a variety of methods including:

- Haematogenous spread
- Direct inoculation (e.g. cat bite abscesses)
- Ascending infections in the urinary tract
- Ascending infections of the common bile and pancreatic ducts
- Migrating foreign bodies (e.g. sublumbar abscesses)
- Inhalation.

The treatment of abscesses usually requires surgical drainage. Systemic antibacterial therapy is always indicated, as bacteraemia often results. Culture and sensitivity testing should be used to guide drug selection. Without such information a mixed population of bacteria, including anaerobes, should be assumed. Combination therapy may be necessary. Cephalosporins, penicillins, lincosamides and metronidazole are all active against most anaerobic bacteria. Fluoroquinolones do not have significant activity against many anaerobes, and potentiated sulphonamides do not penetrate necrotic tissue.

Granulomas

Mycobacteriosis: Infection with some species of mycobacteria can produce a lymphadenopathy and discrete granulomatous masses. Sometimes these masses contain calcified material, which may be apparent during fine needle aspiration. These infections are reviewed in Chapters 6 and 13.

Feline coronavirus: Feline coronavirus can induce an immune-mediated vasculitis that is characterized by the development of small pyogranulomatous lesions. On rare occasions these lesions may be sufficiently large to produce a palpable mass. Histopathology is required to distinguish these masses (which may be few in number) from lymphomas and other tumours. Feline coronavirus infections are discussed fully in Chapter 9.

INFECTIONS ASSOCIATED WITH ANAEMIA

In the UK, infectious agents are a common cause of anaemia in cats though less so in dogs. In warmer climates several infectious agents are major causes of anaemia in dogs (Figure 5.7). Many infections are associated with a mild anaemia of chronic disease, and further investigations should focus on determining the underlying cause. Clinical signs associated with anaemia include:

- Pale mucous membranes
- Lethargy
- Tachycardia and tachypnoea
- Haemic murmurs
- Anorexia
- Pica.

	Cats	Dogs
Viruses	Feline leukaemia virus Feline infectious peritonitis Feline immunodeficiency virus	
Bacteria (including rickettsias)	*Haemobartonella felis* *Ehrlichia* spp.	*Ehrlichia* spp. *Haemobartonella canis*
Protozoa	*Babesia* spp. *Cytauxzoon felis*	*Babesia* spp. *Leishmania* spp.
Helminths		*Ancylostoma caninum*
Major non-infectious causes	Chronic renal disease, haemorrhage, iron deficiency anaemia, anaemia of chronic disease	

Figure 5.7: Infectious causes of anaemia.

Some of these signs are less reliable in the cat (Ramsey and Gould, 1999). Acute severe anaemia results in dyspnoea and extreme lethargy whereas chronic anaemia, despite lower red blood cell parameters, may produce only mild clinical signs.

When investigating anaemias that may be of infectious origin, particular attention should be paid to the following points:

- The FeLV status of a cat and history that might suggest exposure to FeLV (e.g. multicat household)
- Travel abroad – not necessarily in the recent past (*Ehrlichia* may persist even beyond the quarantine period)
- The presence of thoracic or abdominal masses
- The presence of ecchymoses or petechiation – these are often easier to detect on the ventral abdomen and in the mouth
- Ophthalmoscopy is indicated to examine for retinal haemorrhages, evidence of uveitis, etc.

Routine haematology is essential in all cases of anaemia. Adequate samples should be taken before treatment is started. Infections that produce severe anaemias may require blood transfusion before diagnostic procedures (other than blood sampling) are performed. A reticulocyte count and examination of fresh air-dried smears for erythrocytic parasites should be routinely requested. In cats, an FeLV antigen assay or virus isolation should be performed. Tests for FIV and feline coronavirus antibodies are less important as neither virus has been shown to commonly cause severe anaemia. Routine biochemistry is of limited value, although the identification of chronic renal failure is clearly important early in the investigation. Urinalysis will be helpful in detecting haemoglobinuria in cases of anaemia associated with haemolysis, e.g. in *Haemobartonella felis* infections. Further investigations may include radiography, ultrasonography, bone marrow aspiration, Coombs' test and clotting studies.

Viral causes of anaemia

Feline leukaemia virus
Cats with anaemia are at least as likely to be infected with FeLV as those with lymphoma. See above.

Feline coronavirus
About 40% of animals with feline infectious peritonitis (FIP) are anaemic (Sparkes *et al.*, 1991). However, as other clinical signs of FIP are likely to predominate, the anaemia in such cases is not usually the focus of the clinical investigation. See Chapter 9 for details on the diagnosis of FIP.

Feline immunodeficiency virus
Feline immunodeficiency virus (FIV) is a less common cause of anaemia than FeLV and generally the anaemia produced is mild (packed cell volume >0.20 l/l). In one study only 18% of naturally infected cats were anaemic at the time of examination (Sparkes *et al.*, 1993). See below for more information on FIV.

Canine and feline parvoviruses
Both canine and feline parvoviruses may cause anaemia as a result of gastrointestinal losses and septicaemia. Suppression of red blood cell production is not a feature of infection with either virus. The anaemia produced can be severe, but generally other clinical signs will predominate (see Chapter 8).

Bacterial causes of anaemia

Haemobartonella felis
Haemobartonella felis is a parasite of cats. Its life cycle is poorly described. *H. felis* was originally classified as a rickettsial organism but recent work suggests that it is more closely related to mycoplasmas. The importance of *H. felis* as a cause of anaemia has been debated for several years. Some authors regard the parasite as a primary cause of serious anaemia whereas others regard it as an opportunist that only causes serious problems in the immunocompromised individual. FeLV has been shown to be a cofactor in the development of *H. felis*-induced anaemia (Bobade *et al.*, 1995). The role of FIV has not been investigated. In one study, however, 10% of cats naturally infected with FIV had *H. felis* organisms (Sparkes *et al.*, 1993). The parasite can be found in otherwise healthy cats, and the extent of parasitaemia is poorly correlated with the degree of anaemia. Direct haemolysis of erythrocytes by the parasite is probably exceptional, and it is thought that immune-mediated destruction is principally responsible for the development of the anaemia. The role of vectors, such as fleas, has not been demonstrated experimentally but many authors believe they have an important role.

Diagnosis: Parasitaemias can wax and wane on an hourly basis, making diagnosis a haphazard affair. The parasites are best identified on air-dried blood films made at the time of sampling without the addition of anticoagulant. Routine May–Grünwald–Giemsa stains are superior to Giemsa stains, but acridine orange staining is better than either (Figure 5.8). Unfortunately, acridine orange staining requires the slides to be examined with a UV light microscope within a few minutes of being exposed to light. In practice, sending two air-dried blood films taken a few hours apart to a commercial laboratory for examination by a specialist veterinary haematologist is probably the best option. Stain deposits and Howell–Jolly bodies (nuclear remnants) can be confused with *H. felis* organisms by inexperienced people. Thin smears are far preferable to thick smears. *H. felis* is sufficiently common to warrant this procedure in every case of suspected feline anaemia. Although a positive *H. felis* result is

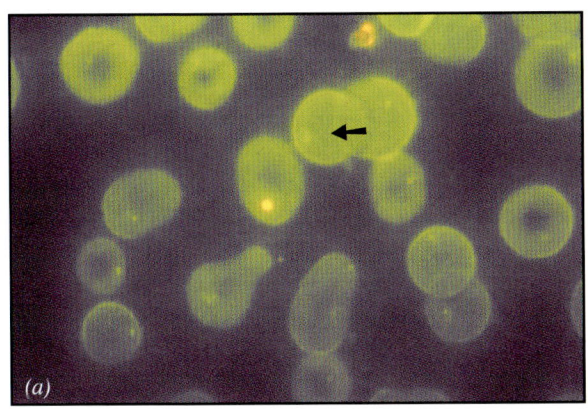

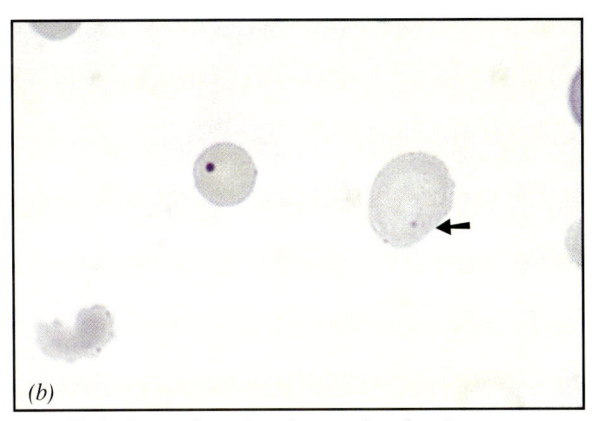

Figure 5.8: Haemobartonella felis *organisms are smaller than Howell–Jolly bodies and are found on, rather than in, the erythrocytes. Two photomicrographs of* H. felis *(arrowed) in blood smears stained with (a) acridine orange and (b) May–Grünwald–Giemsa are shown. Howell–Jolly bodies can be seen in adjacent erythrocytes on both preparations. (Reproduced from Ramsey and Gould (1999)* In Practice, *with permission.)*

diagnostic, a negative result might simply indicate that the cat was aparasitaemic at the time of testing. Samples may have to be taken daily for 7 days to demonstrate the organism.

Recently, the diagnosis of *H. felis* infections by PCR technology has been described in experimentally infected cats (Berent *et al.*, 1998). The value of this technique in the clinical situation has not been established.

Treatment: *H. felis* infection is treated with systemic tetracyclines with or without the addition of immunosuppressive doses of prednisolone. The effect of prednisolone is to suppress erythrophagocytosis and reduce the secondary immune-mediated haemolytic anaemia.

Blood transfusions may be required in a few cases in which the clinical signs produced by the anaemia become life threatening. The severity of the clinical signs and their rate of progression are more important factors than the haematocrit in determining which cats require transfusion. If a blood transfusion is required then it is important to perform a cross match or blood typing beforehand to ensure compatibility.

Haemobartonella canis

Haemobartonella canis is occasionally reported. Its relationship to *H. felis* is not known. Infection can be spread by ticks and blood transfusion. Unless a dog is immunosuppressed or splenectomized then clinical signs are rare. Even in such animals clinical signs tend to be milder than with *H. felis* infection in cats. Diagnosis and therapy are similar to that described for *H. felis*, but *H. canis* tends to form chains across cells more commonly than *H. felis*, making identification a little easier.

Other infectious causes of anaemia

Babesiosis

In Europe, canine babesiosis is caused by the tick-borne intraerythrocytic protozoan parasites *Babesia canis* and, less frequently, *Babesia gibsoni*. In the UK, disease has only been reported in imported animals, including several that have travelled under the Pet Travel Scheme. The pathogenicity of *B. gibsoni* is uniformly high, but that of *B. canis* varies with the strain. *B. canis* var *canis* causes a moderately severe syndrome whereas *B. canis* var *vogeli* causes relatively mild disease. *Dermacentor reticulatus* and *Rhipicephalus sanguineus* ticks transmit canine babesiosis. Although their relative importance varies within Europe, both vectors are found in the UK; *R. sanguineus* has been found in environments around quarantine kennels and *D. reticulatus* in association with cattle in the south west of the UK. Given a large increase in the number of dogs entering the UK, there is a possibility of establishment of babesiosis in the native UK tick population. *B. canis* var *rossi* is found in southern Africa and is highly pathogenic but it is unlikely to be encountered in the UK outside of quarantine establishments.

Peracute, acute, chronic and subclinical syndromes have been described, although an incubation period of 10–21 days is usually described. Subclinically affected dogs may have intermittent periods of clinical disease.

Clinical signs: The severity of the disease varies with the species and strain of *Babesia*, the dog's age and its immune status. Fever, anorexia and lethargy are associated with acute haemolytic anaemia and/or shock. Pale mucous membranes, variable icterus, weakness and tachypnoea are often combined with haemoglobinuria, splenomegaly and hepatomegaly. Collapse, coma and death may follow in susceptible animals. As immune-mediated haemolytic anaemia is part of the pathogenesis of the disease, there may be autoagglutination, and many dogs are Coombs' test positive. Care should be taken to distinguish between autoimmune haemolytic anaemia and babesiosis in dogs returning from endemic countries. Concurrent infection with ehrlichiosis is common as the vectors are shared.

Diagnosis: Diagnosis is based on the demonstration of intraerythrocytic organisms (Figure 5.9) in Giemsa-stained blood films, combined with the clinical picture and a history of travel. Organisms are more easily seen in smears made from peripheral capillaries or from blood below the buffy coat in a centrifuged specimen. Several serological tests are available in Europe, including ELISAs and immunofluorescent antibody tests. These may identify subclinically or chronically affected dogs but will not be positive in acute or peracute cases. PCR tests are able to distinguish *Babesia* genera and strains.

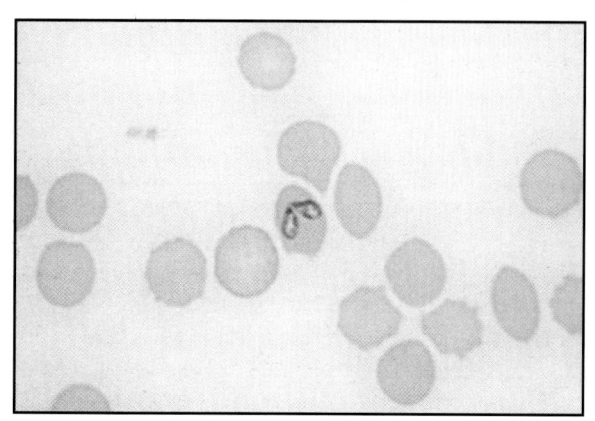

Figure 5.9: Babesia canis *organisms within a Giemsa-stained erythrocyte. (Courtesy of Johannes Schoeman.)*

Treatment and prevention: Current treatment regimens are rarely curative for babesiosis caused by the more pathogenic strains. Persistent subclinical infection followed by recurrence occurs in response to stress, glucocorticoid administration or concurrent disease. In acute haemolytic anaemia, oxygen, fluid therapy and blood transfusions may be necessary.

Imidocarb diproprionate is effective for cases caused by *B. canis* strains but less so for *B. gibsoni*. Reports of doxycycline being effective in babesiosis are now thought to be due to the inadvertent treatment of concurrent ehrlichiosis (see later). However, treatment of ehrlichiosis in coinfected dogs is essential. Infection with the less virulent *B. canis vogeli* can be eliminated by effectively treating the ehrlichiosis.

Vaccination for canine babesiosis is currently available in France but strain variation may limit its efficacy. Use of a reliable acaricide is essential, and to prevent transmission of babesiosis it must kill ticks within 2–3 days of feeding.

Babesia in the cat
Babesiosis is rare in the cat. However, several *Babesia* species affect cats in Africa and Asia. Infected cats show similar but more subtle signs than the dog and rarely develop a haemolytic crisis. They may adapt to the anaemia, but stress may induce signs of weakness and collapse.

Cytauxzoon felis
Cytauxzoon felis is a protozoal infection of cats seen in Africa and certain parts of the USA. It is probably acquired after tick infestation, and the domestic cat is likely to be an aberrant host. The reservoir host may be the bobcat. The outcome of infection varies. Some strains are associated with a fatal disease, whilst others may be less severe or asymptomatic. Affected animals show signs of pyrexia, anaemia and jaundice. The ring-like organisms can be seen parasitizing erythrocytes in the later stages of the disease.

Hookworms
Ancylostoma caninum may produce anaemia due to chronic blood loss. The parasite does not occur in the UK. Other hookworms, such as *A. tubaeforme*, *A. braziliense* and *Uncinaria stenocephala*, are not associated with anaemia (see Chapter 8 for further details).

INFECTIONS ASSOCIATED WITH IMMUNOSUPPRESSION

The immune system is divided into two components:

- The innate immune system: this comprises phagocytes (monocytes, macrophages and neutrophils), plasma proteins (such as complement) and physiochemical barriers (including the skin and mucous membranes). This system should be functional from birth and is capable of responding rapidly to infection
- The antigen-specific immune system: this consists of B and T lymphocytes, antibodies and cytokines. This system develops over the first few months of life, and time is required for each response to develop. It is further divided into humoral immunity and cell-mediated immunity (CMI).

Infections that cause dysfunction of the immune system do so by producing immunodeficiency or immune-mediated disease. The pathogeneses of these conditions are not mutually exclusive and thus some immune-mediated diseases can produce, or arise from, a state of immunodeficiency.

The presence of an immunodeficiency is usually suspected when an animal has:

- Recurrent and/or chronic infections
- Infections at more than one body site
- Opportunistic or unusual infections
- Severe or unusual manifestations of infections
- Delayed, or reduced, response to appropriate antimicrobial therapy
- Adverse reactions to modified live virus vaccines
- Adverse or hypersensitivity reactions to therapeutic agents.

Immunodeficiencies result from defects in one or both parts of the immune system:

- Animals with defective phagocytosis (i.e. innate immunity) may have recurrent infections of the skin, oral cavity or respiratory tract, granulomatous infections or systemic bacterial disease. Chronic infections may lead to systemic amyloidosis, vasculitis and immune complex disease
- Animals with defects in humoral immunity show an increased susceptibility to bacterial infections, whereas deficiencies in CMI tend to result in viral, bacterial (intracellular) and fungal diseases.

Deficiencies may be congenital (primary immunodeficiency) or acquired (secondary immunodeficiency). Primary immunodeficiencies have been identified more often in dogs than in cats. Acquired immunodeficiencies are more common in both species than primary immunodeficiencies (Figure 5.10). It is important to determine whether a secondary immunodeficiency is present before investigating a primary immunodeficiency.

History

Several factors will help to determine whether immunodeficiency is primary or secondary and to find the cause:

- Age: immunodeficiency in young animals most often results from viral infections, transient hypogammaglobulinaemia of infancy or, occasionally, primary immunodeficiency. Disease in older animals is usually secondary to systemic or organic disease, drug administration or neoplasia. The main exception to this is FIV infection, which is seen most often in older cats
- Breed: most primary immunodeficiencies occur in pedigree animals. Some breeds seem to be predisposed to certain infections, and a primary immunodeficiency may be suspected in these cases, e.g. *Mycobacterium avium* infection in Siamese cats
- Sex: some primary immunodeficiencies are sex linked, and only one sex will be affected in these cases
- Coat colour: some defects affect animals with certain coat colours, e.g. cyclic haematopoiesis in grey or beige collie dogs
- Environment of animal: an animal living on its own in a clean and closed environment is unlikely to develop immunodeficiency secondary to infectious disease. However, an animal living in a large heterogeneous group or in unsanitary conditions is more likely to develop a potentially immunosuppressive infection. When environmental contamination is extensive, vaccines may fail to provide adequate protection. This may be misinterpreted as evidence of immunodeficiency

PRIMARY IMMUNODEFICIENCIES
Ciliary dyskinesia (immobile cilia syndrome): Newfoundland, Old English Sheepdog and others
Severe combined immunodeficiency: Basset, Cardigan Welsh Corgi
Selective IgA deficiency: Beagle, Shar Pei, German Shepherd Dog
Cyclic haematopoiesis: Grey collies
Leucocyte adhesion deficiency: Irish Setter
Rhinitis/pneumonia: Irish Wolfhound
Amyloidosis: Shar Pei
Immunoglobulin deficiency: Weimeraner
Lethal acrodermatitis: English Bull Terrier
'Nude' kittens: Birman
SECONDARY IMMUNODEFICIENCIES
Infectious organisms
Canine distemper virus
Canine parvovirus
Feline panleucopenia virus
Feline leukaemia virus
Feline immunodeficiency virus
Demodex
Toxoplasma
Septicaemia
Endogenous hormones
Hyperadrenocorticism
Diabetes mellitus
Hypothyroidism
Hyperoestrogenism
Drugs
Corticosteroids
Antineoplastic drugs
Chloramphenicol (cats)
Oestrogens
Non-steroidal anti-inflammatory drugs
Griseofulvin
Some antibacterials
Age
Neonates
Transient hypogammaglobulinaemia of infancy
Ageing
Others
Barrier damage
Chronic renal failure
Hepatic insufficiency
Malnutrition
Neoplasia, immune-mediated disease, dysproteinaemia
Splenectomy

Figure 5.10: Causes of immunosuppression.

- Siblings: information on the rest of the litter can be helpful in identifying a primary immunodeficiency. However, as most primary immunodeficiencies are recessive, the absence of affected littermates does not exclude the diagnosis
- Vaccination history: a failure to mount an effective immune response after vaccination may suggest an immunodeficiency, although other factors may also be responsible (see Chapter 3)
- Medical history: the medical history of the patient should be examined for evidence of immunosuppressive diseases, e.g. hyperadrenocorticism, diabetes mellitus, immunosuppressive drugs and recent surgical procedures. Prolonged starvation or malnutrition may also reduce immunocompetence. Previous episodes of illness should be reappraised for evidence of immunodeficiency.

Physical examination

Physical examination often reveals evidence of chronic active infections in several different sites, e.g. gingivitis, dermatitis and pneumonia. A full physical examination is essential in determining the extent and severity of disease. It is particularly important to assess the animal's body temperature and to appraise peripheral lymph nodes for size and texture.

Laboratory investigations

Routine haematology

The most obvious indication of a defective immune response is leucopenia in the presence of an active bacterial infection. To determine whether the effect is transient or persistent, blood samples should be collected over the course of several days. Persistent neutropenia can be a feature of overwhelming infection (Figure 5.11). A persistent neutropenia and lymphopenia may suggest immunodeficiency. Persistent leucocytosis is typically associated with an ongoing inflammatory response. It may also be seen with increased concentrations of glucocorticoids (from endogenous or exogenous sources) due to redistribution of the neutrophil pool. When a leucocytosis is combined with a lack of local inflammation or poor pus formation, this may indicate a defect in leucocyte migration. This also occurs with glucocorticoid administration and is a feature of leucocyte adhesion deficiency (LAD) in young Irish Setters.

Leucocyte morphology

The presence and number of immature neutrophils (a 'left shift') indicate the degree of bone marrow responsiveness. A 'degenerate left shift' describes the presence of many immature neutrophils but few mature neutrophils. It is a poor prognostic indicator. Toxic changes, such as swollen nuclei, cytoplasmic basophilia, vacuolation, Döhle bodies and occasionally phagocytosed bacteria, may be seen in severe bacterial infections. Unusual granulation or vacuolation of leucocytes may indicate one of several congenital disorders. Birman cats may have abnormal granulation of their neutrophils as an incidental finding.

Serum globulins

Chronic inflammatory diseases (e.g. FIP, leishmaniasis) usually lead to increased serum globulin concentrations. Low to normal levels, especially in the presence of infection, suggest either external losses or decreased production. External losses may result from haemorrhage or severe protein-losing enteropathy, whereas decreased production is usually associated with chronic liver disease, malnutrition, malabsorption or a primary defect in humoral immunity. Serum protein electrophoresis can be used to identify γ-globulin deficiency. Specific immunological testing is required to determine whether IgA, IgM, IgG or complement fractions are reduced or missing. If required, specialist laboratories can assess immunoglobulin responses to specific pathogens, e.g. in the assessment of response to vaccination.

Other methods of assessing the immune response

Lymph node biopsies and bone marrow aspirates can define the nature of the immunosuppressive disease. The effectiveness of CMI responses can be assessed using delayed-type hypersensitivity testing (which is generally more effective in dogs than cats) or by undertaking specialized lymphocyte stimulation assays. Flow cytometry can be used to differentiate between B and T lymphocytes, determine CD4:CD8 ratios and assess the presence of cell-surface adhesion molecules. A number of disorder-specific assays are available, including molecular analysis to confirm particular gene mutations in primary immunodeficiencies.

Assessment of other body systems

Serum biochemistry profiles and urinalysis enable assessment of renal and hepatic function. They may suggest other metabolic diseases such as endocrinopathies. If enteric disease is present, faecal analysis is required, which may then be followed by endoscopy, with culture and histopathological examination of enteric biopsies. If respiratory disease is present then swabs for respiratory pathogens, culture and cytology of alveolar lavage samples, and radiography may be required. If cutaneous disease is present then skin scrapes, bacterial and fungal cultures, and possibly punch biopsies may be required. Where a particular infectious organism is suspected, its presence can be determined using culture techniques or serological assays.

Abnormality	Causes
Neutrophilia	
Mature cells Moderate increase in total count	Physiological (exercise) Corticosteroids: endogenous ('stress response') or exogenous Stress response (hypoxia, many illnesses) – often seen with increased numbers of lymphocytes in cats and with decreased numbers of lymphocytes and eosinophils and increased numbers of monocytes in dogs
Left shift Moderate increase in total count	Early inflammation
Left shift Marked increase in total count	Established suppurative inflammation – often seen with increased numbers of monocytes in dogs
Marked left shift Marked increase in total count ± toxic neutrophils	Chronic suppurative inflammation – usually seen with increased numbers of monocytes, occasionally with decreased numbers of lymphocytes, especially if stressed
Neutropenia	
Left shift Marked decreased in total count	Overwhelming bacterial infection
Slight or no left shift Moderate decrease in total count	Decreased neutrophil production from bone marrow; normal demand
Mature cells Moderate to marked decrease in total count	Sequestration (usually seen with decreased numbers of lymphocytes) Ineffective granulopoiesis (if stressed; decreased numbers of lymphocytes and eosinophils) Hypoadrenocorticism
Lymphocytosis	Physiological – stress, exercise, transiently after vaccination Hypoadrenocorticism
Lymphopenia	Corticosteroids: endogenous (hyperadrenocorticism, many illnesses) or exogenous (glucocorticoids, etc.) Lymphocyte loss: protein-losing enteropathy (e.g. lymphangiectasia), drainage of chylothorax Reduced lymphopoiesis – primary immunodeficiency, antineoplastic therapy, irradiation
Monocytosis	Excess glucocorticoids in dogs Chronic inflammation/suppuration Granulomatous disease Haemolysis/internal haemorrhage Immune-mediated disease Monocytic leukaemia
Eosinophilia	Type 1 Hypersensitivity – anaphylaxis Parasitism Eosinophilic disease – enteritis/granuloma/pneumonia/bronchitis Eosinophilic leukaemia/mast cell leukaemia Hypoadrenocorticism
Eosinopenia	Excess glucocorticoids – endogenous/exogenous
Basophilia	Type 1 Hypersensitivity Hyperadrenocorticism Hyperlipoproteinaemia (seen in diabetes mellitus, nephrotic disease, chronic liver disease) Basophilic leukaemia

Figure 5.11: Abnormal leucocyte counts and a guide to possible causes.

Feline immunodeficiency virus

Aetiology and epidemiology
FIV is a retrovirus that is common in cat populations throughout the world. The prevalence of FIV infection in the UK is 13-19% of sick cats and 2-3% of healthy cats. Infection is most common in middle-aged to older male cats that have access to the outdoors.

The virus is found in saliva, blood and other body fluids. The major route of transmission is through biting. Those cats exhibiting territorial aggression are therefore most at risk of infection. If fighting does not occur then the rate of horizontal transmission within multicat households is lower but does still occur, probably through mutual grooming. Vertical transmission can occur but its importance in the field is not known.

Pathogenesis
The pathogenesis of FIV infection falls into four phases (Figure 5.12). The acute 'primary phase' begins approximately 3 weeks after infection, when the virus replicates rapidly in lymphoid tissue. Pyrexia, malaise and lymphadenopathy, the last of which may persist for several weeks, are commonly noted, but this phase can be subclinical in some cats. Most infected cats become asymptomatic and remain healthy for an indefinite period. During the asymptomatic phase levels of circulating virus are low, but viral replication continues within infected tissues. Eventually suppression of both T and B lymphocyte functions results in defective CMI and humoral immunity. Lymphopenia, neutropenia and hyperglobulinaemia (predominantly α2- and γ-globulins) are seen. The clinical effects of the immunosuppression induced by FIV are varied. In addition FIV causes some non-immunological diseases, such as neuropathies. The cat eventually becomes terminally ill with opportunistic infections, wasting syndromes or neoplasia.

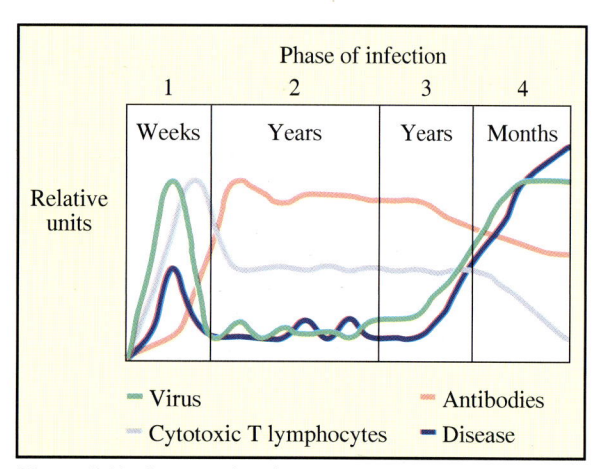

Figure 5.12: Suggested pathogenesis of feline immunodeficiency virus (FIV). The graph shows the relations between the stages of FIV-induced disease, FIV viraemia, the humoral immune response to FIV and the cell-mediated immune response to FIV. The graph is based on experimental and clinical evidence but no single group of cats has been followed from infection to death.

Clinical signs
Clinical signs associated with FIV infections are non-specific and variable, reflecting the variety of opportunistic infections that may arise as a result of the immunosuppression. The following clinical signs are common:

- Weight loss
- Lethargy
- Inappetence
- Lymphadenopathy
- Gingivitis/stomatitis
- Ocular discharge
- Fever
- Chronic nasal discharge
- Chronic diarrhoea.

Although a wide range of other infections have been reported in FIV-positive cats, in some cases the association may be coincidental. Infections that have been shown to be more common or more serious in FIV-positive cats include feline calicivirus (FCV), *Chlamydophila felis* (formerly *Chlamydia psittaci* var *felis*), feline poxvirus and *Microsporum canis*. Associations between FIV and other infections, such as salmonellosis, haemobartonellosis and toxoplasmosis, are largely anecdotal.

FIV may also cause disease in the absence of detectable secondary infections. Cats infected with FIV are reported to have an increased risk of lymphoma (about fivefold). In particular, B-cell lymphomas are more common and this may be related to extensive B lymphocyte proliferation seen in the early stages of infection. Defects in tumour immunosurveillance in FIV-infected cats may also be important, but this has not been investigated. It has been suggested, although not proven, that there may be an increased incidence of squamous cell carcinoma. There has been no other tumour type specifically associated with FIV, but all cats with neoplastic conditions should be tested for antibodies to this virus as its presence may affect treatment options. FIV may also cause neuropathies (see Chapter 15), although these are not common presentations.

The clinical signs of FIV infection can be similar to those associated with FeLV infection. It is important to differentiate these infections, as the prognosis varies with the retrovirus and the particular type of disease that it has produced. Differentiation usually requires specific diagnostic tests, but other features can be helpful (Figure 5.13).

Diagnosis

Clinical laboratory findings: Although clinicopathological abnormalities are common in FIV-infected cats, none is pathognomonic. In the acute phase, many cats show neutropenia and lymphopenia. These usually

	Feline leukaemia virus	**Feline immunodeficiency virus**
Virus	Oncovirus	Lentivirus
Animals in which disease is mainly seen	Young cats (<4 years), especially those living in multicat households	Middle-aged to older, free-roaming males
Transmission	Mainly via licking and mutual grooming. Also vertically transmitted	Mainly by biting
Prevalence of infection in UK	Sick cats: 11-17% Healthy cats: 1-2%	Sick cats: 13-19% Healthy cats: 2-3%
Neoplasia	About 20 × increase compared with uninfected cats	About 5 × increase compared with uninfected cats
Immunosuppression	Common, often fatal	Common, often not fatal if infections treated
Anaemia	Very common in infected cats (at least as common as neoplasia), and often very serious	Usually mild - only about 18% of infected cats
Diagnosis	Test for antigen or whole virus	Test for antibody
Prevention	Vaccine; test and remove	No vaccine; test and remove only
Prognosis	85% of persistently infected cats die within 3 years	May live for years. Once clinical signs become severe or recurrent, prognosis is poor

Figure 5.13: Important differences between feline immunodeficiency virus and feline leukaemia virus infections.

resolve as the cats become asymptomatic but often recur intermittently. Clinically ill cats may show neutropenia, lymphopenia, anaemia, monocytosis or thrombocytopenia (occasionally). Analysis of serum biochemistry often reveals hyperglobulinaemia. Other biochemical abnormalities depend on which body systems are affected by disease; they may include azotaemia, raised liver enzyme concentrations, hypercholesterolaemia, hyperglycaemia or subclinically prolonged coagulation times.

FIV-specific testing: FIV infection is generally confirmed by showing the presence of FIV-specific antibodies (Figure 5.14). In the UK, diagnostic kits are currently based on ELISA or RIM methodologies. The ELISA method detects antibodies to the core protein FIV p24, whereas the RIM method detects antibodies to the envelope protein gp41. Western blotting and immunofluorescence detect antibodies to several different FIV proteins. These tests are available from some commercial laboratories.

Type of test	**What is detected:**	**Comments**
ELISA	Antibody to feline immunodeficiency virus (FIV) p24 and gp41	Rapid and easy to use Possibility of false positive results - should confirm positive results by Western blotting or immunoprecipitation
Rapid immunomigratory test	Antibody to FIV gp41	Rapid and easy to use Possibility of false positive results - should confirm positives by Western blotting or immunoprecipitation
Virus isolation	Infectious virus grown in cell culture from cat's white blood cells	Not readily available. False negative results common
Immunofluorescence	Antibody to all FIV epitopes	Anticoagulant affects results so air-dried smears recommended
Western Blot (Immunoblot)	Antibody to p24, gp41 and gp120	Gold standard if performed by experienced laboratory

Figure 5.14: Tests for feline immunodeficiency virus.

Testing should not be performed until 12 weeks after a bite has been sustained, as the antibody response to FIV may not develop before this time. A test immediately after exposure may be useful to determine whether a cat was negative before being bitten. Kittens born to FIV-infected queens have maternally derived antibody up to 16 weeks of age, and so serological testing should be performed after they are 16 weeks old. As with all serological tests, false-positive and false-negative results occur occasionally. Technical error may result in occasional false-positive results, particularly when whole blood or saliva are used, rather than serum. Ambiguous results should not be over-interpreted, and affected cats should be retested. Up to 10% of FIV-infected cats do not have detectable levels of antibody. This may be due to:

- Early infection (it can take up to 12 weeks for antibodies to develop)
- Terminal immune collapse
- A relative or absolute lack of antibody
- A failure of the test system to identify the antibody.

In cases where FIV infection is strongly suspected but antibody tests prove negative, the virus may be detected using a PCR assay. This assay has recently become commercially available. Alternatively, the virus can be detected using virus isolation (VI) which is available in certain specialist laboratories.

Treatment and management
With the widespread availability of FIV tests, many FIV-infected cats are identified before they develop severe lymphopenia, neutropenia or other markers of immunosuppression. Such cats often respond to appropriate therapy of any infections. Ideally, FIV-infected cats should be kept separate from uninfected animals. This will prevent the spread of virus and reduce the risk of the infected cat being exposed to potential secondary pathogens. Where isolation is not possible, a 'night curfew' is recommended: keeping cats indoors from dusk until dawn greatly reduces the risk of cat-to-cat interactions and so reduces the spread of disease. Neutering male cats may reduce territorial aggression. Vaccination against FIV is not available. A test and remove scheme can be used in multicat households (see Figure 5.15).

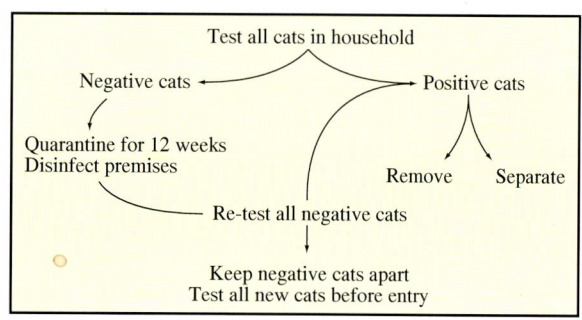

Figure 5.15: Test and remove scheme for feline immunodeficiency virus.

The long-term management of FIV-associated immunodeficiency depends on several factors, such as:

- The type of environment in which the animal has to live
- The willingness of owners to care for their pets.

The long-term care of any immunocompromised animal is not to be undertaken lightly. The animal should be exposed to as few infectious organisms as possible. Ideally, it should be isolated, or at least kept in a small stable group. Exposure to parasites such as fleas and ticks should be prevented as they may act as vectors for other infections, e.g. *Bartonella* spp. and, maybe, *Haemobartonella*. Since stress accentuates immune dysfunction, exposure to stressful situations should be minimized.

Immunosuppressed cats should have regular health checks. Particular attention should be paid to the mouth, skin and body weight. When a secondary infection is noted the causal pathogen should be identified. Appropriate treatment should begin early and be aggressive. Antimicrobial drugs should be chosen carefully, as indicated by culture and sensitivity. Immunosuppressed FIV-infected cats may respond rather slowly, even when given appropriate therapy. The presence of FIV infection does not necessarily preclude a successful outcome, at least in the short term. Prolonged or intermittent courses of treatment may be required. Some immunosuppressive drugs, e.g. griseofulvin, should be avoided (itraconazole may be preferred in an FIV-infected cat with dermatophytosis). Although corticosteroids may seem to be contraindicated, their use in FIV-infected cats often results in clinical improvement. This is possibly due to their anti-inflammatory action on secondary infections. Consideration should be given to the use of non-steroidal anti-inflammatory drugs in such cats. When corticosteroids are used, they should be given at anti-inflammatory doses for the shortest possible time.

Several specific antiviral drugs are available. Treatment with zidovudine or phosphonyl methoxyethyladenine (PMEA) has been associated with improvement of both clinical signs and immune status in many affected cats. However, these drugs are expensive and may cause severe side effects, particularly anaemia. An ever-increasing number of immunomodulating drugs are becoming available. Immunostimulants such as interferon-α, acemannan and *Propionibacterium acnes* may give beneficial results, but side effects are common.

A number of food supplements are claimed to have immune-enhancing effects (e.g. *NN*-dimethyl glycine), but their beneficial effects are unproven in FIV-infected cats.

Recombinant human granulocyte colony-stimulating factor has been used in neutropenic cats and may be helpful in the short-term management of this condition in FIV-positive cats. Long-term use is associated with the development of neutropenia due to the formation of antibodies against this heterologous protein. Treatment for longer than 3 weeks is not recommended.

Hypoglobulinaemic cats may be managed in the short term with plasma transfusions, pooled human immunoglobulins or specific antisera (if available). Their effect is transitory, and there is a small risk of anaphylactic reaction with repeated transfusions. Erythropoietin (epoetin alfa and beta) has been used in some anaemic cats with a non-regenerative anaemia. Antibody formation and expense limit its usefulness.

Care must be taken when vaccinating immunosuppressed animals. Clinically unwell animals should not be vaccinated. Since live attenuated vaccines can induce clinical disease in immunocompromised patients, they should not be used. If exposure to infectious diseases cannot be avoided then killed vaccines and regular boosters are recommended. To prevent exposure to live attenuated viruses, in-contact animals should also be vaccinated with killed vaccines.

There is no specific information on the treatment of FIV-associated neuropathies or lymphomas.

Prognosis
Although the long-term prognosis for an FIV-infected cat is guarded, some will survive many years after diagnosis. An FIV-positive result is not necessarily an indication for euthanasia, even in sick cats, since some will live for many years with appropriate treatment. Currently available tests give no indication as to what stage of disease the cat has reached. However, it is generally true that the more severe and chronic the clinical signs, the worse the prognosis.

Other infectious causes of immunosuppression

Canine distemper virus
Canine distemper virus (CDV) damages lymphoid tissue, resulting in depression of CMI. *In utero* and neonatal infection can result in permanent immunodeficiency. Affected dogs have lymphopenia, hypogammaglobulinaemia and thymic hypoplasia. This is seen as an increased susceptibility to protozoal, viral and fungal infections. When older neonates are infected with CDV, the depression in CMI may be transient. See Chapter 6 for further information.

Canine parvovirus and feline panleucopenia virus
As canine and feline parvoviruses replicate in rapidly dividing cells they cause severe lymphopenia and suppression of the CMI in neonates. Affected animals may develop overwhelming systemic infection by enteric bacteria. Canine parvovirus predisposes unvaccinated puppies to CDV infection. See Chapter 8 for further information.

Canine adenovirus-1
Canine adenovirus-1 (CAV-1) produces severe leucopenia, resulting in immunodeficiency. This may result in opportunistic infections which will adversely affect the prognosis. The leucopenia resolves following recovery. See Chapter 11 for more details on CAV-1.

Feline leukaemia virus
FeLV causes a profound depression of CMI, leading to lymphopenia, neutropenia and hyperglobulinaemia. Latent infections can result in persistent neutropenia. It is thought that more FeLV-positive cats die from immunosuppression than from neoplasia (see above).

Demodex spp.
It is unclear whether disease caused by *Demodex* causes immunosuppression or results from it. Damage to the cutaneous barrier may lead to pyoderma and secondary immune suppression (see Chapter 13).

Toxoplasma
Whereas generalized leucocytosis is seen most commonly, a severe generalized leucopenia may be seen in severely affected individuals (see Chapter 15).

Septicaemia
Severe endotoxaemia can impair CMI, interfere with neutrophil function and reduce complement concentration (see Chapter 7).

INFECTIONS ASSOCIATED WITH IMMUNE-MEDIATED DISEASES

Some infectious diseases are associated with the production of antibodies that are directed against the host's own antigens. These antibodies induce immune-mediated destruction of body tissues that is often more severe than the actual damage caused by the infectious organism. The clinical manifestations of this damage include:

- Polyarthritis
- Haemolytic anaemia
- Thrombocytopenia
- Glomerulonephritis
- Uveitis
- Immune-mediated dermatopathies.

The role of immune-mediated mechanisms in inducing anaemia and other signs listed above is often augmented by direct pathogen-mediated damage. In addition, pyrexia, weight loss and a reactive lymphadenopathy are common non-specific clinical signs of such damage. A list of causes of immune-mediated disease is provided in Figure 5.16.

Infectious cause	Presentations
Viruses	
Feline coronavirus	Immune-mediated vasculitis (see Chapter 9)
Feline leukaemia virus	Thrombocytopenia, anaemia
Feline calicivirus	Polyarthritis (see Chapter 14)
Bacteria (including rickettsias)	
Ehrlichia	Thrombocytopenia, anaemia, polyarthritis
Haemobartonella	Anaemia*
Brucella canis	Uveitis, glomerulonephritis, endophthalmitis
Rocky Mountain spotted fever	Thrombocytopenia?*
Borrelia spp.	Polyarthritis (see Chapter 14)
Fungi	
Coccidioidomycosis	Polyarthritis
Protozoa	
Leishmania	Dermatitis, polyarthritis, panophthalmitis, glomerulonephritis, anaemia
Babesia	Thrombocytopenia, anaemia, polyarthritis
Helminths	
Dirofilaria immitis	Anaemia (see Chapter 7)*
Non-infectious	
Idiopathic	Any of the above
Neoplasia	Any of the above
Drugs, e.g. sulphonamides	Any of the above

Figure 5.16: Causes of immune-mediated disease.
* The role of immune-mediated damage is unclear in this condition. Direct lysis of erythrocytes or platelets may be more important.

The presence of one or more of the clinical manifestations listed above should alert the clinician to the possibility of an underlying infectious disease or neoplastic disease. The diagnosis of primary (i.e. idiopathic) autoimmune diseases, such as systemic lupus erythematosus, relies on the exclusion of underlying causes of immune-mediated disease.

History and physical examination
As several infectious diseases associated with immune-mediated disease are not enzootic to the UK, a history of travel within an endemic area may be very useful. The visit to an endemic area may have occurred several years before the development of clinical signs. Some infections can have long incubation periods or may relapse many years after the initial infection.

A thorough physical examination should be performed to assess the extent of organ involvement. In particular, mucous membranes, joints, eyes and lymph nodes should be carefully inspected.

Laboratory tests
Neutrophilia and hyperglobulinaemia are common and may be pronounced. Urinalysis should be performed in all suspected cases of immune-mediated disease. If proteinuria is present then sediment examination and a protein:creatinine ratio will be useful to assess the severity and source of the protein loss.

Lymph node aspirates should be performed in all cases of lymphadenopathy. Although cytology often only shows a non-specific reaction (characterized by a mixed population of cells with increased numbers of neutrophils and plasma cells) it may show:

- Organisms, such as *Leishmania* spp.
- Neoplasia (particularly lymphoma).

Joint aspirates may produce synovial fluid that is less viscous than normal, with an increased cell count ($>3 \times 10^9$/l; see Chapter 14). Depending on the clinical presentation, Coombs', antiplatelet and antinuclear antibody tests should be considered. Any of these tests may be positive (and with a high titre) as they do not distinguish between primary and secondary causes of immune-mediated disease.

Leishmaniasis
Leishmaniasis is an important disease of dogs that is endemic in the Mediterranean areas of Europe, the Middle East and many tropical and subtropical areas of the world. In Europe, the aetiological agent of canine leishmaniasis is *Leishmania infantum*. Other species of *Leishmania* affect dogs in South America and the Middle East. The agent is transmitted by sand flies (*Phlebotomus* spp.). At present leishmaniasis is restricted in the UK to dogs that have been imported from endemic areas (or that have been in very close contact with such dogs). However, with the lifting of quarantine and increasing mobility of owners and their dogs, the prevalence of this disease in the UK is likely to increase. The long incubation period of the disease (up to 6 years or greater) may divorce the onset of clinical disease from history of quarantine or travel to an endemic area. The vector does not occur in the UK, but should global temperatures increase it is likely that its range will expand to include southern England. Transmission of the disease from an infected imported dog to another that had never been outside the UK has been reported.

Clinical signs
In endemic areas, dogs are exposed at a very early age. Some develop protective immunity, some develop subclinical infections that may relapse later and others develop the classic clinical syndrome. The parasite stimulates an overactive and ineffective B cell response at the same time as suppressing macrophage activation. This allows systemic spread of the parasites

in the face of massive production of immunoglobulins and immune complexes. Both *Leishmania*-specific and non-specific antibodies (including autoantibodies) are produced.

The disease has a waxing and waning course and there is usually a history of non-specific lethargy, polydipsia and anorexia. On physical examination the following are common:

- Pyrexia
- Weight loss
- Generalized lymphadenomegaly
- Pale mucous membranes (due to anaemia)
- Exfoliative dermatitis
- Periocular alopecia
- Hyperkeratosis of the foot pads
- Excessive growth of claws
- Ulcerative and nodular dermatitis (due to vasculitis and granulomatous inflammation)
- Shifting lameness (due to immune-mediated polyarthritis)
- Panophthalmitis.

These systemic signs reflect widespread immune-complex mediated organ damage (Figure 5.17). The cutaneous signs are very common, and the exfoliative dermatitis produces a characteristic silvery scale that is prominent on the dorsum of the nose, periocular region and pinnae.

Diagnosis

A remarkable clinicopathological finding is the significant hyperglobulinaemia, which is due to massive γ-globulin production. A monoclonal or biclonal gammopathy may be seen on serum protein electrophoresis. Affected dogs are often antinuclear antibody positive and Coombs' test positive. Severe proteinuria may be documented due to a protein-losing nephropathy.

Diagnosis is based on the demonstration of the parasite in Giemsa- or Leishman's-stained lymph node and bone marrow aspirates (Figure 5.18) in association with typical clinical signs. Parasites may also be found in Giemsa- or Leishman's-stained skin biopsy samples, and the use of immunohistochemistry increases sensitivity. Serology using IFAT, ELISA, dot-ELISA or agglutination tests supports a diagnosis of disease in non-endemic areas. Because of the relatively long disease incubation period, clinical cases are likely to be antibody positive. PCR testing for leishmaniasis has been developed and is available in the UK. Concurrent ehrlichiosis is common in endemic areas, and care should be taken to eliminate co-infection, particularly in dogs that have bleeding tendencies.

Treatment and prevention

The zoonotic potential of the organism is low but should always be considered, particularly if there is an immunocompromised individual in the household.

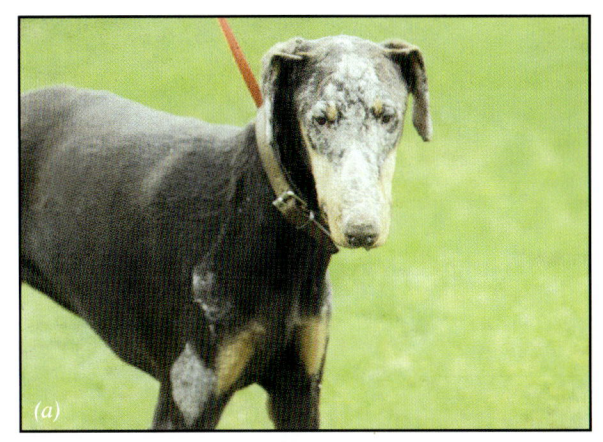

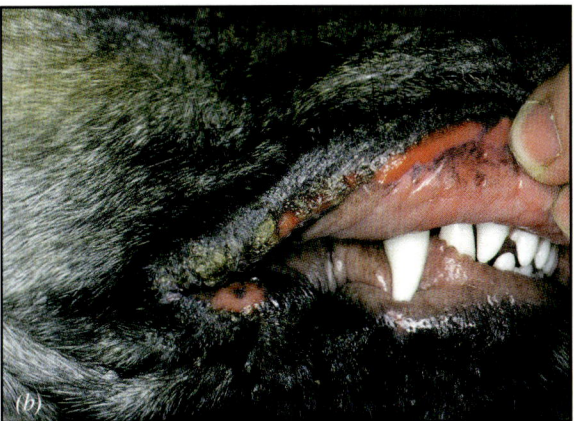

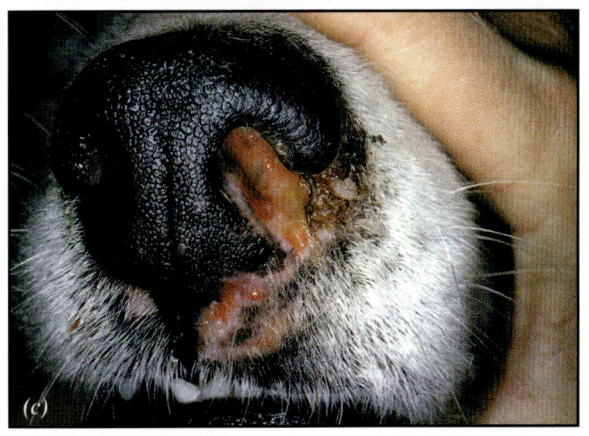

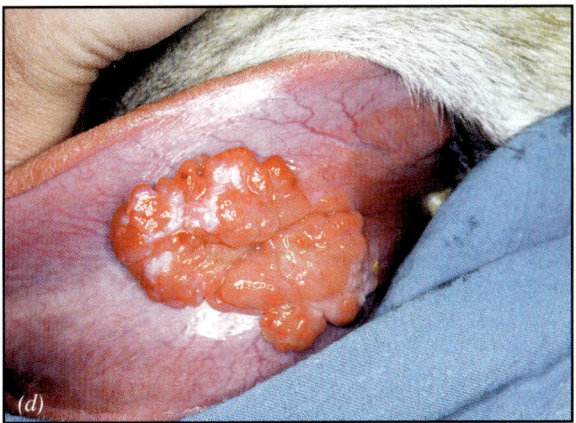

Figure 5.17: Clinical manifestations of leishmaniasis: (a) characteristic 'silvery' exfoliative dermatitis; (b) oral mucocutaneous ulceration; (c) nasal mucocutaneous ulceration; and (d) lingual granuloma formation. (b, c and d courtesy of Dr Artur Font.)

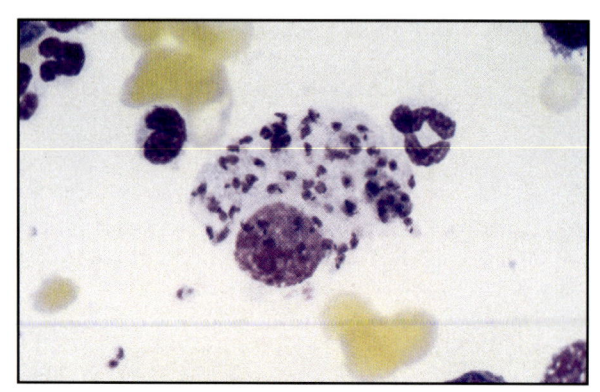

86 Manual of Canine and Feline Infectious Diseases

Figure 5.18: Leishmania infantum *in a Giemsa-stained bone marrow aspirate. (Courtesy of Professor Andrew Nash.)*

The extent of systemic disease should be fully evaluated before therapy is started. Appropriate supportive treatment must be given for each organ system affected.

The basis of treatment is a pentavalent antimonial drug in combination with allopurinol. The antimonial drug that is most commonly used in dogs in Europe is meglumine antimonate. If this drug is used alone, clinical relapse is common and multiple courses are required to maintain remission. This problem has been greatly improved by the concurrent use of allopurinol during induction therapy and its continued use after the antimonial therapy has finished. Allopurinol has been used 'prophylactically' in young dogs that are known to have been exposed to *Leishmania*. The drug is inexpensive, and side effects with long-term therapy have not been reported. Sodium stibogluconante is an alternative to meglumine antimonate but is less available in Europe. Cases that become resistant to antimonials may be treated with amphotericin B, but renal toxicity and lack of well established doses limits its use. Vaccination is not available for leishmaniasis.

Concurrent treatment for ehrlichiosis may be necessary as coinfection is common in Italy, southern France and the Iberian peninsula.

The prognosis ultimately depends on the severity of organ dysfunction at the time of diagnosis. If the dog is a treatment candidate, the prognosis for cure is guarded, although the prognosis for control of the clinical expression of disease is good.

Leishmaniasis in cats

Natural infection and clinical disease in cats caused by *L. infantum* are rare. One case in a cat imported into Britain has been reported. The equivalent of the canine syndrome has been reported rarely; infection is mostly associated with cutaneous nodular lesions.

Ehrlichiosis

Canine and feline ehrlichiosis are caused by intracellular rickettsial organisms of the genus *Ehrlichia*. In dogs, specific ehrlichial species have been identified parasitizing monocytes, granulocytes and platelets. Monocytic ehrlichiosis is an important disease of dogs in southern Europe and other areas of the Mediterranean basin, although its distribution is spreading north. In Europe, the canine disease is primarily caused by *E. canis* and transmitted by the tick *Rhipicephalus sanguineus*. In the UK, it has been reported only in dogs that have travelled through endemic areas. However, should *R. sanguineus* become more prevalent, *E. canis* could become established, as its development is not temperature dependent *per se*.

Acute, subclinical and chronic syndromes have been described for canine monocytic ehrlichiosis. The acute phase has an incubation period of 8–20 days and is followed by clinical remission. However, subclinical infection is common and may persist for years. If an ineffective immune response is mounted, chronic ehrlichiosis develops and is associated with severe bone marrow damage in susceptible animals. Coinfection with *Babesia* sp. and *Leishmania infantum* is common.

In the past 5 years, naturally occurring granulocytic ehrlichiosis has been reported in dogs from Sweden (Egenvall *et al.*, 1997). The ehrlichial species involved is within the *E. phagocytophila* group and is closely related, if not identical, to *E. equi* and the human granulocytic agent of ehrlichiosis. It is transmitted by ticks of the *Ixodes* species, including the common tick infecting dogs in the UK, *Ixodes ricinus*. Although there are reports of *E. phagocytophila* infection in Scotland, the importance of this infection in the UK dog population has yet to be determined.

Clinical signs

In acute monocytic and granulocytic ehrlichiosis, non-specific signs of illness such as fever, anorexia and lymphadenomegaly often occur, along with oculonasal discharge, uveitis and central nervous signs (seizures, stupor). Vasculitis, immune-mediated thrombocytopenia and platelet dysfunction causing petechiation and epistaxis are marked in *E. canis* infection, and leucopenia and variable anaemia occur (Figure 5.19). In granulocytic ehrlichiosis, lameness, joint swelling and limb oedema are more marked. Chronic *E. canis* infection causes pancytopenia due

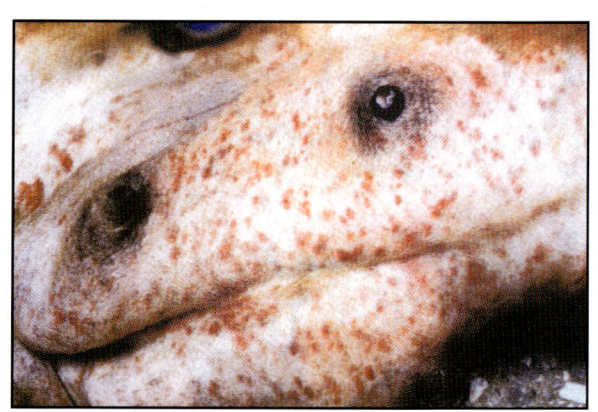

Figure 5.19: Extensive ventral abdominal petechial haemorrhages due to thrombocytopenia caused by Ehrlichia platys. *(Courtesy of Johannes Schoeman.)*

to bone marrow destruction. Varying degrees of non-regenerative anaemia, thrombocytopenia and leucopenia occur that, if left untreated, lead to death through haemorrhage and/or secondary infection. Marked hyperglobulinaemia is a feature. Chronic ehrlichiosis is more severe in certain breeds (e.g. the German Shepherd Dog) and in younger animals. Severity may also depend on the strain of *Ehrlichia* spp. The onset of clinical signs may be triggered by concurrent disease such as leishmaniasis, babesiosis or other tick-transmitted infections. This may present as a complex multisystemic disease.

Diagnosis
The diagnosis is based on appropriate clinical findings and identification of ehrlichial morulae (Figure 5.20) in leucocytes or platelets in buffy coat smears or blood from a capillary vessel. Tissue aspirates of spleen, lung or lymph nodes may also be used. Serological diagnosis was mainly based on IFA testing or immunoblotting, but PCR tests are now available in the UK.

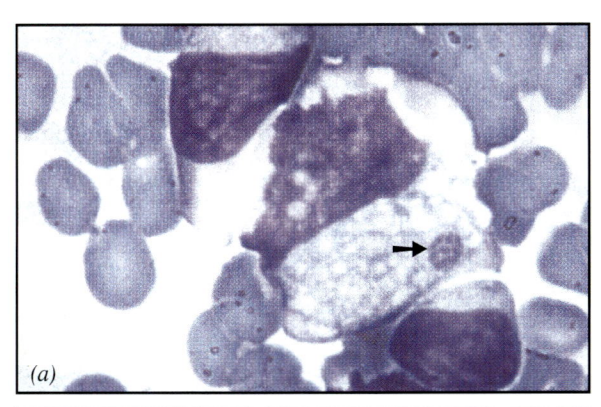

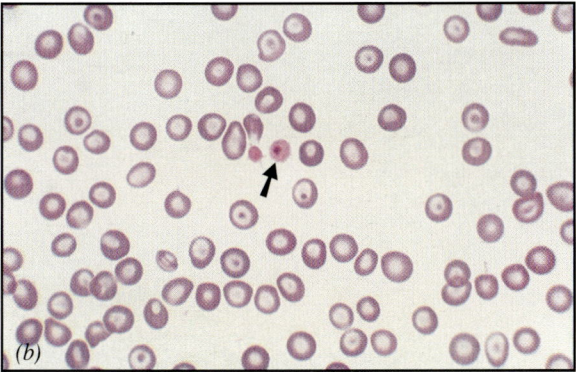

Figure 5.20: (a) Ehrlichia canis morula within a Giemsa-stained monocyte. (b) E. platys inside a platelet. (Courtesy of Johannes Schoeman.)

Treatment and prevention
Supportive therapy with fluids and/or blood transfusions may be required. If life-threatening thrombocytopenia is present, glucocorticoid therapy is rational because of the immune-mediated pathogenesis. Glucocorticoids may also be useful in the immune-mediated arthritis, meningitis and vasculitis of granulocytic ehrlichiosis.

Doxycycline or oxytetracycline therapy is the treatment of choice for ehrlichiosis. In addition, imidocarb can be given for resistant infections.

Vaccination is not available. For travelling dogs, oral tetracycline is prophylactic at 6.6 mg/kg daily in combination with tick control. The time required for transmission from ticks is not known but may be 1–2 days. If so, current means of tick control may not eliminate the risk of contracting disease.

Ehrlichiosis in cats
The species of *Ehrlichia* affecting domesticated and wild cats has not been characterized, but *Ehrlichia*-like bodies have been detected in sick cats in several countries, including France. Clinical signs in affected cats are fever, joint pain, anaemia, dyspnoea and lymphadenomegaly.

Other infections

Rocky Mountain spotted fever
This is a severe disease that is associated with a widespread vasculitis. It is caused by the rickettsial organism *Rickettsia rickettsii* and is transmitted by ticks of the *Dermacentor* genus. Early clinical signs include severe depression, anorexia, lymphadenopathy and oedema of the extremities. Thrombocytopenia is common and is probably due to the direct effects of the organism rather than an immune-mediated destruction. Ecchymoses and petechiae on mucous membranes are seen in approximately 20% of cases. Sequelae in dogs that survive the acute disease include generalized central nervous signs, uveitis, sloughing of peripheral tissues affected by vasculitis, and polyarthritis. The role of immune-mediated mechanisms in the chronic form of the disease is unclear. The disease occurs mainly in the southwestern states of the USA and does not occur in the UK.

Viral diseases
A major proportion of cats with immune-mediated disease are found to be infected with FeLV or FIV or to have developed FIP (see above and Chapter 9).

REFERENCES AND FURTHER READING

Barnes A, Bell SC, Isherwood DR, Bennett M and Carter SD (2000) Evidence of *Bartonella henselae* infection in cats and dogs in the United Kingdom. *Veterinary Record* **147**, 673–677

Berent LM, Messick JB and Cooper SK (1998) Detection of *Haemobartonella felis* in cats with experimentally induced acute and chronic infections using a polymerase chain reaction assay. *American Journal of Veterinary Research* **59**, 1215–1220

Bobade PA, Nash AS and Rogerson P (1995) Feline haemobartonellosis: clinical, haematological and pathological studies in natural infections and the relationship to infection with feline leukaemia virus. *Veterinary Record* **122**, 32–36

Breitschwerdt EB, Kordick DL, Malarkey DE, Keene B Hadfield TL and Wilson K (1995) Endocarditis in a dog due to infection with a novel Bartonella subspecies. *Journal of Clinical Microbiology* **33**, 154–160

Ciaramella P, Oliva G, de Luna R, Gradoni L, Ambrosio R, Cortese L, Scalone A and Persechino A (1997) A retrospective clinical study of canine leishmaniasis in 150 dogs naturally infected by Leishmania infantum. *Veterinary Record.* **141,** 539-543

Cotter SM (1998) Feline viral neoplasia. In: *Infectious Diseases of the Dog and Cat, 3rd edn,* ed. CE Greene, pp. 71-84. WB Saunders, Philadelphia

Court EA, Watson AD and Peaston AE (1997) Retrospective study of 60 cases of feline lymphosarcoma. *Australian Veterinary Journal* **75,** 424-427

Egenvall AE, Hedhammer ÅA and Bjöersdorff AI (1997) Clinical features and serology of 14 dogs affected with granulocytic ehrlichiosis in Sweden. *Veterinary Record* **140,** 222-226

Foley JE, Chomel B, Kikuchi Y, Yamamoto K and Pedersen NC (1998) Seroprevalence of Bartonella henselae in cattery cats: association with cattery hygiene and flea infestation. *Veterinary Quarterly* **20,** 1-5

Giger U and Greene CE (1998) Immunodeficiencies and infectious disease. In: *Infectious Diseases of the Dog and Cat, 3rd edn,* ed. CE Greene, pp. 673-682. WB Saunders, Philadelphia

Harrus S, Aroch I, Lavy E and Bark H (1997) Clinical manifestations of infectious canine cyclic thrombocytopenia. *Veterinary Record* **141,** 247-250

Hartmann K, Werner RM, Egberink H and Jarrett O (2001) Comparison of different in-house tests for rapid diagnosis of feline immunodeficiency and feline leukaemia virus infection. *Veterinary Record* (in press)

Hosie MJ, Robertson C and Jarrett O (1989) Prevalence of feline leukaemia virus and antibodies to feline immunodeficiency virus in cats in the United Kingdom. *Veterinary Record* **128,** 293-297

Jarrett O and Ganiere J (1996) Comparative studies of the efficacy of a recombinant feline leukaemia virus vaccine. *Veterinary Record* **138,** 7-11

Lane SB, Kornegay JN, Duncan JR and Oliver JE Jr (1994) Feline spinal lymphosarcoma: a retrospective evaluation of 23 cats. *Journal of Veterinary Internal Medicine* **8,** 99-104

O'Dair HA, Hopper CD, Gruffydd-Jones TJ, Harbour DA and Waters L (1994) Clinical aspects of Chlamydia psittaci infection in cats infected with feline immunodeficiency virus. *Veterinary Record* **134,** 365-368

Ramsey IK and Gould S (1999) Feline anaemia. *In Practice* **21,** 411-415, 507-517

Robinson A, DeCann K, Aitken E, Gruffydd-Jones TJ, Sparkes AH, Werret G and Harbour DA (1998) Comparison of a rapid immunomigration test and ELISA for FIV antibody and FeLV antigen testing in cats. *Veterinary Record* **142,** 491-492

Sellon RK (1998) Feline immunodeficiency virus. In: *Infectious Diseases of the Dog and Cat, 3rd edn,* ed. CE Greene, pp. 84-96. WB Saunders, Philadelphia

Shelton GH, Grant CK, Linenberger ML and Abkowitz JL (1990) Severe neutropenia associated with griseofulvin therapy in cats with feline immunodeficiency virus infection. *Journal of Veterinary Internal Medicine* **4,** 317-319

Sparkes AH, Gruffydd-Jones TJ and Harbour DA (1991) Feline infectious peritonitis: a review of clinicopathological changes in 65 cases and a critical assessment of their diagnostic value. *Veterinary Record* **129,** 209-212

Sparkes AH, Hopper CD, Millard WG, Gruffydd-Jones TJ and Harbour DA (1993) Feline immunodeficiency virus: clinicopathologic findings in 90 naturally occurring cases. *Journal of Veterinary Internal Medicine* **7,** 85-90

Sparkes AH (1997) Feline leukaemia virus: a review of immunity and vaccination. *Journal of Small Animal Practice* **38,** 187-194

Swenson CL, Kociba GJ, Mathes LE, Hand PJ, Neer CA, Hayes KA and Olsen RG (1990) Prevalence of disease in nonviremic cats previously exposed to feline leukemia virus. *Journal American Veterinary Medical Association* **196,** 1049-1052

Trees A and Shaw S (1999) Imported diseases in small animals. *In Practice* **21,** 482-491

Zeidner NS, Mathiason-DuBard CK and Hoover EA (1995) Reversal of feline leukemia virus infection by adoptive transfer of activated T lymphocytes, interferon alpha, and zidovudine. *Seminars in Veterinary Medicine and Surgery (Small Animal)* **10,** 256-266

CHAPTER SIX

The Respiratory Tract

Kim Willoughby and Susan Dawson

CHAPTER PLAN

Introduction
Respiratory tract defence mechanisms
Aetiology of respiratory tract infections
Diagnosis of respiratory tract infections
    Localizing disease
    Obtaining diagnostic material
Nasal infections
    General historical and clinical features of
        nasal infections
    Acute nasal disease
    Chronic nasal disease
        Rhinitis/sinusitis
        Nasal mycoses
        Parasitic nasal disease
Infections of the upper respiratory tract
    Kennel cough
    Cat flu
    Parasitic infections
Infections of the lower respiratory tract
    Canine distemper
    Feline poxvirus
    Bacterial infections
    Fungal infections
    Protozoal infections
    Parasitic infestation
Pleural and mediastinal infections
    Pyothorax
    Feline infectious peritonitis
    Feline leukaemia virus
    Pulmonary infection/parapneumonic effusion
    Miscellaneous
References and further reading

INTRODUCTION

Infectious respiratory diseases are common in dogs and cats, particularly in those kept in groups. As many cause similar clinical signs, and concomitant infections are often seen, syndromes such as 'kennel cough' and 'cat flu' are often described. Infectious agents generally affect one part of the respiratory tract, although many have the potential to involve adjacent areas. The clinical presentation partly depends on their spread within the respiratory tract.

RESPIRATORY TRACT DEFENCE MECHANISMS

Infectious agents usually gain access to the respiratory tract via the airways. Defence against infection depends on intact humoral and cell-mediated immune systems and physical mechanisms (nasal turbinates and mucociliary apparatus). The mucociliary apparatus, present throughout the entire respiratory tract to the level of the bronchi, comprises ciliated epithelium and a mucous carpet lining. Particulate matter trapped by the mucus is transported by ciliary motion to the pharynx for removal by coughing or swallowing. Coughing allows rapid movement of mucus towards the pharynx and helps clear airways of excess mucus. Foreign particles small enough to reach the alveolus are scavenged by pulmonary macrophages and lymphatic drainage. Conditions or situations that may compromise the physical defence mechanisms, thereby predisposing to opportunistic infections, include:

- Primary respiratory, multisystemic or immunosuppressive infections
- Immunosuppressive therapy, e.g. anti-cancer chemotherapy, corticosteroids
- Thoracic trauma or surgery
- Anatomical/functional disease, e.g. brachycephalic syndrome, tracheal hypoplasia, ciliary dyskinesia
- Gastrointestinal disease that results in dysphagia, regurgitation or vomiting
- Loss of consciousness
- Metabolic diseases causing debility, e.g. diabetes mellitus, Cushing's syndrome, chronic renal failure, hepatic disease
- Iatrogenic factors, e.g. sedation, nasogastric feeding, endotracheal tube placement, tracheostomy tube, assisted ventilation, thoracic or abdominal surgery, indwelling venous catheter, contaminated infusion solutions.

AETIOLOGY OF RESPIRATORY TRACT INFECTIONS

Primary respiratory tract infections are common causes of morbidity; mortality is rare for most of them. Opportunistic infections are almost exclusively limited to bacteria that take advantage of compromised host defence mechanisms. Small numbers of bacteria are normal within the respiratory tract to the level of the mainstem bronchi and are recovered from up to 50% of healthy animals. Numerous species have been isolated (Figure 6.1); some have been associated with disease as opportunistic invaders or occasionally as primary infecting agents. Organisms isolated from the lower respiratory tract are often the same as the oropharyngeal flora, reflecting their aspiration into this area.

DIAGNOSIS OF RESPIRATORY TRACT INFECTIONS

The diagnosis of a respiratory tract infection depends on localizing disease to one or more areas, imaging the respiratory tract, obtaining suitable diagnostic material and applying one or more diagnostic tests to confirm the diagnosis.

Localizing disease

The region of the respiratory tract involved can be determined from historical and clinical information:

- Nasal discharge, sneezing, pain around the nose or nasal deformity indicate nasal disease
- Coughing is a feature of laryngeal, tracheal and bronchial disease; it is not a feature of alveolar or interstitial pulmonary disease
- Dyspnoea and tachypnoea are associated with obstruction anywhere in the respiratory tract, or pulmonary or pleural disease
- Auscultation differentiates diseases of the upper respiratory tract (URT) from those of the lower respiratory tract (LRT) and allows pleural effusion to be detected
- Pyrexia is likely to be associated with pulmonary or multisystemic disease.

Imaging the respiratory tract

Radiography

Radiography enables localization of disease processes to the nose, trachea, lung and pleural cavity, but rarely provides a definitive diagnosis. Specific radiological patterns associated with specific disorders are discussed under each infectious agent.

Organism	Site Dogs	Cats
Staphylococcus spp.	Nasal, oropharyngeal, trachea/lungs	Oropharyngeal, trachea/lungs
Streptococcus spp.	Nasal, oropharyngeal, trachea/lungs	Oropharyngeal, trachea/lungs
Corynebacterium	Nasal, oropharyngeal, trachea/lungs	Oropharyngeal
Micrococcus		Oropharyngeal, trachea/lungs
Haemophilus felis		Trachea/lungs
Bacillus spp.	Nasal, oropharyngeal	
Neisseria	Nasal, oropharyngeal	
Escherichia coli	Nasal, oropharyngeal	Oropharyngeal, trachea/lungs
Enterobacter	Nasal, oropharyngeal	Oropharyngeal, trachea/lungs
Pasteurella multocida	Nasal, oropharyngeal, trachea/lungs	Oropharyngeal
Moraxella	Nasal, trachea/lungs	Oropharyngeal
Proteus	Nasal, oropharyngeal	Oropharyngeal, trachea/lungs
Pseudomonas	Nasal, oropharyngeal	Oropharyngeal, trachea/lungs
Alcaligenes	Nasal, oropharyngeal	
Bordetella bronchiseptica	Nasal, oropharyngeal, tracheal/lungs	Nasal, oropharyngeal
Clostridium spp.	Nasal	
Klebsiella pneumoniae	Oropharyngeal, trachea/lungs	Oropharyngeal, trachea/lungs
Bacteroides spp.	Oropharyngeal	
Propionibacterium spp.	Oropharyngeal	
Peptostreptococcus	Oropharyngeal	
Fusobacterium	Oropharyngeal	
Mycoplasma spp.	Nasal, oropharyngeal, trachea/lungs	Nasal

Figure 6.1: *Bacteria that may be isolated from the respiratory tract.*

Nasal cavity: Lateral and intraoral dorsoventral (non-screen film enhances definition) views of the nasal chamber and a rostrocaudal frontal sinus view are usual, although other views may be helpful.

Lower respiratory tract: Lateral and ventrodorsal views of the thorax are usual, except in cases with suspected pleural effusion, where the first view should be dorsoventral.

Endoscopy

Endoscopy is used to inspect the ventral nasal meatus, nasopharynx, trachea and mainstem bronchi and to obtain appropriate samples. It may show inflammation, neoplasia, polyps, fungal plaques and parasites, but in many cases it does not provide a definitive diagnosis.

Nasal chambers: These can be examined with an endoscope (often a paediatric endoscope is required) placed through the external nares. Arthroscopes and auroscopes can be used, although the latter rarely provide a good view.

Nasopharynx: This may be examined by inserting the endoscope into the oropharynx and retroflexing the endoscope over the soft palate.

Tracheoscopy/bronchoscopy: This allows examination of the URT and LRT. It is preferable to pass the bronchoscope through the lumen of the endotracheal (ET) tube, providing the airway can be maintained. If this is not possible, intravenous anaesthetic agents may be required to maintain anaesthesia, with oxygen or inhalational anaesthesia given via the biopsy channel of the bronchoscope or via a urinary catheter running beside the bronchoscope.

Computed tomography/magnetic resonance imaging

Where facilities are available scanning by computed tomography (CT) or magnetic resonance imaging (MRI) may accurately detect lesions in cases of nasal and frontal sinus disease. Their value in the rest of the respiratory tract is limited owing to respiratory movement.

Obtaining diagnostic material

Several methods are available for obtaining diagnostic material from the respiratory tract for microbiological and cytological assessment.

Swabbing the respiratory tract

Direct swabbing of the nasal cavity, larynx or trachea is used to obtain samples for microbiology. Guarded swabs or a guarded brush system (a brush within a catheter) should be used to prevent contamination of samples with oral commensal bacteria. The larynx and trachea should be swabbed before ET intubation as this may introduce organisms from the oral cavity.

Washings for cytology and microbiology

Aliquots of respiratory tract washings should be placed in EDTA-containing pots. Alternatively, air-dried smears should be made for cytology and placed in a sterile pot or media for microbiological testing; EDTA is bacteriostatic and not recommended for bacterial culture.

Nasal wash: Nasal washing is peformed as follows:

1. Anaesthetize the animal.
2. Insert the catheter into the ventral meatus but not beyond the medial canthus of the eye. A pharyngeal pack and a cuffed ET tube are essential to prevent inhalation of fluid.
3. Introduce warm sterile saline into the nose.
4. Aspirate.

Transtracheal aspiration: This can be performed in a compliant conscious animal but it is not recommended for fractious or nervous animals. It is more difficult to perform in cats than in dogs. Sedatives that interfere with the cough reflex (e.g. butorphanol) should not be used. Transtracheal aspiration is performed as follows:

1. Restrain the animal gently in a normal upright position or in sternal recumbency.
2. Clip the hair over the laryngeal area and scrub. Locate the cricoid and thyroid cartilages – between these lie the cricothyroid ligament.
3. Infiltrate the skin over the cricothyroid ligament with a local anaesthetic. Introduce a through-the-needle catheter through the skin and cricothyroid ligament into the lumen of the trachea.
4. Pass the catheter down the trachea (the animal should be expected to cough, perhaps violently, at this stage). Withdraw the needle and apply the guard to prevent inadvertent sectioning of the catheter.
5. Using a 20 ml (dog) or a 5 ml (cat) syringe, infuse 2–4 ml (dog) or 1–2 ml (cat) of sterile saline (this must not contain a bacteriostatic agent) into the trachea. The animal will cough. Apply suction to recover fluid or mucus. Should only air be obtained, remove the syringe, expel the air and repeat the procedure, up to a maximum of 1 ml saline/kg body weight.
6. Once sufficient material has been obtained, remove the catheter and apply a loose dressing to help prevent bleeding or subcutaneous emphysema, the most common complication of this procedure. Uncommonly, infection at the site, endotracheal haemorrhage or even cardiac arrhythmias may occur.

Endotracheal wash: Endotracheal washing is technically simple, requires minimal equipment and is unlikely to produce adverse reaction, although anaesthesia is required. The major disadvantage is the risk of contamination from oropharyngeal flora. The procedure is as follows:

1. Anaesthetize the animal.
2. Place a sterile ET tube.
3. Place the animal in lateral recumbency and, taking care to prevent contamination of the catheter with oral secretions, introduce a sterile catheter into the lumen of the ET tube and advance it to about the level of the carina.
4. Flush the catheter with sterile saline (5-10 ml for dogs, 2 ml for cats) and aspirate immediately. The procedure may be repeated once on this side. If no sample is obtained, the animal can be placed on the opposite side and washing repeated.
5. If suction is available then a mucus trap is a more efficient method and results in a greater recovery of fluid.

Bronchoalveolar lavage: This requires a sterile, rigid or (preferably) flexible bronchoscope, although a modification using only an ET tube has been described. Figure 6.2 shows the equipment needed to perform bronchoalveolar lavage (BAL). The technique is performed as follows:

1. Pass the bronchoscope into either the left or the right bronchus and direct as appropriate to as low a lung level as possible; in cats this may be the mainstem bronchus, whereas in dogs lobar or even segmental BAL samples can be obtained, depending on both the size of the animal and the bronchoscope. Alternatively, a sterile ET tube can be placed just cranial to the carina, and the washing performed 'blind.'
2. Introduce up to 5 ml/kg (20-100 ml for dogs, maximum 20 ml for cats) of warmed sterile saline (5-10 ml aliquots) into the airway via a catheter placed in the biopsy channel and aspirate immediately.
3. Provide pure oxygen via a fresh catheter placed beside the bronchoscope, and for at least 5 minutes after the sample has been collected.
4. To assist with retrieval of the fluid, it may be helpful to tilt the animal. This technique, particularly if performed blind, carries the risk of perforation of the airway by the catheter, spread of infections further into the respiratory tract and possible acute bronchospasm.

Biopsy material for histopathology/cytology

Biopsy: Biopsy of the respiratory tract mucosa can be carried out endoscopically. The nasal chamber can be biopsied 'blind' by using crocodile forceps placed through the external nares; do not insert beyond the medial canthus of the eye otherwise the cribriform plate may become perforated. This technique results in moderate to severe haemorrhage; a pharyngeal pack and cuffed ET tube are essential. A coagulation screening test, such as measuring whole blood clotting time or activated clotting time, is recommended. In animals with epistaxis further tests, such as measurement of the buccal mucosal bleeding time, are also recommended; epistaxis can also be associated with von Willebrand's disease and performing a biopsy on any animal with a coagulopathy is not recommended.

Fine needle aspiration: This is used to obtain material from lung or nasal masses. If used on lung, iatrogenic pneumothorax or haemothorax may develop. Fine needle aspiration of the lungs should be reserved for use at centres experienced in the procedure, where appropriate facilities are available to manage the complications and where other sampling methods have failed to assist with diagnosis. Ultrasound guidance is often essential for localized masses as their position on radiography varies with the phase of respiration.

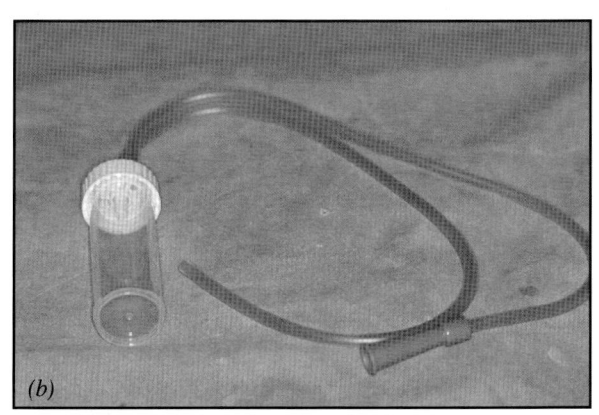

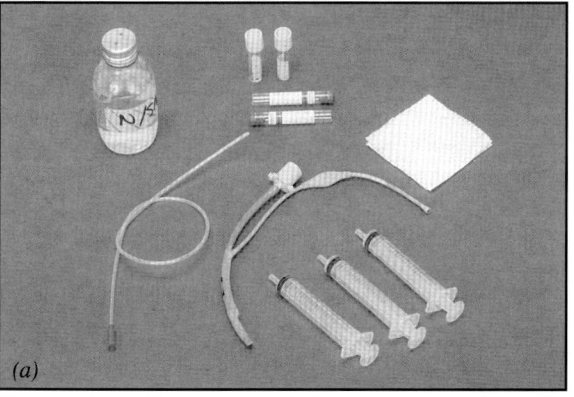

Figure 6.2: *(a) Equipment needed to perform bronchoalveolar lavage (BAL): sterile saline, three 5 or 10 ml syringes, endotracheal tube, canine urinary catheter and sample tubes. A bronchoscope and endoscopic catheter can be used (not shown). (b) Mucus trap used in performing BAL.*

Diagnostic tests

Serum biochemistry and haematology
Serum biochemistry and haematology are of little value in making a specific diagnosis of an infectious respiratory tract disorder. Non-specific features such as a leucocytosis might suggest an inflammatory disorder whereas leucopenia might be found with some viral conditions (e.g. canine distemper virus).

Microbiology

Bacteriology: Bacterial culture and sensitivity is indicated in the diagnosis of primary bacterial infections and to document the extent of secondary bacterial infection. As commensal bacteria may be isolated from the respiratory tract of healthy animals, the importance of an isolate must be considered in the light of the clinical features; the absence of appropriate clinical signs or the presence of another disease process (e.g. fungal rhinitis) suggests the organism is of little or no clinical importance. A heavy and/or pure growth of an organism is likely to be more important than a mixed light growth.

Mycology: Fungal cultures are of value in the diagnosis of nasal, tracheal or pulmonary mycoses. Isolation of any fungus from nasal samples should be interpreted with care as fungi can be present in the noses of normal dogs and cats.

Virology: Virus isolation may confirm a diagnosis. Some viruses, e.g. feline herpesvirus, feline calicivirus, grow readily in cell culture whereas others, e.g. canine distemper virus, parainfluenza virus, are difficult to isolate.

Cytology/histopathology: Cytology is of value in demonstrating bacterial, fungal and neoplastic disorders (Figure 6.3) but is of limited value in confirming

Classification	Mucus	Cytology	Bacteria (culture)	Aetiology
Normal	Small amounts	Low cellularity. Mostly macrophages, some ciliated cuboidal or columnar epithelial cells. Rare neutrophils	Absent or sparse mixed population	Normal
Serous	None	Low cellularity	Absent or sparse mixed population	Allergic nasal disease, viral upper respiratory tract disease, nasal parasites
Mucopurulent	Copious	Largely neutrophils, in high numbers. May be degenerate or have intracellular bacteria. Some epithelial cells and macrophages. Occasionally eosinophils. Bacteria absent or present extracellularly. Fungal hyphae may be present	Absent or sparse to heavy mixed or pure growth. May be culture positive although not observed in smears	Infectious diseases (primary or secondary), including bacteria, fungae, protozoa. Chronic rhinitis/sinusitis. Nasopharyngeal polyps. Nasal neoplasia
Mucohaemorrhagic	Mild to profuse	Red blood cells predominate, inflammatory cells present. Fungal hyphae may be seen	Absent or sparse to heavy mixed growth	Nasal mycosis. Nasal neoplasia. Foreign body. *Linguatula serrata*
True epistaxis	None	Red blood cells predominate	Absent or sparse	Trauma. Bleeding disorders. Nasal neoplasia. Nasal mycosis. Nasopharyngeal polyps
Non-purulent	Varies. May see coils of inspissated mucus	Mixed cell types, one may predominate. Eosinophils, macrophages common. Epithelial cells, perhaps in hyperplastic 'rafts.' Occasional mast cells and neutrophils. Parasitic larvae	Absent or sparse	Allergic tracheobronchitis (feline asthma). Chronic obstructive pulmonary disease (may be secondary). Parasitic disease
Neoplastic		Neoplastic cells rarely observed, usually only in pulmonary carcinoma		Primary or metastatic neoplasia

Figure 6.3: Classification of respiratory wash samples.

viral infections. Exudate may be smeared directly on microscope slides whereas the wash sample should be centrifuged and the sediment used. These should be air dried and stained with Romanowsky-type stains, Ziehl–Neelsen stains or by Gram's method. The type of cell evident and the presence or absence of bacteria may be helpful in classifying the disease process. Histopathology is useful in confirming certain infections.

Serology
This is often of limited value. Demonstration of a rise in antibody titre in paired blood samples can be used to confirm acute infection. *Aspergillus* serology is useful although the sensitivities of available tests vary and all give false negative results.

Parasitology
Parasitic infections can be documented by finding eggs or larvae in nasal/tracheal washes or faeces.

NASAL INFECTIONS

Aetiology
Figure 6.4 lists the infectious causes of nasal disease. Some may be part of widespread respiratory tract infections and are discussed below under upper or lower respiratory tract infections.

Dog
Canine distemper virus (A)
Bordetella bronchiseptica (A)
Canine parainfluenza virus (A)
Aspergillus (C)
Penicillium (C)
Chronic rhinitis/sinusitis (C)
Pneumonyssoides caninum (C)
Rhinosporidium (C)
Linguatula serrata (C)

Cat
Feline herpesvirus (A, C)
Feline calicivirus (A)
Bordetella bronchiseptica (A, C)
Chlamydophila felis (formerly *Chlamydia psittaci* var *felis*) (A)
Mycoplasma spp. (A)
Reovirus (A)
Haemophilus felis (A)
Cryptococcus neoformans (C)
Chronic rhinitis/sinusitis (C)

Figure 6.4: *Infectious causes of nasal disease.*
A = acute disease; C = chronic disease.

General historical and clinical features

Nasal disorders are categorized as acute or chronic. Chronic nasal disease is defined differently in dogs and cats: in the former by the presence of clinical disease for more than 10 days and in the latter by the presence of intermittent or persistent nasal discharge for more than 4 weeks.

The clinical features of acute or chronic rhinitis are variable, non-specific (Figure 6.5) and easily confused with those associated with non-infectious nasal disease.

Sneezing/snorting – most common
Nasal discharge – serous, mucopurulent, serosanguineous
Deformity
Nasal swelling
Depigmentation
Ulceration – nasal planum, nostrils
Coughing
Mouth breathing
Malodorous breath
Pain/irritation

Figure 6.5: *Clinical signs associated with nasal infections.*

Acute nasal disease
Figure 6.4 lists the infectious causes of acute nasal disease; the main non-infectious differential diagnoses are foreign bodies, allergic disease (particularly younger animals) and, less commonly, neoplasia (middle-aged to older animals). Acute infectious nasal disease in the dog is usually recognized in conjunction with generalized upper respiratory tract disease (e.g. kennel cough; see Infections of the upper respiratory tract) or multisystemic disease (e.g. canine distemper; see Infections of the lower respiratory tract); infections presenting with signs of acute nasal disease only are rare. Acute infectious nasal disease in cats is most commonly seen as part of the cat flu complex (see Infections of the upper respiratory tract).

To establish a definitive diagnosis, microbiological sampling is required. As acute infectious nasal disease usually forms part of a wider clinical syndrome, see the URT section for further discussion.

Chronic nasal disease
Non-infectious causes of chronic nasal disease that must be differentiated from infectious causes (see Figure 6.4) are:

- Neoplasia: middle-aged to older animals, dolichocephalic dogs and Siamese and Oriental cats seem more susceptible to nasal neoplasia

- Allergic rhinitis: more likely in younger animals
- Immune-mediated disease
- Palatal defects
- Nasopharyngeal polyps (cats).

Rhinitis/sinusitis

Chronic rhinitis/sinusitis develops subsequent to acute bacterial or viral infections, although the exact mechanisms are unclear. Chronic mucosal damage resulting in mucosal hyperplasia impairs local defence mechanisms allowing commensal bacteria to establish and cause disease. Goblet cell hyperplasia/hypersecretion results in chronic serous nasal discharge. Necrosis of turbinate bones has been shown in cats after feline herpesvirus (FHV) infection and has been suggested as an explanation for chronic rhinitis in these cases. It has been postulated that Irish Wolfhound rhinitis has a similar aetiological basis, although specific agents have not been isolated from cases consistently. Latent viral infections (e.g. feline herpesvirus type 1 (FHV-1)) may show recrudescence (see Infections of the upper respiratory tract) and present as cases of chronic rhinitis.

Although the signalment, history, clinical features (see Figure 6.5) and nature of the discharge are useful in defining a presumptive diagnosis, ancillary tests are required to make a definitive diagnosis:

- Bacterial culture (nasal swabs or nasal flushings) is of limited value, as commensal bacteria are commonly isolated from the nasal cavity, although pure or heavy growth of a single species might be important
- Virus isolation may be of value in confirming FHV-1-associated chronic rhinitis; however, by the time chronic nasal disease has developed, FHV-1 is in the latent stage of infection and infected cats may be missed
- Cytological examination of fluid obtained from the nose often shows an inflammatory response and bacteria but rarely provides a definitive diagnosis
- Radiography often only shows a non-specific diffuse increase in soft tissue opacity within the nasal cavity and sinuses (Figures 6.6 and 6.7)
- Serology is of little value in the diagnosis of bacterial/viral chronic rhinitis, apart from screening for retrovirus (feline leukaemia virus (FeLV) and feline immunodeficiency virus (FIV)) in cats with suspected immunodeficiency.

Chronic rhinitis/sinusitis may respond to antimicrobial therapy for 6–8 weeks, but almost invariably it recurs. Intermittent long-term antimicrobial therapy is often required. Surgical procedures such as turbinectomy have been attempted but usually leave the animal with a chronic serous nasal discharge and may

Disease	Radiological features
Neoplasia	Discrete soft tissue opacities Loss of turbinate pattern Deviation of nasal septum Lytic bone lesions
Fungal disease	Turbinate destruction, increased radiolucency (especially caudally) Punctate lucencies Soft tissue opacities (fungal plaques) Opacity of one or both of the frontal sinuses
Chronic rhinitis/sinusitis	Inconclusive radiographs Increased soft tissue opacity Turbinate pattern masked Turbinate destruction may be seen in cats

Figure 6.6: Radiological features of nasal disease.

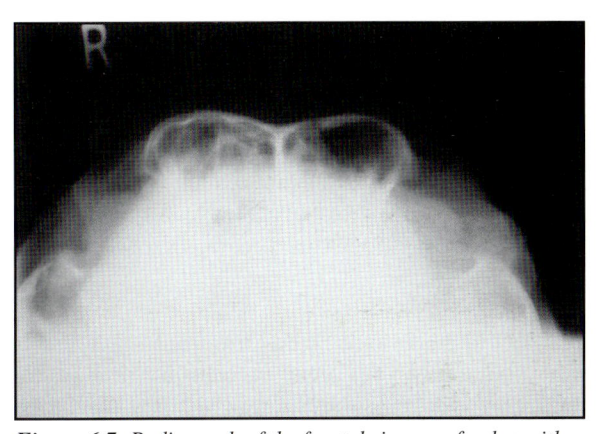

Figure 6.7: Radiograph of the frontal sinuses of a dog with chronic sinusitis. The right sinus shows increased radiodensity.

provide little improvement. Sinus curettage and ablation with an autologous fat graft has been reported to give good results.

Nasal mycoses

Nasal mycoses are rare in cats and uncommon in dogs but there are several fungal species known to be associated with chronic nasal disease in both dogs and cats (Figure 6.8).

Aspergillosis/penicilliniosis: *Aspergillus* spp. and *Penicillium* spp. are ubiquitous saprophytic fungi with a worldwide distribution. *Aspergillus fumigatus* is the most commonly involved fungus in nasal mycosis. Disseminated disease is rare in both dogs and cats; *A. terreus*, *A. deflectus* and *A. flavipes* are usually involved.

Aspergillus spp. can be isolated from the nasal passages of healthy dogs. Unknown factors, perhaps immunosuppression or trauma to the nasal mucosa,

Fungus	Main clinical presentation		Incidence in UK	Diagnosis
	Dog	Cat		
Aspergillus spp.	Nasal disease	Gastrointestinal disease Systemic disease Nasal disease	Most common nasal mycosis of dogs; rare in cats	Cytology, radiography, serology
Penicillium spp.	Nasal disease	Nasal disease Gastrointestinal disease	Less common than aspergillosis	Cytology, radiography, serology
Rhinosporidium seeberi	Nasal disease	Not reported	Not reported	Cytology, histopathology
Cryptococcus neoformans	CNS disease Ocular disease	Respiratory disease, especially nasal Skin disease CNS disease	More common nasal mycosis of cats; rare in dogs	Cytology, culture, biopsy, antigen serology

Figure 6.8: *Fungi associated with nasal infection.*

may trigger pathogenic infection; however, nasal aspergillosis is commonly seen in otherwise healthy dogs with no evidence of immunosuppression or history of trauma to the nose. Suppressed lymphocyte blastogenesis responses reported in dogs with nasal aspergillosis have been suggested by some workers to be caused by, rather than a cause of, the disease. Disease is more common in younger and middle-aged dogs, with half of affected dogs under 3 years old and most under 7 years. Disease is found mainly in dolichocephalic and mesocephalic breeds; brachycephalics are usually spared.

Aspergillosis usually presents as a unilateral mucopurulent nasal discharge that can become bilateral, commonly with blood present. In some cases, true episodes of epistaxis are reported. The discharge is usually profuse, but may not be obvious if the dog constantly licks the nose. Ulceration and depigmentation of the nostrils (Figure 6.9), facial pain, or evidence of pain when eating are often present. Air flow through the affected nasal chamber may occasionally be reduced, although not as commonly as with neoplasia.

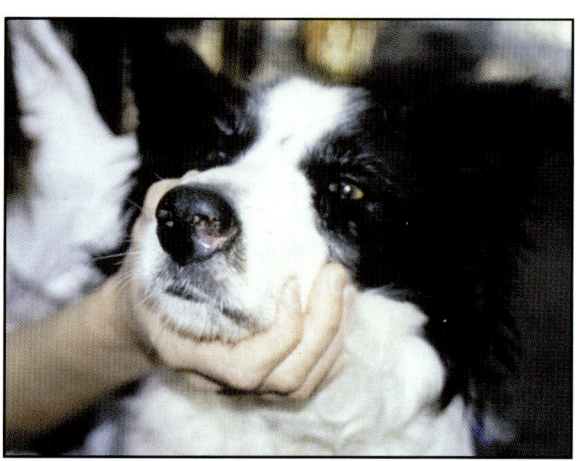

Figure 6.9: *Depigmentation and ulceration of the nares of a dog with nasal aspergillosis.*

Aspergillosis is rare in cats and when it does occur it usually causes systemic disease, although there are reports of nasal disease. Most cats with aspergillosis are immunosuppressed (e.g. concurrent FeLV infection).

Penicillium spp. present with a similar clinical pattern to aspergillosis and the differentiation of the causal organism is by laboratory methods. Treatment is the same for both organisms.

Cryptococcosis: *Cryptococcus neoformans*, a saprophytic yeast-like fungus, causes disease in dogs, cats and humans; it is the commonest nasal fungal infection of cats. It is found worldwide in high concentrations in pigeon droppings and other avian guano and can persist in the environment for several years. Infection in humans is mainly of immunocompromised patients (e.g. those with AIDS). The pathogenesis of the disease is unclear; immunosuppressed cats may be predisposed. The presence of the organism alone in the nose is not sufficient for diagnosis as it may be detected in asymptomatic healthy cats and dogs. Clinical features of cryptococcosis include:

- Respiratory, especially nasal signs, and/or skin lesions and CNS and ocular disease
- Chronic nasal discharge and nasal deformity with infection of the nasal cavity (Figure 6.10)
- Occasionally a polyp-type lesion protruding from the nostril
- Possible nodular or ulcerative lesions elsewhere on the skin and lymphadenopathy
- Weight loss and lethargy, as disease is often chronic.

In dogs, cryptococcosis is rare and, as with other nasal mycoses, tends to occur in younger animals. Nasal and skin disease, similar to the disease in the cat,

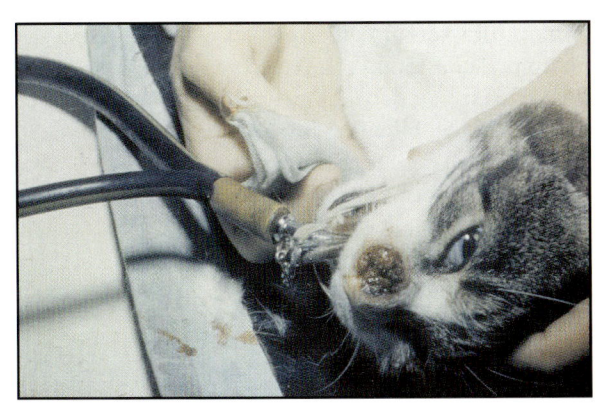

Figure 6.10: Cat with ulcerated nasal swelling associated with Cryptococcus *infection. (© G. Walton.)*

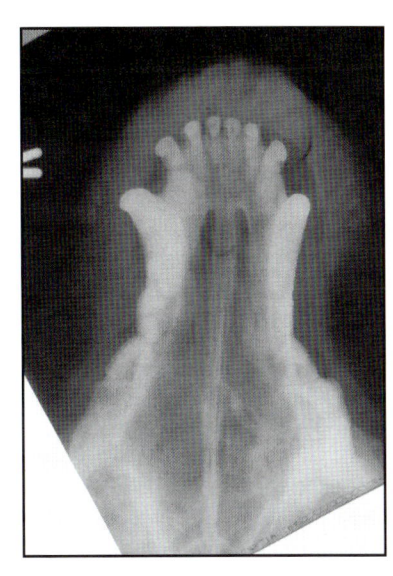

Figure 6.11: Radiograph of the nose in a dog with aspergillosis. The right side of the nose shows loss of turbinate pattern, increased radiolucency (especially caudally) and punctate lucencies.

can occur in dogs but they more often present with CNS or ocular signs, loss of condition and lethargy.

Rhinosporidiosis: *Rhinosporidium seeberi* can cause nasal disease in dogs, but it is not present in the UK. This fungus is sporadically reported from some areas, including North America, and is endemic in India, Sri Lanka and Argentina. Clinical disease is similar to other nasal mycosis, and polyps are a common feature.

Diagnosis of nasal mycoses: The definitive diagnosis of a nasal mycosis requires positive results from several diagnostic tests, e.g. appropriate clinical and radiological features and culture of the fungus; a diagnosis of nasal mycosis should not be based on one test only.

- Radiography may show major changes, but these need to be distinguished from other conditions. Radiography should precede endoscopy as the latter may result in haemorrhage, thereby increasing soft tissue density. Figure 6.6 compares the radiological features of nasal mycosis with those of neoplasia. Features of aspergillosis are illustrated in Figure 6.11
- Endoscopy may show the presence of fungal plaques
- Cytology may show fungal hyphae. *Cryptococcus* spp. are often present in large numbers and easily identified as characteristic budding yeasts with thick capsules that are produced when growing in tissues
- Fungal culture of nasal samples should be interpreted with care as healthy dog and cat nasal cavities can contain fungi
- Fungal serology may show exposure to *Aspergillus* spp. and *Penicillium* spp. (see Chapter 1). The sensitivities of available tests vary, but all can give false negative results. Although the presence of antibodies cannot distinguish a present infection from a previous infection, a positive test result from an animal with appropriate clinical lesions is probably important. ELISA and latex agglutination tests are available for *Cryptococcus* antigen. Serology is positive in the vast majority of cryptococcosis cases.

Treatment of nasal mycoses: The treatment of nasal mycosis is difficult and often unsuccessful. No antifungal agent is licensed for such use in small animals in the UK. For canine nasal mycosis, topical instillation into the nasal cavity and frontal sinuses of either enilconazole or clotrimazole is currently the best form of treatment, and higher success rates are achieved than with systemic therapy. Failure to respond owing to extension of the fungus into adjacent bony and soft tissue is an indication for systemic ketoconazole or fluconazole therapy. Systemic therapy alone often requires prolonged treatment, and recurrence is often a problem.

Two treatment protocols have been described for topical instillation. For both techniques the frontal sinuses have to be trephined. Place tubes bilaterally (feeding tubes are normally used) into the nasal cavities and frontal sinuses (Figure 6.12) as invariably both sides will be affected, although clinical signs may only be evident in one. The two drugs used are:

- Enilconazole: 10 mg/kg instilled into the nasal cavities every 12 hours for 7–10 days. Dilute the solution of enilconazole (100 mg/ml) 50:50 with water (see Appendix 3). The instilled volume

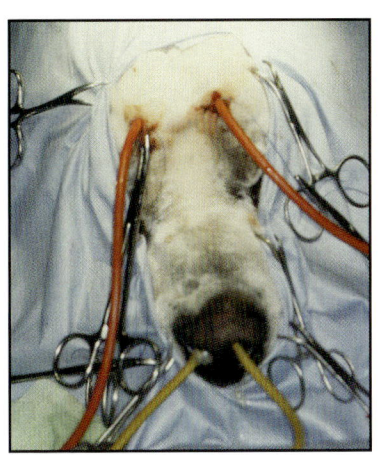

Figure 6.12: Dog with trephine holes in the frontal sinuses and tubes inserted for topical treatment of aspergillosis. (© Mr John Williams.)

should be kept low (<10 ml) to reduce the risk of inhalation, and the tubes should be flushed with an equivalent volume of air. Make up a fresh solution as required. The animal must be admitted to hospital.
- Clotrimazole: a single administration of a 1% solution of clotrimazole solution in a polyethylene glycol base is infused continuously into the nasal cavity for 1 hour (see Appendix 3). Success rates may be increased by repeating the treatment after 6-8 weeks (J. Williams, personal communication). Before infusing the drug, the nasal passages and sinuses are flushed with sterile saline and the external nares and nasopharynx tightly occluded. After treatment the tubes are removed and trephine sites left incompletely sutured to reduce the risk of subcutaneous emphysema. Potential side effects include lingual erythema, transient megaoesophagus and subcutaneous emphysema. To reduce the risk of these ensure that:
  - The nostrils are lower then the nasopharynx during instillation
  - The nasopharynx is tightly packed
  - The trephine holes are only large enough to allow placement of the tubes
  - Pressure is applied to the surrounding area while the drug is given.

After topical treatment, signs should start to resolve within 7 days. If disease recurs or continues after treatment, reassess the dog for fungal disease. If the fungus is still present, systemic therapy or retreatment with a topical drug should be considered. In some cases therapy may not be successful because of involvement of surrounding tissues. As fungi cause major damage to the turbinates, a mild chronic serous/mucopurulent nasal discharge may remain.

For cats with aspergillosis, systemic treatment with ketoconazole or fluconazole should be used. Itraconazole or ketoconazole can be used for cats with cryptococcosis; the former has fewer side effects (see Chapter 2).

Parasitic nasal disease
Several parasites can infect the nasal passages (see Figure 6.4). The incidence of these parasites in the UK is unknown, although they are reported in other European areas, including Scandinavia.

Pneumonyssoides caninum: the nasal mite of dogs is found in the caudal nasal cavity and the frontal sinuses. Infection is usually subclinical, although it can be associated with reverse sneezing and epistaxis. Movement of the mites within the nasal cavity can lead to facial irritation, with affected dogs pawing at the face.

Linguatula serrata: this parasite, belonging to the phylum Pentastomida, infects the nasal passages of dogs and is referred to as the 'tongue worm' because of its appearance. Infection is rare and often subclinical. Where disease occurs, dogs may sneeze and have repeated bouts of epistaxis. Affected dogs may lose their sense of smell.

Capillaria aerophila: see Infections of the upper respiratory tract.

Diagnosis: Parasitic infections can be diagnosed by finding eggs or mites in nasal washes or the eggs of *Capillaria* spp. or *Linguatula* spp. in faeces. Nasal parasites may be seen on endoscopic examination.

Treatment: this may not be required, as a subclinical infestation is common. Fenbendazole and selamectin are likely to be effective against *Capillaria aerophila*. Note that in the UK ivermectin is not licensed for use in cats or dogs and that severe adverse reactions, including death, have been reported after its use in these species.

INFECTIONS OF THE UPPER RESPIRATORY TRACT

Figure 6.13 lists the infectious agents that may cause upper respiratory tract infections (URTIs). Two specific syndromes incorporate the more common infectious causes of URT disease, namely kennel cough and cat flu.

Dog	Cat
Bordetella bronchiseptica	Feline calicivirus
Canine distemper virus	Feline herpesvirus
Canine parainfluenza virus	*B. bronchiseptica*
Canine adenovirus-1 and -2	*Mycoplasma* spp.
Oslerus osleri	*Aelurostrongylus abstrusus*
Canine herpesvirus	*Capillaria aerophila*
Mycoplasma spp.	*Mycobacterium* spp.
Mycobacteria spp.	Reovirus
Reovirus	Cowpox virus
Malassezia pachydermatis	

Figure 6.13: *Organisms that may infect the upper respiratory tract.*

Historical information relating to contact with other animals and vaccination history is important. Most URTIs are acquired where animals are grouped together, such as in boarding kennels or catteries, and younger animals are more susceptible because they generally lack protective immunity.

Figure 6.14 lists the general clinical signs associated with URTIs. They vary with the agent and area most severely affected, e.g. dysphonia with laryngeal disease, coughing with tracheal involvement. The classic presentation in dogs consists mainly of coughing,

> Sneezing
> Nasal discharge
> Coughing
> Gagging
> Submandibular lymphadenopathy
> Pyrexia
> Hypersalivation
> Ocular discharge
> Conjunctivitis
> Dysphonia

Figure 6.14: Clinical signs of upper respiratory tract disease.

with other clinical signs present to variable degrees. In cats, sneezing, nasal discharge, conjunctivitis and hypersalivation are more usual; coughing is not as common a feature.

The nature of a cough may give an indication of the underlying pathology. A productive cough is found with inflammatory disorders whereas a non-productive cough is more common in disease of the larger airways and is often associated with non-infectious disease.

Wheezing or rattling sounds are associated with the narrowing of the airways due to muscle spasm or accumulation of exudates in conditions such as bronchiectasis, chronic obstructive disease and some allergic diseases. Some infectious agents also involve extrarespiratory tissues such as the oral cavity, eye, intestinal tract, skin or CNS.

The presumptive diagnosis of an URTI may be based on historical and clinical signs alone, although it is often difficult to ascribe the clinical picture to a specific aetiology; the features associated with infections overlap with non-infectious aetiologies, and diseases produced by different agents often present similarly. Accurate identification of a specific infectious agent should be attempted where susceptible animals are in contact with an affected case; the specific diagnosis of individual agents is discussed below.

Kennel cough

Kennel cough is a common canine disease syndrome that causes high morbidity but low mortality and is most often, but not exclusively, encountered in dogs kept together, e.g. in kennels. The main infectious agents associated with kennel cough are:

- *Bordetella bronchiseptica*
- Canine parainfluenza virus
- Canine adenovirus (CAV-1 and CAV-2)
- Canine herpesvirus
- Canine reovirus.

Bordetella bronchiseptica

This is a Gram-negative coccobacillus that can act as a primary respiratory pathogen in several species. Originally thought to be an opportunistic pathogen, it is now established as a primary canine pathogen, and is one of the main agents involved in kennel cough. The bacteria attach to ciliated epithelium causing ciliostasis. *B. bronchiseptica* is probably responsible for the more severe manifestations of kennel cough. Dogs are infected for several weeks, possibly months, and remain as a source of infection after clinical recovery.

Canine parainfluenza virus (CPiV)

This is a paramyxovirus implicated in the kennel cough syndrome and is the virus most commonly isolated from cases of URT disease. It replicates in epithelial cells of the respiratory tract and regional lymph nodes; it does not infect other tissues except in immunocompromised dogs. Although the virus may be found in association with lesions in the lung, these are of no clinical importance. Infection occurs after contact with infected oronasal secretions or via aerosols. CPiV alone causes a mild cough and occasionally a serous nasal discharge.

Canine adenovirus

CAV-1 and CAV-2 have been associated with bronchitis, bronchiolitis and focal turbinate and tonsillar necrosis, although CAV-2 is predominantly associated with URT disease; CAV-1 and CAV-2 are serologically related. CAV-1 is associated with multisystemic disease (see Chapter 11), and CAV-2 may be isolated from intestinal tract epithelium, although it is not associated with disease in this tissue. The virus is shed for 8–9 days after infection, and although it can persist in the respiratory mucosa for several weeks, the epidemiological importance of this persistence is unclear.

Canine herpesvirus

CHV is thought only to infect members of the Canidae and is an uncommon component of the kennel cough syndrome. Puppies can be infected in utero, during birth, or by contact with the bitch's saliva. In puppies under 2 weeks of age, the virus may generalize and cause fading puppy syndrome (see Chapter 12). In older puppies and adult dogs, the virus is generally restricted to external mucous membranes of the URT and genital tract, although mild lesions (focal necrosis) may be found anywhere from the nasal and turbinate mucosa to the bronchial epithelium. Clinical signs are usually mild and often restricted to a serous nasal discharge. As with other herpesvirus infections, latent CHV infection develops in recovered dogs and reactivation may occur.

Canine reovirus

This can be isolated from unaffected dogs as well as from those with respiratory disease, and there is serological evidence for all three mammalian serotypes of reovirus in dogs. There is currently no evidence to indicate that they are major pathogens. Reoviruses have been reported to persist in canine lymphatic tissue and are often found in association with other infectious agents. This has led to the suggestion, as yet unproven, that it facilitates infection with other agents by an immunosuppressive effect.

Canine distemper virus
CDV can be involved in the kennel cough complex without causing signs of classic distemper. See the LRT section for a further discussion of CDV.

Influenza virus
This has been isolated from dogs with mild upper respiratory tract disease, but its role as a pathogen in the dog is as yet unproven. Infection is probably acquired from infected humans.

Clinical signs
The different agents cause similar signs, varying from a mild cough and serous nasal discharge to severe coughing, gagging and retching. The cough may be spontaneous or induced and is often exacerbated by exercise, excitement or pressure round the trachea or larynx. A terminal retch may be perceived by the owner as 'something stuck in the throat'. Submandibular lymphadenopathy, pyrexia or ocular discharge may be evident. The severity of the clinical picture is determined by:

- The agent present: *Bordetella bronchiseptica* is associated with more severe disease than the viral agents
- Multiple infections are likely to cause more severe disease
- Areas of the respiratory tract involved
- Immune status: pre-existing immunity ameliorates some or all of the clinical signs
- Opportunistic bacterial infections (see Figure 6.1) that take advantage of damaged defence mechanisms.

Diagnosis
Diagnosis of a viral infection requires that the virus be isolated, that the viral genome be identified with sophisticated molecular or immunological techniques (e.g. PCR, immunostaining) from nasal, oropharyngeal or tracheal material, or that serological evidence of acute exposure using paired titres is available; vaccine titres must be considered when performing serology. Not all viruses can be demonstrated by all of these techniques, and many tests are not commercially available.

Bordetella bronchiseptica and opportunistic bacteria can be isolated from oropharyngeal or nasal swabs, taken into charcoal amies transport medium to maintain bacterial viability. Identification of opportunistic bacterial infections enables accurate selection of appropriate antibacterials.

Treatment
There are no antiviral drugs effective in managing viral URTIs. As many of the signs of URTI are associated with secondary bacterial infection, broad-spectrum antimicrobial cover should be prescribed.

- Antibacterials (clavulanate-potentiated amoxycillin, tetracyclines and potentiated sulphonamides) are generally effective in vitro against canine isolates of *B. bronchiseptica*
- Antitussives are not recommended as the cough mechanism clears excess mucus and should not be prevented
- Expectorants or mucolytics may be helpful
- Methylxanthine bronchodilators (e.g. theophylline) may help prevent bronchospasm
- Nebulization or steam inhalations may also be of benefit
- Rest is a useful adjunctive therapy.

Prevention
Control is based on vaccination and management procedures. Vaccines against CDV and CAV-2 are routinely used, and many multivalent vaccines now include CPiV. Vaccination regimens should follow those recommended in datasheets. Vaccination against *B. bronchiseptica* is recommended when dogs enter boarding kennels, and it may be used in the face of an outbreak.

In situations where vaccination alone may be insufficient to control infectious respiratory disease – either because vaccines are unavailable or carrier animals may be present in multianimal environments – management procedures should be used in conjunction with vaccination programmes (see Chapter 4).

Cat flu
Cat flu is a common syndrome involving several primary infectious agents. It usually causes high morbidity but low mortality. The main infectious agents are:

- Feline herpesvirus type 1 (FHV-1)
- Feline calicivirus (FCV)
- *Bordetella bronchiseptica*
- *Chlamydophila felis* (formerly *Chlamydia psittaci* var. *felis*).

Taken together, FHV-1 and FCV account for about 80% of cases of cat flu. The role of other agents (e.g. reovirus, coronavirus, influenza virus, *Haemophilus felis, Mycoplasma felis*) is unclear.

Feline herpesvirus type 1
FHV-1 is thought only to infect Felidae, although there are sporadic reports of FHV-1-like isolates from dogs. Severe illness and fatalities can occur in young and older cats. Long-term disease, consisting of chronic nasal discharge (see nasal section) or recurrent ocular

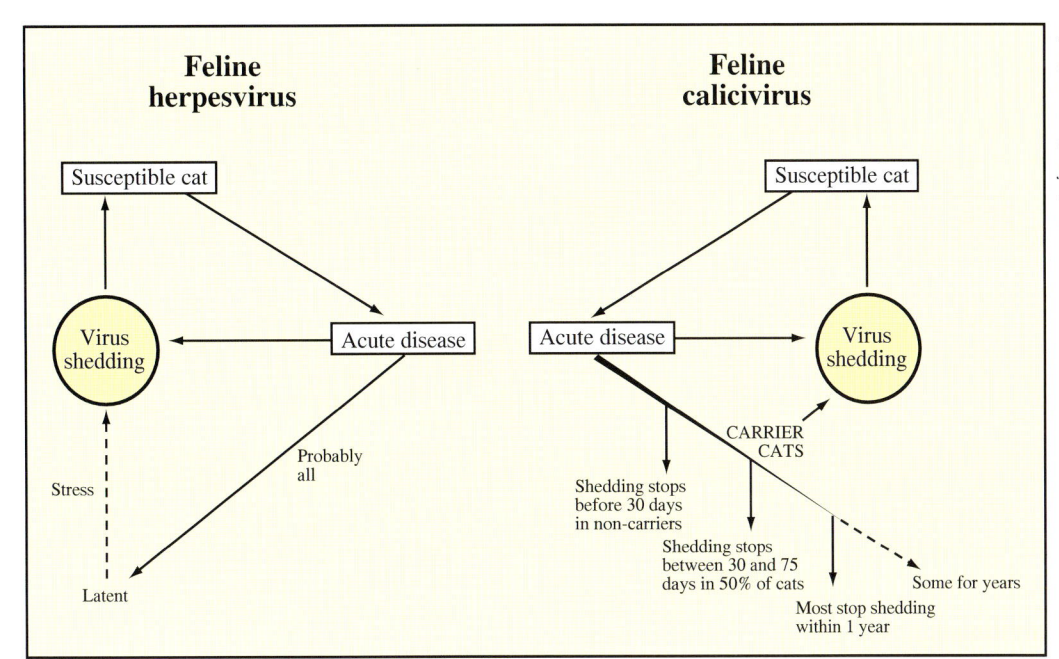

Figure 6.15: *Epidemiological importance of the carrier states associated with feline herpesvirus and feline calicivirus.*

disease (see Chapter 16) may develop. Morbidity is high in a susceptible population.

Transmission is mainly by direct contact. Indirect transmission by fomites and by contact with infected secretions are possible. Herpesviruses possess an envelope that is readily destroyed by disinfectants and drying; the virus persists for about 18 hours in the environment. Indirect transmission is important only in the short term and tends to occur where cats are kept in close confinement. When exposed to field virus, vaccinated cats or those protected by maternally derived antibodies may develop mild disease (mainly sneezing) and may still become carriers.

Irrespective of whether a cat develops chronic disease, probably all cats acutely infected with FHV-1 become lifelong carriers (Figure 6.15). As with other α-herpesvirus infections, this carrier state is characterized by latency interspersed with episodes of shedding, often after a period of stress. Latent virus is present in trigeminal ganglia and possibly other tissues; the mechanisms involved in shedding after stress are not well understood. Shedding commences about one week after stress, for about 10 days. In some cats, this may be associated with recrudescence of disease. Vaccination of known carrier animals does not eliminate latent virus.

Feline calicivirus

FCV is thought to infect only Felidae, although an FCV-like virus has been isolated from dogs with genital vesicles. There is one main serotype but several antigenically distinct isolates, not all of which are protected against by vaccine isolates.

Historically, FHV-1 and FCV have been isolated in equal frequencies from cases of URT disease, but recently an increase in the number of cases of FCV has been reported. This may be due to the large number of different isolates of FCV, which have variable antigenicity and pathogenicity. Oral ulceration found in FCV infection is usually on the surface of the tongue (Figure 6.16) but may be elsewhere in the mouth, nose (Figure 6.17) or other areas. FCV is associated with a shifting lameness syndrome; this is uncommon and is usually seen in kittens.

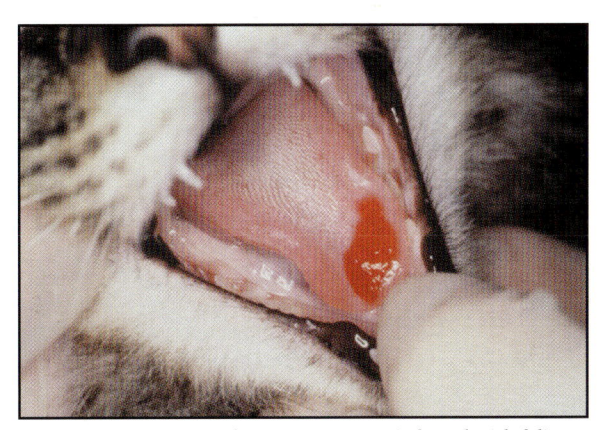

Figure 6.16: *Tongue ulceration in a cat infected with feline calicivirus.*

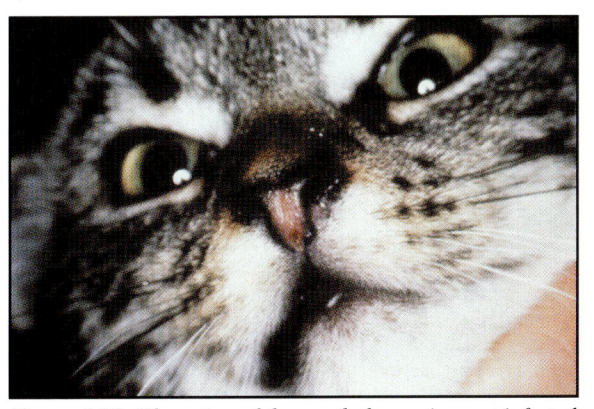

Figure 6.17: *Ulceration of the nasal planum in a cat infected with feline calicivirus.*

102 Manual of Canine and Feline Infectious Diseases

Many cats remain infected with FCV (see Figure 6.15) and are a source of infectious virus to susceptible cats. Most are able to eliminate the virus within a few months, and for the majority the carrier state is not lifelong. Vaccinated cats or those with maternally derived antibodies can also become infected and become carriers; carrier cats need not have a history of disease.

The virus is excreted in oronasal secretions, and the main method of transmission is by direct contact. FCV can survive for up to one week in the environment but is susceptible to low pH and hypochlorite or quaternary ammonium disinfectants. As for FHV, vaccination of known carrier animals neither eliminates the virus nor prevents shedding. Recently reported FCV shedding rates of 25% at cat shows and 19% from a veterinary hospital population are similar to those found in surveys carried out before the advent of vaccination.

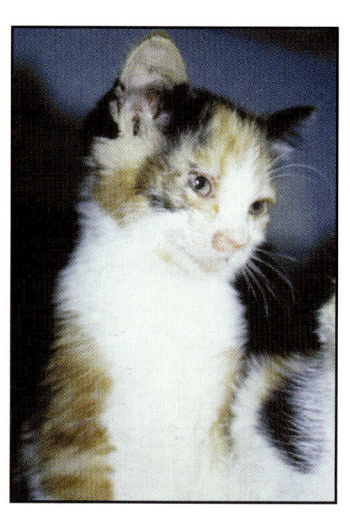

Figure 6.18: Ocular and nasal discharge in a kitten with cat flu. Feline herpesvirus was isolated from this kitten.

Feline reovirus
This has been reported as a cause of URT disease in cats in the USA; however, it is unlikely to be a major cause of URT disease in cats in the UK, as surveys of cats with URT disease and conjunctivitis have failed to isolate the virus.

Feline coronavirus
This is a common infection of cats, usually associated with subclinical infection, diarrhoea or feline infectious peritonitis (see Chapter 9). On rare occasions this virus has been linked to mild URT disease.

Bordetella bronchiseptica
This can be a primary pathogen of cats. Clinical features are summarized in Figure 6.19. Coughing is not as prominent a feature of the disease in cats as it is in dogs. Bronchopneumonia may develop and result in death, particularly in kittens, owing to colonization of the lower respiratory tract. Other pathogens (e.g. FCV, FHV) may facilitate the development of bronchopneumonia. As cats remain infected with *B. bronchiseptica* for several months, possibly longer, they may remain infectious to other animals. In field surveys, 11% of cats are infected with *B. bronchiseptica*, but higher isolation rates are reported from cats in rescue catteries, multicat households and in contact with dogs with respiratory disease. This suggests that there is transmission of this bacterium between dogs and cats.

Chlamydophila felis (formerly *Chlamydia psittaci* var *felis*)
This is predominantly a conjunctival pathogen in cats, causing persistent conjunctivitis, accompanied in some cases by mild URT signs (see Figure 6.18). See Chapter 16 for further discussion on this agent.

Agent	Clinical signs	Diagnosis	Special considerations
Feline herpesvirus	Common: anorexia, pyrexia sneezing, oculonasal discharge, conjunctivitis, hypersalivation. Less common: coughing, ulcerative keratitis. Rare: systemic disease	Acute stage: oropharyngeal swab into virus transport medium for virus isolation Carriers: cannot be detected reliably owing to latency	Clinically recovered cats become lifelong latent carriers, with sporadic shedding episodes
Feline calicivirus	Common: mild respiratory disease, oral ulceration very common, oculonasal discharge, mild pyrexia Less common: shifting lameness	Acute and carrier stage: oropharyngeal swab into virus transport medium for virus isolation	Carriers continuously shed virus from oropharynx. Most cats short-term carriers - some shed for more prolonged periods
Bordetella bronchiseptica	Mild upper respiratory tract disease with sneezing, nasal discharge and possibly coughing. Submandibular lymphadenopathy, adventitious lung sounds	Oropharyngeal or nasal swab into charcoal amies transport medium for culture on selective agar	Prolonged shedding can occur in recovered cats
Chlamydophila felis (formerly *Chlamydia psittaci* var. *felis*)	Common: persistent conjunctivitis Less common: mild respiratory disease	Ocular swab for: isolation (swab in chlamydia transport medium), detection of antigen, polymerase chain reaction	Organism spreads systemically, and cats can remain persistently infected

Figure 6.19: Characteristics of cat flu caused by various agents.

Clinical features

The classic presentation of cat flu consists of nasal discharge (see Figure 6.18), sneezing, conjunctivitis, pyrexia and anorexia, although individual agents present in slightly different ways (see Figure 6.19). The clinical signs and development of disease are often modified by opportunistic bacterial infections.

Diagnosis

Figure 6.19 lists the specific clinical findings to consider when determining the cause of cat flu. Diagnosis of a viral infection requires that the virus be isolated or that the viral genome be identified with polymerase chain reaction technology from oropharyngeal swabs (in virus transport medium if isolating the virus). Serology is not usually helpful in the diagnosis of FHV and FCV, as many cats are vaccinated or have been previously exposed.

Isolation of FCV should be interpreted with care, as a high percentage of healthy cats are carriers (see above). Identification of FHV-1 carrier cats cannot always be made by virus isolation, as shedding of virus is sporadic. It is possible to swab suspected carriers about one week after an episode of natural stress such as kittening or rehousing, although failure to isolate the virus does not prove that the animal is not a carrier. The use of corticosteroids to induce stress is not recommended as some carriers may develop disease, which may be severe.

Bordetella bronchiseptica and opportunistic bacteria can be isolated from oropharyngeal or nasal swabs, taken into charcoal amies transport medium to maintain bacterial viability. Identification of opportunistic bacterial infections enables accurate selection of appropriate antibacterials.

Treatment

There are no systemic antiviral drugs effective in managing viral URTIs. As many of the signs of URTI are associated with secondary bacterial infection and concurrent *Chlamydophila felis* (formerly *Chlamydia psittaci* var. *felis*) or *Mycoplasma* spp. infections, broad-spectrum antimicrobial cover on the basis of in vitro testing is recommended. *C. felis* and *Mycoplasma* spp. are sensitive to tetracycline and doxycycline and *B. bronchiseptica* is usually sensitive to tetracycline, doxycycline and enrofloxacin. Mucolytics (e.g. bromhexine) can be helpful in some cases. Placing cats in warm steamy rooms has been suggested as a form of inhalation therapy. Good nursing/supportive care is important. Hand feeding and fluid therapy may be needed.

Prevention

Control of infectious respiratory disease in cats is based on vaccination and management procedures. Vaccines against FHV-1 and FCV are available in the UK. Vaccination regimens should follow those recommended in company datasheets. In some countries (not the UK) *B. bronchiseptica* vaccines are licensed for use in cats.

In situations where vaccination alone is insufficient to control infectious respiratory disease, either because vaccines are unavailable or because carrier cats may be present in multicat environments, management procedures should be used in conjunction with vaccination programmes. See Chapter 4 for a detailed discussion on disease control in multi-animal environments.

Parasitic infections

Oslerus osleri

The metastrongyloid nematode *Oslerus osleri* (formerly *Filaroides osleri*) causes tracheobronchitis in dogs. Infection is more common where large numbers of dogs are kept together. Infestation usually occurs at a young age, although the parasite may persist in older dogs. The adult worms live in nodules in the area proximal to the tracheal carina, occasionally extending to involve the mucosal lining of the mainstem bronchi. Lower regions of the respiratory tract are only rarely involved.

Adult females lay eggs in the respiratory tract, which hatch into infectious first stage (L1) larvae. These are coughed up and swallowed and either passed out in faeces or expectorated. Puppies are usually infested after ingestion of L1 larvae, which moult to L2 larvae in the intestine, then migrate via the circulation to the respiratory tract, where the adult worms develop.

In most cases, infestation is subclinical. Some dogs show signs of chronic mild non-progressive respiratory disease, with mild to severe inspiratory wheeze, dyspnoea and coughing. Expectorated material is often scanty but may be blood stained, and occasionally is in copious amounts. Occasionally tracheal sensitivity, exercise intolerance and, rarely, debilitation occur. Rarely the parasite causes perforation of the trachea or mainstem bronchi, resulting in pneumomediastinum and pneumothorax.

Oslerus osleri infestation may be diagnosed by:

- Bronchoscopy, which may show cream-coloured nodules, 1–5 mm in diameter, containing visible worms (Figure 6.20)

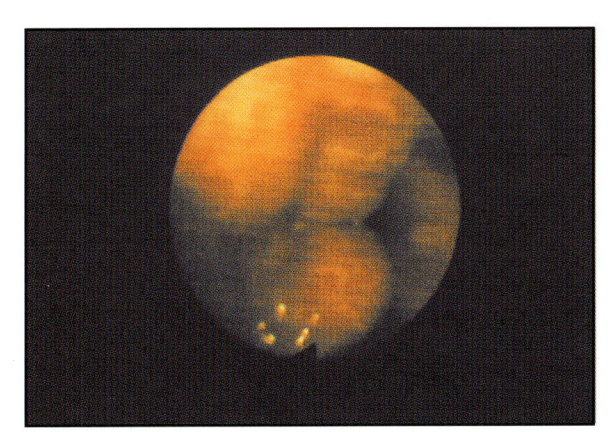

Figure 6.20: Endoscopic appearance of nodules in the trachea of a dog infested with Oslerus osleri. *The parasites are evident within the nodules. (© Dr Bryn Tennant.)*

- Radiography, showing soft tissue density apparently protruding into the tracheal lumen
- The observation of larvae in brushings or biopsy samples of the nodules
- The detection of larvae in faeces or larvae and eggs in sputum.

Tracheal washings or other respiratory samples should be maintained at room temperature and faeces kept fresh or preserved with 10% formalin. The Baermann technique can be used to identify larvae (see Chapter 1). Eggs are 50-80 µm long, thin shelled, colourless and contain larvae; free larvae are 230 µm long, with distinctive kinked tails. Cytology of tracheal washings often shows eosinophils.

Capillaria aerophila
This is a 2-4 cm long nematode that infests the nasal cavity, trachea, bronchi and bronchioles of dogs and cats. Eggs are coughed up, swallowed and passed in faeces. The life cycle is direct. Most infections are asymptomatic. When it occurs, disease consists of a mild cough and nasal discharge if the nasal passages are involved. A secondary bronchopneumonia rarely develops. Diagnosis is confirmed by the presence of eggs (double operculated with asymmetrical plugs, 60 × 35 µm) in a tracheal wash or faeces; shedding is intermittent. Radiography may show a mild bronchial or interstitial pattern.

Treatment
Benzimidazoles such as fenbendazole are usually effective against respiratory parasites. All dogs kept together in kennels should be treated simultaneously. Breeding bitches and puppies should be treated on a regular basis. Surgery for *O. osleri* is occasionally indicated to remove large nodules causing severe obstruction.

INFECTIONS OF THE LOWER RESPIRATORY TRACT

Figure 6.21 lists the organisms that may infect the lower respiratory tract (LRT). Generally LRT infections (LRTIs) are characterized by cough, dyspnoea and sometimes pyrexia. Dyspnoeic animals must be examined carefully to minimize stress that may precipitate a respiratory crisis, and they should not be restrained during examination. Primary physical examination should assess upper and lower airways, lung parenchyma, pleural cavity (effusion, masses), thoracic wall, diaphragm and anaemia. The cause of the dyspnoea should be localized and, if possible, the immediate distress relieved before undertaking a more invasive examination. Emergency treatment of the severely dyspnoeic animal should be instigated before investigating the cause.

General supportive treatment applies to many of the infectious agents and includes:

- Intravenous or other fluid therapy: dehydration interferes with the mucociliary clearance system. Steam inhalations or the use of a nebulizer may be considered. These add water directly to the LRT and assist with maintenance of the mucociliary apparatus
- Nebulization of antimicrobial agents in order that they penetrate the smaller airways; this has been reported to be beneficial by some authors
- Physiotherapy, such as inducing coughing with chest percussion or tracheal manipulation after nebulization; this helps mobilize secretions
- Oxygen therapy: this may be required in severe cases and can be given by simply providing an oxygen-rich atmosphere in an enclosed space, such as an incubator, or by placing a nasal catheter or using clingfilm over an Elizabethan collar. The last two are recommended
- At a higher level of dependency, ventilation or the use of an intratracheal catheter can be considered.

Viral infections

Canine distemper

Aetiology: Canine distemper is a multisystemic disease of dogs caused by canine distemper virus (CDV), a morbillivirus in the paramyxovirus family. It has a lipoprotein envelope and is susceptible to inactivation by standard disinfectants, ultraviolet light, heat and drying. It can survive in the environment under favourable conditions (0-4°C) for, at best, a few weeks. At 20°C in infected tissues it retains infectivity for just a few hours. Although canine distemper is mainly considered a disease of domestic dogs, many other animals are susceptible, e.g. ferrets, badgers. There are reports of suspected CDV infection in exotic Felidae (lions), causing CNS signs, although experimental infections in domestic cats are self-limiting and produce no clinical signs.

The route of infection for CDV is by aerosol/droplet spread to the respiratory membranes (Figure 6.22). The virus spreads to lymphoid tissues where it damages T and B lymphocytes, causing leucopenia. Virus also invades epithelial tissues, notably those of the skin and respiratory and gastrointestinal tracts. The severity of disease depends on the rapidity of development of an immune response. If CDV destroys lymphatic tissues before the development of antibody and adequate cell-mediated immunity (CMI), severe disease occurs.

Dog	Cat
Viral	
Canine distemper virus Canine herpesvirus Canine adenovirus-2 Canine parainfluenza virus	Feline herpesvirus-1 Feline calicivirus Poxvirus Feline leukaemia virus (neoplasia, pleural effusion) Feline coronavirus (effusions, granulomata)
Bacterial	
Bordetella bronchiseptica *Mycobacterium* spp. Opportunistic bacteria (see Figure 6.1)	*Bordetella bronchiseptica* *Mycobacterium* spp. *Haemophilus felis* *Yersinia pestis* Opportunistic bacteria (see Figure 6.1)
Mycoplasmal	
Mycoplasma canis Others	*Mycoplasma felis* Others
Fungal	
Cryptococcus neoformans *Aspergillus* spp. *Histoplasma capsulatum* *Blastomyces dermatitidis* *Coccidioides immitans* *Penicillium* spp.	*Cryptococcus neoformans* *Aspergillus* spp. *Histoplasma capsulatum* *Blastomyces dermatitidis* *Coccidioides immitans*
Protozoal	
Toxoplasma gondii *Pneumocystis carinii*	*Toxoplasma gondii* *Pneumocystis carinii*
Parasitic	
Oslerus osleri *Filaroides milksii, F. hirthii* *Capillaria aerophila* *Crenosoma vulpis* *Toxocara canis* (larva migrans) *Paragonimus kellicotti*	*Aelurostrongylus abstrusus* *Capillaria aerophila* *Paragonimus kellicotti*

Figure 6.21: Organisms that may cause lower respiratory tract disease in the dog and cat.

All affected animals shed virus, some for up to 60 days. Virus is cleared from tissues as antibody levels increase, although it may remain in protected sites (neurological tissue, eye, footpad). After recovery, immunity is considered to be lifelong, although immunocompromise, a virulent high-titre challenge or stress or may overcome this.

Clinical signs: Most affected dogs are 3-6 months of age consequent upon the decline in maternally derived antibody. It is estimated that at least 50% of infections are subclinical, and mild forms of the disease occur. Clinical signs are referable to the tissues affected and vary depending on the infecting strain, host's age, immune status and environment.

In 'classic' distemper, conjunctivitis is usually seen first, followed by the development of a dry cough. The cough progresses to become wet and productive, the ocular discharge becomes mucopurulent and rhinitis develops, with crusting of exudate around the eyes and nose. Auscultation often reveals harsh breath sounds and adventitious noises owing to the production of respiratory secretions. Affected animals are usually pyrexic (>40°C, 104°F), dull and anorectic. The onset of respiratory signs may be followed by gastroenteric signs or opportunistic infections. Ocular lesions (uveitis, optic neuritis and retinal necrosis) are uncommon. Retinal scarring may be present in recovered dogs (see Chapter 16). Animals may die in the acute stage of the disease, but many survive with adequate supportive therapy.

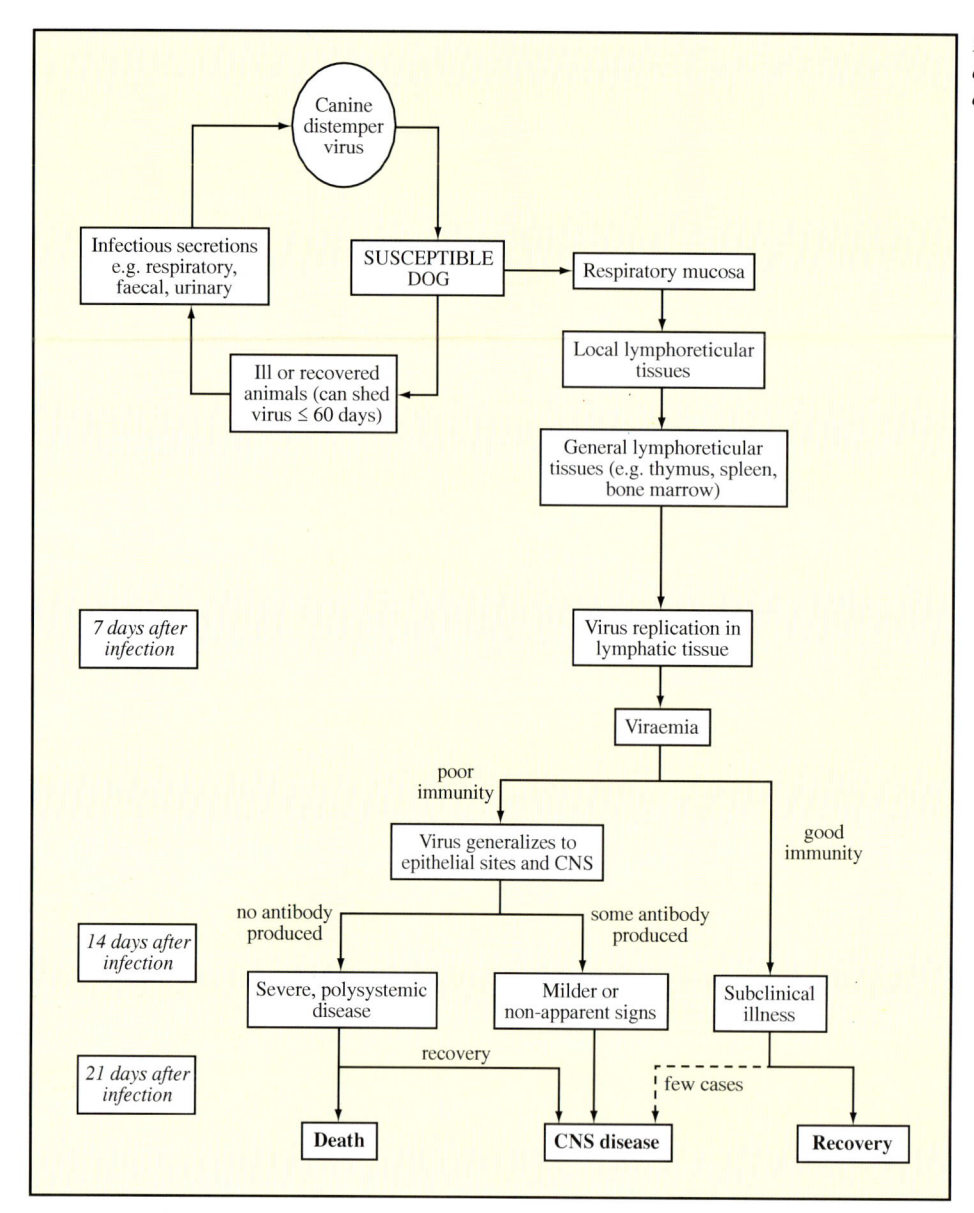

Figure 6.22: *Transmission and pathogenesis of canine distemper virus infection.*

Hyperkeratosis of the nasal planum and footpads is often observed 3-6 weeks after infection and is a useful diagnostic indicator. CDV attacks enamel-producing cells resulting in enamel hypoplasia, another diagnostic indicator of previous CDV infection (Figure 6.23). Some animals, including those subclinically affected, develop neurological signs around 3 weeks after infection. Although neurological signs are more common after severe disease, there is no way of predicting which animals will be affected. Neurological signs, including epileptiform seizures, ataxia, paresis, paralysis and myoclonus may appear suddenly or insidiously, and they can be progressive. Myoclonus may be restricted to one group of muscles or may be extensive and incompatible with a good quality of life. Seizures in less severely affected cases can be managed satisfactorily with anticonvulsant therapy (e.g. phenobarbitone, primidone), but where severe neurological disease is present, many owners will elect for euthanasia.

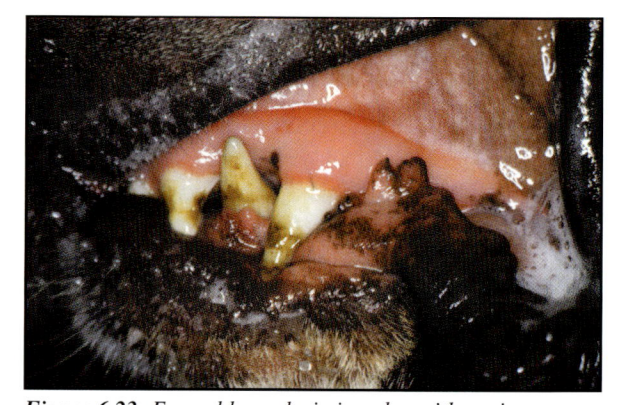

Figure 6.23: *Enamel hypoplasia in a dog with canine distemper. (© Dr Ian Ramsey.)*

Other manifestations of CDV include:

- Abortion, stillbirth or the birth of weakly puppies that may fail to develop normal immune systems (if fetuses are infected transplacentally)

- Neonatal infection at <7 days old has been experimentally associated with a cardiomyopathy and cardiac failure <3 weeks after infection, due to myocardial degeneration, calcification and necrosis
- Metaphyseal osteopathy and hypertrophic osteodystrophy have been associated with CDV infection, although neither has been proven to be caused by this agent.

Diagnosis: This is based on clinical findings, vaccination status, awareness of the incidence of local disease and post-mortem examination. Laboratory investigation of live cases may be non-rewarding. Haematology often shows a non-specific thrombocytopenia and lymphopenia. Inclusion bodies may occasionally be detected in small numbers in leucocytes or erythrocytes (see Chapter 1). No specific biochemical changes are found, although in transplacentally infected puppies hypoglobulinaemia is described. Radiography shows an interstitial pneumonia in early cases, developing through an alveolar or mixed pattern as the pneumonia progresses (Figure 6.24).

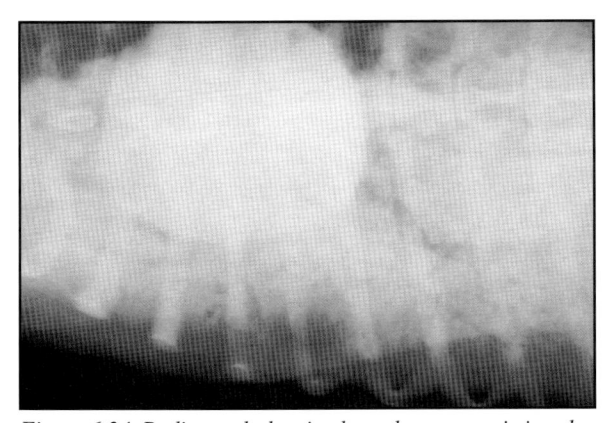

Figure 6.24: Radiograph showing bronchopneumonia in a dog with canine distemper virus infection. (© Dr Bryn Tennant.)

Analysis of cerebrospinal fluid (CSF) is often normal during the acute stage. Where neurological signs are present, the CSF shows both an increased cell count (largely lymphocytes) and protein concentrations (primarily IgG) typical of inflammatory disease. Detection of anti-CDV antibody in CSF is diagnostic, as long as the sample is not contaminated with blood. If such contamination occurs, the serum titre should be compared with that in CSF; a higher titre in CSF suggests active CNS infection.

Immunofluorescence or immunoperoxidase staining for CDV can be performed on cytological preparations of conjunctiva, tonsil, respiratory epithelium, buffy coat, CSF cells, bone marrow or urine sediment. Virus is often not evident, however, since positive test results are usually obtained only early in infection, before the production of virus neutralizing antibody. Some laboratories are able to detect virus antigen in CSF cells via an indirect immunofluorescent antibody test. Other tests, such as immunohistochemical staining, detection of IgM and IgG and lymphocyte transformation studies, are not commercially available in the UK. Definitive diagnosis rests with virus isolation; however, the virus is not easy to culture from infected secretions or tissues.

A CT scan of the brain of an animal with chronic distemper encephalitis may be normal or show focal/multifocal hypoattenuating lesions with a uniform or ring-like contrast enhancement. There is a predilection for the white matter and there may be associated oedema/mass effect. With MRI, T1-weighted images may show hypointense lesions and T2-weighted images hyperintense lesions.

Treatment and prevention: There are no antiviral drugs effective in managing CDV infection. Treatment rests with supportive therapy (expectorants, mucolytics, fluids, antiemetics) and administration of prophylactic antibacterials. Seizures should be controlled with anticonvulsant therapy. Corticosteroids are often used in chronic cases if there is evidence of inflammation, and this often results in a satisfactory response; however, there is a danger that immunosuppression will prevent clearance of the virus in acute cases. Use of free-radical scavengers and antioxidants, e.g. vitamins E and C, may also be useful. Treatment with procainamide or clonazepam is described, although this is often unsuccessful (Tipold *et al.*, 1992). Although euthanasia may be indicated where neurological disease is severe, many dogs can lead nearly normal lives with myoclonus or with seizure control. CDV has been largely controlled in the UK by vaccination.

Prognosis: Affected dogs carry a guarded prognosis.

Feline poxvirus
Poxvirus infection of cats is usually a self-limiting skin disease (see Chapter 13). Rarely, the virus generalizes, particularly in immunosuppressed animals (including those given glucocorticoid therapy for skin lesions), which may result in a fatal pneumonia.

Other viruses
See above for details of CHV, CAV-2, canine parainfluenza virus (CPiV), FHV-1 and FCV.

Bacterial infections
A wide variety of bacteria and mycoplasmas have been implicated in lower airway disease (see Figure 6.21). Most act as secondary or opportunistic pathogens, affecting the LRT by taking advantage of damaged defence mechanisms, although less commonly than for URTIs. They are most often evident in association with chronic inflammatory disorders or immunosuppressive diseases. Although LRT bacterial infections are not usually contagious, transmission to in-contact animals is possible with *Bordetella bronchiseptica*, mycobacterial infections, *Streptococcus zooepidemicus* and *Mycoplasma*-induced disease.

Bacteria can enter the lung by inhalation, haematogenous spread or after direct inoculation (e.g. trauma, bite wound), although such a route usually also involves infection of the pleural space. Pre-existing diseases (non-infectious and infectious) predispose to secondary bacterial invasion. Once bacteria have colonized the LRT, a variety of mechanisms contribute to the development of disease:

- Phagocytosis of bacteria by alveolar macrophages with or without neutrophil assistance
- Adherence to epithelial tissues by bacterial ligands and adhesins
- Failure of mucociliary clearance
- Interference with ciliary movement, e.g. *B. bronchiseptica*, *Pseudomonas aeruginosa*, *Staphylococcus* spp., *Streptococcus* spp., *Mycoplasma* spp.
- Ciliary damage, e.g. CDV, CPiV, CAV-2
- Increased production and viscosity of mucus, making it more difficult for ciliated cells to clear the mucous layer.

The more common agents – some of which may occasionally act as primary pathogens – are discussed below.

Bordetella bronchiseptica
See Infections of the upper respiratory tract.

Streptococcus spp.
Streptococcus spp. can be isolated from tracheal washings of up to 47% of dogs with pneumonia. β-Haemolytic *Streptococcus equi* subsp. *zooepidemicus* (group C) and *S. canis* (group G) are the more important pathogens.

Group C streptococci are carried by dogs and cats, although only in dogs is disease reported. Different strains show marked variation in their virulence, possibly relating to differences in the endotoxins and exotoxins produced. Disease is commonest where large numbers of dogs are kept together. Coughing, dyspnoea, weakness and pyrexia are the major signs; haematemesis and haematuria may also be found. High morbidity and mortality may be reported. Haematogenous spread of the bacteria from the lungs may lead to infection of other tissues, notably joints, heart valves, meninges, kidneys, lymph nodes and spleen. Factors underlying the development of streptococcal pneumonia/septicaemia remain unclear; the organism may be acting as a primary pathogen, or immunosuppression or incompetence may predispose to opportunistic infection.

Streptococcus canis (group G) infection in cats and dogs is implicated in:

- Fading kitten and puppy syndromes (see Chapter 12)
- Cervical lymphadenitis in young cats, after opportunistic infection of the upper respiratory tract.

S. canis (group G) is carried on mucosal surfaces in the upper respiratory and genital tracts and may invade other organs after trauma, surgery, viral infection or immunosuppression. Initial suppurative lesions can result in septicaemia and embolic disease, which may cause pneumonia.

Mycobacteria
Mycobacteria are aerobic non-spore-forming acid-fast bacteria that can survive in the environment for prolonged periods. Different species show wide variation in host affinity and potential to cause disease. They are categorized as:

- Tuberculous mycobacteria: *Mycobacterium tuberculosis* (human bacillus), *M. bovis* (cattle bacillus), *M. microti* (vole bacillus), a newly recognized *M. microti*-like variant and *M. avium* (bird bacillus)
- Lepromatous or non-tuberculous mycobacteria (see Chapter 13)
- Opportunistic mycobacteria (see Chapter 13).

Dogs and cats are variably susceptible to infection by *M. tuberculosis*, *M. bovis*, *M. microti*, *M. microti*-like organisms and *M. avium*; cats have an innate resistance to *M. tuberculosis*. Most cases of tuberculosis are probably subclinical. Classic tuberculosis is caused primarily by *M. bovis* or occasionally *M. tuberculosis*. *M. microti* and *M. microti*-like organisms may be associated with systemic disease in cats, but are most frequently isolated from cutaneous lesions (see Chapter 13). *M. tuberculosis* or *M. bovis* infections are usually acquired from humans. All members of the tubercle group pose potential zoonotic risks; *M. microti* and *M. microti*-like organisms have unknown zoonotic potential. The organism is excreted in sputum or faeces with respiratory or intestinal mycobacteriosis, respectively. Infection is acquired from ingestion of unpasteurized milk, uncooked meat or offal from infected cattle, or from contact with the organism in the environment.

Clinical signs reflect the site of granuloma formation. Whether the organism is contained at these sites or disseminates systemically is determined by host immunity; immunoincompetence promotes dissemination.

Granuloma formation in lung and mediastinal lymph nodes results in a variable cough. Weight loss, pyrexia and anorexia may be present. Occasionally, pleural and pericardial effusions develop. Oropharyngeal granulomas cause dysphagia, hypersalivation and retching. Respiratory infection is more common in the dog than in the cat; cats are more likely to develop intestinal or cutaneous disease. Disseminated mycobacteriosis (rare) presents with splenomegaly, hepatomegaly, pleural or pericardial effusions, generalized lymphadenopathy, weight loss and fever.

Non-specific clinicopathological changes include hyperglobulinaemia and/or hypercalcaemia. Radiography may reveal pulmonary masses, hepatomegaly or splenomegaly, abdominal masses, lymphadenopathy, calcification of lymph nodes and bronchi, osteoproliferation in the skeleton and pleural or peritoneal effusion (Figure 6.25).

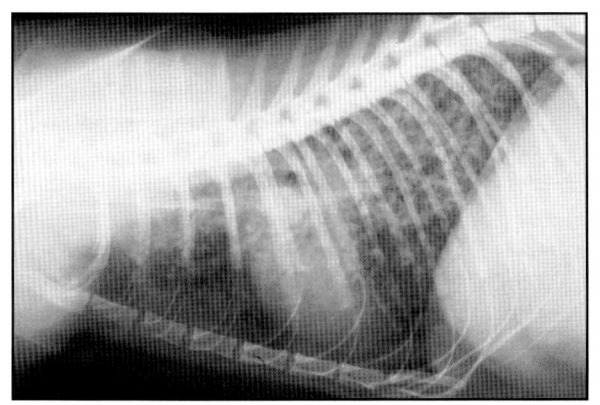

Figure 6.25: Chest radiograph of a cat with tuberculosis (Mycobacterium bovis). *Note the diffuse pulmonary infiltration and enlargement of carinal, mediastinal and perihilar lymph nodes. (© Dr Danièlle Gunn-Moore.)*

A definitive diagnosis relies on demonstrating acid-fast bacilli in leucocytes or biopsy samples and culturing the organism. Intradermal tuberculin testing and specific antibody assays are unreliable in the dog and cat and cannot be recommended.

Before therapy, consider:

- Given the potential zoonotic risk, all members of the affected animal's household should be involved in decision making
- In households inhabited by people with HIV infection or those undergoing chemotherapy or other immunosuppressive therapy, it is strongly advised that treatment should not be considered as an option.

Treatment is long term and can be difficult to maintain because of difficulties in giving the drugs, the inherent toxicity of some drugs and the costs involved. Ideally, treatment consists of two phases:

- The initial phase: at least three drugs are used for at least 2 months; this increases the chance of control and minimizes the development of resistant mycobacteria
- The continuation phase: two drugs are used for at least a further 4–6 months, depending on the extent of disease; in cats where triple therapy is not feasible, treatment should involve two drugs given for 6–9 months.

The rifampicin–isoniazid–ethambutol combination used to treat tuberculosis in man is extremely hepatotoxic to dogs and cats. Mycobacteria are susceptible to fluoroquinolones and variably susceptible to some macrolides (clarithromycin and azithromycin). Clarithromycin, rifampicin and enrofloxacin in the initial phase is probably the safest combination. Rifampicin and either enrofloxacin or clarithromycin are suggested for the continuation phase. In cases where resistance develops, alternative drug combinations have been recommended (Gunn-Moore and Shaw, 1997). For classic tuberculosis, the prognosis is grave to guarded. If treatment is not prescribed, euthanasia should be performed because of the zoonotic risk.

Enterobacteriaceae

Enterobacteriaceae (e.g. *Escherichia coli*, *Klebsiella* spp.) usually enter the LRT from the colonized oral cavity/URT, although haematogenous spread is possible. Endotoxin production may complicate pneumonia, causing severe lung injury and acute respiratory failure. In addition to pneumonia, dissemination of infection to other organs or disseminated intravascular coagulation (DIC) may develop.

Pasteurella spp. and Eugonic fermenter-4

Pasteurella spp. (Gram-negative facultative anaerobic coccobacilli) are frequently isolated from dogs and cats with and without respiratory disease. As part of the normal microflora, they are often isolated from the oral cavities. Entry into the LRT may cause a pneumonia that is difficult to treat successfully and may leave the animal with long-term lung disease, such as lung abscessation.

Pasteurella-like organisms, grouped as Eugonic fermenter-4 (EF-4), have been described as commensals in dogs and cats. They cause severe disease as secondary invaders and have been associated with outbreaks of infectious bacterial pneumonia in cats after inhalation or haematogenous spread. The organism has also been isolated from other sites (often around the head) and may be associated with immunosuppression.

Haemophilus felis

Haemophilus felis (a Gram-negative coccobacillus) can be isolated from the nasopharynx of healthy cats and in mixed or pure culture from cats with respiratory tract infections and conjunctivitis. It seems likely that although *H. felis* is a commensal species, it is capable of causing disease in some circumstances.

Yersinia pestis (plague)

Yersinia pestis has not been described in small animals in western Europe in recent years but is found in other parts of the world. The organism is maintained in wild rodent species and is transmitted by fleas. The disease is mild in dogs, but 50% of affected cats die acutely. There are three forms of the disease: bubonic, septicaemic and pneumonic. The pneumonic form may occur as a sequel to either of the first two forms. Clinical signs of the pneumonic form relate to pneumonia with haemorrhage. Infected cats are a zoonotic risk through droplet spread of respiratory secretions, although there is a greater risk from the infected fleas. Diagnosis is by demonstration of the organism in aspirates, blood or tissues by isolation or polymerase chain reaction, and serology on paired samples can be performed. Control and treatment involves immediate flea control of the affected animal, in-contact animals and the environment and the use of aminoglycoside antibacterials. Suspected cases are a risk to public health and should be reported to the relevant authorities. One quarter of cases of human plague in the USA occur in veterinarians or their technicians.

Mycoplasma spp.

The *Mycoplasma* species of interest in small animals are:

- *M. felis* and *M. gatae* (cats)
- *M. cynos* (dogs).

Mycoplasmas have been isolated from up to 25% of cats with conjunctivitis, and it has been suggested that although *M. gatae* is likely to be a commensal, *M. felis* may be pathogenic. Some studies suggest their involvement in conjunctivitis and URTIs, although further work is required to determine whether this is as a primary or secondary agent.

Mycoplasmas have not been isolated from the LRT of normal cats, but *M. felis* has been isolated from about 25% of cats with chronic bronchial disease. Where *M. felis* has been recovered, the tendency is for prolonged suppurative infection, with early development of bronchiectasis. For this reason antimicrobial treatment is recommended if *M. felis* is recovered from the LRT.

Mycoplasmas are commonly isolated from the LRT of normal dogs and are rarely implicated in disease, except in young puppies or those with underlying disease of the mucociliary apparatus, such as ciliary dyskinesia.

Diagnosis of bacterial infections

Bacterial infections are diagnosed by the demonstration of bacteria in aseptically collected washings or fine needle aspirates and an inflammatory appearance to BAL fluid (Figure 6.26).

Treatment of bacterial and secondary pneumonia

Antibacterial therapy should be based on culture and sensitivity assessment. An initial broad-spectrum treatment regimen is advisable where cytology supports a bacterial infection while awaiting culture results. Intravenous dosing may be indicated where severe or life-threatening bacterial disease is suspected. If Gram-negative rods are evident, trimethoprim-sulphonamide, fluoroquinolone or chloramphenicol

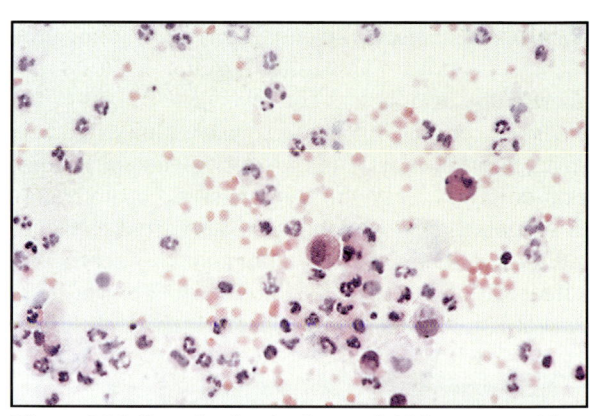

Figure 6.26: Bronchoalveolar lavage fluid from a cat with bacterial pneumonia. The sample contains many erythrocytes and neutrophils. (© Dr Danièlle Gunn-Moore.)

are likely to be effective. Trimethoprim–sulphonamides, chloramphenicol or cephalosporins are indicated for Gram-positive cocci. Many antibacterials do not achieve good penetration into airways, and it may be necessary to give prolonged courses at the high end of the normal dose rate. Chloramphenicol should not be used in dogs or cats unless absolutely necessary.

Fungal infections

Apart from cryptococcosis and aspergillosis (see nasal disease), fungal infections of the respiratory tract (coccidioidomycosis, histoplasmosis and blastomycosis) have not been reported in the UK.

Coccidioides immitans

Coccidioides immitans is a soil organism found in desert areas of North America. In endemic areas most animals and people have been infected, usually subclinically. Disease is restricted to subpleural lung lesions in dogs, causing mild respiratory signs, and skin lesions in cats. Serious disseminated disease may occur, with pyrexia and lethargy. Diagnosis is by cytology or serology, but owing to high exposure rates it can be difficult to confirm.

Histoplasma capsulatum

Histoplasma capsulatum, a yeast-like fungus, is found in North America. In dogs and cats it is primarily a systemic disease, but in cats particularly it may present as respiratory distress, with dyspnoea and tachypnoea; coughing is uncommon. Diagnosis is by cytology of respiratory wash samples or histopathology of affected tissues. Intradermal skin testing is used but considered unreliable in small animals.

Blastomyces dermatitidis

Blastomyces dermatitidis, a yeast-like fungal soil saprophyte, is found mainly in North America, and is more common in dogs than in cats. After inhalation and primary lung infection, dissemination via blood and lymphatics occurs, causing generalized signs, including pyrexia, lethargy, skin lesions and ocular disease. Diagnosis is by cytology or histopathology.

Protozoal infections

Pneumocystis carinii

Pneumocystis carinii, currently classified as a protozoan, is a saprophytic organism known to infect both non-domestic and domestic animals, including man. In dogs, pneumonia due to *P. carinii* probably reflects the presence of other agents or immunosuppression. The disease has been reported in Cavalier King Charles Spaniels in the UK and in long-haired Dachshunds in South Africa and elsewhere. It presents with severe dyspnoea and must be distinguished from congestive heart failure and idiopathic pulmonary fibrosis. Diagnosis is by radiography (Figure 6.27) and cytology. Silver staining of cytological preparations from BAL samples are recommended.

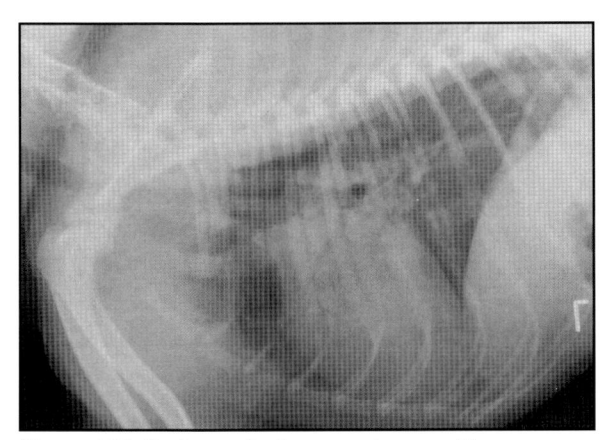

Figure 6.27: Radiograph of pneumonia caused by Pneumocystis carinii. *A dense interstitial pattern is evident. (© Dr Ian Ramsey.)*

Toxoplasma gondii

Toxoplasma gondii may cause pneumonia in complicated or severe cases, although this is a rare manifestation. For further details see Chapter 15.

Neospora caninum

Neospora caninum can manifest as disseminated disease, and the lung may be involved as part of this multisystemic infection. Clinical signs relating to lung damage are not likely to be prominent. For further details see Chapter 15.

Parasitic infestation

A variety of parasites have been associated with LRT disease.

Aelurostrongylus abstrusus

The cat lungworm, *Aelurostrongylus abstrusus*, has a worldwide distribution. Adults are small (<1 cm long) and found in bronchioles. Eggs are deposited in nodules in the lung parenchyma, and first stage (L1) larvae are coughed up, swallowed and passed out in faeces. Intermediate hosts are slugs and snails, and paratenic hosts (small mammals or birds) probably play a role in infecting cats. Asymptomatic infections are common. In heavy infections, major airway inflammation results in nodule formation in lung and pleura that can be present for about 6 months. Clinical signs are similar to those of 'feline asthma,' with mild coughing to severe wheezing.

Poorly defined soft tissue nodular densities resembling metastatic or mycotic disease may be evident radiographically. Mixed bronchial, alveolar and interstitial patterns may be evident. Tracheal wash cytology may show an eosinophilic inflammatory process, occasionally reflected in systemic haematology, although secondary bacterial infection often results in a mixed inflammatory picture. A definitive diagnosis is made by identifying L1 larvae in tracheal wash samples or faeces; L1 larvae are recognized by the presence of dorsal and ventral cuticular spines on their tails. Treatment is indicated in all cats with suggestive clinical signs.

Filaroides spp.

Besides *Oslerus osleri* (see above), other canine filarial worms (*Filaroides milksii, F. hirthi*) are occasionally found in terminal bronchioles and alveoli. Infection is usually asymptomatic, although miliary nodules may be seen at post-mortem examination. Rarely, *F. hirthi* presents with tachypnoea, cough and respiratory distress, especially in immunocompromised animals. Radiography may show a diffuse miliary interstitial or focal nodular pattern. Diagnosis is confirmed by demonstrating larvae or larvated eggs by using zinc sulphate flotation methods (see Chapter 1).

Crenosoma vulpis

Crenosoma vulpis is primarily an infestation of wild species (foxes, badgers) and is important in fox colonies; pet dogs are rarely affected. The parasite is found in the trachea, bronchi and bronchioles. Larvae are coughed up and passed out in faeces. Molluscs are intermediate hosts. Clinical features relate to the development of tracheobronchitis and bronchopneumonia, with coughing, sneezing and nasal discharge reported. Thoracic radiography may demonstrate a mixed lung pattern. Diagnosis is made by identifying larvae in tracheal wash samples or faeces by using the Baermann technique.

Angiostrongylus vasorum and Dirofilaria immitis

A. vasorum and *D. immitis* reside within the pulmonary arteries and right atrium. They may cause respiratory signs (see Chapter 7).

Migration of intestinal parasites

In heavy infestations, migration of *Toxocara canis* larvae through the lung may cause coughing and tachypnoea in puppies (<6 weeks of age). Signs are minor, and usually no treatment is required. During this stage no ova are present in the faeces, but an eosinophilia

112 Manual of Canine and Feline Infectious Diseases

may be evident. *Ancylostoma caninum* and *Strongyloides stercoralis* also migrate through lungs as part of their life cycle, potentially causing coughing.

Paragonimus kellicotti
The lung fluke *Paragonimus kellicotti* is reported in dogs and cats in North America and occasionally causes disease. Infection follows ingestion of the crayfish intermediate host. Adult flukes migrate to the lungs, where air-filled cysts develop around the parasites. Signs relate to inflammation associated with the parasite, secondary infections or pneumothorax or haemothorax as a consequence of cyst rupture. Diagnosis is by identification of single operculated ovoid eggs (80–10 µm long) in tracheal wash samples or faeces.

Treatment of parasitic LRT disease
Aelurostrongylus abstrusus, *Filaroides hirthi* and *F. milksi* infections are often self-limiting or asymptomatic and do not usually warrant treatment. Symptomatic cases may be treated with benzimidazoles (e.g. fenbendazole).

PLEURAL AND MEDIASTINAL INFECTIONS

The pleural cavity is affected by many diseases, most of which are not associated with infectious processes. The commonest infectious conditions are pyothorax and feline infectious peritonitis (see Chapter 9). Other infections that might rarely cause pleural effusion include pulmonary infections/parapneumonic effusion, pyometra and parasites. The mediastinum is occasionally involved in infectious conditions.

Pyothorax

Aetiology
Pyothorax develops when bacteria gain entry to the pleural cavity from pulmonary or extrapleural infection, e.g. oesophageal perforation, migrating foreign body, perforation of the thoracic wall and osteomyelitis (Figure 6.28).

Figure 6.29 lists the bacteria commonly isolated from the pleura of dogs or cats with pyothorax, although any of the bacteria listed in Figure 6.1 may be present and infections may be mixed. Anaerobic infections are common, particularly in the cat. In many cases, bacteria are not isolated.

Clinical features
The clinical features of pyothorax include subacute or acute pyrexia, depression, anorexia, weight loss, dyspnoea and tachypnoea. There may be a history of

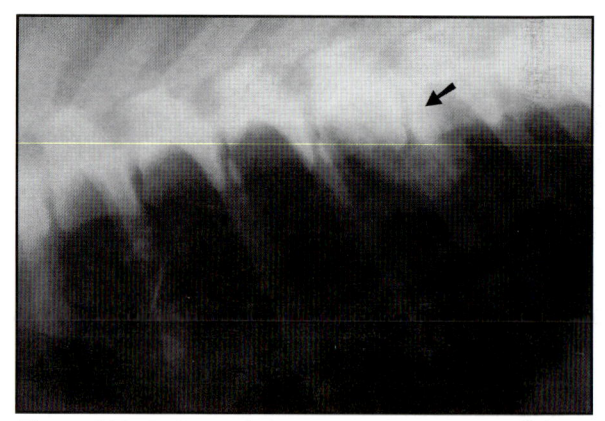

Figure 6.28: Radiographic appearance consistent with osteomyelitis in the rib. The dog had previously been treated for pyothorax. Extension of the infection from the rib into the pleural cavity was considered likely. (© Dr Bryn Tennant.)

Dog	Cat
Fusobacterium	*Fusobacterium*
Actinomyces	*Actinomyces*
Arcanobacterium	*Arcanobacterium*
Corynebacterium	*Corynebacterium*
Streptococcus	*Streptococcus*
Bacteroides	*Bacteroides*
Peptostreptococcus	*Peptostreptococcus*
Pasteurella	*Pasteurella*
Nocardia	*Nocardia*
Escherichia coli	*Mycoplasma*
Klebsiella	Other aerobic/anaerobic bacteria
Other aerobic/anaerobic bacteria	

Figure 6.29: Bacteria that may be isolated from pleura in dogs or cats with pyothorax.

trauma (bite wound or recent surgery) or infection. Pulmonary and cardiac sounds may be dull on auscultation, especially ventrally and perhaps unilaterally. Severe dyspnoea is common, with a marked inspiratory effort.

Diagnosis
Radiography shows a pleural effusion, usually bilateral; unilateral pyothorax can develop (Figure 6.30), particularly if there is mediastinal thickening. Rarely, free gas associated with anaerobic infections or leakage of air from necrotic lung may be evident. Haematologically, an inflammatory response is expected. Grossly, the fluid is expected to be thick, cloudy, yellow/brown, haemorrhagic or dark, containing fibrinous clots. In the case of nocardiosis, sulphur granules may be evident (Figure 6.31). Cytological examination of the fluid will demonstrate a purulent exudate (Figure 6.32). Material must be submitted for aerobic and anaerobic culture. Identification of organisms in the fluid by Gram or acid-fast stains may assist identification.

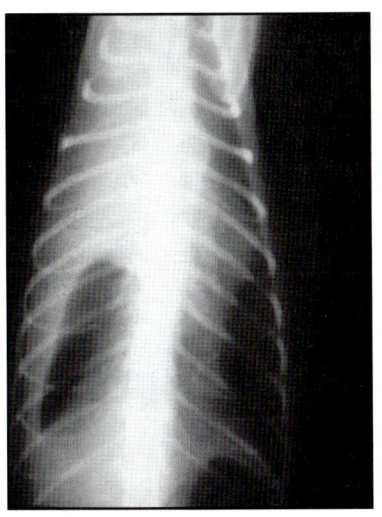

Figure 6.30: Radiograph of a cat with a unilateral pleural effusion, confirmed on thoracocentesis as pyothorax.

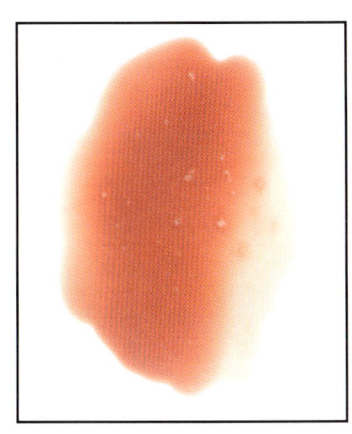

Figure 6.31: Pleural fluid from a dog with pyothorax caused by Nocardia *spp. Note the yellow sulphur granules within the thick red fluid. (© Dr Danièlle Gunn-Moore.)*

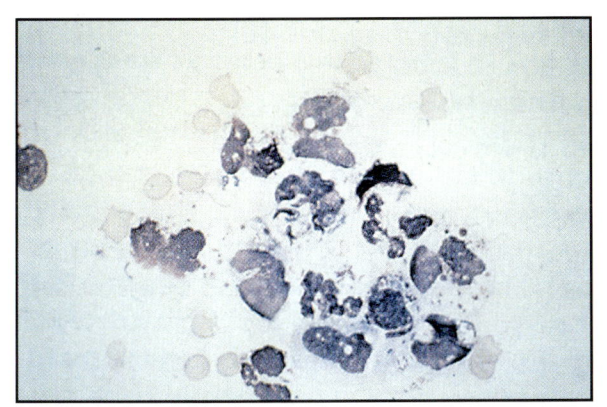

Figure 6.32: Pleural fluid from a cat with pyothorax. Note the highly degenerate, toxic appearance of the neutrophils. (© Dr Danièlle Gunn-Moore.)

Treatment

Pyothorax does not resolve with antibacterial therapy alone. Successful treatment requires systemic antibacterial therapy and effective drainage of the pleural cavity. Unilateral closed-chest pleural lavage with an indwelling chest drain or continuous water seal suction at about 20 cm are the two recommended systems. The latter is the preferred method as it provides a more rapid and complete resolution of the clinical features. Multiple thoracocentesis is not recommended as a first-choice treatment, but it is an alternative if admission to hospital and overnight supervision are not possible.

Restoration of fluid deficits before drainage is recommended to reduce the likelihood of hypotension or apnoea. In many dogs the tube can be placed under local anaesthesia without sedation. If sedation is required, the development of hypoxia due to reduced respiratory function should be borne in mind. General anaesthesia may prove safer than sedation in the dog as intubation allows greater control over respiration; general anaesthesia is essential in the cat.

Thoracostomy tubes are placed in the ventral third of the chest wall, through an intercostal space (usually space 7/8), with the skin incision at least 2 ribs caudally. The drain is secured by suturing or the use of a Chinese finger-trap suture. As much fluid as possible should be drained and the animal radiographed to assess whether a second tube is required on the opposite side to achieve full drainage; rarely is bilateral tube placement required. The drain should be either (a) clamped and a three-way tap attached to the free end of the drain, fixed at closed to prevent iatrogenic pneumothorax (this should be monitored frequently; at least every 3 hours) or (b) attached to a water-seal system for continuous suction; continuous monitoring is required for this.

After drainage, if continuous water-seal suction is unavailable, body temperature, sterile Hartmann's solution (10 ml/kg body weight) is introduced through the drain, gentle coupage applied to the chest and the fluid withdrawn; the use of saline predisposes to the development of hypokalaemia, particularly in cats. Perform this twice daily for at least 7-10 days until cytology and smears treated by the Gram's method suggest the infection has resolved, i.e. presence of non-degenerate neutrophils, reduction in cell numbers and absence of bacteria (bacteria are usually absent by day 3). If continuous water-seal suction is available, intermittent drainage and lavage of the pleural cavity is unnecessary. If hospitalization is not possible, thoracocentesis under general anaesthesia combined with flushing should be repeated every 2 or 3 days. Intermittent thoracocentesis is much less likely to have a successful outcome than is the use of indwelling drains, and referral should be considered early in the course of disease.

Parenteral antibacterial therapy is essential, continued for 6-8 weeks. Sensitivity testing should guide the choice of antibacterial:

- Most organisms are sensitive to the synthetic penicillins ampicillin or amocycillin/clavulanate, and these may be combined with metronidazole or clindamycin
- If nocardiosis is suspected or proven, trimethoprim–sulphonamide is the first-choice antibacterial, followed by aminoglycosides and tetracycline

- Where there is a suggestion of septicaemia or septic shock developing, particularly if Gram-negative bacteria are involved, intravenous aminoglycosides (e.g. gentamicin, amikacin) administered with penicillins, second- or third-generation cephalosporins or fluoroquinolones may be indicated.

Supportive therapy is often required, including intravenous fluid administration and appropriate nutritional support (nasal feeding tube or gastrostomy tube) to counter the marked nutrient loss that develops in these patients. Neither proteolytic enzymes nor intrapleural antibacterials need be used in the lavage fluid.

Failure of the condition to resolve requires further investigation for underlying disease (e.g. FeLV, FIV, foreign body) or for evidence of encapsulated abscess formation in the lung or pleura; this may result from failure to treat promptly or aggressively. Abscess will require removal at thoracotomy.

Feline infectious peritonitis

Feline coronaviral infections are discussed in Chapter 9. Feline infectious peritonitis can present with dyspnoea due to pleural or pericardial effusion.

Feline leukaemia virus

Feline leukaemia virus (FeLV) is covered in Chapter 5 and is mentioned here only with reference to FeLV-positive thymic lymphoma. It is estimated that up to 80% of cats with thymic lymphoma are FeLV-positive. Dyspnoea is a major clinical sign owing to the pleural effusion and compression of intrathoracic structures by the thymic mass. Diagnosis rests with radiography, analysis of the effusion and demonstration of FeLV antigenaemia or virus isolation.

Pulmonary infection/parapneumonic effusion

A sterile inflammatory exudative pleural effusion may develop in patients with pneumonia; the fluid is serous or haemorrhagic rather than purulent. Although this type of effusion may be seen with any bacterial pneumonia, it is reported to be most commonly associated with *Klebsiella* spp. or *Streptococcus* spp. The effusions resolve spontaneously once the pneumonia is managed.

Miscellaneous

Small effusions may be seen in patients with pyometra. The pathophysiology is unclear, and the effusion resolves spontaneously. Pleural effusions with high eosinophil counts are occasionally found and in some cases have been attributed to parasitic (which specific parasite is not stated), hypersensitivity or immunological disorders.

DRUG DOSAGES

See Appendix 3.

ACKNOWLEDGEMENTS

The authors are grateful to Dr Danièlle Gunn-Moore for writing the section on mycobacterial diseases.

REFERENCES AND FURTHER READING

Anderson GI (1987) The treatment of chronic sinusitis in six cats by ethmoid conchal curettage and autologous fat graft sinus ablation. *Veterinary Surgery* **16**, 131-134

Angus JC, Jang SS and Hirsch DC (1997) Microbiological study of transtracheal aspirates from dogs with suspected lower respiratory tract disease: 264 cases (1989-1995). *Journal of the American Veterinary Medical Association* **210**, 55-58

Blunden AS and Smith KC (1996) A pathological study of a mycobacterial infection in a cat caused by a variant with cultural characteristics between *Mycobacterium tuberculosis* and *M. bovis*. *Veterinary Record* **138**, 87-88

Bourdoiseau G, Cadore JL, Fournier C and Gounel JM (1994) Canine oslerosis. *Parasite* **1**, 369-378

Cobb MA and Fisher MA (1992) *Crenosoma vulpis* infection in a dog. *Veterinary Record* **130**, 452

Dawson S and Willoughby K (1999) Feline upper respiratory tract disease – an update. *In Practice* **21**, 232-237

Gartrell CL, O'Handley PO and Perry RL (1995) An update on canine nasal disease: Part I. *Compendium on Continuing Education for the Practicing Veterinarian* **17**, 323-326

Gartrell CL, O'Handley PO and Perry RL (1995) Canine nasal disease: Part II. *Compendium on Continuing Education for the Practicing Veterinarian* **17**, 539-547

Georgi JR (1987) Parasites of the respiratory tract. *Veterinary Clinics of North America: Small Animal Practice* **17**, 1421-1442

Gunn-Moore D and Shaw S (1997) Mycobacterial disease in the cat. *In Practice* 493-501

Keil DJ and Fenwick B (1998) Role of *Bordetella bronchiseptica* in infectious tracheobronchitis in dogs. *Journal of the American Veterinary Medical Association* **212**, 200-207

Marks SL, Moore MP and Rishniw M (1994) *Pneumonyssoides caninum* – the canine nasal mite. *Compendium on Continuing Education for the Practicing Veterinarian* **16**, 577-583

O'Brien RT, Evans SM, Wortman JA and Hendrick MJ (1996) Radiographic findings in cats with intranasal neoplasia or chronic rhinitis: 29 cases (1982-1988). *Journal of the American Veterinary Medical Association* **208**, 385-389

Olsson E and Falsen E (1994) "*Haemophilus felis*": a potential pathogen? *Journal of Clinical Microbiology* **32**, 858-859

Padrid PA, Feldman EF, Funk K, Samitz EM, Reil D and Cross CE (1991) Cytologic, microbiologic and biochemical analysis of bronchoalveolar lavage fluid obtained from 24 healthy cats. *American Journal of Veterinary Research* **52**, 1300-1307

Randolph JF, Moise NS, Scarlett JM, Shin, SJ, Blue JT and Bookbinder PR (1993) Prevalence of mycoplasmal and ureaplasmal recovery from tracheobronchial lavages and prevalence of mycoplasmal recovery from pharyngeal swab specimens in dogs with or without pulmonary disease. *American Journal of Veterinary Research* **54**, 387-391

Randolph JF, Moise NS, Scarlett JM, Shin, SJ, Blue JT and Corbett JR (1993) Prevalence of mycoplasmal and ureaplasmal recovery from tracheobronchial lavages and prevalence of mycoplasmal recovery from pharyngeal swab specimens in cats with or without pulmonary disease. *American Journal of Veterinary Research* **54**, 897-900

Rebar AH, Hawkins EC and DeNicola DB (1992) Cytologic evaluation of the respiratory tract. *Veterinary Clinics of North America: Small Animal Practice* **22**, 1065-1085

Sharp NJH, Harvey CE and Sullivan M (1991) Canine nasal aspergillosis and penicillinosis. *Compendium on Continuing Education for the Practicing Veterinarian* **13**, 41-47

Smith SA, Andrews G and Biller DS (1998) Management of nasal aspergillosis in a dog with a single, non-invasive intranasal infusion of clotrimazole. *Journal of the American Animal Hospital Association* **34**, 487-492

Sparkes A, Wotton P and Brown P (1997) Tracheobronchial washing in the dog and cat. *In Practice* **19**, 257-259

Speakman AJ, Dawson S, Binns SH, Hart CA and Gaskell RM (1999) *Bordetella bronchiseptica* infection in the cat: a review. *Journal of Small Animal Practice* **40**, 252-256

Thrusfield NV, Aitken CGG and Muirhead RH (1991) A field investigation of kennel cough: incubation and clinical signs. *Journal of Small Animal Practice* **32**, 215-220

Tipold A, Vandevelde A and Jaggy A (1992) Neurological manifestations of canine distemper virus infection. *Journal of Small Animal Practice* **33**, 466-470

Willoughby K and Coutts A (1995) Differential diagnosis of nasal disease in cats. *In Practice* **17**, 154-161

CHAPTER SEVEN

The Cardiovascular System

Clive Elwood

CHAPTER PLAN

Introduction
Pericardial infections
Myocardial infections
Endocardial infections
Bacteraemia and septicaemia
Intravascular parasites
    Angiostrongylus vasorum
    Dirofilaria immitis
Pyrexia of unknown origin
    Differential diagnosis
    Diagnostic plan
References and further reading

INTRODUCTION

Infections of the cardiovascular system are rare compared with, for example, gastrointestinal and respiratory infections. The cardiovascular system is shielded from direct environmental challenge by pathogens and also contains blood, which has a high concentration of protective factors such as complement, immunoglobulin and phagocytic cells. In temperate regions such as the UK and northern Europe, certain primary infections of the cardiovascular system are rarer than in tropical and subtropical regions. This probably reflects the lack of arthropod vectors of disease.

Signs of cardiovascular infections vary with the site of infection. Cardiovascular infections may result in dysfunction of the area involved and/or cause disease of organs distal to the point of infection. Thus bacterial endocarditis can cause valvular insufficiency as well as embolic infarction and infection of end arterial tissues such as the kidneys.

PERICARDIAL INFECTIONS

Bacterial infections of the pericardium are rare in dogs and cats and probably arise most commonly as a result of foreign body penetration. Infections are usually well contained within the pericardial sac and lead to a fibrotic pericarditis, fluid accumulation and, ultimately, restrictive pericardial disease. This causes an increase in pericardial pressure until ventricular filling is impaired (cardiac tamponade). Pericardial infections may also develop as extensions of pleural infections or by failure to observe strict asepsis during pericardiocentesis. Viral infections that lead to vascular disease and a serositis can also produce significant pericardial fluid accumulation (e.g. feline infectious peritonitis (FIP), canine herpesvirus-1 infection).

History/clinical signs

Presenting history may include malaise, anorexia, weight loss, abdominal swelling from right-sided congestive heart failure and dyspnoea from pleural effusion. Physical examination findings may include pyrexia, ascites (abdominal enlargement, fluid thrill), prominent pulsating jugular veins, tachycardia, poor peripheral pulses and diminished apex beat.

Careful auscultation of the heart can reveal muffled heart sounds with 'knocks,' thought to occur as a result of rapid diastolic deceleration of blood due to restrictive pericardial disease, and 'pericardial rubs', occurring from contact of the irregular and thickened visceral and parietal pericardial surfaces as the heart beats.

Organisms

In dogs, *Nocardia asteroides* and *Actinomyces* spp. are common, whereas *Pasteurella* spp. are more usual in cats. Some fungal organisms (not found in the UK) have been isolated from pericardial effusions. Viral causes are uncommon, though FIP virus can cause clinically important pericarditis.

Differential diagnosis

Figure 7.1 lists the differential diagnoses for pericardial effusion. Other causes of pericardial fluid accumulation include coagulopathies, uraemia and trauma; however, non-cardiac clinical signs usually predominate in such cases.

> Primary idiopathic pericarditis
> Neoplasia
>   Haemangiosarcoma
>   Chemodectoma
>   Lymphosarcoma
>   Mesothelioma
> Myocardial failure (especially in cats)
> Right-sided congestive cardiac failure
>   Congenital cardiac disease
>   Bacterial endocarditis
>   Endocardiosis
>   Cor pulmonale

Figure 7.1: Differential diagnoses for pericardial effusion.

Diagnostic plan

Clinical pathology
Haematology may reveal a neutrophilic leucocytosis, possibly with a left shift. Increased concentration of hepatic enzymes may be seen as a result of right-sided congestive cardiac failure, and prerenal renal failure may increase urea and creatinine concentrations with hypersthenuric urine. Laboratory analysis of the free abdominal fluid is consistent with a modified transudate.

Radiography
Thoracic radiographs may show a rounded cardiac silhouette with no visible contours and sharply demarcated pericardial borders. In advanced restrictive disease the cardiac silhouette may be much less enlarged. Free abdominal fluid as a result of right-sided congestive cardiac failure may obscure serosal detail.

Electrocardiography
An electrocardiogram (ECG) may show a tachycardia (as a result of fever and reduced cardiac output) and low PQRS voltage. There may also be electrical alternans (variation in the R wave height on alternate beats).

Ultrasonography
Echocardiography will readily reveal pericardial fluid accumulation. It is important when performing echocardiography in such cases to search for neoplastic mass lesions as well as to assess cardiac function. Fibrotic thickening of the pericardium may be seen echocardiographically and should alert the operator to the possibility of infection. Echocardiography may also be used to help guide pericardiocentesis although it is not essential (see below). Cardiac tamponade can result in free abdominal fluid that will be readily visible on abdominal ultrasonograms.

Analysis of pericardial fluid
Definitive diagnosis of bacterial pericarditis requires sampling, cytology and culture of pericardial fluid. Pericardiocentesis is a relatively straightforward technique (Figure 7.2) but should only be performed in cases with a confirmed pericardial effusion. Cytological and microbiological assessment of the pericardial fluid should be performed wthout delay. Large numbers of neutrophils, often with degenerative features, will be present on cytological examination. Smaller numbers of macrophages may be evident, and both types of cell may have intracellular bacteria. In cases associated with FIP, the fluid may contain a more mixed population of leucocytes, and the neutrophils will not have degenerative features.

Treatment
Pericardial infections are so rare in small animals that detailed recommendations are lacking. Treatment of infectious pericarditis requires high doses of intravenous antibacterials as appropriate, based on culture and sensitivity test results, and a subtotal pericardectomy, with subsequent lavage via thoracic drains. While culture and sensitivity test results are pending, broad-spectrum antibacterials covering both anaerobes and aerobes should be provided. If there is major restriction from a fibrotic visceral pericardium, diastolic function is likely to remain poor. In humans, epicardial stripping may be attempted to treat such a fibrotic epicarditis but there are no reports of this in small animals.

MYOCARDIAL INFECTIONS

Infectious myocarditis is rarely diagnosed in adult dogs and cats in the UK, but can be a problem in other areas of the world, e.g. American trypanosomiasis (Chagas' disease) in South and Central America and southern USA.

History/clinical signs
Clinical signs of myocarditis relate to myocardial dysfunction. Myocardial disease can cause cardiac rhythm abnormalities with associated weakness, intermittent collapse and sudden death. Reduced cardiac output can occur as a result of dysrhythmias, reduced myocardial contractility and increased myocardial stiffness. This can cause 'forward failure' (cardiogenic shock) with tachycardia, weak pulses, poor peripheral perfusion and cold, pale mucous membranes and/or congestive cardiac failure with fluid retention, leading to pulmonary oedema and/or ascites.

Organisms
Viral myocarditis used to occur quite frequently in fetuses infected *in utero* or puppies infected in the immediate postnatal period with canine parvovirus. This condition is now considered to be rare. Other viral causes, such as canine herpesvirus (CHV-1) in neonates, are also rare. Various bacterial species

Equipment required
Surgical gloves, surgical scrub, local anaesthetic, long (10 cm) wide-bore (10 G to 16 G) over-the-needle catheter, or pericardiocentesis needle. Some authors introduce a sterile urinary catheter through the over-the-needle catheter to decrease the kinking of the latter.
Method
1. The animal (conscious or sedated) is placed in left lateral recumbency. An intravenous catheter is placed as a precaution. The ventral half of the right chest wall is aseptically prepared in the region of intercostal spaces 4-6
2. Local anaesthetic is infiltrated into the skin and intercostal muscle about two thirds of the way from the sternum to the costochondral junction
3. The pericardiocentesis needle is introduced slowly through the intercostal muscle just cranial to the rib, after tunnelling through the skin by 1-2 cm
4. The needle is advanced, preferably under ultrasound guidance and with a simultaneous ECG tracing, until either the catheter is imaged penetrating the pericardium, or ventricular ectopic beats are seen, or the tip of the needle can be felt scratching against the visceral epicardium
5. Penetration of a fibrotic pericardium may require considerable force and should be performed with appropriate care
6. After penetration, the stylet is withdrawn and gentle suction is applied with a 50 ml syringe, connected via a three-way tap and extension tubing, until fluid is aspirated and can be retrieved in a sterile manner for culture and sensitivity testing, cell counts and cytology
7. A small aliquot should be allowed to stand; if it clots, the fluid includes fresh whole blood and the procedure should be stopped. EDTA and plain samples should be kept
8. The drainage procedure should be continued to completion to minimize the potential for drainage of purulent fluid into the pleural cavity and to relieve constriction of the heart and improve output

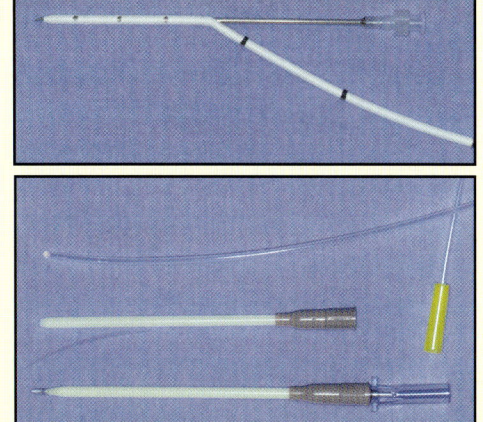

Various pericardiocentesis catheters. (Courtesy of Dr Ian Ramsey.)

Figure 7.2: *Pericardiocentesis.*

could cause myocardial abscessation, and *Borrelia burgdorferi* has been implicated, but not proven, to be a cause of canine myocarditis. Protozoal organisms that can cause specific myocarditis include *Toxoplasma gondii, Neospora caninum, Trypanosoma cruzi* and *Hepatozoon canis*. Fungal organisms such as *Cryptococcus neoformans* and *Aspergillus* spp. can infect the myocardium.

Differential diagnosis

Figure 7.3 lists the differential diagnoses for myocardial dysfunction due to infectious myocarditis. Other causes of sudden onset cardiac rhythm disturbance include myocardial trauma, drugs, myocardial hypoxia and metabolic disease.

Idiopathic cardiomyopathy (most common)
Nutritional cardiomyopathy (carnitine and taurine deficiency)
Immune-mediated myocarditis

Figure 7.3: *Differential diagnoses for myocardial dysfunction due to infectious myocarditis.*

Diagnostic plan

Clinical pathology
In general, the value of haematology in infectious myocarditis is low. Bacterial myocarditis may produce a neutrophilic leucocytosis. Parvoviral myocarditis may be associated with a lymphopenia, though this is not as common as in enteric infections. Biochemistry may reflect the effects of cardiac failure and involvement of other organs in the primary disease process but is generally unhelpful.

Radiography
Acute myocarditis may not be associated with cardiac dilatation. Chronic disease, however, may lead to cardiomegaly on thoracic radiography.

Electrocardiography
An ECG may yield a variety of dysrhythmias, including supraventricular premature complexes, supraventricular tachycardias, atrioventricular block, ventricular premature complexes (unifocal and multifocal) and ventricular tachycardia. Other

possible ECG changes include low-amplitude QRS waves, ST segment abnormalities and T wave inversion.

Ultrasonography
Echocardiography can show reduced cardiac contractility and output, and alterations in myocardial thickness. Echocardiography may also show abscesses and granulomas.

Definitive diagnosis of myocarditis requires histopathological examination of an endomyocardial biopsy, an uncommonly performed technique in canine and feline medicine. Serological tests may be used to confirm toxoplasmosis, neosporosis, cryptococcosis, aspergillosis or trypanosomiasis.

Treatment
Treatment of myocarditis should include antidysrhythmic drugs and/or cardiac pacing as appropriate. In severe acute myocardial dysfunction with forward failure, inotropic support with dobutamine, and afterload reduction with sodium nitroprusside, may be needed. Congestive cardiac failure may be managed with a combination of diuretics, afterload reduction (e.g. angiotensin-converting enzyme (ACE) inhibitors) and inotropic support (e.g. digoxin, pimobendan) as required. If a specific organism is implicated, then appropriate antimicrobial therapy should be given as indicated.

ENDOCARDIAL INFECTIONS

Bacterial endocarditis is an uncommon but well recognized infection of the endocardium including the heart valves (Figure 7.4). It can be extremely difficult to diagnose. Bacterial endocarditis develops as a result of bacteria in the blood becoming lodged in the valve leaflets. Bacteria are more prevalent in the bloodstream of immunocompromised animals, those with concurrent infections (e.g. urinary tract infections) and those that have had non-sterile surgery (e.g. dental procedures). Congenital heart defects may predispose individuals to the development of endocarditis as a result of the altered vascular dynamics. Bacterial endocarditis is rare in cats.

Endomyocardial infection can lead to cardiac rhythm disturbance, valvular insufficiency, bacteraemia, septicaemia, thromboembolism and immune-complex disease. Bacterial endocarditis is a cause of 'pyrexia of unknown origin,' which is described below.

History/clinical signs
Bacterial endocarditis can present with a range of signs, which include:

- Fever
- Malaise
- Shifting leg lameness
- Joint effusion
- Haemostatic abnormalities (including epistaxis and ecchymotic haemorrhages)
- Septic shock
- Neurological dysfunction
- Cardiac murmurs (which may alter in character and/or position)
- Cardiac arrhythmias (conduction blocks and premature rhythms)
- Congestive cardiac failure (right- or left-sided).

Other clinical signs may be present if there is a primary focus for the bacteraemia (e.g. prostatic disease, dental disease). Clinical signs may also develop secondary to immune-mediated or embolic phenomena (e.g. renal infarction, embolic pneumonia). There may be a chronic history of signs relating to a congenital heart defect such as episodic collapse and cardiac murmurs.

Organisms
Bacterial organisms that can cause bacterial endocarditis are varied and include *Staphylococcus intermedius*, *Streptococcus* spp. (particularly β-haemolytic species), *Escherichia coli*, *Pseudomonas aeruginosa*, *Propionibacterium acnes*, *Erysipelothrix rhusiopathiae*, *Pasteurella* spp. and *Corynebacterium* spp.

Differential diagnosis
The differential diagnoses for bacterial endocarditis vary with the clinical presentation but often include the many causes of pyrexia of unknown origin (see below). In addition, bacterial endocarditis can present with signs that might suggest other cardiac disease.

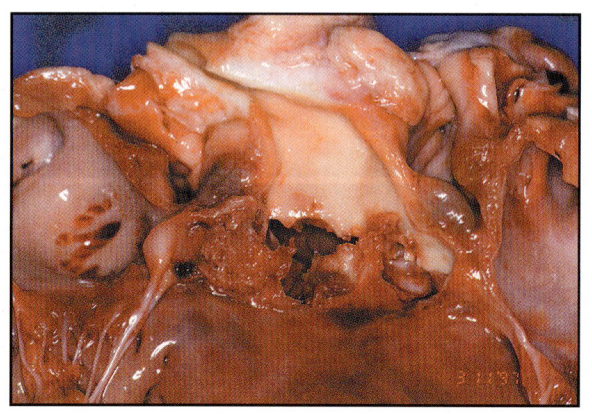

Figure 7.4: Vegetative endocarditis of the aortic valve of a 4-year-old male entire Boxer with bacterial endocarditis. (Courtesy of Dr Ian Ramsey.)

Beside the signs that are produced directly by bacterial endocarditis, signs related to the predisposing causes noted above may also be recognized.

Diagnostic plan
Most cases of bacterial endocarditis present with signs related to pyrexia, and many diagnostic tests may need to be employed to exclude other conditions (see Figure 7.16).

Clinical pathology
Haematology, biochemistry and urinalysis should be routinely performed in suspected cases of bacterial endocarditis. Haematology may show neutrophilia with varying degrees of left shift, monocytosis and lymphocytosis. Biochemistry screens may show hypoalbuminaemia, increased concentrations of liver enzymes, hypoglycaemia (if there is concurrent sepsis), azotaemia, hypercholesterolaemia and hyperglobulinaemia. Urinalysis may show evidence of renal insufficiency and urinary tract infection.

Blood culture
Blood culture should be performed in all suspected cases of bacterial endocarditis. Two or three blood culture samples are obtained with a minimum of 1 hour between samples (Figure 7.5). The isolation of organisms from blood is not always indicative of bacterial endocarditis; however, the isolation of any of the organisms listed above is likely to be important. Blood-borne bacteria from another source (see below), contaminants (from skin) and non-pathogenic organisms may all be isolated on occasions. Coagulase-negative staphylococci, non-haemolytic streptococci, *Micrococcus* spp. and *Acinetobacter* spp. are likely to be skin contaminants. The importance of the isolation of *Clostridium* spp. is unclear, as they have been isolated from healthy dogs.

Prior therapy will reduce the isolation rate and may lead to false negative test results. In general, withholding antibacterial therapy for 24–48 hours is sufficient (depending on the pharmacokinetics of the drug).

Urine culture
Urine culture should be performed in suspected cases of bacterial endocarditis. Urinary tract infection can predispose to, or be secondary to, bacterial endocarditis. The organisms isolated reflect those found in the blood, although the isolation rate is lower. Urine should be obtained by cystocentesis.

Radiography
In most cases thoracic radiography is unremarkable. However, thoracic radiography can show evidence of cardiomegaly, embolic pneumonia (Figure 7.6), cardiac failure and joint effusion.

Equipment required
Surgical gloves, surgical scrub, two hypodermic 21 G needles, 20 ml syringe, spirit and appropriate bottles for aerobic and anaerobic culture.

Method

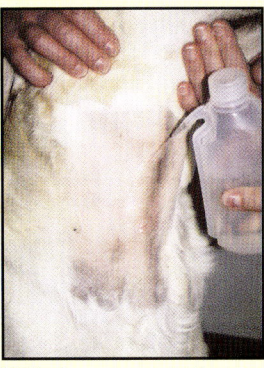

1. An area over the jugular vein is clipped then scrubbed with antiseptic and finally rinsed with spirit
2. Using sterile gloving and a 'no-touch' method, a 20 ml jugular venous blood sample is withdrawn 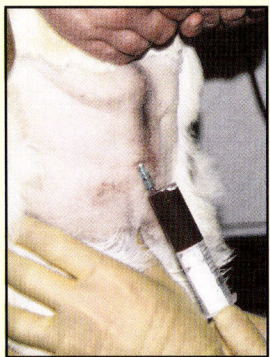
3. To avoid cross-contamination, a new needle is placed on the syringe 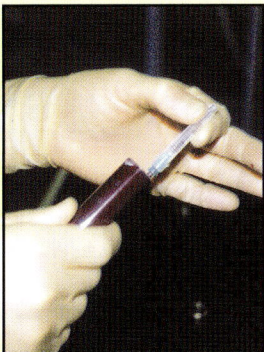
4. The rubber stopper of the blood culture bottle is swabbed with spirit 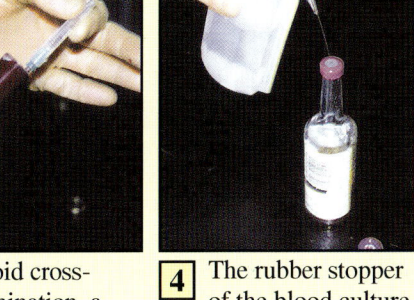
5. The required volume of blood is added to the bottle 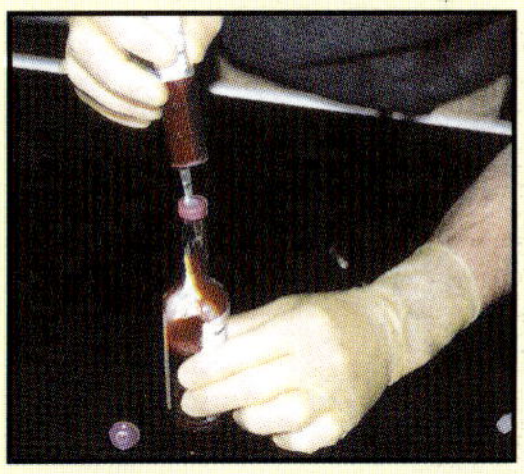
6. Two or three cultures should be obtained with a minimum of 1 hour in between. The bottles are kept at room temperature before transport to the laboratory with minimal delay

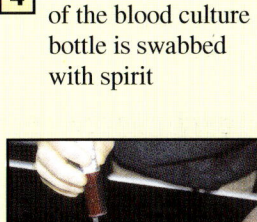

Notes
- It is helpful to get an assistant to raise the jugular vein
- The cephalic vein is inadequate for this procedure

Figure 7.5: Blood culture.

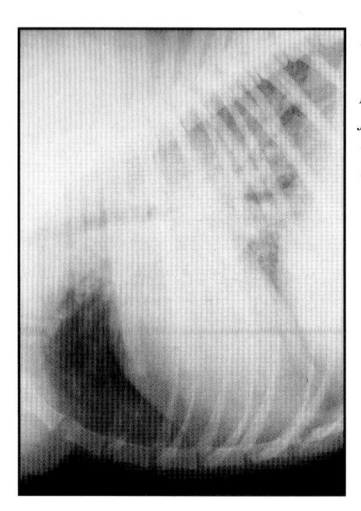

Figure 7.6: Lateral radiograph of embolic pneumonia resulting from bacterial endocarditis. (Courtesy of Dr Ian Ramsey.)

Joint fluid aspirates
Joint fluid aspirates can show either acute septic inflammation or evidence of immune-mediated disease.

Electrocardiography
An ECG can show a variety of dysrhythmias associated with primary damage to the cardiac conduction system from the endocardial infection, with coronary artery embolism or with the metabolic and other effects of cardiac failure and sepsis.

Echocardiography
Conventional two-dimensional echocardiography can be extremely useful to identify endocardial mass lesions either on valves or elsewhere on the endocardium. Doppler echocardiography can help identify and quantify associated valvular stenosis and insufficiency. It can also be used to assess the consequences of bacterial endocarditis on cardiac and valvular function and to look for evidence of predisposing congenital disease (Figure 7.7).

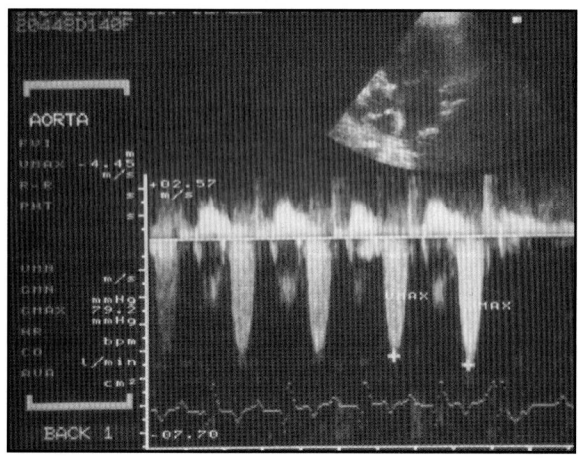

Figure 7.7: Continuous wave Doppler echocardiography of the aorta of a 3-year-old Curly Coated Retriever with bacterial endocarditis. There is a systolic jet of aortic stenosis and a decremental diastolic jet of aortic insufficiency.

Other tests
Tests for possible predisposing infections (e.g. feline leukaemia virus (FeLV), feline immunodeficiency virus (FIV) and feline coronavirus) should be performed as appropriate.

Treatment
Bacterial endocarditis should be treated with intensive cardiovascular and fluid support as indicated by the presence of cardiac failure and/or sepsis. High-dose intravenous bactericidal antibacterials are required to achieve adequate concentrations within the valvular lesions. These should be given for a minimum of 5 days, ideally on the basis of culture and sensitivity test results. If a positive culture and sensitivity spectrum is not available, the author uses a combination of a second generation cephalosporin (e.g. cefuroxime) and either a parenteral aminoglycoside (e.g. amikacin) or a fluoroquinolone (e.g. enrofloxacin). Clavulanate-potentiated amoxycillin is an alternative but should still be given intravenously. There are few suitable drugs in these categories that carry a veterinary licence.

Because of the potential for drug toxicity and interaction, and because of varied systemic consequences of bacterial endocarditis and thromboembolism, the patient should be closely monitored. Septic shock and disseminated intravascular coagulation (DIC) are common complications of bacterial endocarditis. The intravenous treatment should be followed by a long course (4-6 weeks at least) of appropriate oral antibacterials. Vegetation size and character can be monitored during treatment with echocardiography.

BACTERAEMIA AND SEPTICAEMIA

Definitions

- Bacteraemia is the presence of bacteria in the blood
- Endotoxaemia is the presence of endotoxins in the blood (which can cause endotoxic shock)
- Septicaemia is a systemic disease associated with the presence of bacteria or their toxins in the blood.

Bacteraemia can be an asymptomatic event in healthy animals, e.g. during dental procedures, and bacteria can be effectively eliminated by complement, antibody and the monocyte-macrophage system. Chronic bacteraemia (e.g. bacterial endocarditis) can cause a variety of infectious or immune-mediated diseases (Figure 7.8). Severe Gram-negative septicaemia can be associated with endotoxaemia and endotoxic shock. This can also occur when endotoxins enter the bloodstream from other sources, e.g. pyometra, gastrointestinal compromise.

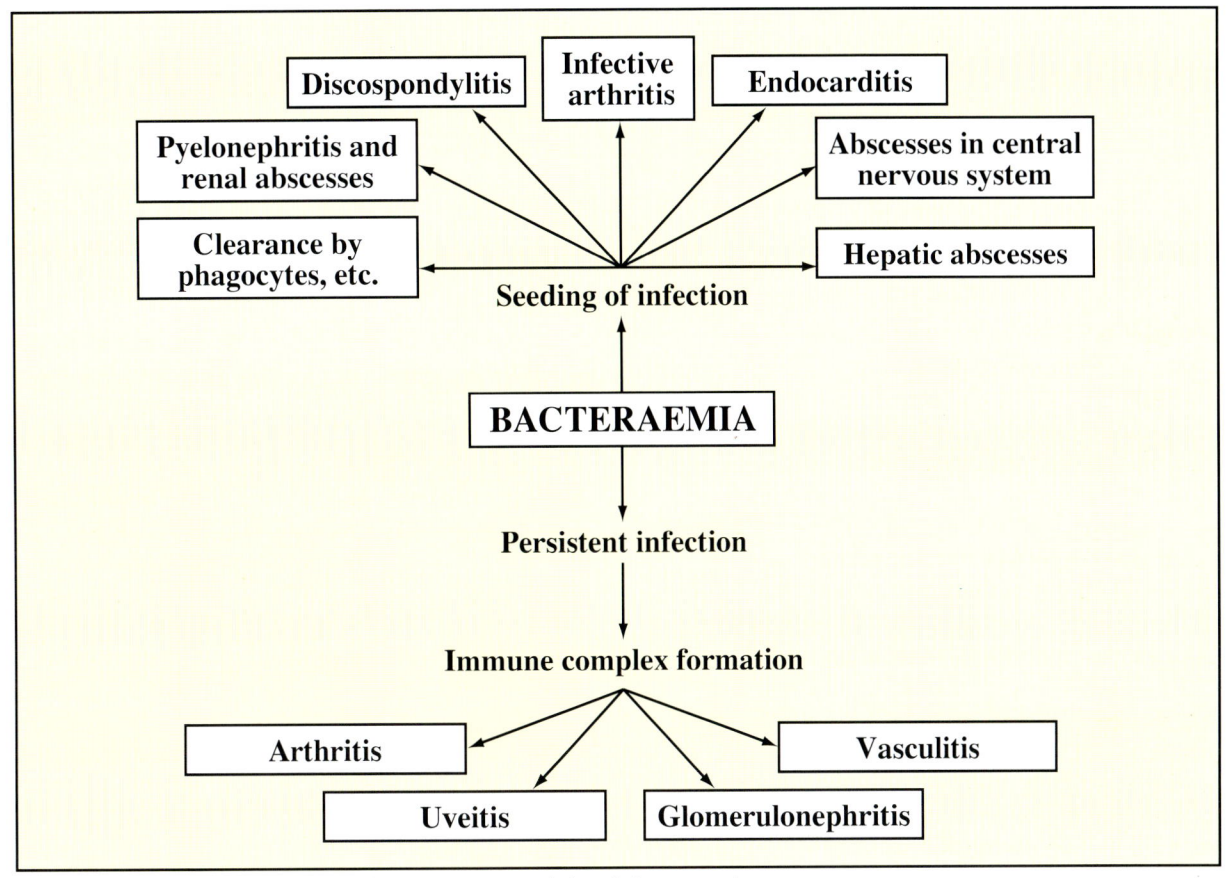

Figure 7.8: Immunological and embolic consequences of chronic bacteraemia.

History/clinical signs
Signs of chronic bacteraemia are similar to signs of chronic bacterial endocarditis. Septic/endotoxic shock causes fever, capillary dilation and vascular pooling, shunting of blood from tissue and activation of immune, clotting and other critical systems. As the condition progresses there is myocardial depression, hypotension and DIC. Hypoglycaemia may develop in some cases.

Clinical signs include:

- Fever and shivering (disordered thermoregulation); ultimately hypothermia develops
- Tachycardia (in response to vascular pooling and hypotension)
- Weak and thready pulses (hypovolaemia)
- Congested mucous membranes (vasodilation)
- Diarrhoea (particularly in dogs)
- Acute respiratory distress (particularly in cats)
- Spontaneous or excessive bleeding (DIC)
- Seizures (hypoglycaemia).

Organisms
Chronic bacteraemia can occur with similar organisms to those isolated from cases of bacterial endocarditis. *Salmonella* spp. are reported as common blood culture isolates in cats (Dow *et al.*, 1989). Gram-negative organisms responsible for bacteraemia and endotoxaemia include *Escherichia coli*, *Klebsiella pneumoniae*, *Enterobacter* spp., *Pseudomonas aeruginosa* and *Proteus* spp.

Differential diagnosis
Chronic bacteraemia can present with similar signs to various neoplastic and primary immune-mediated disease (see Pyrexia of unknown origin, below).

Endotoxic shock should be distinguished from hypovolaemic and cardiogenic shock using the patient's history and early clinical signs. As shock is a final common pathway, the distinction between the various causes of shock can be difficult in the advanced stages on clinical examination alone. However, clinical examination should try to identify primary sources of infection and/or endotoxin production.

Diagnostic plan
For chronic bacteraemia this should include haematology and biochemistry screens, urinalysis and culture, blood culture, survey radiography and ultrasonography, echocardiography and immune tests. For Gram-negative sepsis and endotoxaemia all of the above should be considered, as well as necessary tests to identify and treat serious metabolic imbalances, e.g. blood gas analysis, clotting screens, fibrin degradation products.

Treatment
The source of chronic bacteraemia or endotoxin should be identified and treated or removed.

Therapy in the interim should include:

- Intravenous fluid support
  - Shock doses should be given to maintain circulating blood volume
  - Colloids should be given early
  - Fresh whole blood or fresh frozen plasma may be a valuable addition
  - Hypertonic (7.5%) saline boluses (dog; 4-8 ml/kg, cat; 2-6 ml/kg) are beneficial.
- High-dose intravenous antibacterials
  - As for bacterial endocarditis
- Others
  - Oral nutritional support should be supplied to help maintain gastrointestinal mucosal integrity
  - Anti-endotoxin may sufficiently improve cardiovascular status to allow interventional therapy to treat the primary problem
  - In addition there are several therapies for endotoxic shock, which are controversial and are of minimal benefit or potentially harmful despite proven benefits. Two of these are:
    - Methylprednisolone sodium succinate (MPSS; 30 mg/kg i.v. given as a single dose) has been advocated for treatment of shock and shows benefit in certain models of canine endotoxic shock when given early. There is no proven clinical benefit, however, in using MPSS for canine septic shock, and its use may run the risk of secondary infection. The non-specific use of lower doses of other glucocorticoids given by different routes for the treatment of any form of shock, but particularly endotoxic shock, should be avoided
    - Early antiprostaglandin therapy, e.g. flunixin meglumine, may provide transient benefit but should be used with great caution because of risks of renal failure and gastrointestinal ulceration, especially in the face of tissue hyperperfusion and prior corticosteroid administration, respectively. There is little information on the use of carprofen and other modern antiprostaglandin drugs in endotoxic shock.

INTRAVASCULAR PARASITES

Angiostrongylus vasorum

Angiostrongylus vasorum (the 'French heartworm') is a metastrongylid parasite of canids that has been documented from most areas of England and Wales as well as mainland Europe. No cases have been reported in Scotland. Adult *A. vasorum* live in the pulmonary artery (Figure 7.9) and cause a granulomatous verminous pneumonia. Haemorrhages into the lungs and subcutaneous tissues result from a low-grade consumption of clotting factors (Ramsey *et al.*, 1996). Angiostrongylosis has also been associated with glomerulonephritis (D. Connolly, personal communication). *Angiostrongylus* requires a terrestrial mollusc (snail or slug) as an intermediate host. Dogs that have access to such invertebrates (e.g. kennelled dogs) are at a higher risk of developing an infestation.

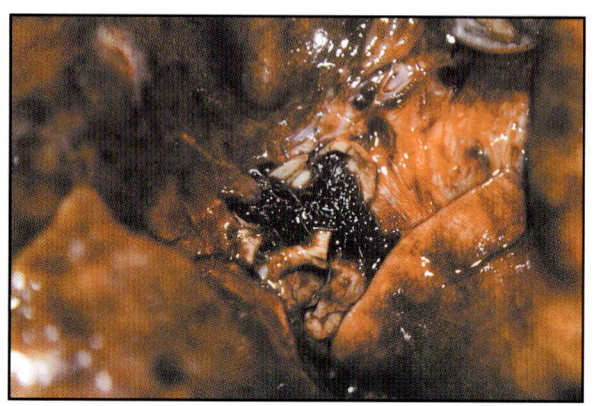

Figure 7.9: *Infestation of the pulmonary artery of a 2-year-old Boxer dog with* Angiostrongylus vasorum. *The dog died suddenly with central nervous system signs, presumed consequent to aberrant migration of worms or haemorrhage.*

History/clinical signs

Angiostrongylosis is most common in young dogs and can present with any of the following signs:

- Haemoptysis
- Coughing
- Dyspnoea
- Weight loss or poor growth
- Subcutaneous haemorrhages
- Weakness
- Collapse.

Hindlimb paralysis and other diverse manifestations have also been found owing to widespread haemorrhage. A history of ingestion of slugs or snails or shared territory with wild foxes may be apparent.

Diagnosis

Haematology may show an eosinophilia. Coagulation tests, such as whole blood clotting time and activated clotting time, will indicate a haemostatic problem in many cases. More specific tests usually yield a coagulopathy resulting from the deficiency of several factors. Fibrin degradation products may be increased.

Thoracic radiography in angiostrongylosis typically shows a bronchointerstitial pattern located in the dorsocaudal lung fields, sometimes with right-sided cardiac enlargement (Figure 7.10). Tracheobronchoscopy will often show major intrabronchial haemorrhage (Figure 7.11). Confirmation of infestation is by demonstration of larvae in bronchial washings (Figure 7.12) or in faeces by the Baermann method. Species identification should be performed by an appropriately experienced person.

Differential diagnosis
Figure 7.13 lists the differential diagnoses for angiostrongylosis.

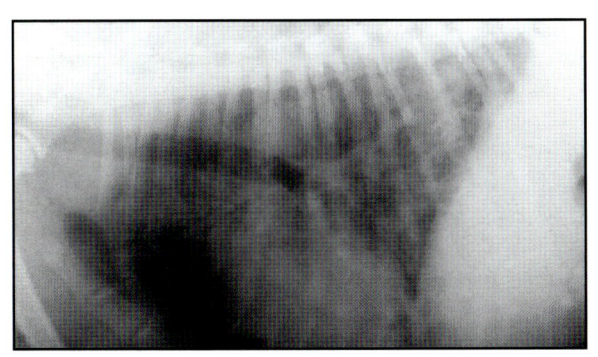

Figure 7.10: Right lateral thoracic radiograph of a 6-year-old female Border Collie with dyspnoea, haemoptysis and weight loss. There is a diffuse interstitial pattern. This dog had a verminous pneumonia caused by Angiostrongylus vasorum, *confirmed by tracheal wash cytology and faecal larval speciation.*

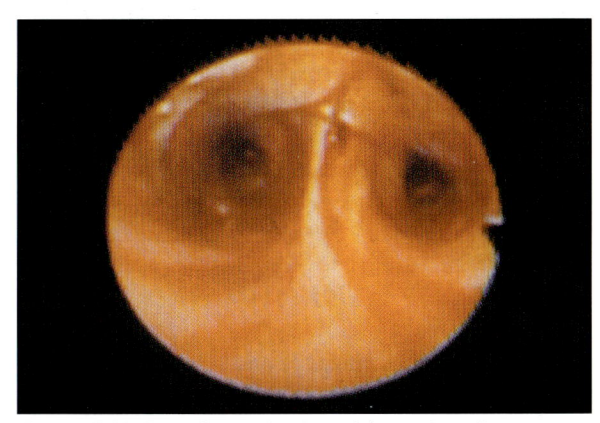

Figure 7.11: Bronchoscopic view of the carina of an 8-month-old Irish Wolfhound with haemoptysis due to Angiostrongylus vasorum *infestation. Fresh blood is visible in the lumen of the airway.*

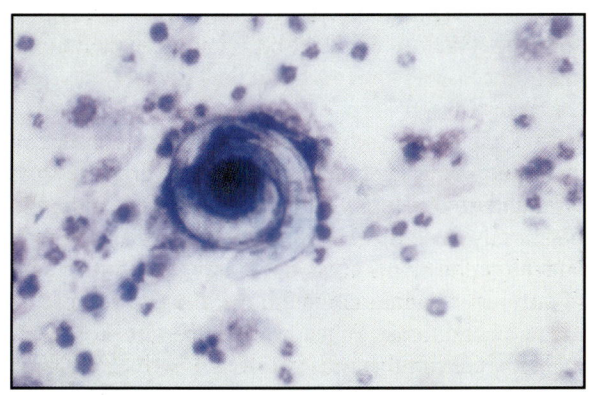

Figure 7.12: An Angiostrongylus vasorum *larva in a direct smear of a bronchial wash sample from a 4-month-old Shih Tzu that presented with coughing.*

Infectious pneumonias
Eosinophilic bronchitis
Congenital immunodeficiency (e.g. ciliary dyskinesia)
Acquired coagulopathies (including rodenticide poisoning)
Hereditary coagulopathies

Figure 7.13: Differential diagnoses for angiostrongylosis.

Treatment
Fenbendazole is effective. The prolonged course at this low dose is thought to reduce the risk of pulmonary thromboembolism subsequent to massive worm death. Other treatments, although often effective, carry the risk of complications.

Dirofilaria immitis
Dirofilaria immitis ('heartworm') is a filarial helminth that is endemic in much of the tropical and subtropical world, including southern parts of Europe and most of the USA. The adults are 10–35 cm long, the females being larger than the males. They are found predominantly in dogs, though feline infestation does occur occasionally. Cases of heartworm disease in the UK are confined to imported animals. Although the species of mosquito which can transmit the disease are found in the UK, the average ambient temperature is too low for the parasite to multiply in its vector. It is therefore unlikely that the disease will become endemic in the UK in the near future.

D. immitis causes pulmonary end-arteritis with intimal proliferation, eosinophilic pneumonia, pulmonary hypertension and cor pulmonale with right-sided congestive cardiac failure. Normal blood flow helps the worms maintain their position within the pulmonary arteries. The increase in pulmonary pressure is normally slight as the arterial lumen dilates. Heavy infestations may result in obstruction of the right atrium and cause acute severe tricuspid regurgitation (the 'caval syndrome'). Figure 7.14 shows the life cycle of *D. immitis*.

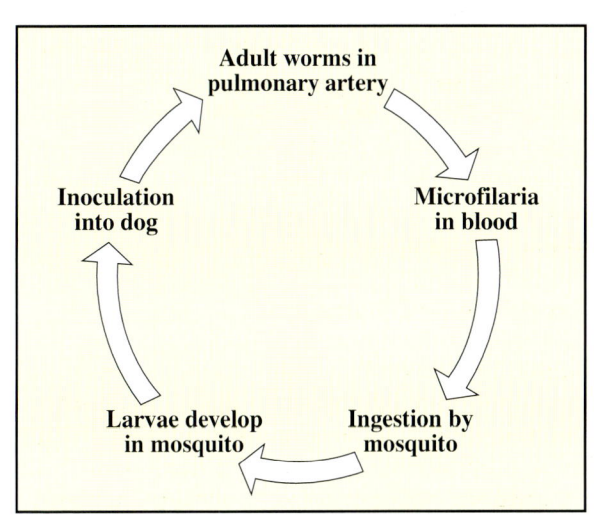

Adult worms in pulmonary artery → Microfilaria in blood → Ingestion by mosquito → Larvae develop in mosquito → Inoculation into dog → (Adult worms in pulmonary artery)

Figure 7.14: Life cycle of Dirofilaria immitis.

History/clinical signs
Heartworm occurs in adults and many light infestations are asymptomatic. Clinical signs in dogs include:

- Coughing
- Lethargy
- Weight loss
- Dyspnoea
- Abdominal distension
- Sudden death (due to embolization).

In cats, heartworm can manifest as vomiting, coughing, dyspnoea and anorexia. Migrating immature worms may be found in almost any location, particularly in the cat, and therefore may produce atypical signs. Heartworm has also been associated with glomerulonephritis (due to the deposition of immune complexes).

Differential diagnosis
Figure 7.15 lists the differential diagnoses for dirofilariasis. In cats, feline asthma (feline allergic bronchitis) is a major differential diagnosis.

Acquired heart disease
Congenital heart disease
Bacterial inhalational pneumonia
Chronic bronchitis
Eosinophilic bronchitis
Ciliary dyskinesia

Figure 7.15: Differential diagnoses for dirofilariasis.

Diagnosis
In symptomatic heartworm disease thoracic radiographs typically show pulmonary artery enlargement, tortuosity and 'pruning,' with an interstitial lung pattern. Echocardiography may identify the worms in some severe burdens. Eosinophilia, basophilia and a mild non-regenerative anaemia are often seen on haematology.

Heartworm infestation may be shown by identification of a microfilaraemia by using concentration tests (e.g. a modified Knott's test) or by identification of adult antigens using an enzyme-linked immunosorbent assay (ELISA). Serology is insensitive and non-specific. Blood smears can be examined for microfilaria but this is not a very sensitive test and 20-30% of infected dogs are amicrofilaraemic. Furthermore, experience is required in distinguishing the microfilaria from the harmless helminth *Dipetalonema reconditum*.

Treatment
The treatment of heartworm infestation has four components:

1. Management of the consequences of infestation (e.g. aspirin for pulmonary arteritis, corticosteroids for eosinophilic pneumonia, therapy of congestive heart failure)
2. Adulticide therapy (thiacetarsemide or melarsomine)
3. Microfilaricide treatment (levamisole, ivermectin or milbemycin)
4. Prophylaxis (ivermectin, milbemycin, moxidectin).

Adulticide therapy alone is insufficient, and reinfestations will occur. After adulticide treatment, strict rest is advised to avoid thromboembolic complications. Several of these drugs are not available in the UK, and the current regulations on their importation should be obtained from the Veterinary Medicines Directorate. If possible, ivermectin should be avoided in dogs (especially collie types) as the therapeutic index is lower than in other species. The use of adulticides may result in more complications in cats and, as the worms do not live as long in this species, symptomatic therapy is often all that is given while waiting for the adults to die (about 2 years).

Prophylaxis is routine in endemic areas. Note that the dose of ivermectin for prophylaxis is much lower than the treatment dose. Prophylaxis should be continued after importation as only some stages of the life cycle are treated by the drugs. Diethylcarbamazine is no longer widely used and should only be given to uninfected animals. Cats may given ivermectin for prophylaxis.

The treatment of caval syndrome requires urgent removal of the adult worms from the right side of the heart. This is usually accomplished by a jugular venotomy and gentle removal with long forceps. The complication rate is high and many dogs die of DIC or pulmonary thromboembolism.

PYREXIA OF UNKNOWN ORIGIN

Pyrexia is the commonest clinical sign of infectious diseases. It is associated with the depression and inappetence found in many of the conditions described in this manual. Pyrexia should always be distinguished from hyperthermia, which is an increased body temperature without an alteration in hypothalamic set point. Pyrexia, unlike hyperthermia, does not require emergency therapy to reduce body temperature. Pyrexia has been shown to have several beneficial effects, and animals with sepsis have been shown to have a higher mortality if they do not develop a febrile response. The use of non-steroidal anti-inflammatory drugs to treat mild and moderate fevers is usually unnecessary and potentially harmful. It is tempting to equate pyrexia with infection alone; however, it is also a common sign of various immune-mediated, neoplastic and inflammatory conditions. When pyrexia persists for more than 3 weeks and the cause of the pyrexia remains undiagnosed after repeated physical examinations and routine laboratory tests, the condition is referred to as pyrexia of unknown origin.

Differential diagnosis
Figure 7.16 lists the conditions associated with pyrexia of unknown origin.

Diagnostic plan
When faced with a case of pyrexia for which there is no apparent cause, it is helpful to perform a series (often quite extensive) of diagnostic tests (Figure 7.17). The clinical signs shown by an animal should be used to determine the most appropriate order for these tests.

DRUG DOSAGES

See Appendix 3.

Infectious diseases	
Bacterial endocarditis Bacteraemia (from any source) Localized soft tissue infections (e.g. lung, pleura, peritoneum, liver, kidney, prostate) Discospondylitis Feline infectious peritonitis Haemobartonellosis	Leptospirosis Infections secondary to immunosuppression (e.g. feline immunodeficiency virus) Rickettsial, protozoal and disseminated fungal infections (imported animals) Lyme disease
Immune-mediated diseases	
Immune-mediated polyarthritides (several types) Immune-mediated thrombocytopenia Immune-mediated haemolytic anaemia	Polysystemic immune-mediated diseases (e.g. systemic lupus erythematosus)
Neoplastic disease	
Lymphoproliferative diseases, particularly leukaemias, plasma cell myelomas and feline leukaemia virus-related diseases	Myeloproliferative disease Large or necrotic solid tumours
Miscellaneous diseases	
Metaphyseal osteopathy Hepatic portosystemic shunt (bacteraemia)	Panosteitis Pansteatitis (cats)

Figure 7.16: Conditions associated with pyrexia of unknown origin.

Test	Diagnostic information
Signalment	Breed-associated diseases (e.g. leucocyte adhesion deficiency of Irish Setter dogs) Sex-associated diseases (e.g. pyometra)
History	Onset and course of disease Clinical signs Disease in 'in-contacts' Exposures Responses to treatment
Physical examination (include rectal and ophthalmic examination)	Localization of clinical signs Evidence of pain/dysfunction Evidence of mass lesions/lymphadenopathy
Haematology	Examine for haematological malignancy and bone marrow disorders Evidence of responses to infection/inflammation
Biochemistry	Localization of organ disease Examine for severe systemic consequences
Urinalysis	Examine for urinary disease and help determine renal function
Urine protein/creatinine ratio	Examine for significant proteinuria
Urine culture	Examine for urinary infection
Faecal culture	Examine for enteric infection

Figure 7.17: Applicability of diagnostic testing to the investigation of pyrexia of unknown origin. (continues overleaf)

Test	Diagnostic information
Blood culture	Examine for bacteraemia
Thoracic radiography	Examine for pneumonia, pleural effusion, intrathoracic masses
Abdominal radiography	Examine for organomegaly, ascites, peritoneal disease, mass lesions
Skeletal radiography	Evidence for discospondylitis, panosteitis, metaphyseal osteopathy, hypertrophic osteodystrophy, osteomyelitis, polyarthritis, bone metastases, multiple myeloma
Echocardiography	Examine for endocarditic mass lesions
Abdominal ultrasonography	Examine liver, biliary tract, gastrointestinal tract, peritoneum, urogenital tract, pancreas
Thoracic ultrasonography	Examine extracardiac thoracic tissue
Aspirate effusions/masses	Culture and cytology
Aspirate lymph nodes	Examine for lymphosarcoma. Evidence for other disease
Joint taps	Examine for arthritis
Bone marrow biopsy	Examine for bone marrow disease
Serology	Examine for infections (e.g. feline leukaemia virus, feline immunodeficiency virus, feline infectious peritonitis, toxoplasmosis, neosporosis, leptospirosis, cryptococcosis, borreliosis) and autoimmune diseases (e.g. rheumatoid arthritis, systemic lupus erythematosus, immune-mediated haemolytic anaemia, immune-mediated thrombocytopenia)

Figure 7.17 continued: Applicability of diagnostic testing to the investigation of pyrexia of unknown origin.

REFERENCES AND FURTHER READING

Anderson CA and Dubielzig RR (1984) Vegetative endocarditis in dogs. *Journal of the American Animal Hospital Association* **20**, 149-152

Bennett D, Gilbertson EMM and Grennan D (1978) Bacterial endocarditis with polyarthritis in two dogs associated with circulating autoantibodies. *Journal of Small Animal Practice* **19**, 185-196

Boswood A (1996) Resolution of dysrhythmias and conduction abnormalities following treatment for bacterial endocarditis in a dog. *Journal of Small Animal Practice* **37**, 327-331

BSAVA Scientific Committee (1998) Heartworm disease. *Journal of Small Animal Practice* **39**, 407-409

Calvert CA (1982) Valvular bacterial endocarditis in the dog. *Journal of the American Veterinary Medical Association* **180**, 1080-1084

Calvert CA (1983) Treatment of heartworm in dogs. *Canine Practice* **18**, 13-28

Calvert CA, Greene CE and Hardie EM (1985) Cardiovascular infections in dogs: epizootiology, clinical manifestations and prognosis. *Journal of the American Veterinary Medical Association* **187**, 612-616

Cobb MA and Fisher MA (1990) *Angiostrongylus vasorum*: transmission in south east England. *Veterinary Record* **126**, 529

Dow SW, Curtis CR, Jones RL and Wingfield WE (1989) Bacterial culture of blood from critically ill dogs and cats: 100 cases (1985-1987). *Journal of the American Veterinary Medical Association* **195**, 113-117

Dow SW and Jones RL (1989) Bacteraemia: pathogenesis and diagnosis. *Compendium on Continuing Education for the Practicing Veterinarian* **11**, 432-443

Dunn JK and Gorman NT (1987) Fever of unknown origin in dogs and cats. *Journal of Small Animal Practice* **28**, 167-181

Elwood CM, Cobb MA and Stepien RL (1993) Clinical and two-dimensional echocardiographic findings in 10 dogs with vegetative bacterial endocarditis. *Journal of Small Animal Practice* **34**, 420-427

Martin MWS, Ashton G, Simpson VR and Neal C (1993) Angiostrongylosis in Cornwall: clinical presentations of eight cases. *Journal of Small Animal Practice* **34**, 20-25

Murdoch DB (1984) Heartworm in the United Kingdom. *Journal of Small Animal Practice* **25**, 299-305

Patteson MW, Gibbs C, Wotton PR and Day MJ (1993) *Angiostrongylus vasorum* infection in seven dogs. *Veterinary Record* **133**, 565-570

Ramsey IK, Littlewood JD, Dunn JK and Herrtage ME (1996) The role of chronic disseminated intravascular coagulation associated with a case of canine angiostrongylosis. *Veterinary Record* **138**, 360-363

Thomas WP, Reed JR, Bauer TG and Breznock EM (1984) Constrictive pericardial disease in the dog. *Journal of the American Veterinary Medical Association* **184**, 546

CHAPTER EIGHT

The Alimentary Tract

Bryn Tennant

CHAPTER PLAN

Introduction
Defence mechanisms of the alimentary tract
The oral cavity, pharynx and salivary glands
   Historical and clinical features
   Diagnosis
   Causes and treatment of infections
The oesophagus
   Historical and clinical features
   Infectious causes of disease
   Diagnosis
   Treatment
The stomach
   General historical and clinical features
   Causes of infection
The intestine
   Historical and clinical features
   Bacterial enteritides
   Viral enteritides
   Treatment of bacterial and viral infections
   Helminth diseases
   Protozoal diseases
   Mycotic diseases
   Rickettsial diseases
References and further reading

INTRODUCTION

Infections of the oral cavity, oesophagus, stomach and intestinal tract are some of the most important infectious and zoonotic diseases encountered in small animal medicine. They can be common, particularly in animals kept in groups or where a large susceptible population exists.

Some agents that cause similar clinical signs are discussed under a general category, e.g. pharyngitis. For other agents, particularly those involving the stomach and intestinal tract, the pathogenesis, clinical features and diagnosis of specific agents are dealt with individually. Most of the infectious agents discussed below generally affect only the alimentary tract and are often restricted to one area. Some are associated with multisystemic infections or have the potential to cause systemic infections.

DEFENCE MECHANISMS OF THE ALIMENTARY TRACT

Infectious agents gain access to the alimentary tract after ingestion or by a haematogenous route. Defence against infection depends on:

- Intact humoral (local and systemic antibody production) and cell-mediated immune systems
- Physical mechanisms - gastrointestinal motility, gastric acid, biliary and pancreatic secretions, mucous layer, constant turnover of mucosal cells and normal gut flora.

Conditions or situations that compromise these defence mechanisms predispose to infections. They include:

- Reduced gastrointestinal motility
- Immunosuppressive therapy, e.g. antineoplastic chemotherapy, corticosteroids
- Defective local immunity, e.g. secretory immunoglobulin A (IgA) deficiency
- Gastrointestinal surgery
- Anatomical/functional disease, e.g. exocrine pancreatic insufficiency, obstructive disorders, malabsorptive/maldigestive disorders
- Ingestion of foreign material that may abrade the mucosa
- Metabolic diseases causing debility, e.g. diabetes mellitus, hyperadrenocorticism, chronic renal failure, hepatic disease
- Protein-energy malnutrition resulting in villus atrophy and reduced immunocompetence.

THE ORAL CAVITY, PHARYNX AND SALIVARY GLANDS

Historical and clinical features

Disease of the oral cavity, whether due to infectious agents or non-infectious disorders, may be associated with abnormal food prehension, unwillingness to eat,

130 Manual of Canine and Feline Infectious Diseases

dysphagia, excessive movement of the tongue, abnormal mastication, pain, ulceration and drooling of saliva. Occasionally saliva may be blood tinged. Involvement of teeth is often associated with pain. Infectious disorders of the salivary glands may present with swelling of the salivary gland and, if the zygomatic gland is affected, epiphora and exophthalmos.

Diagnosis

If there is no evidence of systemic disease, examination of the oral cavity under general anaesthetic is required. It is essential that all oral and pharyngeal mucosal surfaces are examined. Confirmation of a diagnosis relies on demonstrating the presence of an infectious agent and histopathological changes in affected tissues. Swabs taken for bacterial culture are rarely of value, as a mixed growth of normal commensal bacteria is usually obtained. It is important to rule out non-infectious causes of oral inflammation (see below).

Causes and treatment of infection

Oral inflammation and/or granuloma formation develop as a consequence of many disease processes, including immune-mediated disease, renal failure, endocrinopathies, feline eosinophilic granuloma complex, neoplasia, trauma and a variety of primary infectious conditions (Figure 8.1). Of these only feline calicivirus (FCV) in the cat (see Chapter 6) is seen frequently. Secondary bacterial infections are very common. Systemic infections that might predispose to secondary infections of the oral cavity include feline leukaemia virus (FeLV), feline immunodeficiency virus (FIV), canine distemper virus (CDV) and feline panleucopenia virus (FPV). Treatment relies on managing the primary infectious or non-infectious disease. Resolution of the primary disease should result in resolution of the secondary infection. Antibacterial use for secondary bacterial infections is rarely warranted except in those that are chronic and deep seated, or where dental disease is the primary problem.

Feline calicivirus
Feline immunodeficiency virus
Papillomavirus (dogs)
Candida albicans (dogs, cats)
Miscellaneous bacteria, e.g. mycobacteria

Figure 8.1: *Infectious agents associated with oral inflammation.*

Candidiasis

Candida spp. are yeasts found as part of the normal mucosal flora. Of the nearly 200 *Candida* spp. only a few may occasionally act as opportunistic pathogens; the most important are *C. albicans* and *C. tropicalis*. Candidiasis is mainly a disease of keratinized epithelium. It is seen in immunosuppressed animals and those with pre-existing chronic oral and mucocutaneous ulcerative diseases. A white pseudomembranous covering or greyish mucoid plaques develop on mucosal surfaces, with irregular ulcers within areas of mucosal inflammation (Figure 8.2). Cutaneous, systemic and intestinal candidiasis have been rarely described in dogs and cats, with signs of fever, pleural effusion, anterior uveitis, osteomyelitis, diarrhoea and dermatitis reported. *C. albicans* can be recognized by demonstrating budding yeasts, pseudohyphae or true hyphae in cytology or histopathology preparations. Cutaneous or mucocutaneous candidiasis can be treated with topical antifungal agents (e.g. miconazole, clotrimazole, amphotericin B). Lesions within the oral cavity require systemic administration of amphotericin B, ketoconazole or itraconazole.

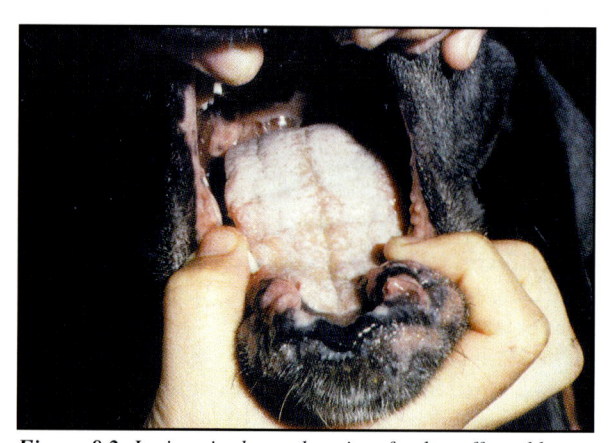

Figure 8.2: *Lesions in the oral cavity of a dog affected by* Candida *spp. (© Dr Susan Shaw.)*

Viral stomatitis

Viral stomatitis/gingivitis in the cat is principally associated with coinfection with FCV (see Chapter 6) and FIV (see Chapter 5). Ulceration and hyperplasia of the oral mucosa develop (Figure 8.3). Feline calicivirus can be cultured from oropharyngeal swabs submitted in virus transport medium. Caliciviruses have been isolated from dogs in association with glossitis, although their significance is unknown.

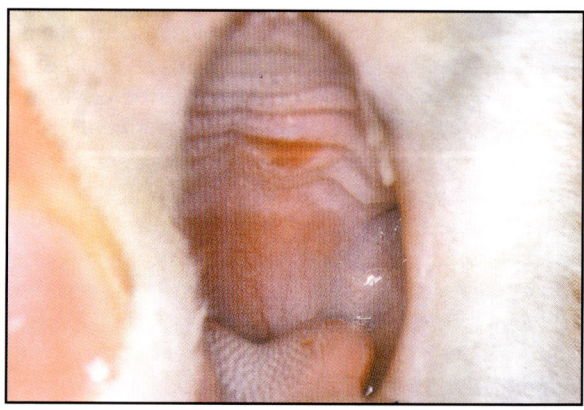

Figure 8.3: *Oral ulceration associated with feline calicivirus infection in a cat. (Courtesy of Dr Ian Ramsey.)*

Papillomatosis

Papillomavirus induces the formation of single or multiple fibropapillomas or dysplastic plaques, usually greater than 1 cm in diameter anywhere on the body including the oral cavity (Figure 8.4). Confirmation of papillomavirus requires demonstration of the virus using immunohistochemistry (not commercially available) or electron microscopy. Papillomas can be surgically removed. They have a tendency to recur. No specific treatment is available. Papillomas in young dogs may show spontaneous regression as the dogs grow.

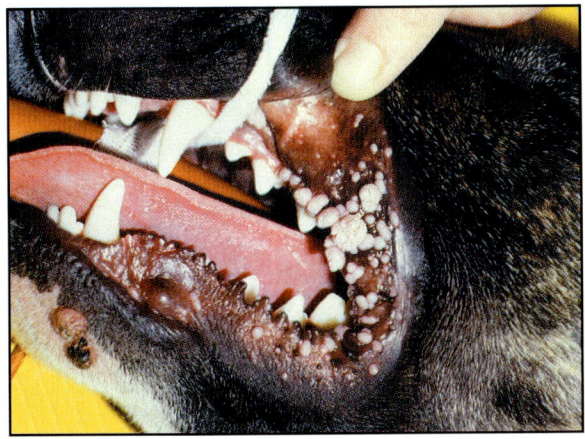

Figure 8.4: Papillomas in the oral cavity of a dog associated with papillomavirus. (© Dr Susan Shaw.)

Infectious agents and dental disease

The role of infectious agents in the development of dental disease is complex. Bacterial plaque formation plays a major part in the development of gingivitis and periodontitis. The oral bacteria that are present are poorly characterized, and individual species have yet to be correlated with specific dental diseases. Mature plaque reduces the oxygen tension at the gingival margin and sulcus thereby promoting the colonization of anaerobic bacteria that produce enzymes and toxins. These initiate inflammation in in-contact tissues. Gingivitis develops, which if left unchecked progresses to periodontitis. With the development of periodontal disease, deepening of the gingival sulcus and periodontal pocket formation results in the development of an anaerobic environment. This favours the growth of motile Gram-negative anaerobic rods, predominantly *Bacteroides* spp., *Fusobacterium* spp. and *Peptostreptococcus anaerobius*, in contrast to the normal oral flora of non-motile Gram-positive aerobic cocci. Other influencing factors include the efficacy of the local immune response, the presence of systemic disease (e.g. renal failure, endocrinopathies such as diabetes mellitus), immunosuppressive disorders and physical factors that influence plaque formation (e.g. overcrowding of teeth, reduced saliva production, soft diet, tooth anomalies).

Antibacterials are indicated in the management of periodontal disease either acutely (hours) to control iatrogenic bacteraemia at the time of the dental procedure or chronically (days to weeks) to manage specific severe periodontal disease. The antibacterials of choice are ampicillin, amoxycillin, clindamycin or metronidazole.

Sialoadenitis

Sialoadenitis may develop as an extension of infection from surrounding structures. Salivary gland abscessation has been reported but is extremely rare. Distemper virus causes inflammation of salivary glands, although this is usually not clinically evident. Non-infectious conditions of the salivary gland, e.g. mucocoele, infarction and neoplasia are more common diseases of this organ.

Tonsillitis/pharyngitis

Tonsillitis/pharyngitis is recognized occasionally, particularly in young dogs. The aetiology is unclear. Suggested causes include chronic regurgitation/vomiting, periodontal disease, chronic disease of the upper respiratory tract (e.g. rhinitis, sinusitis), foreign bodies and brachycephalic obstruction syndrome. Tonsillitis with or without pharyngitis can develop in young dogs without the involvement of any other area of the upper respiratory tract and presents with coughing and gagging. Currently infectious agents are not considered as primary agents in the development of tonsillitis, although bacteria may play a secondary role.

THE OESOPHAGUS

Historical and clinical features

Infectious conditions of the oesophagus result in oesophagitis and/or megaoesophagus. Signs of oesophageal inflammation vary; mild damage may be self-limiting and clinically silent whereas severe disease results in anorexia, dysphagia, excess salivation and regurgitation. Regurgitated saliva may be blood tinged. Palpation of the cervical oesophagus may elicit pain. The presence of glossitis/pharyngitis raises the possibility of trauma or ingestion of caustic material causing oesophagitis.

Causes of infection

Primary infections of the oesophageal mucosa have been reported but are extremely rare as causes of symptomatic oesophagitis (Figure 8.5). Opportunistic infections may, however, gain access to the submucosa as a result of oesophagitis resulting from ingestion of irritant (e.g. acids, alkalis, corrosive drugs) or traumatic materials (e.g. foreign body), or after anaesthesia, endoscopy or the use of naso-oesophageal tubes.

132 Manual of Canine and Feline Infectious Diseases

Candida albicans
Papillomavirus
Phycomyces
Feline calicivirus (see Chapter 6)
Secondary bacterial infection

Figure 8.5: Infectious agents associated with oesophagitis.

Infectious causes of megaoesophagus are listed in Figure 8.6. These agents cause various systemic signs and are discussed elsewhere; megaoesophagus is rarely a major clinical feature with these infections. Extra-oesophageal manifestations of infectious diseases may compress the oesophagus thereby causing regurgitation, e.g. FeLV-induced thymic lymphosarcoma.

Clostridium botulinum (see Chapter 15)
Clostridium tetani (see Chapter 15)
Trypanosoma cruzi – not in UK
Distemper virus (see Chapter 6)

Figure 8.6: Infectious agents associated with megaoesophagus.

Diagnosis
Endoscopy allows confirmation of oesophagitis. Specific features such as the presence of fungal plaques, or multiple mucosal vesicles or ulcers suggestive of calicivirus may be evident. Culture from swab material or histological assessment of oesophageal mucosal biopsies may be helpful.

Treatment
The need for antibacterials to manage non-specific secondary opportunistic bacterial infections depends on the degree of damage. With moderately severe or extensive mucosal damage or where deep oesophageal ulceration or aspiration pneumonia are suspected broad-spectrum antibacterial therapy is indicated. For most cases of oesophagitis, oesophageal rest (feed through a gastrostomy tube) and the use of mucosal protectants, e.g. sucralfate and H$_2$-blockers, such as ranitidine to combat the effects of gastro-oesophageal reflux, are indicated. If *C. albicans* is identified then systemic amphotericin B, itraconazole or ketoconazole can be considered.

THE STOMACH

General historical and clinical features
Historical and clinical signs associated with infectious and non-infectious gastric disorders are non-specific and include vomiting (chronic or acute), anorexia, depression, cranial abdominal pain, haematemesis, hypersalivation, pica and weight loss. There are no pathognomonic signs of gastritis that suggest an infectious disorder in preference to a non-infectious one.

Infectious conditions
Helicobacter spp.
Pysaloptera spp.
Viral infections, e.g. canine parvovirus, canine distemper virus (see section on intestine)
Pithiosis (not UK)
Roundworms (see section on intestine)
Ollulanus tricuspis
Cyathospirura spp.
Gnathostoma spp.

Non-infectious conditions
Diet – allergy/intolerance, spoiled food, foreign body, bacterial toxins
Ingestion of toxins
Drugs – non-steroidal anti-inflammatory drugs, corticosteroids
Neoplasia – mast cell tumour, gastrinoma, primary gastric tumours
Liver failure
Renal failure
Inflammatory bowel disease
Hypoadrenocorticism
Hypovolaemia
Pyloric gastropathy

Figure 8.7: Conditions that may result in signs of gastric disease.

Causes of infection
Of the many disorders that present with signs of a gastric disorder, the vast majority are not associated with infectious agents (Figure 8.7).

Helicobacterosis
Helicobacter spp. are spiral Gram-negative urease-positive bacteria found in the stomach and small intestine. *H. pylori* causes persistent active chronic gastritis and gastric ulceration in humans and has been associated with the development of gastric adenocarcinoma. Other species of gastric spiral organisms (GSOs) have been isolated from animals, including *H. felis* (dogs and cats) and *H. mustelae* (ferrets). Information on the importance of *Helicobacter* spp. in dogs and cats is lacking. Demonstration of inflammatory cell infiltrates concomitantly with GSOs in the gastric mucosa of dogs and cats is uncommon in the UK. In the dog, *Helicobacter* spp. are thought to cause gastritis, although asymptomatic infections are probably more common. GSOs can be isolated from cats, but the recovery rates are independent of gastrointestinal signs. Oral–oral and faecal–oral transmission is possible.

Endoscopy is the diagnostic modality of choice, allowing inspection of the mucosa and the taking of biopsy specimens and brushings for culture and cytology. A presumptive diagnosis of helicobacterosis may be made by demonstrating the presence of GSOs or by demonstrating urease activity in biopsy specimens of the gastric mucosa that also show inflammation histologically. The presence of GSOs alone without mucosal inflammation is insufficient to make a diagnosis of GSO-induced gastritis as they are commensals of the normal stomach. A definitive diagnosis of helicobacterosis requires isolation and characterization of the bacteria from gastric material; not all GSOs are *Helicobacter* spp. Historical information relating to drug therapy, ingestion of inappropriate or spoiled foods or signs consistent with systemic disorders such as renal, hepatic or adrenal failure may suggest a non-infectious cause. Serum biochemistry is rarely of value in identifying infectious disorders of the stomach. An inflammatory response may be seen on haematology, but is often absent.

Single antibacterials are ineffective at eliminating *H. pylori* in humans. Triple therapy using a combination of two antibacterials with a bismuth compound or an acid blocker such as cimetidine, ranitidine or omeprazole is prescribed. The antibacterial combinations most commonly recommended are amoxycillin/metronidazole or tetracycline/metronidazole. The recommendation for the use of triple therapy for *Helicobacter* infection in dogs and cats has been extrapolated from infections in humans and may not necessarily be required or effective.

Parasitic gastritis
Nematodes may infest the stomach but are rare causes of disease:

- *Ollulanus tricuspis* is a small trichostrongyle that inhabits the stomach of cats and pigs. Third stage larvae are excreted in vomit. The parasite lies beneath the mucous layer or partly in gastric glands. Infection is associated with increased numbers of lymphoid follicles, connective tissue and leucocytes in the mucosa. Heavy burdens result in mucous metaplasia and hyperplasia of gastric glands causing the stomach surface to be thrown into thickened convoluted folds resembling idiopathic hypertrophic gastritis in dogs. It is most commonly a problem in catteries where there is close contact between cats. The organism is transmitted in vomit
- *Physaloptera* spp. that infect the stomach include *P. praeputialis* (cat), *P. rara* (dogs, cats and wild canidae and felidae) and *P. canis* (dog). These nematodes utilize arthropod intermediate hosts. They resemble small ascarids and may be free in the lumen or embedded in the mucosa. They can induce lymphocytic/plasmacytic infiltration or ulceration at the site of insertion. Infection is often asymptomatic, although heavy burdens have the potential to cause major damage and protein loss. There are no reports of it occurring in the UK
- *Cycliospirura felineus* may be found in the stomachs of members of the Felidae. They are usually found in submucosal nodules. Pathogenicity is low and, there are no reports of it occurring in the UK
- *Cyathospirura* spp. have been reported in the stomachs of members of the Felidae. They are usually found free in gastric lumen. Pathogenicity is low, and there are no reports of it occurring in the UK
- Ascarids, hookworms and tapeworms may occasionally migrate into the stomach from the small intestine, causing irritation and nausea
- *Capillaria putorii* has been reported in the stomach of cats. It probably migrates from the intestine and is of little if any significance
- Gnathostomiasis is a rare problem in certain parts of the USA but more common in Asia and Australia. It has not been reported in Europe. *Gnathostoma* spp. are associated with the formation of a gastric mass that may be asymptomatic, mild gastritis or gastric perforation. This may be seen in dogs in more temperate areas imported from endemic areas
- Pseudomyiasis occurs when animals eat fly larvae, a rare problem.

P. rara may be identified endoscopically, although immature parasites are easily overlooked because of their size (2-3 mm long). *O. tricuspis* may be seen on microscopic examination of vomit or gastric juice/brushings either directly or after concentration using the Baermann technique (see Chapter 1). Faecal examination is unrewarding for demonstrating *Physaloptera* or *Ollulanus* infections.

Physaloptera may be treated using pyrantel or fenbendazole. Treatment of *Ollulanus* is difficult but fenbendazole may be effective. Single parasites of *Physaloptera* and fly larvae may be removed endoscopically. With gnathostomiasis surgical removal of the mass and associated parasite is recommended.

THE INTESTINE

Historical and clinical features
Signs of infectious enteritis are variable and similar to those of non-infectious enteritis; there are no pathognomonic signs indicative of specific infectious disorders. Signs include:

- Diarrhoea - this is invariably a feature; acute or chronic, watery, mucoid or haemorrhagic
- Vomiting, dehydration, pyrexia, inappetence, depression, increased vocalization, abdominal pain and signs of shock may be evident.

Large intestinal disease is usually associated with less severe signs than small intestinal disease, typically faecal tenesmus is seen and a mucoid diarrhoea that may contain fresh blood.

Bacterial enteritides

Many bacterial species are associated with enteritis (Figure 8.8). These represent some of the more major zoonoses; dogs and cats may act as reservoirs for human infection. Four general methods are recognized by which bacteria cause intestinal disease:

- Enterotoxigenic bacteria (e.g. enterotoxigenic strains of *Escherichia coli* (ETEC)) produce enterotoxins that stimulate intestinal epithelial cell secretion or directly damage the cell membrane of enterocytes. There may be no or very little associated inflammation. A secretory diarrhoea develops, which is large in volume and rich in electrolytes
- Cytotoxigenic bacteria (e.g. *Clostridium* spp., shiga-toxin producing strains of *E. coli* (STEC)) produce cytotoxins that damage enterocytes resulting in their loss and inflammation. The presenting picture is similar to enteroinvasive pathogens, although the bacteria itself does not invade or attach
- Enteropathogenic bacteria, also known as attaching and effacing bacteria (e.g. enteropathogenic strains of *E. coli* (EPEC)), attach to the surface of enterocytes and efface microvilli without invading the epithelial surface. Some may produce cytotoxins. The reduction in the surface area of the small intestine results in maldigestion and malabsorption
- Enteroinvasive bacteria (e.g. *Salmonella* spp., *Campylobacter* spp., *Yersinia* spp., enteroinvasive strains of *E. coli* (EIEC)) invade intestinal epithelial surfaces causing direct mucosal damage. Acute enterocolitis characterized by inflammation, exudation, hypersecretion and a mucoid, sometimes haemorrhagic diarrhoea develops. This is often accompanied by abdominal pain and pyrexia. Some organisms invade the submucosa and spread systemically via lymphatics and blood vessels. These bacteria may produce enterotoxins.

Bacteria	Viruses	Helminths
Salmonella spp.	Canine parvovirus-2	*Toxocara canis*
Campylobacter spp.	Canine distemper virus	*Toxocara cati*
Clostridium difficile	Canine adenovirus	*Toxascaris leonina*
Clostridium perfringens	Canine coronavirus	*Ancylostoma* spp.
Mycobacterium spp.	Canine rotavirus	*Uncinaria stenocephala*
Yersinia enterocolitica	Canine parvovirus-1	*Dipylidium caninum*
Yersinia pseudotuberculosis	Feline parvovirus	*Taenia* spp.
Bacillus piliformis	Feline coronavirus	*Echinococcus* spp.
Escherichia coli	Feline rotavirus	*Diphyllobothrium* spp.
Aeromonas hydrophila	?Feline astrovirus	*Spirometra* spp.
Plesiomonas shigelloides	?Reovirus	*Mesocestoides* spp.
?*Brachyspira* spp.	?Calicivirus	*Trichuris* spp.
Staphylococcal food poisoning	?Enterovirus	*Strongyloides* spp.
?*Chlamydophila felis*	?Torovirus	*Alaria* spp.
?*Lawsonia intracellularis*	?Herpesvirus	*Heterophyes heterophyes*
		Metagonimus yokagawi
		Echinochasmus perfoliatus
Protozoa	**Fungi/yeasts**	**Rickettsia**
Isospora spp.	*Aspergillus* spp.	*Neorickettsia helminthoeca*
Cryptosporidium parvum	*Pythium* spp.	*Neorickettsia elokominica*
Toxoplasma gondii	Mucoraceae	
Caryospora spp.	Entomophoracetes	
Neospora caninum	*Candida* spp.	
Hammondia spp.	*Histoplasma capsulatum*	
Eimeria spp.	*Prototheca* spp.	
Besnoitia spp.		
Sarcocystis spp.		
Frenkelia spp.		
Giardia intestinalis		
Pentatrichomonas hominis		

Figure 8.8: *Organisms that may infect the intestine of the dog and/or cat.*
A question mark indicates an organism that has not been proven to cause intestinal disease in the dog or cat.

Salmonellosis

Salmonella spp. are Gram-negative rod-shaped bacteria with a worldwide distribution. Infection may occur in all animals, and it is an important zoonosis. There are many *Salmonella* serotypes of varying pathogenicity. They may be acquired through contact with contaminated water or food and from exposure to infected faecal material. The organism multiplies rapidly in moist foodstuffs stored at room temperature or in foodstuffs inadequately cooked. *Salmonella* can survive in the environment for prolonged periods, especially where the temperature and humidity are high. Higher incidences of infection are reported in kennels and breeding establishments. This may relate to higher stocking densities, poor hygiene or animal attendants spreading infection via hands, boots, clothing or food bowls.

Salmonella spp. may be intermittently isolated from non-diarrhoeic faeces over prolonged periods and from colonic mucosa and mesenteric lymph nodes from asymptomatic animals, indicating the existence of carrier animals. Its true incidence in clinical disease is unclear. Transmission is via the faecal–oral route. *Salmonella* is an invasive bacterium and may spread to mesenteric lymph nodes. If the nodes are unable to contain the organism, septicaemia develops, and the infection may become established in other tissues (including placenta, conjunctiva, joints and meninges). Septicaemia may occur without signs of gastroenteritis. Carrier animals may exhibit gastrointestinal signs when subjected to stress or concurrent disease. Old, young and sick animals are more likely to be affected.

Acute gastroenteritis is the commonest clinical manifestation of salmonellosis:

- Diarrhoea, anorexia and depression with or without vomiting may be evident
- Dehydration may develop as a consequence of water and electrolyte losses
- Septicaemic animals are often pyrexic and show signs of pneumonia, meningitis, abortions, stillbirths or vaginal infection
- Mortality is greatest when septicaemia develops, but is uncommon with gastroenteritis (as long as supportive therapy is instituted).

Salmonella infection is confirmed by culture from faeces. If possible, samples of food should also be cultured to determine the source of infection. Blood cultures can be helpful in septicaemic patients and, if an animal dies, then samples from the small intestine, liver, kidney and lung should be submitted for bacteriology. All *Salmonella* isolates should be referred to a reference laboratory for precise identification of the serotype involved as this has zoonotic implications. The veterinary surgeon is under an ethical obligation to discuss with the owner the public health implications when salmonellosis has been confirmed in a dog or cat.

Treatment of affected animals depends on the severity of infection:

- Septicaemic animals require rapid and effective treatment comprising intravenous fluids and appropriate antibacterial therapy based on the culture and sensitivity. *Salmonella* spp. may show multidrug resistance
- Enteric salmonellosis is self-limiting and there is no indication for antibacterial drugs in the management of the acute uncomplicated case. Oral antibacterials do not reduce the severity of clinical signs, the rate of excretion or the likelihood of the carrier state developing. Fluoroquinolones are the exception to this rule (see below). Where there is evidence of gastrointestinal ulceration, systemic antibiosis is indicated
- Supportive therapy using oral rehydration or intravenous fluid therapy is required (see general treatment of bacterial and viral enteritides below).

Once clinical signs have resolved, reculturing on several occasions is recommended to ensure that the animal is not continuing to shed the bacteria. Recovered animals may excrete the bacteria for several months, posing a risk to other animals and humans. Fluoroquinolones have been shown to clear some carriers of the organism, although their routine use for this cannot be recommended in most cases. They have to be given for prolonged periods (possibly weeks), favouring the development of resistance in the intestinal flora and in the *Salmonella* isolate.

The prognosis is good in uncomplicated cases but guarded if septicaemia is present. Although *Salmonella* spp. are zoonotic agents, human infection from pet animals is rare; it usually follows the development of diarrhoea in the pet with contamination of the environment. As children are particularly at risk owing to their poor levels of hygiene, they should be kept away from diarrhoeic pets and increased attention paid to regular washing of the hands, especially prior to eating. Occasionally, pets will be affected concomitantly with other members of the household after introduction of a common infected foodstuff. Protective clothing should be worn by animal handlers in contact with the animals and they should wash thoroughly after handling infected patients and contaminated material. Where clinical disease has occurred, all infected material, including faeces, bedding and other contaminated material, should be incinerated and disinfection of the premises carried out. *Salmonella* is readily destroyed by desiccation, modern disinfectants and others such as phenolic compounds or a 1:32 bleach solution.

Campylobacteriosis

Campylobacter spp. are thin curved Gram-negative motile rods, evident in Gram smears as S-shaped, seagull-shaped, long spiral or coccoid bacteria. Many are commensals of the oral cavity, genital tract and intestinal tract and some non-pathogenic species are saprophytes in the environment. Their role as primary pathogens in companion animals has not been fully elucidated. *C. jejuni*, *C. coli*, *C. laridis* and *C. upsaliensis* can be isolated from diarrhoeic and non diarrhoeic dogs and cats. *C. jejuni* is isolated most commonly from diarrhoeic animals. They are opportunistic organisms and probably act synergistically with other infectious or non-infectious causes of enteritis. Any derangement in the gut flora may allow commensal *Campylobacter* spp. to overgrow and contribute to the disease state. For example, *C. jejuni* is more likely to cause disease in young animals where stressful conditions such as overcrowding and poor hygiene are present.

Campylobacter spp. are spread by the faecal-oral route through contact with undercooked/raw food (liver, chicken, raw tripe and unpasteurized milk), contaminated water, faeces from infected animals and contaminated food/water bowls or other implements. Infection is commonest in groups of animals in kennels. *Campylobacter* spp. may survive in water for long periods, resisting chilling and freezing.

Accurate figures for the incidence of *Campylobacter* infection in symptomatic companion animals have not been published. In colonies, up to 100% of dogs may be asymptomatic excretors of *Campylobacter* spp. The prevalence in colonies of cats has not been reported.

Campylobacter spp. have been associated with watery or mucoid diarrhoea, occasionally haemorrhagic, faecal tenesmus, dullness and inappetence. Illness is more often recognized in animals under 6 months old. Pyrexia reflecting systemic invasion and vomiting is rarely reported. *C. jejuni* produces an adhesin, a cytotoxin and a heat-labile toxin, of which the last two account for the clinical signs. Infection is generally self-limiting, and affected animals recover within 10 days. After infection a secretory IgA response develops that protects against subsequent colonization. Campylobacteriosis may rarely be associated with abortion as a consequence of fetal septicaemia.

Diagnosis of campylobacteriosis relies on demonstrating the organism in the presence of appropriate clinical signs:

- *Campylobacter* spp. may be detected by dark-field or phase contrast microscopy or on Gram-stained faecal material. These tests are of low sensitivity and cannot indicate the species
- Isolation of the organism from fresh (less than 24 hours old) faeces or rectal mucosal scrapes are reliable methods of diagnosis. Selective media are required
- Detection of *Campylobacter* spp. genetic material using polymerase chain reaction (PCR) technology is available; however, such tests have yet to be validated for companion animal species
- All *Campylobacter* spp. isolates from animals should be assumed to be potentially zoonotic and be fully identified
- As a carrier state exists a positive isolation of a *Campylobacter* spp. alone is not diagnostic for campylobacteriosis.

As campylobacteriosis is self-limiting and rarely develops into a systemic infection, therapy does not affect the clinical outcome. Antimicrobial treatment reduces the duration and severity of diarrhoea, minimizing the risk to humans and other animals. Erythromycin, chloramphenicol and fluoroquinolones are all effective; oral erythromycin for 10 days is the antibacterial agent of choice, whereas the use of fluoroquinolones should be reserved for resistant cases. Routine in vitro sensitivity testing using the disc diffusion method is unreliable for *Campylobacter* spp. as the activity of many antibacterials is affected by the high environmental carbon dioxide level required to culture the organism. Most *Campylobacter* species produce β-lactamases and are therefore resistant to penicillins and cephalosporins.

Some *Campylobacter* spp. are zoonotic agents and therefore:

- Infected material should be disposed of by burning or burial after disinfection
- Hands should be thoroughly disinfected after contact with infected animals or bedding; the organism is sensitive to most disinfectants
- Affected animals should not be mixed with susceptible ones
- Dogs with diarrhoea should be kept away from children and isolated from food preparation areas. Scrupulous hygiene and disinfection should be carried out.

Clostridiosis

Clostridium spp. are anaerobic Gram-positive spore-forming bacteria. They are commensal organisms in the intestinal tract. The two main isolates of concern are *C. perfringens* and *C. difficile*, both of which have been implicated in intestinal disease. Dual infection with *C. piliforme* and feline panleucopenia virus, causing enterocolitis in kittens, has been reported.

In humans a severe colitis has been reported after administration of certain antibacterials (e.g. clindamycin, lincomycin, ampicillin and cephalosporins) and is related to colonic overgrowth of cytotoxin-producing clostridia, particularly *C. difficile*. A similar severe ulcerative colitis has been suspected in dogs. The presence of the organism does not relate to the presence of disease. If colitis due to *C. difficile* is suspected, diagnosis requires:

- Demonstration of the cytotoxin in faeces (available from human hospitals)
- Isolation of the organism.

Mild cases respond to cholestyramine (a toxin-binding agent), whereas in severe cases metronidazole or tetracyclines may be required.

C. perfringens has been associated with peracute necrotizing haemorrhagic enteritis (HGE), a non-specific chronic mucoid diarrhoea and nosocomial diarrhoea. It may act as an opportunistic pathogen, contributing to disease associated with other conditions, e.g. parvoviral enteritis. There are five toxigenic types of *C. perfringens* (types A to E). Several are causes of enteric clostridiosis in herbivores. They are differentiated on the basis of which of the alpha, beta, epsilon and iota toxins they produce. The strains of *C. perfringens* associated with HGE in dogs are untyped. Type A strain (alpha toxin only) has been recorded in dogs with recurrent diarrhoea. Multiple serotypes of clostridia have been associated with hospital-acquired, usually non-fatal, small intestinal enteritis in dogs.

Features of HGE include very rapid development of clinical signs, and sudden death without premonitory signs can occur. Massive loss of extracellular fluid into the lumen of the gastrointestinal tract results in severe hypovolaemic shock and an increase in PCV. Signs of intracellular fluid loss, e.g. abnormal skin turgor, are usually not apparent at the acute stage. Serum biochemistry and other haematological variables are usually unremarkable, in contrast to canine parvoviral enteritis.

Chronic mucoid diarrhoea associated with *C. perfringens* presents as a typical large bowel diarrhoea with mucous, fresh blood and increased frequency of defecation. Pain and difficulty in defaecating may be apparent. Weight loss is not a feature. There are no pathognomonic signs associated with this presumed manifestation of clostridiosis. Faeces from cases of nosocomial diarrhoea associated with enterotoxigenic *C. perfringens* vary from watery to mucoid; haemorrhagic diarrhoea is rare. Diarrhoea lasts for a few days.

A presumptive diagnosis of clostridiosis relies on:

- Isolating the bacteria
- Demonstrating large Gram-positive rods associated with endospores in Gram's smears from faeces
- Demonstrating *C. perfringens* enterotoxin in faeces (although *C. perfringens* may be isolated from symptomatic and asymptomatic animals, its enterotoxin is only found in animals with diarrhoea); commercial assays are available for alpha, beta and epsilon toxins
- Leucocytes are expected in cytology preparations from faeces.

Treatment of HGE:

- Systemic antibacterials are required to manage opportunistic secondary infections that take advantage of intestinal mucosal ulceration. Clavulanate-potentiated amoxycillin (preferred antibacterial), ampicillin, metronidazole, clindamycin, aminoglycosides or cephalosporins are suggested
- Fluid replacement (e.g. Hartmann's solution) at a high flow rate for the first hour (up to 70 ml/kg/h may be required), subsequently reducing the flow rate to balance continued losses
- Hypoproteinaemia may develop requiring plasma transfusion if available.

Treatment of chronic mucoid diarrhoea:

- Oral antibacterials (ampicillin, metronidazole, clindamycin, tylosin) reduce clostridial bacterial numbers
- A high fibre diet alters the colonic microenvironment, reducing clostridial bacterial numbers
- Cholestyramine may be helpful
- In relapsing cases tylosin may be required long term.

Mycobacteriosis

Mycobacteriosis is covered in detail in Chapter 6. *Mycobacterium* spp. may affect the gastrointestinal tract, resulting in a granulomatous enteritis that manifests with vomiting, diarrhoea, mesenteric lymphadenopathy and ascites. Diagnosis relies on demonstrating acid-fast bacteria in fluid or intestinal biopsies.

Yersiniosis

Yersinia enterocolitica is a motile Gram-negative rod that causes chronic enterocolitis and occasionally bacteraemia in humans. Dogs have been shown to be carriers, and rarely young dogs may develop clinical signs of haemorrhagic mucoid diarrhoea, increased frequency of defecation and tenesmus in association with the organism.

Y. pseudotuberculosis infections in cats results in a disseminated pyogranulomatous condition primarily involving the gastrointestinal tract, mesenteric lymph nodes and liver. Clinical signs include vomiting, diarrhoea, weight loss, depression, pyrexia and jaundice. It is usually fatal.

Yersinia infection may be confirmed by isolation of the organism from faeces. *Y. enterocolitica* is usually susceptible to trimethoprim–sulphonamide, tetracycline, chloramphenicol and aminoglycosides, although sensitivity profiles from cultures should be used. Treatment of cats affected by *Y. pseudotuberculosis* is often unrewarding.

Bacillus piliformis (Tyzzer's disease)

Bacillus piliformis is a pleomorphic Gram-negative spore-forming obligate intracellular bacillus. Rodents are the main reservoir of the bacteria. It is a rare cause of haemorrhagic necrotizing enterocolitis and hepatic necrosis, with young animals most likely to be affected. It is rapidly progressive and invariably fatal. The disease may develop as a complication of other infectious conditions, e.g. parasitism, canine parvovirus, canine distemper virus. Diagnosis can be confirmed histologically; the bacteria cannot be cultured in routine media.

Escherichia coli

Pathogenic strains of *E. coli* fit into one of five main groups:

- Enteropathogenic strains (EPEC) - associated with disease in young dogs
- Enterotoxigenic strains (ETEC) - associated with disease in young dogs
- Enteroinvasive strains (EIEC) - not reported in dogs or cats
- Cytotoxin (vero or shiga toxins) producing strains (VTEC or STEC) - isolated from healthy and diarrhoeic cats and dogs; their significance is unclear
- Enteroaggregative (EAggEC) strains - not reported in dogs or cats.

Data relating to the role of *E. coli* as a cause of disease in cats are lacking.

The clinical signs associated with *E. coli* vary with the specific strain involved (see classification of bacterial infections earlier). Acute diarrhoea that may be haemorrhagic, and/or associated with vomiting, is expected. Anorexia, depression and pyrexia may be seen; pyrexia is most likely if systemic invasion occurs. Dehydration is expected with severe disease, and death can occur rapidly.

As *E. coli* is a commensal organism in the intestinal tract its isolation in routine cultures is to be expected. Differentiation of pathogenic from non-pathogenic strains relies on:

- Demonstrating the presence of toxins. Toxins produced by isolates pathogenic for the dog and cat have not been characterized. Although assays used in human medicine have not been validated for canine/feline isolates, they may be of some value
- Detection of genes that code for toxins or the ability to attach and efface enterocytes. Commercial assays are unavailable
- Serotyping. Serotypes isolated from dogs are different from those found in humans and other animals and thus cannot be identified in current assays
- Histology. Demonstrating the organism attached to enterocytes in biopsy samples is helpful; this is likely to be performed only as part of a post-mortem examination.

Miscellaneous bacteria

Various other bacteria may be isolated from diarrhoea (some require selective media). These include:

- *Aeromonas hydrophila* - this is associated with small bowel diarrhoea in dogs, particularly puppies, although its role as a primary cause of enteritis is unclear
- *Plesiomonas shigelloides* - this may be isolated from the faeces of dogs, particularly puppies, presented with small bowel diarrhoea. Its significance is unclear
- *Brachyspira* spp. - these have recently been isolated from cases of diarrhoea in dogs, although their role as pathogens is still unclear. Several isolates with different cultural and morphological characteristics have been defined. The organism may be a commensal spirochaete that overgrows secondary to other intestinal disorders. *Brachyspira* spp. are recognized causes of colitis in humans and pigs
- Staphylococcal food poisoning - this is a well recognized cause of enterotoxigenic diarrhoea in humans but has not been well described in dogs
- *Chlamydophila felis* (formerly *Chlamydia psittacci* var *felis*) - this is a rare cause of intermittent vomiting and diarrhoea in the cat. Ocular signs may be present as well (see Chapter 16)
- *Lawsonia intracellularis* - there is one report of diarrhoea in a puppy being associated with this agent. It is a cause of intestinal disease in other species, including guinea pigs, pigs and horses.

Viral enteritides

Many viruses (see Figure 8.8) play a part in the development of gastroenteric disease either as primary enteric pathogens or as part of a multisystemic disorder.

Canine parvovirus type 2

Epizootiology and pathogenesis: Canine parvovirus type 2 (CPV-2) appeared as a pathogen of dogs in 1978. The original CPV-2 strain was replaced between 1979 and 1981 by CPV type 2a, which in turn has largely been replaced by CPV type 2b. Although CPV-2 was only able to infect members of the Canidae, type 2a and type 2b replicate efficiently in cats, and about 10% of isolates from cats with natural parvovirus disease are antigenically indistinguishable from these strains (Truyen *et al.*, 1996). CPV-2 has a worldwide distribution and is far more commonly recognized than CPV-1 (see below). The current incidence of CPV-2 infection is unknown, although seroprevalence is high owing to widespread vaccination. Transmission is via contact with infected dogs or cats or environmental virus; CPV-2 may survive for months to years in the environment. Persistent or periodic faecal shedding from infected dogs does not seem to be a feature of CPV-2 infection; viral shedding ceases no later than 14 days post infection. CPV infects all cells although viral replication and therefore disease is only evident in tissues with high mitotic rates, e.g. lymphoid system, bone marrow and crypt epithelia of the intestinal tract. Infection may result in lymphoid depletion, leucopenia and intestinal crypt necrosis, respectively. In puppies under 4 weeks of age CPV-2 has an affinity for myocytes, and the resulting myocarditis can cause cardiac failure (although this is now very rare).

After ingestion or inhalation, CPV probably enters through pharyngeal or gut-associated lymphoid tissue and replicates in systemic lymphoid tissue. Viraemia from day 3 or 4 post infection distributes virus to all cells. Viraemia is terminated when virus neutralizing antibodies appear, usually days 5-7 post infection. Clinical signs are evident between days 4-7 post infection. Virus excretion increases up to the fifth and sixth days post infection as clinical disease progresses and ceases by days 7-14 post infection. Serum antibodies can be detected in all dogs by day 7, increasing to maximal titres by days 7-10. After recovery, high titres are maintained in dogs for at least 2 years.

Clinical features: Dogs of any age can be infected, although the incidence of disease is highest in those under 1 year of age. The severity of clinical signs after CPV infection depends on several factors including:

- Maternally derived antibodies (MDA). These protect puppies or reduce the severity of disease up to 12 weeks of age (in some cases MDA are non-protective by 8 weeks or less). The incidence of CPV myocarditis is low because of the protective influence of MDA
- Vaccination status
- Stress factors, e.g. overcrowding, poor hygiene
- Presence of other enteric pathogens, e.g. canine coronavirus, *Salmonella*, *Campylobacter*, *Clostridium*, intestinal parasites
- 'Gut stress.' The high incidence in puppies that have been recently rehomed may relate in part to 'gut stress.' Puppies may be reluctant to eat in their new environment, resulting in reduced enterocyte turnover. Once they start eating, enterocyte turnover increases, providing a more favourable situation for CPV-2 infection to establish itself
- The magnitude and duration of the viraemia.

Parvoviral enteritis presents acutely or peracutely with anorexia and depression followed within a few hours by vomiting and profuse, usually haemorrhagic, diarrhoea; occasionally mild non-haemorrhagic diarrhoea is reported. Pyrexia, depression that is often severe, anorexia and dehydration are expected. Oral ulceration is a rare feature. Damage to the intestinal mucosa permits bacterial translocation and overgrowth that can result in endotoxic shock characterized by signs such as hypothermia, disseminated intravascular coagulation (DIC) and jaundice. Death occurs in severe cases and particularly in young animals as a consequence of dehydration, endotoxic shock, electrolyte imbalances or overwhelming secondary bacterial infection. Mortality is as high as 7-10% of treated puppies but does not generally exceed 1% of the adult population. Mild or inapparent infections are common, particularly in dogs over 6 months of age.

Diagnosis: Parvovirus can be suspected from the clinical signs and history of exposure. Panleucopenia is present in 85% of affected dogs within 72 hours of the onset of enteric signs. Neutropenia results from CPV-2-induced marrow necrosis and depletion of circulating mature neutrophils as a consequence of their migration into the inflamed intestinal mucosa. An increase in the white cell count is an indicator of recovery. Occasionally a reactive lymphocytosis is seen. The normal or slightly reduced PCV helps to distinguish parvoviral enteritis from haemorrhagic gastroenteritis (see clostridiosis above). At post-mortem examination marked intestinal inflammation is evident (Figure 8.9).

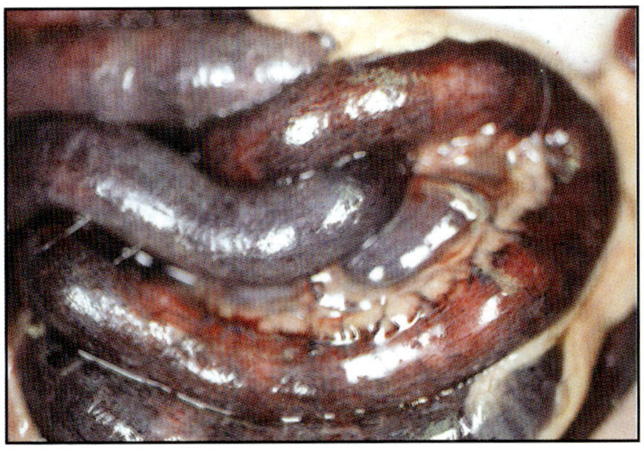

Figure 8.9: Markedly inflamed small intestine associated with canine parvovirus infection. (© Dr Bryn Tennant.)

Various diagnostic tests are available to attempt to confirm CPV-2 infection:

- Histopathology is useful in confirming parvoviral enteritis
- Demonstration of the virus in faeces using a haemagglutination assay, an enzyme-linked immunosorbent assay, electron microscopy or virus isolation. This is often unrewarding as virus excretion may cease once clinical signs develop

- Serology. This is of limited value as a significant rise in antibody titre over the course of the disease may be difficult to demonstrate once clinical signs have developed. High antibody titres are often already present by day 7 post infection prior to or consequent with the development of clinical signs
- Demonstration of anti-CPV-2 IgM is indicative of a recent infection (unavailable in the UK)
- Viral antigens may be demonstrated in tissues using immunocytochemical methods, although this is not commercially available.

Treatment and prevention: There is no specific treatment for CPV-2 infection. Supportive therapy is required (see general treatment of bacterial and viral enteritides). Very effective and safe modified live vaccines are available to prevent CPV infection. They induce a long lasting immunity and a consistent response. The timing of primary and booster vaccinations is a matter of debate. Puppies are protected against CPV for the first few weeks of life by MDA. The duration of this immunity is highly variable, with some puppies becoming susceptible to infection at 6 weeks of age whereas others may be protected for up to 18 weeks. Low levels of MDA may interfere with vaccine virus reducing its efficacy but may not protect against infection or disease. This has led to suggestions that puppies whose immune status is unknown should be vaccinated every 3 weeks from 6 weeks to 18 weeks of age. Many vaccines now contain high titre virus, which enables them to overcome MDA and therefore induce immunity before protection from MDA is lost; the use of such vaccines often only requires two doses. Immunity after the use of a modified live vaccine lasts from 1-3 years. Currently annual boosters are recommended to ensure that all dogs are protected, although it is accepted that not all dogs require annual boosters. Assessment of serum antibody levels can be used to determine whether booster vaccination is required. Titres greater than or equal to 1:80 are considered protective.

Animals with suspected parvovirus infection should be isolated. Waterproof protective clothing and protective footwear that can be disinfected or disposed of should be worn by all individuals in contact, and they should wash thoroughly after handling the patients and contaminated material to prevent spreading the virus. All infected material, including faeces, bedding and other contaminated material, should be incinerated and disinfection carried out. Several commercial disinfectants and sodium hypochlorite (household bleach, diluted 1:32) are effective for killing parvoviruses.

Canine distemper virus
Canine distemper virus (CDV) affects the epithelial surfaces of respiratory, alimentary and urogenital tracts, skin and CNS. There is only one serotype of CDV but many strains that vary in their tissue tropism and pathogenicity. Clinical signs are highly variable, often severe and may be restricted to one organ system or present with multisystemic involvement. See Chapter 6 for a discussion of the pathogenesis, diagnosis and management of CDV infection.

Gastrointestinal localization of CDV results in gastroenteritis characterized by vomiting and a mild to severe, often haemorrhagic, diarrhoea 10-20 days post infection. As with CPV-2, pyrexia, endotoxic shock and secondary bacterial infections may complicate the clinical picture. When enteric signs predominate it can be difficult clinically to distinguish CDV from CPV-2 infection. More commonly, respiratory and/or neurological signs are present concomitantly with enteric signs, allowing CPV-2 to be excluded. There is no specific treatment for CDV. Supportive therapy is required (see below). The prognosis is guarded and depends largely on the severity of signs and the extent of multiorgan involvement. Mortality often approaches 50%.

Canine adenovirus
Canine adenovirus-1 (CAV-1) has a tropism for hepatocytes and endothelial cells. Haemorrhagic diarrhoea may be seen because of vascular endothelial damage in the intestine. Adenoviruses serologically similar to but genetically distinct from canine adenovirus-2 (CAV-2) have been isolated from diarrhoeic faeces. CAV is discussed in detail in Chapter 11.

Canine coronavirus

Epizootiology and pathogenesis: Canine coronavirus (CCV) has a worldwide distribution, with a seroprevalence of 54% in family dogs and 100% in some kennel populations. Dogs of all ages and breeds are susceptible to infection. The virus can be isolated from diarrhoeic and non-diarrhoeic faeces. Its role as a primary pathogen is equivocal. Although CCV is isolated in association with disease, particularly in dogs aged 6-12 weeks, it may be acting as a secondary pathogen.

Lysis of CCV-infected enterocytes causes epithelial loss and villus atrophy; crypt cells are unaffected. Colonic and alveolar epithelium and mesenteric lymph nodes may be infected, although this seems to be clinically insignificant. The incubation period is from 1-7 days. Viral shedding persists for at least 16 days post infection and virus neutralizing antibodies are detected by day 5 post infection.

Clinical features: CCV infection is usually associated with very mild or subclinical disease. When diarrhoea develops it is usually watery. Very occasionally more severe signs of acute onset depression and anorexia followed by vomiting and diarrhoea are seen. Haemorrhagic diarrhoea, pyrexia and leucopenia are not associated with uncomplicated CCV infections; the presence of such findings reflects the presence of other concomitant infections. Dual infections of CCV and CPV-2 have been reported in up to 25% of animals with enteritis (Evermann et al., 1989). CCV may increase the severity of disease associated with CPV-2, as loss of epithelial cells from villi after CCV infection stimulates replication of crypt cells making them more susceptible to parvoviral infection. Spontaneous recovery occurs over 7-10 days, although occasionally diarrhoea has been reported to persist for several weeks. Mortality is very rare and is most often seen after neonatal infection. The prognosis for a complete recovery is good.

Diagnosis: As clinical signs are mild and dogs respond well to symptomatic treatment, confirmation of the diagnosis is usually unnecessary. A definitive diagnosis can be made by:

- Demonstrating virus particles, either by electron microscopy or virus isolation, in fresh diarrhoeic faeces examined or cultured within 48 hours. False negative results are common as coronaviral particles are fragile and are easily disrupted with prolonged storage
- Paired serology showing a fourfold rise in antibody titres allows the diagnosis to be made retrospectively. This is not available commercially; however, with slight modification, the commercially available feline coronavirus serology tests can be used.

Treatment and prevention: There is no specific treatment for CCV. Supportive therapy may be required (see below). Protection against CCV infection is provided by mucosal IgA, stimulated by infection of the intestine. Systemic antibodies induced by parenteral vaccination do not protect against infection probably because vaccination does not induce an appropriate mucosal immune response. Oral vaccination is more likely to induce protection, although, given the low incidence of disease and the mild clinical presentation, CCV vaccination is not indicated.

Canine rotavirus

Rotaviruses are major pathogens in humans and farm animals and have been isolated from dogs with diarrhoea. Seropositive rates of up to 84% of the canine population indicate that canine rotavirus (CRV) is widespread. However, CRV has not been proven to be a significant enteric pathogen in the dog. Infection of puppies under 4 weeks of age has been associated with a self-limiting mild watery to mucoid diarrhoea. Rare fatalities have been reported, although whether this was due to rotavirus is unclear. Clinical disease is more likely in overcrowded unhygienic conditions, when concomitant infections with other enteric pathogens may complicate rotavirus infection. In dogs over 6 months of age only subclinical infection occurs. The incubation period ranges from 1-7 days.

Diagnosis is by detection of virus in faeces using polyacrylamide gel electrophoresis (PAGE), ELISA (detects some rotaviruses), electron microscopy or virus isolation. Serology is of little value and is not currently available in the UK. There is no specific treatment for CRV. Supportive therapy may be required.

Canine parvovirus-1

Canine parvovirus type-1 (CPV-1), also referred to as the 'minute virus of canines' (MVC) was long thought to be of no or minimal pathogenicity. Recently it has been associated with mild to severe illness involving the intestinal tract (diarrhoea), the respiratory tract (bronchitis and interstitial pneumonia) and fetal resorption and abortion. One survey reported a seroprevalence for MVC of 50% in adult dogs from across the USA. Its prevalence in the UK is unknown. Confirmation of infection by this virus is difficult as there are no serological assays available in the UK and its isolation is difficult.

Feline parvovirus

Epizootiology and pathogenesis: Feline parvovirus (feline panleucopenia virus; FPV) is a highly contagious infection of cats including domestic and wild cats. It has a worldwide distribution and is a cause of enteritis, panleucopenia, fetal death, cerebellar disease and possibly myocarditis and idiopathic cardiomyopathy. The disease has become uncommon in the UK since the advent of effective vaccines. Cats are also susceptible to strains of FPV that are almost identical to CPV-2. These cause disease very similar to that associated with FPV and transmission from dogs is possible.

Transmission is via direct contact with infected cats or environmental virus. Virus may persist in recovered cats for several months and in kittens infected *in utero* for up to a year. It persists in secretions in the environment for months to years.

After ingestion, the virus replicates in pharyngeal or gut-associated lymphoid tissue. Following viraemia FPV infects all cells, although viral replication and therefore disease is only evident in tissues with high mitotic rates, including:

- Crypt epithelia in the intestinal tract. The virus causes intestinal crypt necrosis
- Lymphoid tissue (lymph nodes, spleen and thymus) and bone marrow. The virus destroys lymphocytes and leucocyte stem cells; red cell stem cells seem to be less affected or unaffected
- Placental and fetal tissue, particularly the cerebellum, causing cerebellar hypoplasia
- Myocardium, causing myocarditis and idiopathic cardiomyopathy.

The incubation period ranges from 2-10 days. Cats of any age can be infected, although the incidence is highest in young cats. The severity of clinical signs after FPV infection can be influenced by other factors but to a lesser extent than with CPV-2 infection:

- MDA may protect kittens or reduce the severity of disease up to 8 weeks of age
- Vaccination status
- Stress factors, e.g. overcrowding, poor hygiene
- Presence of other enteric pathogens, e.g. feline coronavirus, *Salmonella*, *Campylobacter*, *Clostridium*
- The magnitude and duration of the viraemia
- The development of virus neutralizing antibodies, usually by day 7, limits any further viraemia.

Clinical features: Clinical disease varies from peracute to subclinical:

- Peracute disease is characterized by severe depression, subnormal temperature and death within 24 hours
- Acute disease is characterized by acute pyrexia, anorexia, depression and abdominal pain. Vomiting and diarrhoea develop 24-72 hours after the initial signs are seen and the diarrhoea may be profuse and watery or haemorrhagic (diarrhoea may not be seen early in the disease). Cats often appear to be thirsty but do not drink, and dehydration develops. Damage to the intestinal mucosa permits bacterial translocation and overgrowth that can result in endotoxic shock. Mortality ranges from 25-90%
- Subacute infection presents with mild depression, pyrexia and enteritis. Clinical signs are present for up to 3 days. Recovery is rapid and uncomplicated. Death is not expected
- Subclinical infection is common, particularly in adult cats. Mild leucopenia and pyrexia may develop, which are often not appreciated; no other signs of illness are evident
- *In utero* infection. Fetal death and resorption occur if dams are infected in the first third of gestation. Maternal infection from the middle third through to the immediate postnatal period may result in cerebellar hypoplasia (feline ataxia syndrome) (see Chapter 15).

Diagnosis: Feline parvovirus infection can be suspected from the clinical signs and history of exposure. Panleucopenia is present in most affected cats. After about 7 days post infection a neutrophilia with a left shift may be evident, indicating recovery is in process. Confirmation of FPV infection may be made on the basis of:

- Histopathological assessment of jejunum, ileum, mesenteric lymph node and spleen
- Demonstration of the virus in faeces, spleen, mesenteric lymph node or ileum using a CPV ELISA (faeces only), electron microscopy or virus isolation
- Serology - this is of limited value as a significant rise in antibody titre over the course of the disease may be difficult to demonstrate.

Treatment and prevention: There is no specific treatment for FPV. Supportive therapy is required (see below). Very effective modified live vaccines are available to prevent FPV infection. The timing of primary vaccinations varies with the antibody status of the dam and the risk of exposure. Kittens are protected against FPV for the first few weeks of life by MDA. The duration of passive immunity is highly variable and some kittens may become susceptible to infection by 6 weeks of age whereas other may be protected for up to 12 weeks.

Immunity after the use of a modified live vaccine has been suggested to last for 3 years or more in many, but not all, cats. Annual revaccination may not be necessary; although, to ensure immunity is maintained, annual vaccination is suggested. Assessment of serum antibody levels may be used to determine whether a booster vaccination is required. Titres of 1:80 or greater are considered protective.

Animals with suspected FPV should be isolated. Precautions should be as for canine parvovirus above.

Feline coronavirus

Enteric infections with this virus seem to be common, with the virus being shed by many normal cats. After infection cats may develop a self-limiting acute small intestinal diarrhoea sometimes with mild vomiting, lasting up to 4 days. Fatal peracute haemorrhagic gastroenteritis in an adult cat has been associated with coronavirus infection; however, this would seem to be a very rare presentation of this agent. Coronaviruses have been suggested as the cause of chronic diarrhoea in FIV-infected cats, but this remains unproven. Feline coronavirus (FCoV) infection is covered in more detail in Chapter 9.

The main significance of enteric strains of FCoV is that they induce a systemic antibody response that cannot be differentiated from antibodies induced by strains of FCoV that cause feline infectious peritonitis. Confirmation of enteric coronavirus infection is rarely warranted given the self-limiting nature of the disease. There is no specific treatment for FCoV. Supportive therapy may be required (see below).

Feline rotavirus

Rotavirus may be demonstrated in faeces from normal and diarrhoeic faeces of kittens and 28% of cats; however, its significance as an enteropathogen is unclear. Very mild self-limiting small intestinal diarrhoea has been associated with rotavirus infection in young kittens. Diagnosis is by detection of virus in faeces using PAGE, ELISA (detects some rotaviruses), electron microscopy or virus isolation. Serology is of little value and is currently unavailable in the UK. There is no specific treatment for rotavirus infection. Supportive therapy may be required.

Miscellaneous viruses
The following viruses have been detected in diarrhoeic and/or normal faeces; however, their role as enteropathogens has not been elucidated:

- Feline astrovirus has been associated with watery diarrhoea lasting 4–14 days, occasionally accompanied by vomiting, pyrexia, depression and vomiting
- Reoviruses have been found in healthy dogs and cats and from those showing a variety of clinical signs, including diarrhoea, respiratory signs and conjunctivitis
- Caliciviruses (see Chapter 6) have been detected in dogs and cats. Enteric feline calicivirus may be associated with chronic diarrhoea (unproven)
- Enteroviruses
- Feline torovirus has been linked with, but not proven to be responsible for, a syndrome of diarrhoea and prolapse of the nictitating membrane
- Feline herpesvirus-1 (see Chapter 6) causes alimentary tract lesions, the clinical significance of which is unreported. A virus antigenically related to FHV-1 has been isolated from dogs with diarrhoea; the descriptions of lesions have not been reported
- Canine herpesvirus (see Chapter 12) can cause focal necrosis in the intestine as part of a systemic syndrome.

Treatment of bacterial and viral enteric infections

In many cases of gastroenteritis a definitive diagnosis is not made. This is not necessarily a problem when treating the individual, as many patients improve spontaneously or require non-specific supportive therapy. Morbidity and mortality due to gastroenteritis most commonly develop as a consequence of dehydration, sepsis, acidosis or electrolyte imbalances. Various treatments are available to manage gastroenteritis:

- Dietary modification is an effective treatment, irrespective of the cause. Withholding food for up to 48 hours allows mucosal regeneration, prevents an osmotic diarrhoea and reduces faecal water loss. Subsequently food should be reintroduced, even if diarrhoea is still present. Only in exceptional circumstances, e.g. parvovirus infection, when the whole villus/crypt unit is damaged and healing takes longer, should food be withheld for longer than 48 hours. Early refeeding results in a more rapid resolution of damage. Prolonged food restriction is unnecessary and may be counterproductive when enterocyte damage is mild. Suitable foods include highly digestible low fat foods such as cottage cheese or boiled chicken and rice or commercial low fat or selected protein diets
- Antidiarrhoeal protectants and adsorbents are often prescribed on the mistaken assumption that they coat the inflamed and damaged gastrointestinal mucosa and absorb, bind or otherwise limit the effects of toxins and other noxious substances. Given the large surface area and volume of the gastrointestinal tract the small volumes administered are very unlikely to be effective. They may increase morbidity by enhancing faecal sodium excretion. Thus, mixtures containing pectin or kaolin are not indicated for cases of enteritis. Bismuth is sometimes indicated for gastric disease because of its antimicrobial action (bismuth is active against GSOs) and suggested anti-inflammatory and antisecretory action. Long-term bismuth use is not recommended due to toxicity unless bismuth chelates are used (e.g. tripotassium dicitratobismuthate)
- Opiate antidiarrhoeal drugs (diphenoxylate and loperamide) may be indicated to reduce faecal water content and the severity of diarrhoea. They act by reducing water excretion in the crypts and increasing absorption by villi. Their use as motility modifiers is not indicated. In many cases of gastroenteritis hypomotility rather than hypermotility is present and further depression of gut motility is an unwanted effect of these drugs
- Intravenous balanced electrolyte solutions (e.g. Hartmann's solution), sometimes with potassium supplementation (at rates < 0.5 mmol/kg/h) are required when severe fluid/electrolyte losses or volume contraction are present. Oral rehydration protocols are indicated for mild fluid deficits
- If hypoglycaemia develops (more likely in young animals), 20% dextrose solutions should be given slowly intravenously through a jugular catheter
- Where severe blood loss or a marked hypoproteinaemia (plasma protein <45 g/l) develops, e.g. with parvovirus infection, blood or plasma transfusion respectively are indicated
- Oral antibacterials are only indicated to manage known specific infections such as campylobacteriosis. The routine use of oral preparations containing neomycin or sulphonamides in association with motility modifiers and absorbents is not recommended in

the management of most cases of non-specific gastroenteritis. Recovery in dogs receiving such polypharmacy is coincidental. The indiscriminate use of antibacterials, particularly neomycin, ampicillin and erythromycin, may delay recovery or induce diarrhoea, through their effect on the colonic flora. Their use may result in a decrease in short chain fatty acids, an increase in colonic carbohydrates and the potential development of an osmotic diarrhoea. There is also concern relating to the development of antibacterial resistance
- Systemic antibacterials are indicated if secondary systemic bacterial infection is present or considered to be impending because of pyrexia, leucopenia/neutropenia, shock, DIC or where the mucosal barrier has been compromised as indicated by vomit or faeces containing blood. Parenteral fluoroquinolones, cephalosporin or clavulanate-potentiated amoxycillin with or without an aminoglycoside are suggested where therapy is undertaken to manage an assumed bacteraemia. Where a specific bacterial infection (e.g. *Salmonella* septicaemia) is identified, antibacterial use should be determined by the specific organism and results of sensitivity tests
- Antiemetic therapy with metoclopramide or other agents may be indicated if vomiting is a significant feature
- Corticosteroids. Shock doses of corticosteroids have been advocated in the initial management of endotoxic shock. No clear advantage of this treatment has yet been demonstrated, and their use is not recommended
- Non-steroidal anti-inflammatory drugs (NSAIDs) are not indicated in the management of any form of gastroenterocolitis, owing to the increased risk of gastrointestinal ulceration
- Administration of immunoglobulins against CDV, CPV and several *Salmonella* spp. may be helpful in ameliorating the severity of these specific diseases. To be effective they must be given before or immediately after infection. Once a viraemia/bacteraemia has occurred and target organs have been affected, immunoglobulins will only have a limited effect on ameliorating disease
- All cases of gastroenteritis should be assumed to be infectious until proved otherwise, and animals must be housed in kennels away from other patients. All personnel handling infected animals must wear protective clothing and use appropriate disinfectants such as hypochlorite solutions diluted 1:32 with water (kills CPV and other agents) to disinfect contaminated areas
- Motility modifiers such as cisapride, ranitidine and erythromycin are not indicated in acute gastroenteritis. If motility disorders subsequently develop therapy may be indicated.

Helminth diseases

Helminths that inhabit the intestinal tract of the dog and cat are listed in Figure 8.8. Most of these cause disease under some circumstances, although in many cases asymptomatic infections are common.

Ascaridiasis

Toxocara canis infests dogs. Infestation is most commonly acquired *in utero*. Arrested *Toxocara* larvae in muscles of the bitch become reactivated during pregnancy and migrate to the placenta and invade the fetus. The factors that activate these quiescent larvae are unclear. Puppies may become infested from the bitch's milk (transmammary migration). *Toxocara* eggs appear in the puppies' faeces within 3 weeks of birth. Infestation may then be acquired after ingestion of embryonated eggs or a paratenic host, although larvae have to undergo systemic migration (most commonly liver to lung) to establish a patent infection. Infections may remain patent for several months, but eventually acquired immunity prevents further patent infections from developing. Repeated exposure once immunity has been acquired often results in arrest of larvae in somatic tissues rather than the development of a patent infection. In males and neutered bitches these arrested larvae are of no clinical consequence and are considered a 'dead-end' stage. Larvae can only be passed vertically by breeding bitches. Figure 8.10 shows the lifecycle of *T. canis*.

Toxocara cati infests cats. Infestation is most commonly acquired from milk-borne infection. Arrested *Toxocara* larvae in muscles of the queen become reactivated during pregnancy and migrate to the mammary gland. The factors that activate these quiescent larvae are unclear. *Toxocara* eggs appear in the kittens' faeces within 3 weeks of birth. Infestation may be acquired after ingestion of embryonated eggs or a paratenic host, although larvae have to undergo systemic migration (most commonly liver to lung) to establish a patent infection. Unlike dogs, cats do not develop an age-related immunity and adult cats may carry adult ascarids in their intestinal tract. Figure 8.11 shows the lifecycle of *T. cati*.

Toxascaris leonina infests cats and dogs. It is acquired by ingestion of embryonated eggs or an intermediate host such as small mammals. Prenatal infections do not occur. Migration is confined to the intestinal wall; systemic migration does not occur.

Clinical signs: Inapparent infection is common. In young animals moderate to heavy burdens can cause diarrhoea, vomiting, abdominal discomfort, pot-bellied appearance, unthriftiness, lethargy, weakness and poor growth. Occasionally partial or complete intestinal obstruction may develop, with large tangled masses of worms (Figure 8.12) that predispose to intussusception or ulceration.

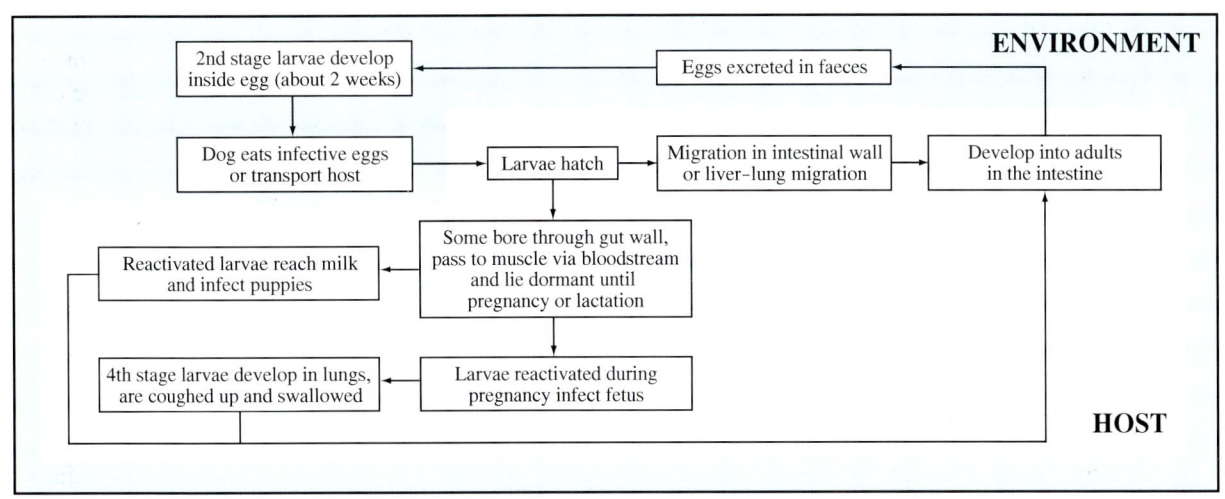

Figure 8.10: Lifecycle of Toxocara canis.

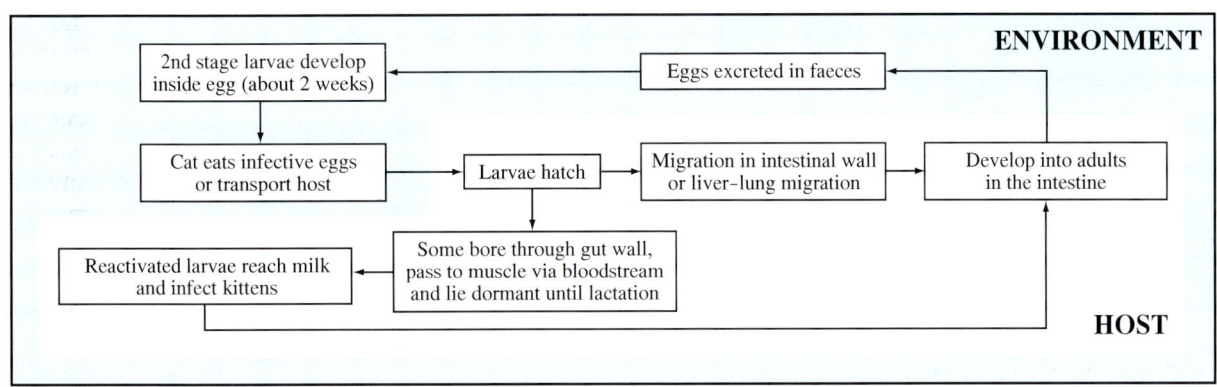

Figure 8.11: Lifecycle of Toxocara cati.

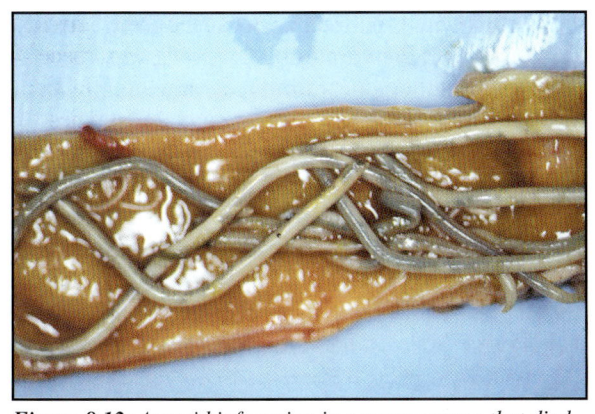

Figure 8.12: *Ascarid infestation in a young puppy that died owing to intestinal obstruction secondary to intussusception. (© Dr Bryn Tennant.)*

Diagnosis: This relies on demonstrating the presence of eggs (Figure 8.13) using faecal flotation techniques (see Chapter 1) or by observation of the adults in vomit or faeces. Occult infections, i.e. prepatent helminth infection, will not be detected using these techniques.

Treatment and control: Many anthelmintics are effective against roundworms. Which drug is used is likely to be determined by economics, the need to treat other parasitic infestations and ease of dosing. Treatment of puppies and kittens is recommended from 2 weeks of age, before eggs are first passed in faeces, and then continued every 2 weeks until 8 weeks. Treatment of the dam is recommended to control *T. canis* and *T. cati*. Fenbendazole 50 mg/kg every 24 hours from day 40 of gestation until 2 weeks post-partum, reduces perinatal roundworm and hookworm burdens. Newborn puppies may be treated with fenbendazole 100 mg/kg for 3 days to provide a 90% kill of prenatally acquired larvae.

Public health aspects: *T. canis* is the cause of toxocaral visceral larva migrans (VLM), a potentially serious but rare disorder in humans, particularly in children. It results from invasion of visceral tissues by migrating *T. canis* larvae. There is a need for routine worming of all dogs, although *T. canis* excretion rates are extremely low (less than 1 in 1000 diarrhoeic faecal samples show evidence of *T. canis* infection; B. Tennant, unpublished observation).

Hookworms

Several hookworms infest dogs or cats:

- *Ancylostoma caninum* is endemic in tropical, subtropical and warm temperate zones of Africa, Australia, Asia and North America. It is not present in the UK. Infestation is usually acquired

146 Manual of Canine and Feline Infectious Diseases

Egg sizes

12 x 10μm	10 x 15μm	36 x 30μm	37 x 32μm	42 x 35μm	60 x 40μm	70 x 35μm	72 x 45μm	80 x 38μm
Toxoplasma gondii	*Giardia*	*Isospora canis*	*Taenia* sp.	*Isospora felis*	*Ancylostoma caninum*	*Capillaria aerophila*	*Uncinaria stenocephala*	*Trichuris vulpis*

75 x 65μm	82 x 70μm	87 x 75μm	97 x 30μm	105 x 63μm	45 x 45μm	2.2mm x 34μm
Toxocara cati	*Toxascaris leonina*	*Toxocara canis*	*Paragonimus*	Grain mite egg (non-parasitic)	*Dipylidium caninum* 1-63 eggs/packet	*Strongyloides stercoralis*

Figure 8.13: Schematic diagram indicating the relative sizes of different worm eggs and protozoal cysts that may infest the intestinal tract of the dog and cat. By kind permission of Intervet UK Ltd. Reproduced from BSAVA Manual of Small Animal Clinical Pathology.

by penetration of the skin by larvae, ingestion of infective larvae or paratenic hosts, milk-borne infection (quiescent larvae in bitch's tissues are activated and migrate to the mammary gland) and occasionally prenatal transplacental transmission. It is a major pathogen causing anaemia, ill thrift and haemorrhagic diarrhoea.
- *Uncinaria stenocephala* occurs in cool temperate regions of Europe (including the UK) and North America. Infestation is usually acquired through skin penetration or ingestion of infective larvae. It is mildly pathogenic
- *Ancylostoma braziliense* occurs in dogs and cats in the tropics and subtropics and is of mild pathogenicity
- *Ancylostoma tubaeforme* infests cats and is a very mild pathogen
- *Ancylostoma ceylanicum* is found in dogs and cats in South East Asia.

Larvae develop within the small intestine but may rarely be found attached to the colonic mucosa. Those that penetrate the skin migrate to the lung before colonizing the intestine. Milk-borne infestation only occurs where bitches have migrating somatic larvae from a previous infestation. Free-living larvae may survive for up to 4 weeks in a warm moist environment but are killed by drying, sunlight or cold.

The parasites inhabit the small intestine. *A. caninum* may penetrate deeply into the mucosa, causing severe mucosal damage and persistent blood flow (the result of an anticoagulant). Clinical signs include tarry or haemorrhagic diarrhoea, with vomiting, inappetence, pallor due to anaemia, weakness, emaciation and dehydration. *U. stenocephala* is relatively non-pathogenic, although large numbers of the parasite may cause diarrhoea; anaemia does not occur. Solar dermatitis is a feature of *Uncinaria* infestation.

Diagnosis relies on demonstrating the presence of eggs (see Figure 8.13) using a faecal flotation technique (see Chapter 1). Occult infections, e.g. prepatent helminth infection, will not be detected using these techniques. Several anthelmintics are effective. In very young puppies, pyrantel is likely to be the safest drug. Puppies should be dosed at 2, 4, 6 and 8 weeks in hookworm endemic areas. Blood transfusions may be required by severely anaemic patients.

Tapeworms
Several tapeworms can parasitize the intestines of dogs and cats:

- *Dipylidium caninum*, the commonest tapeworm of small animals in the UK, is acquired through the consumption of fleas and lice infested with *Dipylidium* cysticercoids. It may be associated with anal irritation as the proglottids crawl around the perineal area. The organism is relatively non-pathogenic

- *Taenia* spp. are acquired by consuming infected tissues of intermediate hosts such as rabbits, rodents and sheep. *Taenia pisiformis*, *T. multiceps*, *T. serialis* and *T. ovis* are found in the dog and *T. taeniaeformis* in the cat. They rarely cause clinical signs, although very heavy burdens might cause intestinal obstruction or mild diarrhoea. Their main importance is not because of the effect they have on the adults of the carnivorous host but rather the effects of their metacestodes or larval forms in intermediate hosts
- *Echinococcus granulosus* uses the dog and some other Canidae as its definitive host. In intermediate hosts, metacestodes are found in hydatid cysts, usually in sheep, but humans may be affected. In the dog little or no inflammatory response accompanies infestation
- *Echinococcus multilocularis* uses mainly foxes as its definitive host, although dogs and cats may be infected in enzootic areas such as central and western Europe (not the UK). Ingestion of eggs by the intermediate host results in hydatid cyst development. Humans may be affected after consumption of eggs shed by infected carnivores. In the definitive host it rarely causes clinical signs. Dogs travelling to Europe under the PETS scheme must be treated for *E. multilocularis* prior to returning to the UK (see Appendix 2)
- Several other rare cestode infestations are seen outside the UK, including *Diphyllobothrium* spp., *Spirometra* spp. and *Mesocestoides* spp. (found in Europe). Dogs infested with *Mesocestoides* may develop diarrhoea.

The diagnosis is made by the observation of tapeworm segments (see Figure 8.13) in faeces. Eggs are not usually detected with faecal flotation as they are confined to the segments. The exception is *Echinococcus* spp., where ova may be detected. Occult (prepatent) infections will not be detected with these techniques. Praziquantel is effective against all tapeworm species and is preferred to older drugs (niclosamide, bunamidine). Prevention of *Dipylidium caninum* infection also involves controlling flea and louse infestations.

Whipworms

Trichuris spp. inhabit the caecum and occasionally colon. *T. vulpis* infests the dog, whereas *T. serrata* and *T. campanula* have been described in cats. The last two usually cause asymptomatic infestations. *T. vulpis* eggs are shed, embryonate after 10 days or more and, after ingestion, hatch in the small intestine. Larvae burrow into the mucosa for 2 to 10 days before emerging and attaching to the caecal and occasionally ascending colonic mucosa. Embryonated eggs can persist for several years in the environment but are killed by direct sunlight. Infection is most commonly found in kennels or where dogs are exercised on grass runs.

The development of clinical signs relates to tunnelling of the adult worm into the mucosa, where localized inflammation, hyperplasia and occasionally granulomatous changes develop. The parasite feeds on tissue fluid, blood and cellular debris. The severity of clinical signs depends on:

- The worm burden – heavy infestation is associated with severe often haemorrhagic typhlitis or typhlocolitis
- Localization within the large bowel – with heavy infestations the parasite can overflow from the caecum to involve the whole of the colon and sometimes rectum
- Extent of the inflammatory process – infestations limited to the surface epithelium cause little morphological alteration in the mucosa and no disease, whereas infestations that breach the lamina propria can induce a moderate mixed inflammatory response
- Degree of anaemia and hypoproteinaemia that may develop
- Nutritional status
- Presence of other infectious agents.

Clinical signs are often intermittent and are typically those of a large bowel diarrhoea with fresh blood and mucus present. Very occasionally severe signs including abdominal pain, inappetence, weight loss, excess protein loss, dehydration, prerenal azotaemia, hyponatraemia, hyperkalaemia, hyperglycaemia, hypochloraemia and hypercalcaemia may develop. Why such severe disease should develop is unclear.

Diagnosis relies on demonstrating the presence of ova (see Figure 8.13) using a salt faecal flotation technique. The presence of *T. vulpis* can be intermittent, and assessment of several samples on consecutive days is indicated. Occult (prepatent) infection will not be detected using these techniques. Colonoscopy may allow observation of the parasites.

Many drugs are active against adult *T. vulpis*, including oxfendazole, fenbendazole, mebendazole, dichlorvos and febantel. Treatment of affected dogs should be repeated after 3 weeks and 3 months. As dogs are often returned to contaminated grassed areas, reinfection is common, and continual retreatment is indicated.

Strongyloides

Strongyloides spp. are found in warm tropical areas (whether they occur in southern Europe is unclear) and are only likely to be seen in animals imported into temperate regions. Infection is acquired by penetration of skin by third stage larvae or by ingestion:

- *S. stercoralis* affects dogs and cats. It burrows into the proximal small intestinal mucosa causing severe villous atrophy and heavy mononuclear cell infiltrates. It may present as haemorrhagic enteritis
- *S. felis* may cause focal granulomatous or eosinophilic interstitial pneumonia in response to lung migration and local adenomatous hyperplasia in the duodenum. Diarrhoea is very uncommon
- *S. planiceps* reported in cat duodenum is of limited pathogenicity
- *S. tumefaciens* infects the colon, causing submucosal nodules. It has been rarely associated with chronic diarrhoea.

Diagnosis is made by demonstrating free larvae (see Figure 8.13) in faeces using the Baermann technique (see Chapter 1). Fenbendazole is effective at clearing *Strongyloides* infection.

Trematodes (flukes)

Various trematodes may infest the dog and cat, including *Alaria* spp. (worldwide but not reported in the UK), *Heterophyes heterophyes* (Mediterranean area), *Metagonimus yokagawi* (Far East) and *Echinochasmus perfoliatus* (Eurasia). Infestations with *Alaria* spp. are acquired from eating frogs or other amphibians and other trematode infestations are acquired from eating fish. Infections are usually asymptomatic although *Echinochasmus* and *Alaria* may be associated with mild enteritis.

Protozoal diseases

Coccidiosis

Coccidians are intracellular parasites. They commonly replicate in the intestinal mucosa in the definitive host but some, e.g. *Toxoplasma* and *Neospora* (see Chapter 15), and *Caryospora* (see Chapter 11) may infect other tissues in intermediate hosts causing systemic disease. In the dog and cat *Isospora* and *Cryptosporidium* have been associated with enteric disease whereas infections with *Hammondia*, *Eimeria*, *Besnoitia*, *Sarcocystis* and *Frenkelia* are usually asymptomatic; very heavy burdens of *Hammondia* have been associated with diarrhoea.

Isosporiasis

Isospora spp. are the commonest coccidial agents found in dogs and cats. They are species-specific:

- *I. canis*, *I. ohioensis* and *I. burrowsi* infect dogs
- *I. neorivolta*, *I. felis* and *I. rivolta* infect cats.

Infection occurs after ingestion of sporulated oocysts or consumption of a paratenic host (e.g. mouse).

Isospora oocysts (Figure 8.14) are often recognized in diarrhoeic samples from puppies and kittens but their role as a primary pathogen is unclear. They may act as opportunistic pathogens in the presence of other primary infections, malnutrition or immunoincompetence. Where animals are exposed to large numbers of *Isospora* oocysts, as may occur in kennels with poor hygiene, a mild to severe, occasionally haemorrhagic, diarrhoea may develop. Blood loss may occasionally be marked.

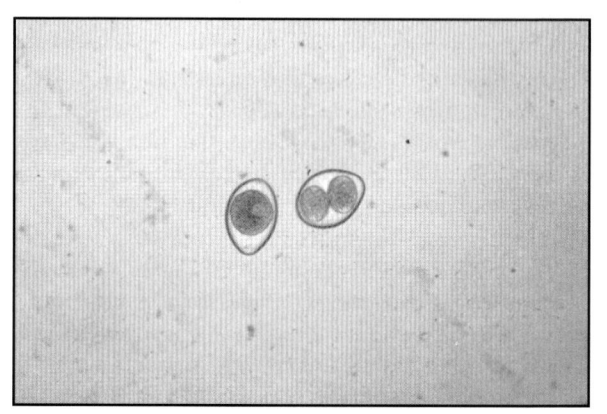

Figure 8.14: Isospora felis *oocysts from an 8-week-old kitten. (© Dr Bryn Tennant.)*

Cryptosporidiosis

Cryptosporidiosis is caused by *Cryptosporidium parvum*. It is generally considered to be an asymptomatic infection in most dogs and cats although associations between infection and clinical signs have been reported, particularly in cats. Whether the parasite acts as a primary or opportunistic pathogen is unclear. Different strains may have varying pathogenicities. Clinical signs associated with cryptosporidiosis include acute profuse watery diarrhoea, and chronic unresponsive diarrhoea. Mesenteric lymphadenopathy is reported to be a feature. Immunocompromised animals, those with intercurrent infections, e.g. CDV and FeLV, or young animals seem to be most at risk of developing clinical signs with cryptosporidial infections.

Diagnosis: Faecal flotation techniques using centrifugation methods (see Chapter 1) may detect coccidial oocysts (see Figures 8.13 and 8.14). Confirming a diagnosis of cryptosporidiosis is difficult as *Cryptosporidium* oocysts are small (one-tenth the size of *Isospora* oocysts) and are often shed in low numbers. Use of carbol fuchsin-negative staining, modified acid-fast staining or fluorescent labelling (phenol/ auramine) is recommended for *Cryptosporidium*. An ELISA is available to detect *Cryptosporidium* antigen in faeces. PCR technology may demonstrate *Cryptosporidium* spp. but may also lead to overdiagnosis of the infection as a cause of disease.

Treatment: Most infections are self-limiting. Sulphonamide drugs given for 3 weeks are usually effective in controlling *Isospora* infections. Treatment of bitches immediately post-whelping may prevent infection passing to the puppies. Tylosin may be effective against *Cryptosporidium* spp. The prognosis for recovery is usually good, although the presence of intercurrent problems including other infections, malnutrition and immunoincompetence will affect the outcome. *Cryptosporidium parvum* is not host-specific and may infect humans. In severely immunocompromised people cryptosporidiosis may be fatal. Good hygiene and environmental use of strong ammonium hydroxide or boiling water reduces oocyst numbers; bleach is ineffective.

Giardiasis

Giardia intestinalis (also termed *G. lamblia* and *G. duodenalis*) is a pear-shaped binucleate flagellated protozoan parasite that infects the proximal small intestine of the dog and cat. It has a worldwide distribution. *Giardia* damages mucosal cells, interfering with mucosal function and causing villous atrophy. It also deconjugates bile acids and possibly interferes with intestinal motility. Prevalence varies between 1 and 36%. Although classed as a small bowel parasite, *Giardia* may be associated with large bowel signs. Two forms of the parasite are found: the motile trophozoite that attaches to the brush border surface or lies within the mucous layer of the duodenum (dog) or jejunum/ileum (cat); and the cyst. Trophozoites may be found in diarrhoeic samples but never in formed faecal material, whereas the infective cyst can be found in either. *Giardia* has a direct life cycle, with infection occurring after ingestion of contaminated food or water. Cysts may persist for long periods in the environment.

Most *Giardia* infections are subclinical. If clinical signs develop they are expected within 1 to 2 weeks of initial infection and are most commonly recognized in young animals. Chronic subclinical infections may become symptomatic if there is concurrent infection of the intestinal tract with other pathogens. The severity of disease is also determined by the presence of other pathogens. Immune deficiency predisposes humans to clinical giardiasis, although whether this is important in animals is unclear.

Clinical features include a watery to semi-solid foul-smelling pale diarrhoea, steatorrhoea and weight loss. Diarrhoea may be acute or chronic, persistent or self-limiting and continuous or intermittent. Melaena is not usually a feature. Large bowel signs associated with giardiasis may relate to concurrent infection or the presence of irritating malabsorbed nutrients and deconjugated bile acids in the colon.

Diagnosis relies on demonstrating the presence of cysts or trophozoites. The organism is not easily demonstrated. The most reliable method is through finding *Giardia* cysts (Figures 8.13 and 8.15) using a zinc sulphate flotation technique (see Chapter 1). As excretion of the parasite is intermittent, a minimum of three samples from consecutive days should be examined. Fresh saline smears from diarrhoea can be used to look for motile trophozoites. An ELISA to detect *Giardia intestinalis* antigen is available, although its sensitivity and specificity in the clinical setting have yet to be evaluated. Duodenal cytology and washes are also useful for demonstrating *Giardia* spp. Some empirical treatments (e.g. barium, some antibacterials, antacids, laxatives, enemas and antidiarrhoeals) reduce the level of *G. intestinalis* in faeces. If *Giardia* cannot be identified, a therapeutic trial can be used to provide a presumptive diagnosis. A 5-day course of fenbendazole is the treatment of choice and is effective in 100% of cases, whilst metronidazole is effective in 67% of cases. The prognosis for recovery is good, although some infections may require long-term therapy.

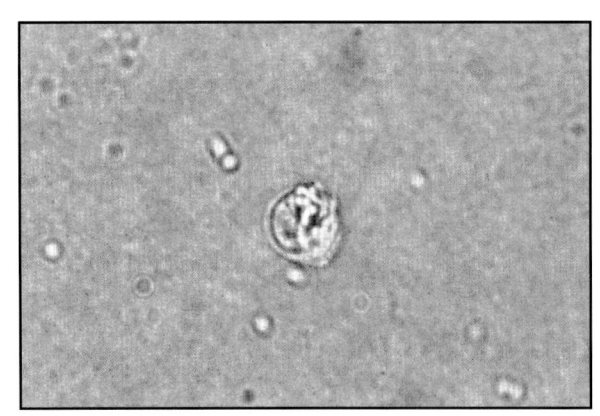

Figure 8.15: Giardia intestinalis *oocysts (8–12 × 7–10 μm) from a dog. (© Dr Bryn Tennant.)*

Pentatrichomonas hominis

Pentatrichomonas hominis is a motile pear-shaped protozoan that infects the large intestine of dogs. It has not been conclusively shown to be a pathogen in dogs and cats. Large numbers of trichomonads may be seen in diarrhoea.

Mycotic diseases

Mycotic invasion of the gastrointestinal tract is seen as an uncommon sequel to other diseases or lesions affecting the mucosa. One or more of the following are required for opportunistic mycotic diseases to become established:

- Heavy fungal challenge
- Disruption of the normal flora (e.g. secondary to antibacterial therapy)
- Primary local lesions allowing fungi access to deeper layers of the gastrointestinal wall
- Lowered host resistance. Spores are probably carried across the mucosa by macrophages in the normal animal. If phagocytic or neutrophil function is compromised these spores germinate.

Organisms associated with alimentary tract disease include *Aspergillus*, *Pythium*, Mucoraceae (e.g. *Absidia*, *Mucor*, *Rhizopus*), entomophthoracetes (e.g. *Basidiobolius*, *Coniobulus*), *Candida* spp. and *Histoplasma capsulatum*.

- Mycotic ileitis and colitis (most often *Aspergillus* spp.), characterized by haemorrhagic necrotic foci are occasionally seen as a sequel to FPV infection. Sometimes multifocal mycotic emboli localize in lung. Mycotic enteritis is a rare complication of CPV enteritis
- Pythiosis is a disease of tropical and subtropical areas, where it may cause diarrhoea in dogs and less commonly cats
- Gastrointestinal entomophthoromycosis causing ulcerative stomatitis, gastritis and enteritis has been reported in a few dogs
- Candidiasis is a very rare cause of gastrointestinal disease; it is more commonly associated with oral cavity disease
- *Histoplasma capsulatum* is a cause of disease in parts of the USA but not in the UK. Diarrhoea and weight loss develop.

Diagnosis of mycotic alimentary tract disease requires culture and identification of the organism from swabs, scrapes or biopsy material. Treatment is difficult. Systemic amphotericin B, ketoconazole or itraconazole are required.

Algae

Prototheca zopfi and *Prototheca wickhamii* are algae acquired from the environment that may invade tissue. Colonic involvement causes signs of colitis, and a colonic biopsy is required for diagnosis. The disease is rare in the USA and has not been reported in the UK.

Rickettsial diseases

Salmon poisoning disease

Salmon poisoning disease is caused by *Neorickettsia helminthoeca* and *N. elokominica*. Disease is geographically limited by the distribution of the intermediate host to coastal areas of Washington, Oregon and California. It is characterized by pyrexia, anorexia, vomiting, diarrhoea, weight loss, lymphadenopathy and splenomegaly. Nasal and ocular discharge is seen in some dogs. Death in untreated cases occurs within 7-10 days. Diagnosis is by demonstration of intracytoplasmic inclusion bodies in lymph nodes. Tetracycline is the treatment of choice.

DRUG DOSAGES

See Appendix 3.

REFERENCES AND FURTHER READING

Beutin L (1999) *Escherichia coli* as a pathogen in dogs and cats. *Veterinary Research* **30**, 285-298

Carmichael LE, Schlafer DH and Hashimoto A (1994) Minute virus of canines (MVC, canine parvovirus type-1): pathogenicity for pups and seroprevalence estimate. *Journal of Veterinary Diagnostic Investigation* **6**, 165-174

Cruikshank J (1986) *Salmonella* and *Campylobacter* infections - an update. *Journal of Small Animal Practice* **17**, 673-681

Drolet R, Fairborther JM, Harel J and Helie P (1994) Attaching and effacing of enterotoxigenic *Escherichia coli* associated with enteric colibacillosis in the dog. *Canadian Journal of Veterinary Research* **58**, 87-92

Evermann J, McKiernan A and Eugster A (1989) Update on canine coronavirus infections and interactions with other enteric pathogens of the dog. *Companion Animal Practice* **19**, 6-12

Ford RB and Schultz RD (2000) Vaccines and vaccinations: issues for the 21st century. In: *Current Veterinary Therapy XIII*, ed. RW Kirk, pp. 250-253. WB Saunders, Philadelphia

Hammermueller J, Kruth S, Prescott J and Gyles C (1995) Detection of toxin genes in *Escherichia coli* isolated from normal dogs and dogs with diarrhoea. *Canadian Journal of Veterinary Research* **59**, 265-270

Happonen I, Linden J and Westermarck E (2000) Effect of triple therapy on eradication of canine gastric heliobacters and gastric disease. *Journal of Small Animal Practice* **41**, 1-6

Harrison LR, Stryer EL, Pursell AR, Carmichael LE and Nietfeld JC (1992) Fatal disease in nursing puppies associated with minute virus of canines. *Journal of Veterinary Diagnostic Investigation* **4**, 19-22

Holland RE, Walker RD, Sriranganathan N, Wilson RA and Ruhl DC (1999) Characterisation of *Escherichia coli* isolated from healthy dogs. *Veterinary Microbiology* **70**, 261-268

Ikegami T, Shrota K, Goto K, Takakura A, Itoh T, Kawamura S, Une Y, Nomura Y and Fujiwara K (1999) Enterocolitis associated with dual infection by *Clostridium piliforme* and feline panleucopenia virus in three kittens. *Veterinary Pathology* **36**, 613-615

Meurs KM, Fox PR, Magnon AL, Liu S and Towbin JA (2000) Molecular screening by polymerase chain reaction detects panleucopenia virus DNA in formalin-fixed hearts from cats with idiopathic cardiomyopathy and myocarditis. *Cardiovascular Pathology* **9**, 119-126

Mochizuki M, Horiuchi M, Hiragi H, San Gabriel MC, Yasuda N and Uno T (1996) Isolation of canine parvovirus from a cat manifesting signs of feline panleucopenia. *Journal of Clinical Microbiology* **34**, 2101-2105

Parrish CR, Aquadroa CF, Strassheim ML, Evermann JF, Sgro JY and Mohammed HO (1991) Rapid antigenic-type replacement and DNA sequence evolution of canine parvovirus. *Journal of Virology* **65**, 6544-6552

Quinn P, Carter M, Markey B and Carter L (1994) *Campylobacter* species. In: *Clinical Veterinary Microbiology*, ed. P Quinn et al., pp. 268-272. Wolfe, London

Smith KA, Kruth S, Hammermueller J, Gyles C and Wilson JB (1998) A case control study of verocytotoxigenic *Escherichia coli* infection in cats with diarrhoea. *Canadian Journal of Veterinary Research* **62**, 87-92

Tennant BJ (1989) *Studies on the epizootiology and pathogenesis of canine coronavirus in the dog*. PhD Thesis, University of Liverpool

Tennant BJ, Gaskell RM, Chalmers S and Baxendale W (1990) The development of a vaccine to canine coronavirus in the dog. Clinical Research Abstract, BSAVA Congress

Truyen U, Evermann JF, Vieler E and Parrish CR (1996) Evolution of canine parvovirus involved loss and gain of feline host range. *Virology* **215**, 186-189

Turk J, Fales W, Miller M, Pace L, Fischer J, Johnson G, Kreeger J, Turnquist S, Pittman L, Rottinghaus A, et al (1992) Enteric *Clostridium perfringens* infection associated with parvoviral enteritis in dogs: 74 cases (1987-1990). *Journal of the American Veterinary Medical Association* **200**, 991-994

Turk J, Maddox C, Fales W, Ostlund E, Miller M, Johnson G, Pace L, Turnquist S and Kreeger J (1998) Examination for heat-labile, heat-stable and Shige-like toxins and for the *aeA* gene in *Escherichia coli* isolates obtained from dogs dying with diarrhoea: 122 cases (1992-1996). *Journal of the American Veterinary Medical Association* **212**, 1735-1736

Wada Y, Kondo H, Nakaoka Y and Kubo M (1996) Gastric attaching and effacing *Escherichia coli* lesions in a puppy with naturally occurring enteric colibacillosis and concurrent canine distemper virus infection. *Veterinary Pathology* **33**, 717-720

Woldehiwet Z, Jones J, Tennant B and Jones D (1990) Serotypes of *Campylobacter jejuni* and *C. coli* isolated from dogs. *Journal of Small Animal Practice* **31**, 382-384

CHAPTER NINE

The Peritoneal Cavity

Danièlle Gunn-Moore and Diane Addie

CHAPTER PLAN

Introduction
Aetiology and pathophysiology of peritonitis
Septic peritonitis
    History and clinical signs
    Diagnosis
    Clinical pathology
    Imaging the peritoneal cavity
    Treatment
Feline infectious peritonitis
    Aetiology
    Pathogenesis
    Clinical features
    Differential diagnoses
    Diagnosis
    Treatment
    Prognosis
    Control and prevention
References and further reading

INTRODUCTION

Peritonitis describes inflammation of part of, or the entire, peritoneal cavity. It can be associated with infectious and non-infectious conditions. Infectious causes of peritonitis are uncommon in dogs and cats, but when they do occur they are often associated with severe disease and high mortality. The peritoneal cavity itself is not usually a primary target for infection; it is diseases of the structures and organs surrounding or contained within the peritoneum that result in peritonitis. Multisystemic infections that may involve the peritoneal cavity are covered in detail elsewhere in this book.

AETIOLOGY AND PATHOPHYSIOLOGY OF PERITONITIS

Localized peritonitis often occurs without infection and may develop after:

- Abdominal surgery (e.g. gastropexy, gastrostomy) (Figure 9.1)
- Trauma
- Pancreatitis
- Perforation of the intestine, where omentum walls off the inflammatory process.

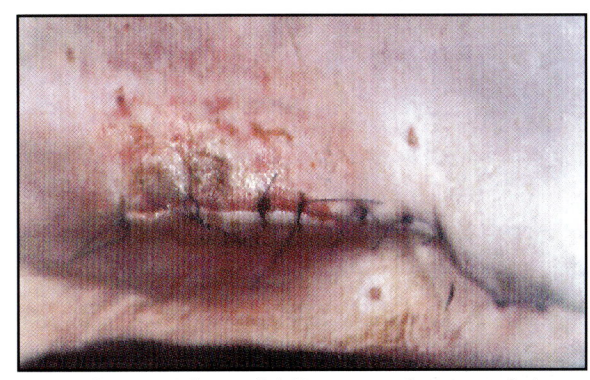

Figure 9.1: Partial wound dehiscence and some exudation associated with the development of bacterial peritonitis in a cat that had undergone abdominal surgery (© Dr Ian Ramsey).

Generalized peritonitis is diffuse inflammation affecting most of the surfaces in the peritoneal cavity. It should be considered an emergency. It may develop:

- After the release of irritant material into the body cavity (e.g. bile, gastric fluid, pancreatic secretions, urine)
- Due to the presence of an infection within the peritoneal cavity. Figure 9.2 lists the main infectious aetiologies recognized in the UK. Some of these are primarily associated with disease of other organ systems and are discussed in detail elsewhere
- Due to inflammation extending from intra-abdominal organs or tissue (vasculitis, pancreatitis, lymphocytic cholangitis, feline infectious peritonitis (FIP))
- Secondary to neoplasia
- When irritant peritoneal effusions, even if aseptic, cause ileus, intestinal irritation, dilation and sometimes ischaemia of the intestinal tract. The last can result in compromise of the intestinal wall and translocation of bacteria from the gut lumen into the body cavity, thereby turning an initially aseptic process into a septic disorder.

152 Manual of Canine and Feline Infectious Diseases

Infection	Comments
Canine adenovirus-1 (infectious canine hepatitis)	Ascites, if present, is part of a multisystemic disease (see Chapter 11 for further discussion on CAV-1) *The ascitic fluid is typically serosanguineous or haemorrhagic*
Feline infectious peritonitis (FIP)	Caused by infection with feline coronavirus (FCoV). Found mainly in young cats, often pedigree breeds, coming from multicat households *The ascitic fluid is non-purulent, highly proteinaceous, viscous, usually yellow-to-gold in colour, clots on standing and contains a low to moderate number of neutrophils in a high-protein background*
Feline leukaemia virus (FeLV)-associated lymphosarcoma	Persistent feline FeLV infection is found mainly in young cats. FeLV-induced lymphosarcoma may be associated with ascitic fluid production when neoplasia develops within abdominal organs (liver, spleen, kidney or mesenteric lymph nodes). See Chapter 5 for further discussion on FeLV *The ascitic fluid may be variable in nature, from a transudate that quickly becomes modified, to chyle or possibly pseudochyle, to a serosanguineous exudate*
Toxoplasmosis (cats more commonly than dogs)	Toxoplasmosis may be associated with ascites in transplacentally infected kittens. It is found only rarely in young puppies. Ascites, if found, is part of severe multisystemic disease. See Chapter 15 for further discussion on toxoplasmosis *The ascitic fluid is typically serosanguineous*
Neonatal streptococcal infection (cats more commonly than dogs)	Group G and B streptococcal infections occasionally cause septicaemia, pneumonia, hepatitis, pyelonephritis or peritonitis in neonatal kittens and puppies. Group G infections in kittens acquired via the umbilicus are associated with omphalophlebitis, septic peritonitis and septicaemia. See Chapter 12 for further discussion on this *The ascitic fluid is purulent*
Actinomycosis (dogs more commonly than cats)	*Actinomyces* spp. are endogenous saprophytes found in the environment and the oral cavity of dogs and cats. The organisms cause disease when inoculated into tissue with other bacteria. Actinomycosis is found mainly in young to middle-aged large-breed dogs that live outside. Migrating grass awns are believed to be a common route by which the infection gains entry. The infection is less common in cats, where it usually arises secondary to bite wounds; in cats, it rarely results in peritonitis. When infection results in a pyogranulomatous peritoneal infection it is usually secondary to migrating plant material. It usually produces chronic disease. *The ascitic fluid is serosanguineous to purulent and commonly a reddish brown. It may contain numerous yellow-tan granules ('sulphur granules'), which are small soft macroscopic colonies of bacteria*
Nocardiosis (dogs more commonly than cats)	*Nocardia* spp. are ubiquitous soil saprophytes. Infection is opportunistic, occurring either through inhalation or inoculation of puncture wounds. Nocardiosis is uncommon in the dog and rare in the cat. Only very rarely is it associated with peritonitis. It produces ascitic fluid similar to that described for actinomycosis above. See Chapter 6 for further information on nocardiosis
Mycobacteriosis	Rarely, *Mycobacterium* spp. can disseminate from intestinal, respiratory or cutaneous sites to involve body cavities. See Chapters 6 and 13 for further discussion of mycobacteriosis
Intra-abdominal bacterial infections (dogs, cats)	Bacterial peritonitis may arise as a complication of gastrointestinal perforation, severe ulcerative gastroenteritis, foreign body migration, rupture of intra-abdominal abscesses (e.g. prostatitis), penetrating abdominal wounds or surgery (e.g. laparotomy, enterotomy, gastrotomy). Ascitic fluid may become secondarily infected from haematogenous, lymphogenous or transmural migration of bacteria from the gastrointestinal tract or from iatrogenic contamination during paracentesis. The type of bacteria involved depends on the source, i.e. enteric organisms with perforation, Gram-positive organisms if secondary to surgery and anaerobes if due to a bite wound. Anaerobic bacteria predispose to the development of abscesses, whereas aerobic bacteria predispose to sepsis and death *The ascitic fluid is purulent*
Yersinia enterocolitica (cats)	*Y. enterocolitica* is thought to be a natural intestinal commensal of dogs and cats. It has occasionally been isolated from chronic peritonitis in cats. See Chapter 8 for further information on yersiniosis *The ascitic fluid is purulent*
Rhodococcus equi (cats)	*R. equi* is a soil-borne bacterium most typically associated with suppurate infections in livestock. It has occasionally been isolated from cats with peritonitis, associated with infection of the liver and mesenteric lymph nodes *The ascitic fluid is purulent*

Figure 9.2: *Infectious agents found in the UK that can cause peritonitis.*

Peritoneal irritation or inflammation results in:

- Vasodilation and increased vascular permeability, which promotes influx of protein and fluid into the abdominal cavity resulting in the development of a high protein exudate
- Infiltration by white blood cells
- Stimulation of pain fibres, causing pain.

Other factors that contribute to the development of clinical signs include:

- Hypovolaemia, as a result of fluid loss into the peritoneal cavity or, in cases complicated by ileus, fluid lost into the intestinal lumen
- The presence of fibrin in the exudate; this promotes the development of adhesions and visceral immobility
- The presence of bacteria and toxic factors such as bacterial toxins, gastric contents and bile salts in the peritoneal cavity; this may contribute to the development of bacteraemia and endotoxaemia, which often complicate peritonitis
- Metabolic acidosis, which may be a sequel to hypovolaemia, the primary disease process and hypoxia
- The development of hypoglycaemia in septic patients
- Reduced renal perfusion and poor cardiac output, which result in the accumulation of nitrogenous waste, toxins, hydrogen ions and potassium
- The development of disseminated intravascular coagulation (DIC) and thromboembolization within kidney, liver and lung. This occurs secondary to hypovolaemia, sludging of blood cells in smaller vessels as a consequence of a reduction in blood flow and platelet activation by toxins and cellular debris.

SEPTIC PERITONITIS

History and clinical signs
Disease within the peritoneal cavity should be suspected in any animal presenting with abdominal distension and/or abdominal pain. Abdominal distension may result from organomegaly or an abnormal accumulation of fluid or gas (Figure 9.3). The severity of clinical signs depends on the nature of the underlying disease and the speed with which distension has occurred. The signalment of the animal is unhelpful as there is no age, sex or breed predilection for septic peritonitis. Historical information that may be of use includes:

- Trauma, suggesting a penetrating wound
- Acute onset vomiting and diarrhoea followed by collapse, suggesting bowel perforation
- Pre-existing infectious diseases, suggesting extension to the peritoneum
- Recent abdominal surgery or wound breakdown followed by collapse, suggesting iatrogenic infection.

Physical examination may reveal:

- Evidence of trauma or a penetrating wound
- Abdominal pain, free abdominal fluid and/or gas, an abdominal mass or enlarged organs (e.g. uterus, prostate, liver)
- An increased, normal or subnormal rectal temperature. Subnormal temperature is a bad, often terminal, sign
- Dry and 'muddy' mucous membranes owing to haemoconcentration and sepsis, or dry and pale mucous membranes owing to hypovolaemia. Slow capillary refill suggests poor peripheral perfusion, hypovolaemia or shock
- Fever and abdominal pain after vomiting and diarrhoea, which could indicate gastrointestinal perforation.

Recognizing septic peritonitis as a complication of abdominal surgery is difficult. Abdominal discomfort and dullness from surgery are expected, and the routine use of analgesics is advisable. In such cases, monitoring of peripheral haematology and repeated abdominal ultrasonography (see below) are indicated.

The clinical features of septic peritonitis relate to:

- The inflammatory response, which results in the formation of a highly cellular exudate comprising macrophages and neutrophils
- Pain due to stimulation of pain fibres lining the peritoneal cavity
- An increase in vascular permeability, which allows large exchanges of fluid and electrolytes, resulting in severe acid–base disturbances and protein influx into the abdominal cavity
- Fibrin deposition, which results in the adherence of serosal surfaces to each other.

The severity of the lesions varies with the severity of the inflammation (local or general), duration and underlying aetiology. Thus, clinical signs may vary from mild depression to septic shock (e.g. 'muddy' mucous membranes, slow capillary refill time, cool extremities). Hypovolaemic shock and dehydration develop early in generalized peritonitis. This is a consequence of an absolute fluid deficiency due to vomiting, diarrhoea, pyrexia and insensible losses, coupled with functional unavailability of fluids owing to sequestration of fluid in the abdominal cavity, the development of oedema in inflamed tissues and splanchnic pooling secondary to endotoxaemia.

Fluid accumulation (ascites)	
Transudate*	Hypoproteinaemia: glomerular disease, intestinal malabsorption or protein loss, severe chronic liver disease Congestive heart failure Neoplasia: obstruction of lymphatic drainage/lymphangectasia
Modified transudate	Feline infectious peritonitis (FIP) Congestive heart failure Portal hypertension/obstruction of posterior vena cava Hepatic disease: cirrhosis, neoplasia, lymphocytic cholangitis (in cats) Neoplasia: obstruction of blood vessels and/or lymphatics
Non-septic exudate	Bile or urine peritonitis Pancreatic peritonitis Hepatitis (particularly lymphocytic cholangitis in cats) Diaphragmatic or pericardial hernia Steatitis Neoplasia
Purulent exudate	Extension of infection from elsewhere Intestinal perforation/bowel rupture Ruptured pyometra Penetrating wound Migrating foreign body Haematogenous spread
Haemorrhagic effusion	Organ or major blood vessel rupture; associated with trauma or secondary to ruptured neoplasm Perforation of stomach or intestine Bleeding disorder: warfarin poisoning, thrombocytopenia Splenic or gastric torsion Thrombosis
Bile	Ruptured biliary tract (because bile is irritant it usually results in a secondary serosanguineous exudate)
Urine	Ruptured urinary tract (because urine is irritant it usually results in a secondary serosanguineous exudate)
Chyle	Ruptured lymphatic drainage Obstruction of lymphatic drainage/lymphangectasia Congestive heart failure (especially in cats) Neoplasia Steatitis
Other abdominal causes	
Weak abdominal wall	Hyperadrenocorticism
Organomegaly	Hepatomegaly/renomegaly/splenomegaly Mesenteric lymphadenopathy Gastric distension/bladder distension/advanced obstipation Pregnancy/pyometra Neoplasia Obesity
Gas accumulation (pneumoperitoneum)	Traumatic penetration of abdominal wall Rupture of the stomach or bowel Gas-forming bacterial infection Extension from pneumomediastinum or pneumothorax

Figure 9.3: Causes of abdominal distension.
* *When present for any length of time, a transudate will become modified. This is particularly true of transudates that develop slowly, such as those associated with congestive heart failure or portal hypertension. Modified transudates are therefore more common than unmodified ones.*

Diagnosis

The diagnosis of septic peritonitis depends on determining the nature of the peritoneal effusion and localizing its origin. The diagnostic plan depends on the clinical signs:

- If abdominal distension is the main presenting problem, the first step is to determine its cause, i.e. organomegaly, an abnormal accumulation of fluid or gas, or weakness of the abdominal wall
- If the clinical picture suggests an abdominal catastrophe (i.e. peracute abdominal pain, fever and depression) it is more important to define the nature of any effusion and to assess damage to abdominal organs.

Although physical examination, abdominal palpation, ballottement and percussion may be helpful, radiography, ultrasonography and abdominal paracentesis are the major tools of assessment. Routine haematology, serum biochemistry, urinalysis and serology may be required to characterize the extent of systemic involvement.

Clinical pathology

Clinical pathology rarely defines the underlying cause of peritonitis, although it is always indicated to look for underlying or secondary metabolic disorders that may complicate the clinical picture and to help with monitoring.

Serum biochemistry

Serum biochemistry is useful for assessing metabolic status and abdominal organ involvement. Some changes are of prognostic importance (e.g. increased concentration of bilirubin, azotaemia) but others may be non-specific (e.g. increased concentration of alkaline phosphatase, hyperglobulinaemia).

Haematology

Haematology is likely to show a profound neutrophilia with a left shift, or a neutropenia owing to sequestration of neutrophils in the abdominal cavity. Toxic neutrophils suggest a suppurative process. Chronic infection may be associated with a monocytosis and neutrophilia. Thrombocytopenia, hypofibrinogenaemia and the presence of fibrin degradation products suggest DIC.

Biochemical analysis

Biochemical analysis of ascitic fluid is rarely helpful in septic peritonitis. The fluid is expected to have a high protein content that may contain bilirubin if there is damage to the biliary tree, amylase in cases of pancreatitis and creatinine if the urinary tract is ruptured (although serum and fluid levels equilibrate within 24 hours).

Where there is concern over possible iatrogenic septic peritonitis, e.g. after abdominal surgery, white blood cell variables and peripheral blood smears should be monitored for a few hours. In these patients, routine use of analgesics reduces pain, and the physical signs may be muted.

Cytology and histopathology

Assessment of ascitic fluid is essential in its classification as a transudate, modified transudate, exudate, chylous effusion (Figure 9.4) or blood. The colour, specific gravity, protein content, packed cell volume (PCV), nucleated cell count, white cell morphology and presence of free or phagocytosed bacteria (Figure 9.5) and neoplastic cells should be determined.

Bacteriology

Bacterial culture of ascitic fluid is indicated if inflammation is evident cytologically. Any bacteria isolated from ascitic fluid are of importance, although care must be taken to ensure that skin commensals do not contaminate the sample. The fluid should be assessed for aerobic and anaerobic bacteria. Culture requires a

	Transudate	Modified transudate	Exudates	Chylous effusion
Clarity	Clear	Clear-cloudy	Variable	Cloudy*
Colour	Colourless to pale yellow	Yellow or pink	Variable	White to pale pink
Cell types	Predominantly mesothelial cells	Macrophages, mesothelial ± PMN ± neoplastic cells	PMN ± macrophages ± neoplastic cells	Predominantly small lymphocytes
Cell count (× 10^6/l)	<1000	<5000	>5000	Variable
Protein content	<20 g/l	20-30 g/l	>30 g/l	20-30 g/l
Specific gravity	<1.015	1.010-1.030	>1.018	1.010-1.030

Figure 9.4: Analysis of ascitic fluid samples.
The figure is meant only as a guide. Many effusions do not fit neatly in a particular group. PMN, polymorph nucleocytes (neutrophils). *Biochemically rich in triglycerides. Can be differentiated from a pseudochylous effusion by measuring triglyceride concentrations or performing an ether-clearance test. The addition of ether or chloroform usually causes clearing of a chylous fluid but not a pseudochylous one. Pseudochylous effusions are rare, but may be seen with neoplasia or occasionally infection.

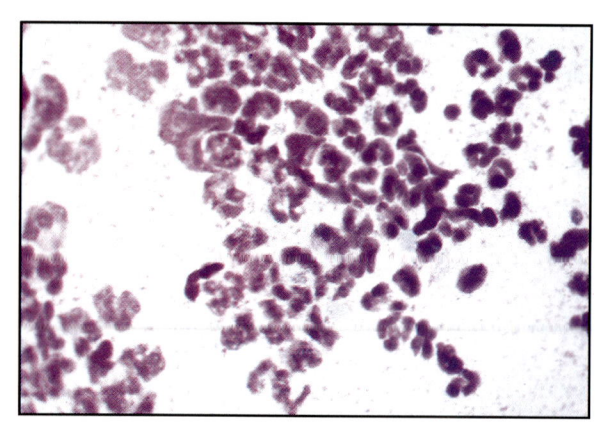

Figure 9.5: Degenerate neutrophils with intracytoplasmic bacteria from a case of peritonitis associated with intestinal rupture (© Elizabeth Villiers).

plain sterile container. The tube should be filled to the top and all residual air removed if anaerobic culture is to be performed (the use of vacuum tubes are ideal); the sample should not be placed in a pot containing anticoagulants (e.g. EDTA, citrate, heparin) as they are bactericidal or bacteriostatic for many bacteria. Ideally, all fluids should be assessed for both aerobic and anaerobic bacteria and fungi.

Paracentesis

Abdominal paracentesis is usually performed after ascites has been confirmed by radiography and/or ultrasonography; in healthy animals the peritoneal cavity contains little free fluid. Figure 9.6 describes a technique for paracentesis.

If no fluid is obtained by paracentesis, some authors recommend diagnostic peritoneal lavage; however, others consider this technique to be of little value. It is safer to identify small amounts of free fluid or pockets of fluid by ultrasonography. Figure 9.7 describes the technique for diagnostic peritoneal lavage.

Imaging the peritoneal cavity

Radiography, ultrasonography and computed tomography (CT) can be used to image the peritoneal cavity. Imaging does not diagnose septic peritonitis but allows identification of free fluid and may allow the identification of any underlying primary disorder.

1. Place the patient in lateral recumbency and clip and aseptically prepare the ventral abdomen over the whole area to be sampled (see below)
2. Catheterize and empty the urinary bladder or, if unable to catheterize the bladder, empty it by cystocentesis (this is not necessary if using ultrasound to guide the needle)
3. Place a 20 or 22 gauge 2.5–5 cm needle through the body wall caudal to the umbilicus and in the midline into the peritoneal cavity. Allow abdominal fluid to drip into a sterile tube. Gentle abdominal pressure may encourage the fluid to flow. Prior instillation of local anaesthetic into the abdominal wall is rarely necessary
4. If necessary, attach a 5 ml syringe to the needle to apply gentle negative pressure; do not apply excessive negative pressure. Alternatively an over-the-needle intravenous catheter can be used in place of the needle, the stylet being removed once the catheter has been inserted into the abdominal cavity, and a syringe attached to the catheter hub. This method reduces the risk of iatrogenic organ laceration, but care must be taken to prevent the catheter becoming kinked at the abdominal wall
5. A four quadrant tap is often recommended. This involves four separate punctures made cranial and caudal to the umbilicus and lateral to the midline on each side; ensure an appropriate area is clipped and aseptically prepared. If a negative tap is obtained, alter the animal's position by standing it up or rolling it before repeating the taps
6. When draining larger volumes of fluid it may be useful to use a three-way tap attachment

Figure 9.6: Technique for abdominal paracentesis.

1. For diagnostic peritoneal lavage, a large-diameter soft sterile catheter or human dialysis catheter is required. If the catheter has only a single opening, other holes can be cut along its length; do not make these too large, as the catheter may become kinked
2. Prepare the animal as for paracentesis (sedation may be required), and apply a local anaesthetic to the body wall
3. Make a small stab incision, and insert the catheter through this incision in a caudal direction; a channel may need to be made by blunt dissection through the abdominal musculature with a haemostat
4. Samples for analysis may be collected directly or secondary to lavage. The latter entails the instillation of about 20 ml/kg body weight of warm sterile saline followed by gentle abdominal massage and rolling the animal from side to side. After the fluid has circulated through the abdomen, a sample can be collected
5. It is not necessary to remove all of the fluid that has been instilled
6. Remove the catheter once samples have been obtained

Figure 9.7: Technique for diagnostic peritoneal lavage.

Radiography

Radiography may reveal organomegaly or abnormal distribution of gas or fluid. Gas may be contained within the gut (e.g. in ileus associated with perforation by a foreign body or inflammatory peritonitis) or be free in the abdominal cavity (see Figure 9.3). Small accumulations of intraperitoneal fluid may be seen as areas with a 'ground-glass' appearance (Figure 9.8). Their presence may help to localize disease, as loss of serosal detail in the:

- Cranial third of the abdomen suggests liver involvement
- Middle third of the abdomen suggests kidney or splenic involvement
- Caudal third of the abdomen suggests prostatic, urinary bladder or uterine disease
- Cranial right quadrant suggests pancreatitis.

Ileus and intestinal dilation may be evident, and these suggest generalized peritonitis. Because a large accumulation of fluid results in extensive loss of abdominal detail, radiography is generally less helpful in cases with marked ascites, although it may allow assessment of liver size.

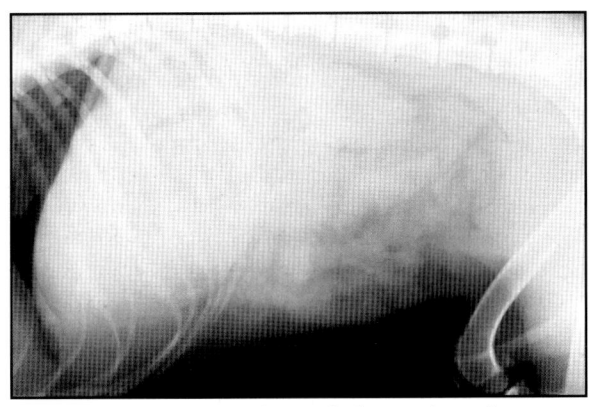

Figure 9.8: Abdominal radiograph showing loss of contrast consistent with accumulation of intraperitoneal fluid.

Ultrasonography

Ultrasonography can be used to assess the size, structure and integrity of intra-abdominal structures and to determine whether fluid or gas is present. Because different parenchymatous organs have differing echogenicities, ultrasonography can also be used to detect changes in cellularity and stromal composition. Ultrasonography shows the extent of any fluid accumulation and may also indicate the nature of the fluid. For example, the echo pattern may detect flocculent particles within an exudate. Ultrasound guidance can be useful when collecting samples of fluid or tissue by fine-needle aspiration or needle biopsy.

Computed tomography

CT scanning can accurately identify alterations to organs and may indicate the primary disorder underlying septic peritonitis.

Treatment

Resolution of peritonitis involves successful correction of the underlying condition, management of the bacterial infection and correction of metabolic disturbances.

Fluid therapy

Fluid therapy aims to correct hypovolaemia and to manage acidosis, electrolyte abnormalities, hypoglycaemia and any reduction in renal blood flow through:

- Intravenous infusion of Hartmann's solution at rates of up to 150 ml/kg/day
- Intravenous administration of potassium and glucose in some cases; concentrated potassium solutions should not be given rapidly intravenously – maximum rate of 0.5 mmol/kg/h is advised.

Where there is concern that iatrogenic septic peritonitis may develop or may be developing, supportive care such as fluid therapy should be instituted early.

Antibacterial therapy

Where possible, antibacterial therapy should be selected according to culture and sensitivity. Although some antibacterials may seem to be a good choice, they may fail to gain therapeutic concentrations within purulent exudate (see Chapter 2). To treat septic peritonitis effectively, drugs active against Gram-positive and Gram-negative aerobic and anaerobic bacteria and that achieve sufficient concentration within the peritoneal cavity are required. The following should be considered in both dogs and cats:

- Clindamycin or amoxycillin–clavulanate, with enrofloxacin, gentamicin or a third-generation cephalosporin (cefoxitin). If an aminoglycoside such as gentamicin is to be used, hypovolaemia must be corrected first to reduce the risk of nephrotoxicity (see Chapter 2)
- Metronidazole for the management of anaerobic infections
- A long course of high-dose ampicillin for actinomycosis
- Ampicillin for streptococcal infections
- A prolonged course of trimethoprim-sulphonamide for nocardiosis
- Tetracyclines, cephalexin or trimethoprim-sulphonamide for *Yersinia* infections.

Analgesic and anti-inflammatory drugs

Septic peritonitis is painful, and narcotic analgesics, e.g. morphine, pethidine, buprenorphine, are often required (see Appendix 3). The use of anti-inflammatory agents such as non-steroidal anti-inflammatory drugs (NSAIDs) and corticosteroids are not indicated, as the inflammatory process is required for healing, and there is no evidence that excessive inflammation is a problem. The use of NSAIDs rather than narcotic analgesics to control pain in septic peritonitis cannot be recommended, as they are less effective analgesics and all NSAIDs have the potential to cause gastrointestinal ulceration or renal papillary necrosis, particularly in hypovolaemic patients; newer NSAIDs are associated with far fewer adverse effects.

Some authors believe that corticosteroids are of benefit although any effects are unproven. Others indicate that corticosteroids are absolutely contraindicated because of their deleterious effects on the immune system. It is the authors' and editor's view that corticosteroids should not be used.

Surgery

Where bacterial infection results from perforation of the intestine or a ruptured abscess (e.g. pyometra, prostatic abscess), the damaged organ must be surgically repaired or drained. Abdominal lavage at laparotomy with 200-300 ml/kg of warmed isotonic saline is indicated to remove debris and to dilute toxins. Open abdominal drainage is indicated in some cases, although such cases require intensive postoperative management. The technique is described in general surgery texts (e.g. Greenfield, 1998). If unable to carry out this technique, immediate referral is recommended. Patients managed with open abdominal drainage carry a much better prognosis than those in whom the abdomen is closed. Factors used to decide whether open abdominal drainage is necessary include:

- Severity of the illness - the more severe the illness the greater the need for open abdominal drainage
- The extent of peritoneal contamination
- An assessment of the extent to which all contaminated material was removed by lavage
- An expectation that the septic process will continue after removal of the debris.

FELINE INFECTIOUS PERITONITIS

Aetiology

Feline infectious peritonitis (FIP) was first recognized in 1963. The causal agent, a coronavirus, was initially named feline infectious peritonitis virus (FIPV). Subsequently it was shown that many healthy cats were seropositive to this coronavirus, and it was postulated that they were infected with an avirulent coronavirus, named feline enteric coronavirus (FECV). At that time it was believed that FECV lived solely in the intestine and caused only mild diarrhoea in kittens; however, later studies showed that many healthy cats were viraemic, indicating that FECV was not confined to the intestine. Epidemiological studies have shown that FIP develops in up to 10% of cats seropositive for coronavirus. It is now thought that virulent FIPV arises by mutation of FECV within an individual cat, which may then go on to develop FIP. Since FIPV and FECV can no longer be considered as separate virus groups, the broader term of feline coronavirus (FCoV) has been adopted. There are many strains of FCoV, which differ widely in virulence; however, there is no reliable method of distinguishing virulent from avirulent strains.

Prevalence

Many cats, especially those in multicat households, are infected with FCoV. The percentage of cats seropositive for FCoV is:

- 82% at cat shows
- 53% of pedigree cats
- 28% of domestic cats in multicat households
- About 15% of healthy domestic cats in single cat households.

Up to 10% of FCoV infected cats living in large multicat groups develop FIP, whereas it is rarely seen in cats kept either singly or in small stable groups.

Pathogenesis

Transmission of FCoV occurs mainly via the faeco-oral route. After oronasal infection, the virus initially replicates in pharyngeal, respiratory or intestinal epithelial cells. Most infections at this stage are asymptomatic. Signs of mild enteritis may be present, although chronic and severe diarrhoea have also been reported. The virus is then eliminated by mosts cats, which never develop FIP.

In some cats, after replication in epithelial cells, viraemia develops, resulting in infection of the target cell, the macrophage. Virus-specific antibody may increase the infectivity of the virus for macrophages: cats with FIP often have high anti-FCoV antibody titres. Virus binds to antibody to form immune complexes. These are deposited in the walls of small blood vessels where they activate the complement and co-agulation cascades and establish an immune-mediated vasculitis. Two clinical situations may then arise. First, involvement of many blood vessels results in increased vascular permeability and leakage of a protein-rich exudate into body cavities and potential spaces, including occasionally the pericardial sac and the scrotum. This gives rise to the effusive or 'wet' form of FIP. Second, when fewer blood vessels are affected, the course of FIP is more chronic, and discrete pyogranulomas form throughout the body. This gives rise to the non-effusive or 'dry' form of FIP.

Factors that determine whether a cat exposed to FCoV develops the disease include:

- Strain - different strains of FCoV vary in their virulence

- Dose – exposure to higher titres of virus increases the risk of FIP developing
- Stress – cats that develop FIP usually have a history of stress 3–6 weeks before the development of effusive FIP and 3 weeks to several months before the development of non-effusive FIP
- Genetic susceptibility – some breeds of cat seem to be more susceptible to the development of FIP. This suggests that there is a genetic predisposition to developing FIP, possibly relating to certain major histocompatibility gene (MHC) loci.

Clinical features

History

Effusive ('wet') and non-effusive ('dry') FIP present in distinct ways. As they represent different ends of the same clinical spectrum, some cases show features of both forms. The historical and clinical signs of FIP are highly variable, depending on the form of FIP. In addition to obtaining routine historical information, several factors are particularly relevant in the diagnosis of FIP:

- Has the cat come from a cat breeder, multicat rescue establishment or boarding cattery within the previous weeks or months? In these situations it is more likely to have been exposed to FCoV
- Has the cat been stressed in previous weeks, e.g. rehoming, surgery? Effusive FIP, the acute form of FIP, usually occurs within 3–6 weeks of a stressful event in a cat's life
- What age is the cat? Although cats of any age may develop FIP, 80% are less than 2 years old. Both sexes are equally affected
- What breed is the cat? Although any breed can develop FIP, pedigree cats form a disproportionately large percentage of those affected
- Has there been a history of diarrhoea, coughing or sneezing in the past few weeks? For both forms, diarrhoea and mild upper respiratory disease may precede the development of fulminant FIP
- Is there any history of exposure to cats, particularly littermates, affected by FIP?

Physical examination

Effusive or 'wet' FIP: The predominant clinical and physical signs consistent with effusive FIP are:

- Ascites and/or pleural effusion
- Bright and eating or dull and anorexic
- Mild pyrexia in some cases; this tends to fluctuate
- Dyspnoea if a pleural effusion present
- Weight loss
- Palpably enlarged mesenteric lymph nodes and liver
- Extension of the disease process to involve other abdominal organs (this results in clinical signs relating to their dysfunction, e.g. hepatopathy, renal failure, pancreatic disease)
- Ocular and CNS involvement – these may accompany effusive FIP, although they are more commonly associated with non-effusive FIP.

Non-effusive or 'dry' FIP: The clinical features are often vague, non-specific and variable; this condition is one of the more difficult to diagnose. Common presenting signs include:

- Weight loss
- Inappetence.

Other clinical signs depend on which organs have been affected and how much damage has been done. They include:

- Eye – uveitis, keratic precipitates, aqueous or vitreous flare, retinal vessel cuffing and pyogranulomata on the retina
- CNS – pyogranuloma formation and the development of hydrocephalus results in nystagmus, vestibular signs (e.g. head tilt), seizures, cerebellar ataxia, cranial nerve dysfunction, paresis, proprioceptive loss, urinary incontinence or signs of behavioural changes. Neurological signs occur in 10% of dry FIP cases (Kline *et al.*, 1994)
- Intestine – thickened colonic wall
- Mesenteric lymph node – palpably enlarged
- Liver – jaundice and hepatomegaly
- Kidneys – pyogranulomas may be palpable.

Differential diagnosis

Figure 9.9 lists the main differential diagnoses for effusive FIP and indicates how to differentiate them from effusive FIP. The effusive form of FIP and the inflammatory disease lymphocytic cholangitis can be particularly difficult to differentiate. Both can present with similar clinical signs of weight loss, anorexia and ascites. They produce a similar ascitic fluid (see Figure 9.4), and they both show similar changes in serum biochemistry and haematology, although cats with FIP are more likely to have a non-regenerative anaemia. Other clinical signs can help differentiate these conditions, e.g. uveitis or a thoracic effusion in FIP. Generally, cats with lymphocytic cholangitis are brighter than those with FIP, and they may occasionally be polyphagic. Where differentiation is not possible from clinical findings, histopathological examination of a liver biopsy may be required.

Figure 9.10 lists the main differential diagnoses for non-effusive FIP.

Condition	How to differentiate from FIP
Cardiomyopathy	Transudate with low protein content (<35 g/l). Radiography may reveal enlarged or globular heart. Ultrasonography of heart
Liver disease (lymphocytic cholangitis, cholangiohepatitis, cirrhosis)	If ascites is a modified transudate rather than an exudate, FIP is ruled out. However, in some liver conditions associated with post-hepatic vascular obstruction, the effusion may have a high protein content like that of FIP. Reverse transcriptase-polymerase chain reaction of the effusion is useful; if unavailable, exploratory laparotomy and biopsy may be necessary. Bile acid stimulation test may be helpful in documenting cirrhosis
Liver tumour	As above, ultrasonography may also help by detecting masses
Purulent serositis	Foul-smelling opaque effusion containing bacteria and high white blood cell count with degenerate neutrophils
Lymphosarcoma (LSA)	If thymic LSA, then radiography of lateral thorax may reveal a mass cranial to the heart and possible elevation of the oesophagus. If abdominal LSA, organomegaly may be found. Fluid analysis typically reveals fluid with a low protein content, and the cell population consists mainly of lymphocytes rather than neutrophils and macrophages
Pregnancy	Abdominal palpation, unable to draw fluid on paracentesis, kitten in uterus on radiography or ultrasonography
Obesity	Abdominal palpation, unable to draw fluid on paracentesis, absence of ascites on radiography or ultrasonography

Figure 9.9: Differential diagnoses for effusive feline infectious peritonitis (FIP) and methods for differentiating them. The conditions are listed in order; the most common disease misdiagnosed as FIP is first and the least common is last.

Clinical sign	Differential diagnosis
Chronic weight loss, anorexia, mild pyrexia	Feline leukaemia virus (FeLV), feline immunodeficiency virus (FIV), neoplasia, hyperthyroidism in older cat
Intraocular signs	FIV (uveitis), FeLV, toxoplasmosis, fungal infection, idiopathic
Icterus	Cholangiohepatitis, *Haemobartonella felis*, biliary obstruction, autoimmune haemolytic anaemia
Neurological signs	Trauma, portosystemic shunt, FeLV, FIV, toxoplasmosis, neoplasia, feline spongiform encephalopathy

Figure 9.10: Differential diagnoses for the various clinical signs associated with non-effusive feline infectious peritonitis (FIP).

Diagnosis

Despite many claims to the contrary, there is no simple way to diagnose FIP in a living cat other than by biopsy and histopathology of affected tissues or granulomas. Most available tests demonstrate exposure to a FCoV, whereas reverse transcriptase-polymerase chain reaction (RT-PCR) detects a feline coronavirus (see later). No test can distinguish virulent from avirulent field strains of FCoV, although some tests differentiate laboratory isolates. In most cases, a diagnosis of FIP (either form) in a cat with appropriate historical and clinical features requires consideration of several different diagnostic tests, which fit together to suggest FIP. These include:

- Clinical pathology to assess for specific organ involvement
- Analysis of thoracic or abdominal effusions
- Serology to demonstrate exposure to the virus
- RT-PCR assays to demonstrate the presence of the virus
- Histopathological examination of affected tissues; this is the only means of definitively diagnosing FIP.

Figure 9.11 lists the different diagnostic tests and the samples suitable for each assay. Figure 9.12 summarizes the tests currently available for the detection of FCoV and anti-FCoV antibody and indicates the clinical situations for which each type of test is indicated.

Laboratory test	Samples required
Immunofluorescent antibody test	Whole blood, serum, plasma or effusion
Reverse transcriptase-polymerase chain reaction	Faeces, rectal swabs, effusion, saliva swabs or blood
Analysis of effusion	Effusion in plain tube
Immunohistochemistry	Pieces of organs, especially kidney, in 10% formalin
Histopathology	Pieces of organs, especially kidney, in 10% formalin

Figure 9.11: Laboratory tests that may be used in the diagnosis of feline infectious peritonitis (FIP) and recommended samples required for each.

Test detects	Tests available	Clinical situations when tests are indicated
Antibody	Immunofluorescent antibody test (IFAT) ELISA (e.g. IDEXX Snap)* Immunocomb® Rapid immunomigration*	Diagnosis of feline infectious peritonitis (FIP) (in conjunction with other tests and clinical signs) Screening a cat that has been in contact with a cat that developed FIP to assess whether or not it might be infectious Screening a cat before mating Screening a household for the presence of FCoV Screening cats before entry into FCoV-free households
Virus	Reverse-transcriptase-polymerase chain reaction	Diagnosis of effusive FIP when performed on effusion Screening a cat that has been in contact with a cat that developed FIP to assess whether it is infectious; multiple tests required Screening a household of cats for the presence of FCoV Screening cats before entry into FCoV-free households; multiple tests required
Virus in tissues	Immunohistochemistry	Definitive diagnostic technique, especially if histopathology result is equivocal
Pathological changes	Histopathology	Definitive diagnostic technique

Figure 9.12: List of diagnostic tests that can be used to demonstrate exposure to, or infection with, feline coronavirus (FCoV), and the clinical situations in which their use is recommended.
*Not recommended by the authors; in their experience the results do not correlate with the gold standard assay (IFAT).

Clinical pathology

Serum biochemical abnormalities depend on the organs involved and the duration of the clinical problem. Hyperglobulinaemia (occasionally monoclonal gammopathy) and increased α1-acid glycoprotein (AGP) concentrations are consistent features (see below). Non-specific haematological abnormalities that may be present include neutrophilia (often with a left shift), lymphopenia and non-regenerative anaemia. Such changes are more likely to be found with non-effusive FIP. A coagulopathy may be evident.

Nature of the effusion

The technique for abdominal paracentesis is described in Figure 9.6. Analysis of the effusion is helpful in demonstrating abnormalities consistent with FIP and for ruling out FIP. The following major features may be associated with an effusion from an animal with FIP:

- Usually straw-coloured and always sterile
- High total protein content (>35 g/l), froths when shaken (Figure 9.13) and may clot if left to stand at room temperature for a few hours
- If the albumin:globulin ratio of the effusion is below 0.4, FIP is likely; above 0.8 FIP is unlikely; and between 0.4 and 0.8 FIP is possible but not certain
- AGP >1500 mg/ml (Duthie *et al.*, 1997) is consistent with FIP
- Total nucleated cell count of <5000 cells/ml (mainly neutrophils and macrophages)
- May be reverse transcriptase-polymerase chain reaction-positive for virus RNA (see later).

Figure 9.14 shows cytology consistent with FIP.

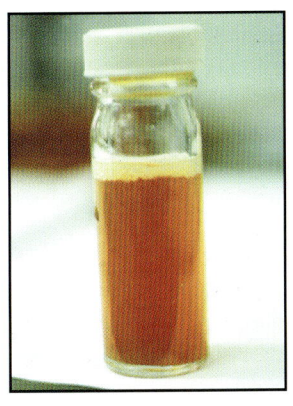

Figure 9.13: Straw-coloured frothy fluid from a cat with feline infectious peritonitis (© Dr Bryn Tennant).

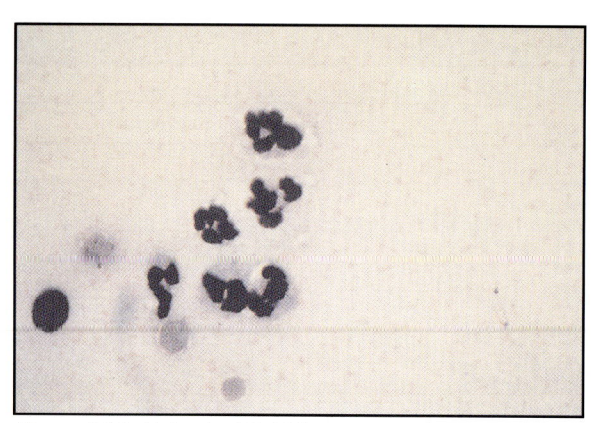

162 Manual of Canine and Feline Infectious Diseases

Figure 9.14: Abdominal fluid from a cat with FIP. Note the proteinaceous background and the presence of the neutrophils.

Serology

Serology is used:

- In the diagnosis of cats with suspected FIP
- To assess for exposure when a cat has been in contact with a cat suspected of excreting FCoV
- When a cat breeder has requested testing
- For screening a household of cats for the presence of FCoV
- For screening a cat before allowing it to mix with FCoV-free cats.

Serological testing presents problems of interpretation as:

- A cat with a clinically similar condition may coincidentally be seropositive, especially pedigree cats; therefore, although a high antibody titre in a cat with suspect clinical signs is consistent with a diagnosis of FIP, it is not diagnostic
- Some cats with effusive FIP have low antibody titres or are seronegative, probably because antibody is bound to the huge amount of virus within the cat and therefore unavailable to bind to the virus in the antibody test.

Serological tests may detect antibody without giving a titre (e.g. Rapid immunomigration tests, Snap tests), whereas others (e.g. Immunocomb®, immunofluorescence) provide an antibody titre. Results expressed as a titre may be useful when monitoring individual cats or households of cats for elimination of FCoV.

Interpretation of serology results in ill cats

Effusive FIP: Although serology is useful in the diagnosis of effusive FIP, it should only be used where the clinical signs, albumin:globulin ratio, AGP concentration and cytology of the effusion are appropriate.

Cats with effusive FIP vary from being seronegative to having high antibody titres. Those with conditions other than FIP can coincidentally have anti-FCoV antibodies, especially those from multicat households or those who have come from a cat breeder or rescue organization within the past 6-12 months.

Non effusive FIP: The anti-FCoV immunofluorescent antibody titres in non-effusive FIP are generally 640 or higher. A titre of less than 160 nearly always rules out non-effusive FIP. A positive FCoV antibody test result in a healthy cat should not be misinterpreted as an early form of non-effusive FIP.

Interpretation of serology results in healthy cats

Screening healthy in-contact cats: Screening healthy cats that have been in contact with a case of FIP or a FCoV excretor is usually done for one of the two reasons detailed below. In either case, it should be made clear to the owner before testing that it is highly likely that the cat will be seropositive. Almost all cats exposed to FCoV become infected. This does not indicate a poor prognosis as less than 10% of cats infected with FCoV develop FIP; most eventually eliminate the virus and become seronegative.

In the situation where the owner wishes to replace a cat that has died of FIP and needs to know if an exposed cat is shedding FCoV:

- If the exposed cat is seronegative it is highly unlikely to be infected and therefore will not be shedding virus; it is safe to get another cat
- If the exposed cat is seropositive (i.e. has an antibody titre of 1:10 or more) there is a 1 in 3 chance that it is shedding FCoV and so it would be unwise to get another cat (unless it has antibodies indicating that it has been exposed). The cat should be retested after 3-6 months to determine if its antibody titre has fallen. Most cats that eliminate FCoV infection lose their antibodies between 3 months and several years. Ideally, seropositive cats should be separated from seronegative ones in the household. As soon as a seropositive cat becomes seronegative, it should be added to the seronegative group to prevent it becoming reinfected by the other cats.

Where the owner wants to know the prognosis for the exposed cat:

- If the cat is seronegative it most probably is not infected and so will not develop FIP
- If the cat is seropositive there is a low probability (less than 1 in 10) that the cat will develop FIP.

Screening breeding cats: Cat breeders often request that their cats be screened for FCoV before mating. In this situation:

- If the cat is seronegative it is unlikely to be infected so will not be excreting FCoV and can be safely mated, with a seronegative mate
- If the cat is seropositive it would be wise to find a seropositive mate to reduce the risk of introducing FCoV into a coronavirus-free cattery. The isolation and early weaning procedures outlined in Figure 9.15 should then be followed to prevent infection of the kittens.

Screening a cattery for FCoV: A random sampling of three or four cats living together will show whether FCoV is endemic, because the virus is highly contagious. Households of fewer than 10 cats and those where the cats are isolated from each other in groups of three or less often lose their FCoV infection eventually. Testing every 6-12 months establishes when this is occurring, as antibody titres fall and an increasing proportion of cats becomes seronegative. It is helpful to separate seronegative cats from seropositive ones to prevent reinfection.

Screening a cat that is to be introduced into a FCoV-free household: Only seronegative cats should be introduced into coronavirus-free catteries. Cats with antibody can be isolated and retested after 3-6 month intervals until they become seronegative.

Reverse transcriptase-polymerase chain reaction
Reverse transcriptase-polymerase chain reaction (RT-PCR) amplifies a selected part of the viral nucleic acid to detectable concentrations (see Chapter 1). The technique is sensitive, but stringent precautions must be taken to avoid contamination that can result in false positives. Some laboratories claim to have a RT-PCR that is diagnostic of FIP and even predictive of the development of FIP in a healthy cat; however, at the time of writing, genetic sequence analysis of several FIPV and FECV strains has failed to demonstrate a consistent mutation responsible for virulence. Because of the variability of the FCoV genome, it is unlikely that an assay will ever be available that can consistently discriminate between 'avirulent' and 'virulent' strains (Horzinek, 1997). The technique can be used on faeces, blood, saliva or effusions, although monitoring salivary virus excretion is not useful as saliva excretion stops long before faecal virus shedding ceases.

RT-PCR may be used in the diagnosis of FIP:

- The presence of FCoV RNA in an effusion is probably but not definitively diagnostic of FIP
- An RT-PCR-positive blood test result is not conclusive of a diagnosis of FIP as healthy cats and those with conditions other than FIP may be RT-PCR positive
- An RT-PCR-negative blood result does not rule out a diagnosis of FIP as cats with FIP may be RT-PCR negative.

RT-PCR can be used to monitor virus shedding in households in which FCoV control is being attempted. Three types of cat may be identified:

- Most FCoV-infected cats shed virus for a while, seroconvert, cease shedding, lose their antibodies and become reinfected, and then the cycle restarts
- A small group of cats are virus carriers, shedding virus continually (Foley *et al.*, 1997)
- A small group of cats seem to be resistant to virus shedding.

Preparation of kitten room	1. Remove all cats and kittens one week before confining the queen 2. Disinfect room by using 1:32 dilution of sodium hypochlorite (Domestos or Milton) 3. Dedicate litter trays, food and water bowls to this room and disinfect with sodium hypochlorite 4. Introduce queen 1-2 weeks before she is due to give birth
Avoidance of indirect transmission of virus	1. Deal with the kitten room before tending other cats 2. Clean hands with disinfectant before going into kitten room 3. Have shoes and coveralls dedicated to the kitten room
Early weaning and isolation of kittens	1. Test queen for antibodies to FCoV either before or after kittening 2. If queen's antibody titre is greater than zero, the kittens should be removed to another clean room when they are 5-6 weeks old 3. If the queen has an antibody titre of zero, she can remain with the kittens until they are older 4. Take care to socialize isolated kittens when they are 2-7 weeks old to accustom them to humans
Testing kittens	1. Test kittens for antibodies to FCoV at over 10 weeks of age to ensure that they are seronegative

Figure 9.15: Protocol for prevention of feline coronavirus (FCoV) infection in kittens.

Gross pathology/histopathology

Serosal surfaces are often covered in white fibrinous plaques, 1-2 mm in diameter (Figure 9.16). Large granulomas may be evident in solid organs. Miliary tumours and other infections (e.g. mycobacteriosis) may present with similar appearances. Liver, omentum and intestinal tract can be biopsied at a laparotomy, whereas these tissues together with eyes and CNS can be obtained at a post mortem examination. Histology allows a definitive diagnosis.

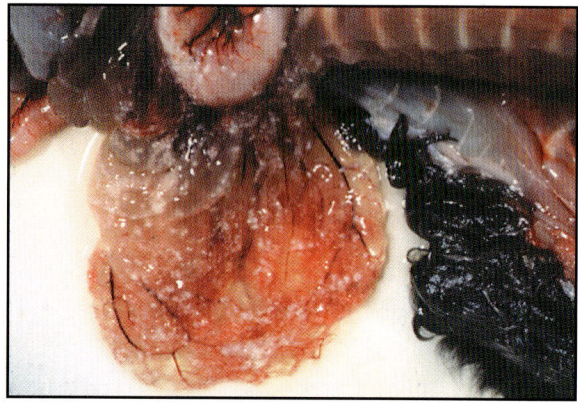

Figure 9.16: Multiple white nodules in the omentum of a cat with feline infectious peritonitis.

Immunohistochemistry

Immunohistochemistry is a further aid to diagnosis in cases where histopathology cannot clearly identify FIP (see Chapter 1).

Treatment

FIP is usually fatal and no treatment has proved to be reliable. Therapy is therefore largely symptomatic, consisting of fluid replacement and nutritional support. Since FIP is an immune-mediated disease, treatment is often aimed at moderating the immune response to the virus. Although several authors claim to have found suitable treatment protocols, caution should always be applied when interpreting these results because FIP is notoriously difficult to confirm in the live animal. Typically, immunomodulation is attempted with immune suppressants or immune stimulants, either alone or in combination:

- Immunosuppressants include corticosteroids (e.g. prednisolone) or cyclophosphamide. The readily available cyclophosphamide tablets (50 mg) do not lend themselves to the dosing regimen; 25 mg tablets are available for importation (see Chapter 5 for further information on therapeutic options for immunosuppression) (see Appendix 3 for doses)
- Many compounds may have non-specific immunostimulant, anti-inflammatory or antioxidant properties that may be of benefit in the management of FIP; however, their usefulness has not been proven. Of the many compounds suggested, those that may potentially be beneficial and are least likely to do harm include: human α-interferon; aspirin (salicylic acid); vitamin C (ascorbic acid); vitamin B1 (thiamine); and anabolic steroids. See Appendix 3 for doses.

For an extensive review of treatment for FIP see Weiss (1994).

Prognosis

The prognosis for FIP is always poor as it is almost invariably fatal. Cats with effusive FIP may survive for days to weeks. Some cases may develop non-effusive FIP, following resolution of the effusion with treatment. Cats with non-effusive FIP may survive up to a year with treatment, provided that the disease is diagnosed early in its course before anorexia or neurological signs are evident.

Control and prevention

Preventing infection of kittens

FCoV does not normally cross the placenta, and kittens are usually protected by maternally derived antibody until they are 5-6 weeks old. Therefore in colonies where FCoV is endemic, pregnant queens should be isolated from all other cats in the household from just before birth until their kittens are 5-6 weeks old. The litter should then be removed and kept in complete isolation until sold. Infected kittens may not seroconvert until 10 weeks of age, therefore they should not be tested for antibodies before this time. Figure 9.15 gives a step-by-step protocol of the isolation and early weaning procedure (Addie and Jarrett, 1992).

Eradication of FCoV from a cattery

In most closed households with less than 10 cats, FCoV is spontaneously eliminated. The cats cease to shed virus and their antibody titres eventually decline towards zero; loss of infection may take months to years. Where owners wish to eradicate FCoV from their catteries, all the cats must be tested every 3-6 months with a reliable immunofluorescence antibody test and/or RT-PCR of the faeces. Two or more groups of cats should be established: a seronegative group and a seropositive group. When a seropositive cat becomes seronegative it should be moved into the seronegative group. It is preferable for the cats to be split into stable groups of two or three cats. All the cats in most catteries should stop shedding virus because the separation of seropositive from seronegative cats breaks the cycle of infection to immunity to loss of immunity to reinfection.

A small percentage of chronic FCoV shedders do, however, exist. At present there is no way of identifying these carrier cats except by isolation of the cat and

Reduce the numbers of cats in any area
Owners should keep no more than 6–10 cats
Cats should be kept in stable groups of up to 3 or 4
Cats should be kept singly in rescue facilities
In a FCoV eradication programme, cats should be kept in small groups according to their antibody or virus excretion status: antibody- or virus-negative cats together, antibody- or virus-positive cats together
Avoid introducing virus to uninfected cats: antibody or virus testing
Incumbent cats should be tested before introducing new cats or before breeding
Only antibody- or virus-negative cats should be introduced into FCoV-free catteries
It is safer to introduce antibody-positive cats than antibody-negative cats into FCoV-infected households, but there is still a risk of feline infectious peritonitis in both the newcomer and the incumbent cats
Prevent infection of kittens: early weaning and isolation
Both cat breeders and rescuers of pregnant cats should follow the protocol outlined in Figure 9.15
Reduce faecal contamination of environment
Have adequate numbers of litter trays – one tray for 1 or 2 cats
Litter trays should be 'declumped' at least daily
Remove all litter and disinfect litter tray at least once a week
Site litter trays away from the food area
Vacuum around litter trays regularly
Clip fur off hindquarters of longhaired cats
Vaccination (where available)
If new cats must be introduced into a household with endemic infection, they should receive a full course of Primucell vaccine before introduction
Where economically possible, rescue catteries should vaccinate all new cats with Primucell

Figure 9.17: Protocol for minimizing introduction or spread of feline coronavirus (FCoV) in a cattery.*
* Based on recommendations from working groups of the international feline enteric coronavirus and feline infectious peritonitis workshop (Pedersen et al., 1995).

repeated monthly RT-PCR testing of its faeces. If the cat continues to shed virus for more than 8 months, despite being removed from any sources of reinfection, it is likely to be a carrier. Figure 9.17 gives a step-by-step protocol for obtaining and maintaining a FCoV infection-free household.

Prevention of FIP in healthy FCoV-infected cats
There is no certain way to prevent an infected cat from developing FIP, but the following may help:

- Minimize stress for the cat: do not rehome seropositive cats, delay non-essential surgery until the cat is seronegative, avoid putting the cat into a cattery by having the cat cared for in its own home while the owners are on holiday.
- Where possible do not breed from seropositive cats: because a cat's genetic makeup plays an important part in determining which FCoV-infected cat goes on to develop FIP, matings that previously produced kittens that developed FIP should not be repeated. Ideally, any cat that has produced kittens that have developed FIP should never be bred from again.
- Avoid immunosuppressive drugs, e.g. corticosteroids, progestogens.

Vaccination
Only one vaccine is available against FCoV at the time of writing; it is available in parts of Europe but not in the UK. It is a temperature-sensitive modified live vaccine containing an FCoV that replicates only at the lower temperature of the nasopharynx and not at the higher body temperature. The principle of the vaccine is that it induces immunity at the first site to be challenged by FCoV, the oropharynx, thereby preventing colonization of the body by the virus. It promotes local (an IgA response), systemic humoral (the cat becomes positive on serological tests) and cell-mediated immunity. The vaccine is ineffective in a cat that has already been exposed to FCoV and in which FIP has begun. It has an efficacy of 50–75% (i.e. of 100 cats infected with FCoV 10 would be expected to develop FIP, but if all 100 cats had been vaccinated, then only 2–5 would develop FIP). The vaccine is only licensed for use in kittens over 16 weeks of age; however, many pedigree kittens will already be infected with FCoV by this time. It is important to safeguard young kittens from infection by keeping them in isolation and weaning them early, and by breeding from the least susceptible cats.

DRUG DOSAGES

See Appendix 3.

REFERENCES AND FURTHER READING

Addie DD and Jarrett O (1992) A study of naturally occurring feline coronavirus infection in kittens. *Veterinary Record* **130**, 133-137

Addie DD and Jarrett O (1998) Feline coronavirus infection. In: *Infectious Diseases of the Dog and Cat*, 3rd edn, ed. CE Greene, pp. 58-68. WB Saunders, Philadelphia

Davidson M, Else R and Lumsden J (1998) *Manual of Small Animal Clinical Pathology*. BSAVA, Cheltenham

Duthie S, Eckersall PD, Addie DD, Lawrence CE and Jarrett O (1997) Value of α1-acid glycoprotein in the diagnosis of feline infectious peritonitis. *Veterinary Record* **141**, 299-303

Fehr D, Holznagel E, Bolla S, Hauser B, Herrewegh AAPM, Horzinek MC and Lutz H (1997) Placebo-controlled evaluation of a modified life virus vaccine against feline infectious peritonitis: safety and efficacy under field conditions. *Vaccine* **15**, 1101-1109

Foley JE and Pedersen NC (1996) The inheritance of susceptibility to feline infectious peritonitis in purebred catteries. *Feline Practice* **24**, 14-22

Foley JE, Poland A, Carlson J and Pedersen NC (1997) Patterns of feline coronavirus infection and fecal shedding from cats in multiple-cat environments. *Journal of the American Veterinary Medical Association* **210**, 1307-1312

Greene CE (1998) Gastrointestinal and intra-abdominal infections. In: *Infectious Diseases of the Dog and Cat*, 3rd edn, ed. CE Greene, pp. 595-614. WB Saunders, Philadelphia

Greene CE and Prescott JF (1998) Streptoccocal and other Gram-positive bacterial infections. In: *Infectious Diseases of the Dog and Cat*, 3rd edn, ed. CE Greene, pp. 205-213. WB Saunders, Philadelphia

Greenfield CL (1998) Open peritoneal drainage for peritonitis. In: *Current Techniques in Small Animal Surgery, 4th edn*, ed. M. Bojrab, pp. 330-335. Williams and Wilkins, Baltimore

Herrewegh AAPM, Mahler M, Hedrich HJ, Haagmans BL, Egberink HF, Horzinek MC, Rottier PJM and de Groot RJ (1997) Persistence and evolution of feline coronavirus in a closed cat-breeding colony. *Virology* **234**, 349-363

Herrewegh AAPM, Smeenk I, Horzinek MC, Rottier PJM, de Groot RJ (1998) Feline coronavirus type II strains 79-1683 and 79-1146 originate from a double recombination between feline coronavirus type I and canine coronavirus. *Journal of Virology* **72**, 1508-1514

Horzinek HC (1997) Update on feline infectious peritonitis. *Feline Focus* **5**, 1-4

Kline KL, Joseph RJ and Averill DR (1994) Feline infectious peritonitis with neurologic involvement: clinical and pathological findings in 24 cats. *Journal of the American Animal Hospital Association* **30**, 111-118

Pedersen NC (1995) An overview of feline enteric coronavirus and infectious peritonitis virus infections. *Feline Practice* **23**, 7-20

Pedersen NC, Addie D and Wolf A (1995) Recommendations from working groups of the international feline enteric coronavirus and feline infectious peritonitis workshop. *Feline Practice* **23**, 108-111

Shelly SM, Scarlett-Kranz J and Blue JT (1988) Protein electrophoresis on effusions from cats as a diagnostic test for feline infectious peritonitis. *Journal of the American Animal Hospital Association* **24**, 495-500

Vennema H, Poland A, Foley J and Pedersen NC (1998) Feline infectious peritonitis viruses arise by mutation from endemic feline enteric coronaviruses. *Virology* **243**, 150-157

Weiss RC (1994) Feline infectious peritonitis virus: advances in therapy and control. In: *Consultations in Feline Internal Medicine 2*, ed. JR August, pp. 3-12. WB Saunders, Philadelphia

CHAPTER TEN

The Urinary System

Bryn Tennant

CHAPTER PLAN

Introduction
Urinary tract infections
    Routes of infection
    Urinary tract defence mechanisms
    Aetiology
    Clinical features
    Diagnostic plan
    Treatment
Renal infections
    Feline coronavirus
    Leptospirosis
    Canine herpesvirus
    Septicaemia/bacteraemia
    FIV
    FeLV
References and further reading

INTRODUCTION

The urinary tract comprises the kidneys, ureters, bladder, urethra and prostate. Infections of these organs are major causes of disease. This chapter is divided into two parts: the first is concerned with the general approach to the diagnosis of urinary tract infection, and the second is concerned with specific primary infections of the kidney. As infections at one site often affect adjacent structures of the urinary tract, the urinary system is here considered as a single entity. Prostatitis is covered in Chapter 12.

URINARY TRACT INFECTIONS

Urinary tract infection (UTI) is a common cause of morbidity but rarely of mortality in the dog and cat. Its manifestation depends on:

- The site(s) of the urinary tract affected
- The infecting organism.

UTIs comprise infections of the lower urinary tract (cystitis, prostatitis and urethritis) and those of the upper urinary tract (pyelonephritis and ureteritis). An infection established in one area of the urinary tract can pass relatively easily to adjacent areas.

Routes of infection

Infectious agents primarily gain access to the urinary tract via:

- Ascending infection – migration of infectious agents up the urethra is the commonest route of infection, and perineal, rectal and genital bacterial flora are the principal bacterial reservoirs. Infections may ascend to the kidney resulting in pyelonephritis.
- Haematogenous infection – haematogenous seeding of bacteria into the urinary tract is a potential cause of UTI, but is rare. This possibly reflects resistance of the renal cortices to infection (only 0.01% of blood-borne bacteria lodge in the kidney (Osborne *et al.*, 1995)) and the lower bacterial burden when compared with the potential burden from the perineal area.

Urinary tract defence mechanisms

In addition to systemic cell-mediated immunity and humoral immunity, the urinary tract has an array of local defence mechanisms (Figure 10.1), any defect of which predisposes to the establishment of infection. A wide range of commensal non-pathogenic organisms, particularly Gram-positive bacteria and mycoplasma, are present in the distal urethra and lower genital tract (Figure 10.2). Such bacteria protect against infection by pathogenic organisms by preventing adhesion to the mucosa. The remainder of the genitourinary tract is normally sterile.

Aetiology

With the exception of some primary renal infections, most UTIs are opportunistic, developing secondarily to compromise of the urinary tract defence mechanisms. Classifying UTIs as acute or chronic is useful when determining therapy and providing a prognosis, although it gives no indication as to the cause. The terms uncomplicated or simple and complicated or

168 Manual of Canine and Feline Infectious Diseases

> **Micturition:** Frequent and complete voiding reduces the burden of infectious agents
> **Anatomical structures:** Muscle tone in the urethra, urethral length and peristalsis, ureterovesicular flaps
> **Mucosal defence barriers:** Prostatic secretions (antibacterial activity and immunoglobulins), local antibody production, surface glycosaminoglycans, exfoliation of cells, interference by commensal bacteria in distal urethra
> **Antimicrobial properties of urine:** High/low pH, high osmolality, high urea concentration, presence of organic acids, low molecular weight carbohydrates and Tamm-Horsfall mucoprotein
> **Systemic immunity:** Cell-mediated and humoral immunity

Figure 10.1: List of defence mechanisms that protect the urinary tract against infection.

Organism	Distal urethra	Prepuce	Vagina
Acinetobacter spp.		✓	✓
Bacteroides spp.			✓
Bacillus spp.		✓	✓
Citrobacter spp.			✓
Corynebacterium spp.	✓	✓	✓
Enterococcus spp.			✓
Enterobacter spp.			✓
Escherichia spp.	✓	✓	✓
Flavobacterium spp.	✓	✓	✓
Haemophilus spp.	✓	✓	✓
Klebsiella spp.	✓	✓	✓
Micrococcus spp.			✓
Moraxella spp.		✓	✓
Mycoplasma spp.	✓	✓	✓
Neisseria spp.			✓
Pasteurella spp.		✓	✓
Proteus spp.		✓	✓
Pseudomonas spp.		✓	✓
Staphylococcus spp.	✓	✓	✓
Streptococcus spp.	✓	✓	✓
Ureaplasma spp.	✓	✓	✓

Figure 10.2: List of commensal non-pathogenic organisms and where they may reside in the distal urethra and lower genital tract of dogs.

difficult have recently been suggested to describe the clinical situation more accurately (Senior, 2000).

Uncomplicated or simple infections
Uncomplicated or simple refers to infection of a normal healthy urinary tract subsequent to a temporary reduction in host defences (e.g. after catheterization). Bacteria attach to the uroepithelium and trigger an inflammatory process that may ultimately result in haematuria, dysuria, stranguria and pollakiuria. After appropriate antibacterial therapy, the invading bacteria are cleared, host defence mechanisms are restored and the animal remains free of infection.

Complicated or difficult infections
Complicated or difficult refers to infection by: bacteria resistant to antibacterial drugs; infections that are deep seated within the mucosa; or infections that recur because of permanent or prolonged compromise of the host defence mechanisms. Bacteria isolated from complicated UTIs are often opportunistic bacteria of low virulence that do not attach to the mucosa and do not elicit a marked inflammatory process. Identifiable abnormalities that predispose to complicated UTI are listed in Figure 10.3.

Abnormal micturition
Obstruction to urinary outflow
Uroliths, strictures, prostatic enlargement, urethral/cystic neoplasms
Incomplete emptying of the bladder
Neurological disorder, e.g. intervertebral disc disease, spinal trauma, reflex dyssynergia, anatomical defects, e.g. persistent urachus
Incontinence
Anatomical defects
Congenital/inherited
Ectopic ureters, persistent urachus, primary vesicoureteral reflux
Acquired
Secondary vesicoureteral reflux, urethral surgery
Mucosal abnormalities
Trauma
Catheterization, palpation, trauma, urolithiasis
Metaplastic changes
Oestrogen induced, e.g. iatrogenic, testicular neoplasm
Neoplasia
Presence of cytotoxic drugs, e.g. cyclophosphamide metabolite
Altered urine volume and composition and frequency of urination
Voluntary or involuntary retention of urine
Glucosuria, e.g. diabetes mellitus
Dilute urine (predisposes to urinary tract infection)
Immunodeficiency
Iatrogenic, e.g. administration of corticosteroids, immunosuppressant drugs
Acquired disorders, e.g. hyperadrenocorticism, uraemia, ?feline immunodeficiency virus/feline leukaemia virus
?Congenital immunodeficiency

Figure 10.3: Identifiable abnormalities that predispose to the development of urinary tract infection.

Infectious agents

Figure 10.4 lists the infectious agents that affect the urinary tract. Of these, bacteria are the commonest causes of disease.

Bacteria
Escherichia coli
Staphylococcus spp.
Streptococcus spp.
Pasteurella spp.
Proteus spp.
Pseudomonas spp.
Klebsiella spp.
Enterobacter spp.
Fungi
Candida spp.
Aspergillus spp.
Trichosporon spp.
Cephalosporium spp.
Cryptococcus spp.
Blastomyces spp. (not in UK)
Torulopsis spp. (not in UK)
Histoplasma spp. (not in UK)
Helminths
Capillaria feliscati in cats (not in UK)
Viruses (suggested but not proven causes of UTI in cats)
Feline calicivirus
Feline syncytium-forming virus
Bovine herpesvirus-4 (feline herpesvirus-2) (USA only)
Mycoplasma/Ureaplasma (suggested but not proven causes of UTI)
Mycoplasma felis
Mycoplasma gateae
Ureaplasma spp.

Figure 10.4: Infectious agents associated with urinary tract infection (UTI) in the dog and cat.

Bacterial UTIs: Bacterial genera isolated from the urinary tract are predominantly commensals of the intestine and skin reflecting the perineal region as the main source of bacteria. Whether a specific bacterium can cause disease is determined by virulence factors, which allow colonization and growth on the urinary tract epithelial surface, and the number of bacteria.

Virulence factors include:

- Adhesion factors (enable bacteria to adhere to mucosal surfaces)
- Capsular antigens (inhibit phagocytosis)
- Haemolysins (increase the amount of free iron and cause tissue damage)
- Growth-promoting proteins
- Plasmids containing antibacterial resistance genes
- Ureases.

Mycoplasma spp. and *Ureaplasma* spp. can be isolated from cats with UTI and from clinically normal cats. Their role in UTI is unclear.

Fungal UTIs: Fungal UTI is rarely described. *Candida albicans* is the commonest isolate, although others have been identified (see Figure 10.4). Fungal infection may cause disease in immunodeficient animals or where host defences are impaired.

Viral UTIs: The role of viruses in feline urinary tract disease (except feline coronavirus) is unclear. There is little evidence that immunosuppressive viruses such as feline immunodeficiency virus and feline leukaemia virus predispose to UTIs.

Feline herpesvirus-2 (FHV-2), serologically distinct from feline herpesvirus-1, was apparently isolated from the urine of a cat with feline urological syndrome. Antibodies to the original isolate have been detected in 30% of cats in the USA but not in cats in the UK. FHV-2 is identical to bovine herpesvirus-4 (BHV-4), and experimentally it is reported to establish a persistent UTI in cats, but this infection remains clinically silent. As the European strain of BHV-4 does not infect cats (Gaskell and Bennett, 1996) and antibodies to it have not been found in the UK, it is probable that this virus plays little if any part in feline urinary tract disease.

Feline syncytium-forming virus, a member of the foamy virus group, has been isolated from many tissues in the cat, including those of the urinary tract. It has never been shown to be pathogenic.

Urethral obstruction has been observed in cats experimentally exposed to feline calicivirus (FCV; Osborne *et al.*, 1995). However, failure to isolate the virus for more than 4 days, lack of an antibody response and the lack of isolation of FCV from the urinary tract of clinically affected cats with urethral obstruction suggests that this virus plays little if any part in feline urinary tract disease.

Clinical features

UTIs may be symptomatic or asymptomatic. Clinical signs of UTI are variable, depending on the causative organism, the presence and type of predisposing factors, the response of the urinary tract to infection and the duration and site of infection. Clinical signs include pollakiuria, dysuria, stranguria, pain on urination, abnormal urine (e.g. haematuria) and urge incontinence. Systemic signs are rarely seen unless the kidney or prostate is involved, in which case polyuria/polydipsia (renal involvement), pyrexia, depression and anorexia may be reported. Although historical and clinical features may localize a problem to the urinary tract, there are no signs that are pathognomonic for an infectious disorder.

170 Manual of Canine and Feline Infectious Diseases

A particular problem with UTIs is recurrence of clinical signs owing to relapse, reinfection or superinfection.

Relapse
Relapse occurs with persistent infections. The recurrence occurs within weeks of cessation of therapy and involves the same organism. Figure 10.5 lists the potential causes.

Ineffective antibacterial used
Antimicrobial sensitivity testing not performed
Improper sensitivity tests undertaken or misinterpretation of results
Failure to attain therapeutic concentrations in urine or other sites in urinary tract
Improper use of an effective drug
Antibacterial not prescribed for long enough
Inappropriate dose prescribed
Inappropriate frequency of administration or timing of dosing in relation to meals
Lack of owner compliance in giving antibacterial
Proper use of an effective drug
Mixed infections not detected during routine culture
Premature assessment of response
Starting therapy too late in the course of the disease
Development of antibacterial resistance

Figure 10.5: Potential causes of relapsing urinary tract infections.

Reinfection
Reinfection is defined as a recurrent infection involving a different organism and occurring some weeks to months after the initial problem. Figure 10.6 lists the potential causes of reinfection. Contamination of urine during sampling results in a false positive diagnosis of reinfection.

Dysfunction of defence mechanisms due to:
Persistence of a known previous problem
Modification of defences by surgery, e.g. urethrostomy
Inappropriate management of, or failure to recognize, a predisposing cause
Iatrogenic infection, e.g. after catheterization
Spontaneous reinfection

Figure 10.6: Potential predisposing causes of reinfection of the urinary tract with different bacteria.

Superinfection
Superinfection occurs when an additional organism gains entry to the urinary tract while the patient is receiving antibacterial therapy. It is found most commonly in patients with indwelling urinary catheters.

Canine chronic prostatitis is a common cause of recurrent UTI. Relapses relate to poor penetration of antimicrobial drugs into prostatic secretions, and reinfection may be associated with persistent abnormalities in prostatic defence mechanisms.

Diagnostic plan
Assessment of urine is essential in the investigation of an animal with suspected UTI. The urine sample should be assessed biochemically, cytologically and by culture. It is recommended that urine should always be obtained by cystocentesis to minimize bacterial contamination and should be transported in a sterile sealed container. Urine obtained by catheterization may be contaminated by commensal bacteria and cells of the lower urinary and genital tract. Catheterization runs the risk of introducing infection into the urinary tract and causing trauma. A free catch sample runs a high risk of bacterial contamination from the distal urethra, lower genital tract and perineum. Storage of urine has many deleterious effects on sample quality and therefore in-practice analysis is important, even if sending to a commercial laboratory.

Urinalysis
Urinalysis, including microscopic examination of a wet preparation, should be performed in all animals with suspected UTI. The presence of protein, blood and an alkaline pH are consistent with bacterial UTI. These changes are non-specific. It is the combination of abnormal results that indicates possible UTI rather than any single result. Glucose in the urine suggests diabetes mellitus or renal tubular damage, either of which may be associated with a bacterial UTI. Certain drugs used as urinary acidifiers, e.g. ascorbic acid, may cause false positive results for glucose when using standard dipsticks.

Urine cytology
Examination of urine sediment is indicated in all cases of suspected UTI. The following observations may be made:

- An active urine sediment characterized by significant numbers of white cells (>5 white blood cells/high power field). This suggests an inflammatory disorder. There are several urinary tract conditions, many of which are non-infectious, that result in an active sediment (Figure 10.7)
- The presence of a major number of bacteria and inflammatory cells (Figure 10.8). This suggests that the inflammatory lesion is caused or complicated by bacterial infection
- The presence of bacteria in the cytoplasm of inflammatory cells. This indicates an active infection within the urinary tract rather than contamination after sampling

Infectious urinary tract disease
Prostatitis
Urolithiasis/feline lower urinary tract disease
Neoplasia
Mucosal hyperplasia
Interstitial cystitis in cats
Trauma, e.g. catheterization

Figure 10.7: Possible causes of inflammation of the urinary tract.

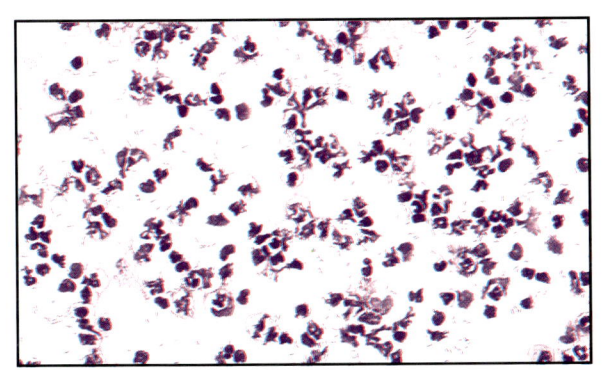

Figure 10.8: Giemsa-stained smear of an active urine sediment, showing many neutrophils and bacteria.

Too few bacteria (<10^4 rods/ml or <10^5 cocci/ml)
Prostatitis
Non-bacterial infections, e.g. mycoplasma, fungi
Previous antimicrobial therapy

Figure 10.9: Reasons for an active urinary sediment in the absence of bacteriuria.

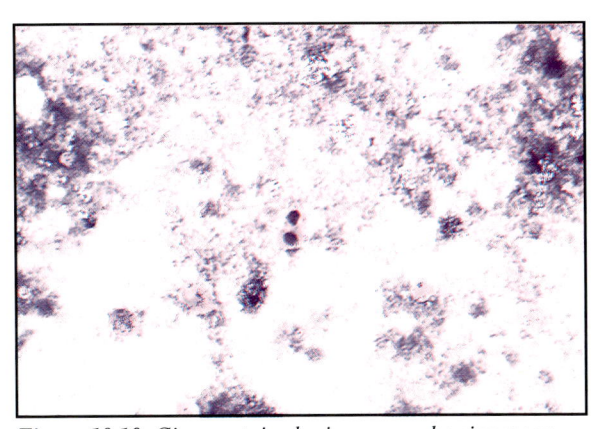

Figure 10.10: Giemsa-stained urine smear showing many bacteria but no inflammatory cells. This appearance is consistent with contamination of urine after collection.

- An inflammatory appearance to the urine sediment in the absence of bacteria. This does not rule out an infection (Figure 10.9)
- The identification of bacteriuria in the absence of white cells (Figure 10.10). This suggests contamination and subsequent growth of bacteria after the sample had been collected
- The presence of crystals. This increases the possibility of urolithiasis underlying a bacterial UTI although the presence of crystals does not confirm the presence of uroliths. Crystals may develop spontaneously in urine stored overnight
- The presence of sheets of morphologically normal transitional epithelial cells or clumps of atypical cells. This suggests mucosal hyperplasia or neoplasia, respectively. Presence of prostatic epithelial cells suggests prostatic disease.

Urine culture
Urine culture is essential for a definitive diagnosis of bacterial UTI. It should be obtained before initiating antibacterial therapy; if this has already started, antibacterials should be suspended for as long as possible (minimum 3-5 days).

Urine should be cultured as soon as possible after collection as it is a good medium for bacterial growth when kept at room temperature. If culture is delayed, refrigeration reduces the rate of bacterial growth. Fastidious bacteria may not survive if storage is prolonged. Boric acid should not be used as a preservative for urine as it may have a deleterious effect on any bacteria present.

Qualitative urine culture identifies bacteria in urine. However, it can be difficult to distinguish between a major isolate and contaminant solely by using qualitative methods. Isolation of a single species is likely to be an important finding, whereas a mixed growth suggests, but does not prove, contamination. About 75% of bacterial UTIs in dogs are caused by a single species, 18% by two species and 6% by three or more species.

Quantitative urine culture identifies bacterial species and quantifies the number of bacteria by counting colonies in serial dilutions. This is useful when samples can be cultured within 1-2 hours of collection. High counts of a single species probably indicate a bacterial UTI, moderate counts of a single species possibly indicate a bacterial UTI and low counts suggest contamination.

The numbers of bacteria per millilitre of urine that constitute high, moderate or low levels have been suggested to be (Lulich and Osborne, 1995):

- Cystocentesis: (dogs and cats) high >10^3/ml, moderate 10^2-10^3/ml, low <10^2/ml
- Catheterization: (dogs) high >10^4/ml, moderate 10^3-10^4/ml, low <10^3/ml; (cats) high >10^3/ml, moderate 10^2-10^3/ml, low <10^2/ml
- Free catch: (dogs) high >10^5/ml, moderate 10^4-10^5/ml, low <10^4/ml; (cats) high >10^4/ml, moderate 10^3-10^4/ml, low <10^3/ml.

False negative results occur occasionally, i.e. bacterial UTI is present although only low numbers of bacteria are isolated. False positive results may occur when there is a long delay (greater than a few hours) in culturing urine, and high bacterial counts can occasionally be obtained from free catch samples in dogs without bacterial UTI. When attempting quantitative culture, urine should be obtained by cystocentesis or catheterization. During catheterization the external genitalia should be cleansed with an appropriate non-irritant solution to reduce the potential for contamination. Where results are equivocal, serial cultures should be performed.

Treatment

Management of underlying causes

As bacterial UTI often develops when host defences are compromised, any therapeutic plan must address the underlying problem rather than rely solely on antimicrobial agents. The risk of iatrogenic UTI should be reduced by avoiding indiscriminate use of urinary catheterization, by using closed rather than open indwelling systems, by using appropriate antibacterial drugs and by considering the effect surgical techniques have on the defence mechanisms. Figures 10.3 and 10.5 list the predisposing causes of UTI, and each of these should be considered in individual animals before or during appropriate antibacterial therapy.

Antibacterial therapy

Antibacterial therapy is the cornerstone of therapy for UTI. Chapter 2 indicates those suitable for managing UTIs. Bacterial culture of urine and antibacterial sensitivity testing is essential:

- Where antibacterial drugs for a UTI or other infection have been prescribed in the past 6 weeks
- Where there is a high risk of UTI developing secondary to other diseases, e.g. diabetes mellitus, renal failure, hyperadrenocorticism, immunosuppressive therapy, urinary outflow obstruction or neurological disorders affecting urination
- After the use of indwelling urinary catheters. It has been suggested that when using such catheters, antibacterials should only be given once the catheter has been removed
- When recurrent or complicated UTI is confirmed
- Where clinical signs deteriorate or persist for more than 5 days after initiation of antibacterial therapy.

Some texts suggest that antibacterials may be prescribed empirically for the management of uncomplicated bacterial UTI, without resorting to culture and sensitivity testing, as long as the patient has not received antibacterials within the preceding 6 weeks. However, it is this author's recommendation that culture and antibacterial sensitivity testing in vitro should always be used to guide the antibacterial choice, as multiresistant strains of certain bacteria (*Escherichia coli*, *Proteus* spp., *Pseudomonas aeruginosa*) may be involved. A failure to recognize and appropriately treat such infections may lead to complications such as cystic mucosal hyperplasia, fibrosis and extension to other areas of the urinary tract.

Fluoroquinolones reliably cover all the agents but should not be used as a first-line treatment; their use should be restricted to resistant infections. The least expensive, least toxic and most effective antibacterial is indicated, and the indiscriminate administration of multiple antibacterial drugs should be avoided.

As animals empty their bladder about 3–5 times a day, administration of antibacterials at least every 8 hours and if possible immediately after micturition or before a period of confinement (e.g. overnight), may be beneficial. Single-dose therapy as used in humans has not proven to be effective in treating ongoing UTI in animals.

Resistant bacterial infections, particularly those caused by *Proteus* spp. and *Pseudomonas aeruginosa*, are difficult to deal with and may require aggressive therapy. Intravesicular administration of an aminoglycoside and penicillin (e.g. gentamicin and clavulanate-potentiated ticarcillin – not mixed in the same syringe) once or twice daily for 2–3 weeks can be helpful and removes the risk of nephrotoxicity associated with systemic aminoglycosides. This strategy is only effective when the bladder alone is involved, which is the minority of cases. Systemic use of antipseudomonal penicillins (see Chapter 2) is also advocated, although expensive.

Antibacterial therapy must be continued until the organism has been eliminated and the host defence mechanisms have recovered sufficiently to prevent recurrence. Bacteriuria may be eliminated within 2 days of initiating treatment. However, as bacteria often invade the mucosa, treatment should be maintained for at least 10 days after the first episode of UTI and for 4 weeks or more for recurrent infections.

Remission of clinical signs is not synonymous with eradication of infection; it is necessary to monitor response to therapy by serial urinalysis and culture as well as elimination of clinical signs. Therapy must anticipate the potential consequences of the UTI such as the risk of recurrence and the development of potentially irreversible changes (e.g. mucosal hyperplasia), which might develop with a progressive disease.

Ancillary therapy

Other therapeutic agents used in the management of UTI include:

- Urine acidifiers (e.g. ascorbic acid)
- Urine antiseptics (e.g. hexamine)
- Drugs that alter urine volume
- Drugs that alter the storage and voiding of urine.

None of these has been shown to be of any value in the immediate management of UTI. Promoting diuresis may worsen infections of the lower urinary tract. However, in cases caused by incontinence, phenylpropanolamine reduces the recurrence rate. Similarly, bethanecol and phenoxybenzamine have their place in cases with bladder or urethral dysfunction.

Monitoring therapy
The following are guidelines, which may not apply in every case:

- Urine can be collected by cystocentesis 3–5 days after initiating therapy, at which time no bacteria should be present. If bacteria remain, treatment is likely to be ineffective
- Urine can be assessed by culture and microscopy 3–5 days before the planned cessation of therapy to ensure that urine is sterile and that an inactive sediment is present
- Urine can be cultured one week after cessation of therapy to assess for a relapse
- Urine can be cultured 4 weeks after cessation of therapy to detect reinfection. Repeated cultures on a monthly basis may be indicated in animals where reinfection is considered likely.

Managing recurrent infections
Where irreversible changes have developed in the mucosa, i.e. mucosal hyperplasia or fibrosis after chronic infection, host defences are often so damaged that recurrence owing to reinfection or relapse frequently occurs. In such cases continuous antibacterial therapy with a reduced dose (one third to one half the routine dose) of an antibacterial excreted in high concentrations in urine given once daily, usually at night, for an indefinite period (often years) has been advocated as a means of controlling clinical signs. Urine should be cultured monthly and if bacteria are isolated therapeutic doses of an appropriate antibacterial should be prescribed. Once the organism has been eradicated, the animal may be returned to the preventive course of therapy. Once urine cultures are consistently sterile, usually within 6–12 months, the antibacterial can be withdrawn on a trial basis. If the defences have been repaired, UTI may not recur.

It has been suggested that the antibacterial be changed every 3 months to reduce the risk of resistance. However, this strategy has not been proven to have any effect on the development of antibacterial resistance in companion animals. When choosing an antibacterial for long-term therapy, those with low toxicity should be chosen, e.g. a penicillin or nitrofurantoin. Aminoglycosides, fluoroquinolones, trimethoprim–sulphonamide or chloramphenicol should not be used long term (see Appendix 3). A relapsing infection should be treated with a narrow-spectrum antibacterial, and constant reinfection with different bacteria should be treated with a broad-spectrum drug.

Managing persistent bacteriuria
Long-term antibacterial therapy has no value in the management of asymptomatic persistent bacteriuria. It may lead to the development of antibacterial resistance.

RENAL INFECTIONS

Tubulointerstitial disease
Infection or inflammation that primarily involves the renal interstitium and tubules is classified as interstitial nephritis or pyelonephritis.

Interstitial nephritis may be: acute or chronic; focal or generalized; and suppurative or non-suppurative. Infection is haematogenous. Many infectious agents have the potential to cause interstitial nephritis, including *Leptospira* spp., canine herpesvirus and *Encephalitozoon cuniculi* (see below), but in most cases a specific infection is not identified. Acute interstitial nephritis, particularly if embolic suppuration is present, may present with acute renal failure. In many cases the presence of interstitial nephritis is not suspected until chronic renal failure develops, at which time small shrunken kidneys are present.

Urogenous infection of the kidney results in pyelonephritis (inflammation of the renal pelvis and parenchyma). It is rare for pyelonephritis to develop as an extension of a primary renal septic process. Factors that influence the development of ascending lower urinary tract infections are discussed earlier in this chapter. Organisms isolated from cases of pyelonephritis reflect those found in the lower urinary tract. Clinical features of pyelonephritis might include polyuria/polydipsia, pyrexia, depression, abdominal pain and a leucocytosis. If both kidneys are affected, acute renal failure may also develop. However, the renal involvement is usually occult, with clinical signs limited to recurrent lower urinary tract infection. Chronic bilateral pyelonephritis leads to chronic renal failure.

Acute interstitial nephritis and pyelonephritis are difficult to confirm. Diagnosis relies on demonstrating an active urine sediment, persistently dilute urine, positive urine culture and ultrasonographical features such as hyper- or hypoechoic cortical areas, dilation of the renal pelvis and decreased corticomedullary demarcation. Renal biopsy is required to make a definitive diagnosis.

If identified early, antibacterial therapy based on culture and sensitivity testing is indicated. With chronic disease, the infecting agent may have been cleared and treatment is directed at managing the subsequent chronic renal failure.

Leptospirosis

Leptospirosis is discussed in detail in Chapter 11. *Leptospira interrogans* serovar. *canicola* is the predominant serovar associated with renal disease; it is a cause of acute oliguric/anuric renal failure. *L. interrogans* serovar. *icterohaemorrhagiae* can also cause renal disease. Clinical features associated with *L. canicola* include pyrexia, anorexia, dehydration, polydipsia and vomiting. Diagnosis and treatment are discussed in Chapter 11.

Canine herpesvirus

Canine herpesvirus is a cause of fading puppy syndrome and is discussed in detail in Chapter 12. As part of its multisystemic effects, it causes acute renal damage in neonatal pups.

Feline immunodeficiency virus (FIV)

Glomerular and tubulointerstitial lesions associated with proteinuria and occasionally renal failure are described in FIV-infected cats. It has been suggested that FIV may play a direct role in the induction of renal damage. See Chapter 5 for more detailed discussion of FIV.

Feline leukaemia virus (FeLV)

FeLV infection can result in lymphoid neoplasia that may involve the kidney (renal lymphoma). This virus is discussed in detail in Chapter 5.

Feline coronavirus

Feline infectious peritonitis (FIP) commonly involves the kidney, resulting in a granulomatous nephropathy and severe renal dysfunction. A detailed discussion of FIP is presented in Chapter 9.

Encephalitozoon cuniculi

Encephalitozoon cuniculi is an obligate intracellular microsporidian parasite. It is a supposedly rare cause of diffuse interstitial nephritis and granulomatous encephalitis in dogs. However, the incidence of subclinical disease is unknown and clinical disease is almost certainly underdiagnosed because of the difficulty in confirming infection. One serosurvey of stray dogs in the UK reported a seroprevalence of 13%. A report from South Africa indicated that 23% of dogs with chronic renal disease were seropositive for *E. cuniculi* compared to 2% of control dogs.

The organism is acquired transplacentally or following consumption of infected rodents or rabbits. Puppies are most at risk of disease. Brain, kidney and vascular endothelium are most commonly infected, with liver and heart occasionally involved. Acute renal disease may be subclinical, but the renal damage is severe enough to lead ultimately to chronic renal failure. Focal hepatic necrosis and myocardial necrosis may develop. Nervous system lesions are those of a widespread non-suppurative meningoencephalitis. The severity and nature of the clinical signs are unpredictable, varying with the area of the CNS affected. The main differential diagnoses for the neurological signs are *Neospora caninum* and *Toxoplasma gondii* infections.

Confirming encephalitozoonosis relies on demonstrating the presence of the organism. This is difficult in chronic infections. Infected dogs may develop a lymphocytosis and hypergammaglobulinaemia. Methods for isolating the organism and immunohistochemical methods of identification are not commercially available. Serology is available from many human hospitals.

Helminths

Migrating *Toxocara canis* larvae may result in small granulomata in the renal cortex. These are of no clinical significance.

Capillaria plicata can be found in the lumen of the renal pelvis, ureter or bladder. It has a wide geographical distribution but is an uncommon parasite. Infections are usually clinically silent, although haematuria and dysuria have been reported.

Dioctyphyma renale is the giant kidney worm. It has a worldwide distribution but its incidence is unknown. It is predominantly a pathogen of fish-eating mammals such as mink, foxes, dogs and cats. The life cycle involves an intermediate host (mud-worms); fish and frogs are paratenic hosts. Adult worms live in the renal pelvis and cause a haemorrhagic pyelitis that becomes suppurative. The renal parenchyma is progressively destroyed until the capsule contains only the worm and exudate. *D. renale* has been reported to entwine liver lobes, causing erosion of the hepatic capsule and haemoperitoneum.

DRUG DOSAGES

See Appendix 3.

REFERENCES AND FURTHER READING

Davidson M, Else R and Lumsden J (1998) *Manual of Small Animal Clinical Pathology.* BSAVA, Cheltenham

Gaskell RM and Bennett M (1996) Feline herpes virus type 2 infection. In: *Feline and Canine Infectious Disease*, p. 119. Blackwell Science, Oxford

Hollister WS, Canning EU and Viney M (1989) Prevalence of antibodies to *Encephalitozoon cuniculi* in stray dogs as determined by an ELISA. *Veterinary Record* **124**, 332-336

Lulich J and Osborne C (1995) Bacterial infections of the urinary tract. In: *Textbook of Veterinary Internal Medicine*, ed. S Ettinger and E Feldman, pp. 1775-1788. WB Saunders, Philadelphia

Osborne C, et al. (1995) Feline lower urinary tract diseases. In: *Textbook of Veterinary Internal Medicine*, ed. S Ettinger and E Feldman, pp. 1805-1832. WB Saunders, Philadelphia

Senior D (2000) Management of difficult urinary tract infections. In: *Current Veterinary Therapy XIII*, ed. RW Kirk, pp. 883-886. WB Saunders, London

Stewart CG, Reyers F and Snyman H (1988) The relationship in dogs between primary renal disease and antibodies to *Encephalitozoon cuniculi*. *Journal of the South African Veterinary Association* **59**, 19-21

CHAPTER ELEVEN

The Liver, Pancreas and Spleen

Bryn Tennant

CHAPTER PLAN

The hepatobiliary system
  Extrahepatic sepsis
  Bacterial cholangiohepatitis
  Leptospirosis
  Liver abscessation
  Bacillus piliformis (Tyzzer's disease)
  Canine adenovirus
  Canine herpesvirus
  Feline coronavirus
  Acidophil cell hepatitis
  Toxoplasmosis
  Miscellaneous infections
Pancreatitis
Splenitis
References and further reading

Common
Dogs
Extrahepatic sepsis
Bacterial cholangiohepatitis
Leptospirosis
Canine adenovirus-1 (infectious canine hepatitis)
Canine herpesvirus
Cats
Extrahepatic sepsis
Bacterial cholangiohepatitis
Feline coronavirus (see Chapter 9)
Uncommon or rare
Dogs
Liver abscess (several bacterial species)
Bacillus piliformis (Tyzzer's disease)
Toxoplasmosis (see Chapter 15)
Mycobacteriosis (see Chapters 6 and 13)
Hepatozoon canis (see Chapter 5)
Leishmaniasis (see Chapter 5)
Babesiosis (see Chapter 5)
Cytauxzoonosis (see Chapter 5)
Ehrlichiosis (see Chapter 5)
Neosporosis (see Chapter 15)
Capillaria hepatica
Opisthorchis felineus
Metorchis conjunctus
?? Bartonellosis (see Chapter 5)
Metorchis conjunctus
Cats
Liver abscess (several bacterial species)
Bacillus piliformis (Tyzzer's disease)
Toxoplasmosis (see Chapter 15)
Mycobacteriosis (see Chapters 6 and 13)
Yersiniosis (see Chapter 8)
Opisthorchis felineus
Rhodococcus equi

Figure 11.1: Infections that may result in hepatic disease.

Toxic hepatopathy: Griseofulvin, trimethoprim-sulphonamide, ketoconazole, paracetamol, tetracycline, blue-green algae, heavy metals
Metabolic disorders: Acute pancreatitis, acute haemolytic anaemia, hepatic lipidosis
Trauma, hypoxia, thermal injury: Abdominal trauma, heat stroke, liver lobe torsion
Extrahepatic bile duct obstruction due to tumour or acute pancreatitis can resemble leptospirosis

Figure 11.2: Examples of some acute non-infectious differential diagnoses for infectious hepatopathies.

THE HEPATOBILIARY SYSTEM

The liver is a primary target for infection by bacteria and viruses. Such agents readily gain access to the liver via blood vessels, lymphatics and the biliary tract. The hepatobiliary system may be affected alone or as part of a multisystemic infection. Its defence mechanisms to infection depend on intact humoral and cell-mediated immune systems and the presence of macrophages (Kuppfer cells) lining sinusoids. Clinical signs of hepatobiliary infection relate to cellular damage and dysfunction. Figure 11.1 lists the main infectious agents that may cause hepatobiliary disease in the dog and cat. One of the major clinical challenges when dealing with a case of suspected hepatopathy is distinguishing infectious from non-infectious causes (Figure 11.2).

Clinical and historical findings
Clinical and historical features of acute hepatobiliary disease are often vague and non-specific (Figure 11.3).

Anorexia	Jaundice	Polyuria/
Vomiting	Ascites	polydipsia
Diarrhoea	Ptyalism (cat)	Constipation
Pyrexia	Hepatomegaly	Depression

Figure 11.3: The more common non-specific presenting signs associated with liver infection.

Information that may be of value includes:

- History of infectious hepatopathy
- Age
- Exposure to potential toxins
- Exposure to animals with infectious hepatopathies, rats or standing or stagnant water
- Trauma
- Lack of recent vaccination.

Information relating to these factors may allow certain diagnoses to be ruled out or a tentative diagnosis to be made. However, as most infectious liver diseases do not generally present with specific signs (exceptions are discussed below), ancillary testing is required for a definitive diagnosis. Some infectious hepatopathies may be associated with chronic hepatic disease or present with multisystemic signs (e.g. feline coronavirus or canine adenovirus-1 infection) and need to be distinguished from the various non-infectious chronic hepatopathies.

Diagnostic tests

Clinical pathology
Routine serum biochemistry, haematology and urinalysis are often the initial diagnostic tests used to evaluate suspected hepatopathy. These document the presence of hepatic disease but rarely if ever provide a definitive diagnosis.

Serum biochemistry
Non-specific serum biochemical changes that may be expected with infectious hepatopathies include:

- Increased concentrations of alanine aminotransferase (ALT), aspartate aminotransferase (AST), γ-glutamyltransferase (GGT) and alkaline phosphatase. These are indicators of liver damage
- Increased concentrations of bile acids and bilirubin. These are indicators of liver dysfunction
- Increased concentrations of serum globulins and often decreased concentrations of albumin with acute infections. These reflect the switch to the production of acute-phase proteins.

Haematology
Haematological changes may include:

- A leucocytosis, usually a neutrophilia, which may indicate an inflammatory disorder; there may be a concurrent lymphopenia (particularly in stressed cats or those with FIP)
- Neutropenia and thrombocytopenia, which are features of some infections (e.g. CAV-1)
- Anaemia of chronic disease (non-regenerative anaemia) with chronic infections (e.g. cholangiohepatitis, FIP)
- Morphological red cell changes, although these are usually restricted to non-infectious hepatopathies.

Urinalysis
Urinalysis may show:

- Bilirubinuria indicative of conjugated hyperbilirubinaemia or reduced bilirubin-protein binding before jaundice is visible
- Tubular casts, inflammatory cells, red cells and increased protein if there is urinary tract involvement.

The *BSAVA Manual of Small Animal Clinical Pathology* gives a more detailed discussion on clinicopathological changes associated with liver disease.

Imaging
Radiography is important for assessing liver size, e.g. microhepatica might suggest chronic liver disease. Free abdominal fluid may be found on radiography or ultrasonography. Ultrasonography may demonstrate hepatic abscesses, lesions associated with gas-forming bacteria or biliary tract changes consistent with cholangiohepatitis. Both of these diagnostic modalities are, however, rarely useful in confirming an infectious hepatopathy.

Serology
Serology is discussed later for specific agents.

Histopathology and cytology
Histological assessment of a liver biopsy sample is often helpful in providing a diagnosis. The increased anaesthetic risk associated with acute liver failure may preclude obtaining such biopsies by laparotomy. However, Trucut biopsy samples of enlarged livers can be useful and may be obtained without resorting to general anaesthesia. Fine-needle aspirates of the liver parenchyma can be readily obtained without general anaesthesia. When stained with a Romanowsky-type stain (e.g. Giemsa) the aspirates may demonstrate suppurative inflammatory diseases, whereas Gram or acid-fast (see Chapter 1) stained smears can help identify bacterial types. In peracute infectious disorders, specific histological changes may not be apparent.

Extrahepatic sepsis
Extrahepatic septic foci have been associated with intrahepatic cholestasis. The hepatic lesions are mild,

non-specific and characterized by intrahepatic cholestasis. Although lymphocytes, macrophages and neutrophils may be present, severe necrosis and inflammation are not features. The disorder may result from haematogenous spread of bacteria from the primary site to the liver, injury due to hypoxia or pyrexia or endotoxin-induced structural or functional disturbances that inhibit excretion of conjugated bilirubin. Increased concentrations of serum ALP, bile acids and bilirubin are often evident, and the serum ALT concentration may be increased.

Cholestasis secondary to extrahepatic bacterial infection should be considered whenever there is biochemical evidence of cholestasis concurrent with a known septic process or where clinical signs suggest a septic process. It is important from a diagnostic and therapeutic standpoint to recognize that this mild hepatopathy may develop and that the hepatic damage does not require specific treatment; it will resolve once the primary septic process resolves.

Bacterial cholangiohepatitis

Cholangiohepatitis is an inflammatory condition that affects the biliary system and hepatic parenchyma and which may in some cases be initiated by bacteria. It is more common in cats than in dogs.

Aetiology

Two forms of cholangiohepatitis are recognized: suppurative and non-suppurative. Ascending bacterial invasion of the biliary tract by enteric organisms may be facilitated by bile stasis, anatomical anomalies of the gall bladder and cholelithiasis. Concurrent inflammatory bowel disease or chronic pancreatitis may be seen. Many bacteria may be isolated from affected animals, including *Escherichia coli* (commonest isolate), *Clostridium* spp., *Bacteroides* spp., *Actinomyces* spp., *Rhodococcus equi* and *Enterococcus* spp. Non-suppurative cholangiohepatitis may have an immune-mediated basis or may develop as a chronic sequel to the suppurative form.

Clinical features

Clinical features, including inappetence, depression, pyrexia, weight loss, vomiting and jaundice, may develop acutely or chronically and may be persistent or intermittent. Haematologically a neutrophilia with a left shift and a mild anaemia may be evident. The anaemia is thought to be one of chronic disease. Serum biochemistry reflects damage to the biliary tract and hepatocytes. Hyperbilirubinaemia is common, with concentrations of liver enzymes often moderately increased, and bile acids ranging from normal to markedly increased. The development of cirrhosis is often associated with other serum biochemical abnormalities such as hypoalbuminaemia and reduced urea concentration.

Diagnosis

Ultrasonography of the liver and biliary system may demonstrate choleliths or sludging of bile, but it does not provide a definitive diagnosis. A presumptive diagnosis of suppurative cholangiohepatitis is suggested by a history of pyrexia and jaundice that respond to antibacterials. A definitive diagnosis requires histopathological examination of a liver biopsy sample. If the sample is taken via a laparotomy, bile should also be obtained by fine needle aspiration for aerobic and anaerobic culture. Bile may also be obtained using ultrasound-guided fine-needle aspiration of the gall bladder, but the animal must be well sedated for this procedure.

Treatment

Suppurative cholangiohepatitis requires antibacterial therapy. Antibacterial choice should be based on culture and sensitivity if possible. If this is unavailable, a broad-spectrum antibacterial with activity against Gram-negative and anaerobic bacteria, which is excreted in bile and is non-toxic to the liver, is required (see Chapter 2). Ampicillin or clavulanate-potentiated amoxycillin would be good first-choice antibacterials. If anaerobic bacteria are suspected, metronidazole may be used alone or in combination with a penicillin.

Other therapies include:

- Prednisolone – this is primarily used in the management of non-suppurative inflammation, although it is useful in cases of suppurative cholangiohepatitis when the response to antibacterials is poor
- Ursodeoxycholic acid – this may be of benefit if bile sludging is present.

Prognosis

The prognosis for suppurative cholangiohepatitis is variable. Many treated animals show a good short-term response, but in the longer term, recurrence is likely.

Leptospirosis

Leptospirosis is a worldwide disease affecting many species of animals, although cats are generally resistant to infection. *Leptospira* spp. are motile spirochaetes. Figure 11.4 lists the leptospires that have been associated with disease in the dog. *Leptospira icterohaemorrhagiae*, *L. canicola* and *L. grippotyphosa* are the predominant serovars associated with disease in the dog, primarily causing hepatic and renal damage. *L. canicola* is host-maintained in the dog. Widespread vaccination has virtually eradicated it. *L. icterohaemorrhagiae* is acquired from rats and other serovars from their respective hosts. Other serovars, including *L. interrogans* serovars *pomona* and *bratislava*, have been found in clinical cases, but they are probably rare causes of disease. The organism survives for weeks or months in damp environments but is killed by drying.

178 Manual of Canine and Feline Infectious Diseases

Serovar	Maintenance host
Predominant	
L. interrogans serovar *icterohaemorrhagiae*	Rat
L. interrogans serovar *canicola*	Dog
L. kirschneri serovar *grippotyphosa*	Rodents
Rare	
L. interrogans serovar *pomona*	Pigs, wildlife, cattle
L. interrogans serovar *bratislava*	Pigs, bison, dogs
L. interrogans serovar *australis*	Unknown

Figure 11.4: Leptospires that may infect the dog, showing their maintenance hosts.

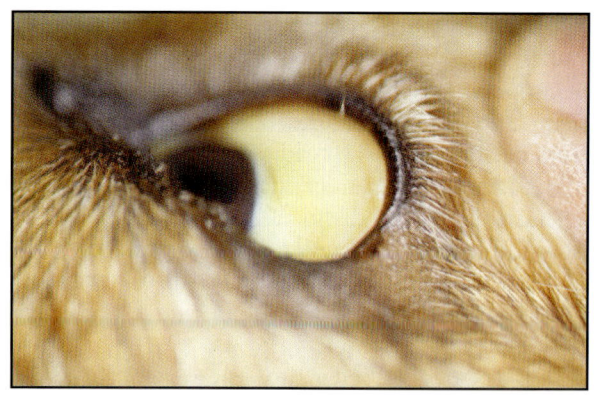

Figure 11.5: Profound jaundice in a dog infected with Leptospira interrogans *serovar* icterohaemorrhagiae. (© Dr Bryn Tennant.)

Pathogenesis

Leptospires can be transmitted by direct contact with urine from infected animals or indirectly through environmental contamination, especially in damp conditions or where there is stagnant water. The bacteria are able to penetrate mucosal surfaces and damaged skin. The bacteria replicate in blood, renal tubular epithelium and liver, resulting in damage to many solid organs, particularly kidney and liver.

Clinical signs

The development of specific clinical signs depends on factors, including:

- Dose of bacteria
- Age and level of immunity; pre-existing antibodies protect against disease, and seronegative dogs are at risk of developing severe disease
- Virulence and tropism of the serovar; *L. icterohaemorrhagiae* is primarily associated with hepatic damage, *L. canicola* is more likely to cause acute renal failure, *L. grippotyphosa* has been associated with hepatic and renal disease and *L. australis* may be associated with the development of chronic hepatitis (as yet unproven).

Leptospiral infections may be divided into three groups:

- Peracute disease – characterized by massive leptospiraemia, pyrexia, muscular pain, shock and death
- Subacute disease – clinical features relate to the organs involved. Non-specific findings include pyrexia, anorexia, dehydration, polydipsia, congested mucous membranes, petechiation and vomiting. With hepatic involvement, jaundice is a feature (Figure 11.5), whereas renal involvement results in the development of oliguric/anuric acute renal failure. Animals that recover from the disease may develop chronic renal failure secondary to extensive renal damage
- Chronic disease – chronic leptospirosis is associated with vague signs of pyrexia and progressive renal or hepatic disease.

Diagnosis

Non-specific alterations in clinical pathology may include:

- A leucocytosis and thrombocytopenia
- Increased concentrations of liver enzymes, bile acids, bilirubin, urea and creatinine, reflecting the extent of hepatic or renal damage. Variable electrolyte abnormalities are also common.

Various ways of demonstrating leptospiral infection have been described. These include:

- Isolating the bacteria from urine – this is feasible with specific media; however, it is not commercially available and is technically difficult
- Demonstrating the bacteria in urine by using dark-field microscopy – this is technically difficult and has low specificity
- Demonstrating the bacteria in renal or hepatic tissues by using Warthin–Starry stain – this has a low sensitivity and low specificity
- Serology – a single titre in excess of 1:800 in a dog with clinical signs consistent with leptospirosis could be considered diagnostic. Alternatively demonstrating a fourfold increase in antibody titres in paired samples taken 3 weeks apart indicates recent infection; antibacterial therapy may reduce the serological response
- Fluorescent antibody testing to detect leptospires in urine (currently unavailable in the UK). Antibacterials that eliminate leptospiruria produce false negative results
- Use of polymerase chain reaction (PCR) technology allows individual serovars to be identified (not yet commercially available). The technique is specific and sensitive although false positives may occur.

Gross findings at post mortem examination vary with the serovar involved, for example:

- *L. icterohaemorrhagiae* – swollen, friable liver and widespread petechiation and jaundice
- *L. canicola* – renomegaly; jaundice is generally not a feature
- *L. grippotyphosa* – hepatic fibrosis/cirrhosis and/or renomegaly
- *L. australis* – possibly hepatic fibrosis/cirrhosis.

The main differential diagnoses for acute leptospirosis are non-infectious causes of acute renal failure, non-infectious acute hepatopathies and CAV-1 infection. Distinguishing between these conditions is difficult and can often only be achieved after demonstration of leptospires.

Treatment
Penicillin is effective in terminating leptospiraemia and is not contraindicated in hepatic or renal disease. The carrier state in pet animals should be eliminated if possible. Tetracycline or doxycycline should be given during recovery to prevent establishment of the carrier state. Renal haemodynamics should be supported with intravenous fluids (0.9% saline or 0.45% saline with 2.5% dextrose). If required, diuresis should be induced with frusemide (with or without concurrent dopamine infusion), mannitol or glucose. Management of the gastrointestinal effects of acute renal failure may include the use of histamine H_2-receptor antagonists (e.g. cimetidine), omeprazole, sucralfate, misoprostol or metoclopramide. Central venous pressure (CVP) should be monitored, particularly if oliguria persists, and fluid administration discontinued if CVP rises above 8–12 cm H_2O. Acid–base status should be assessed if available.

The prognosis is guarded. The response to therapy is variable, with some dogs recovering rapidly but others dying even when prompt and appropriate therapy was instituted. The best prognostic indicator for recovery from renal leptospirosis is the rate of serum creatinine decline following treatment.

Prevention
Vaccines containing inactivated *L. canicola* and *L. icterohaemorrhagiae* are available. These protect against disease but not necessarily against either subclinical infection or infection with other serovars. Frequent vaccination is required to ensure protective titres are maintained, as the duration of immunity after vaccination is less than a year in many cases.

Zoonotic potential
Leptospira species are infectious to humans; suspect cases must be handled appropriately, and contact with dog urine should be avoided. Post-mortem examinations should be done with great care.

Liver abscessation
Liver abscessation in the dog and cat is rare. Bacteria may pass to the liver: haematogenously (portal vein, hepatic artery, umbilical vein in the neonate) from extrahepatic septic foci; via the biliary or lymphatic system; or after penetration of the abdominal cavity. Hepatic trauma, neoplasia and immunosuppressive infections (e.g. feline leukaemia virus, feline immunodeficiency virus) or metabolic diseases (e.g. diabetes mellitus) predispose to hepatic abscessation. Hepatic hypoxia may promote growth of dormant anaerobic bacteria, e.g. *Clostridium* spp., although this is unproven.

Abscessation can take the form of a single large discrete abscess or multifocal microabscesses. The causative organisms include *Staphylococcus* spp., *Streptococcus* spp. (mainly cats), *E. coli*, *Salmonella* spp., *Nocardia asteroides*, *Klebsiella pneumoniae*, *Enterococcus* spp. and *Clostridium* spp. Concurrent infections may be identified in other tissues, including the biliary tract, endocardium, spleen, blood, lung, prostate, peritoneum, lymph nodes, salivary gland or brain.

Clinical and physical features
Clinical and physical features associated with hepatic abscessation include anorexia, depression, vomiting, hepatomegaly, cranial abdominal pain and occasionally ascites, although an underlying primary disease process may be clinically more obvious. Rupture of a hepatic abscess results in peritonitis, septic shock and often death.

Diagnosis
Diagnosis of hepatic abscessation is difficult, but the following points may be helpful:

- Haematologically there will be neutrophilia, usually with a left shift although neutropenia may develop after rupture of an abscess
- Increased concentrations of liver enzymes reflect the degree of ongoing hepatocyte destruction; this may be minimal with a discrete established abscess and thus the concentrations of serum enzymes may occasionally be unremarkable
- Liver function as assessed by concentration of serum bilirubin and bile acid is expected to be normal with a solitary liver abscess but may be compromised with multifocal abscessation
- Hyperglobulinaemia may develop as a consequence of the inflammatory process
- Radiography may show diffuse or focal hepatomegaly and/or splenomegaly, poor abdominal detail possibly owing to a local peritoneal effusion and, rarely, radiolucent areas reflecting gas production by bacteria

- Ultrasonographically hypoechoic or anechoic areas can be found; these can be difficult to distinguish from cysts or haematomas but can usually be distinguished from neoplasia. Care must be taken to identify the gall bladder before diagnosing hepatic abscessation. Ultrasound-guided fine-needle aspiration can be used to obtain samples for cytology and culture
- Where ultrasonography is unavailable, hepatic abscesses are usually diagnosed by laparotomy
- Abscess contents should be cultured aerobically and anaerobically. A Gram and acid-fast stain of the contents may provide an indication of the bacterial type (see Chapter 1).

Treatment
Antibacterial therapy should be initiated as soon as samples have been obtained.

- Metronidazole, penicillin or clindamycin will be effective against anaerobes such as *Clostridium* spp.
- An aminoglycoside with clavulanate-potentiated amoxycillin would be indicated if Gram-negative organisms predominate. Aminoglycosides should not be used until any prerenal azotaemia and hypovolaemia have been corrected.

Prognosis
The prognosis for liver abscess is guarded and depends largely on whether there are unifocal or multifocal abscesses present and the type of infecting organism. Unifocal abscess should be treated surgically (full or partial liver lobectomy) and medically (antibiosis). A full recovery can be expected if prompt aggressive therapy is instituted. Surgery for multifocal abscessation is less likely to be feasible. Clostridiosis carries a poor prognosis and is often only diagnosed at post mortem examination.

Bacillus piliformis (Tyzzer's disease)
Bacillus piliformis is a pleomorphic Gram-negative spore-forming obligate intracellular bacillus. It may rarely cause multifocal hepatic necrosis and haemorrhagic necrotizing enterocolitis, which are invariably fatal.

Clinical signs are acute in onset and include abdominal pain, depression, lethargy and anorexia, progressing to death within 48 hours. Successful therapy has not been reported. See Chapter 8 for further details.

Canine adenovirus-1 (infectious canine hepatitis)

Aetiology
Canine adenovirus-1 (CAV-1) is a DNA virus that causes hepatocellular necrosis and vasculitis. Although once common, CAV-1 is now a rare clinical problem because of the widespread use of effective vaccines. It is antigenically related to CAV-2 (see Chapter 6), and cross-protective immunity between these viruses occurs. CAV-1 is a moderately resistant virus, surviving for months in the environment; infectivity is lost under conditions of high humidity and temperature. The virus is completely inactivated at 56°C, and steam cleaning or the application of quarternary ammonium compounds can be used for disinfection (see Chapter 4).

Asymptomatic infection is common in dogs with high serum neutralizing antibody titres. Those with low or negative antibody titres may develop acute fatal disease. It has been suggested that dogs with intermediate titres may develop chronic hepatitis or cirrhosis when exposed to the virus.

Pathogenesis
Following infection via the oronasal route, CAV-1 infects and replicates in regional lymphoid tissues, including tonsil. Subsequent to a viraemia, hepatocytes and reticuloendothelial cells in other organ systems become infected and secondary replication occurs. Release of viral particles results in cell lysis, and this cellular necrosis is responsible for the clinical signs. During acute infection the virus can be isolated from faeces, urine, oropharyngeal secretions and blood. Later in the course of disease the virus localizes in renal tubular cells and can be shed in urine for up to one year. Environmental contamination is the predominant source of infection rather than contact with infected animals.

Clinical signs
The incubation period is 4–7 days, and any seronegative dog is susceptible to disease. An initial pyrexia usually declines after 24 hours, and in mild cases recovery is rapid. In moderate or severe cases the low-grade pyrexia worsens after 24–48 hours, corresponding to the development of viraemia. This is associated with more pronounced depression, lethargy and reluctance to move. Figure 11.6 lists the clinical features attributable to cellular damage within target organs found from this stage onwards. The presence of multisystemic signs carries a guarded prognosis. Occasionally, peracute disease and sudden death occurs before the development of clinical signs.

Pyrexia
Lethargy, depression, anorexia
Hepatomegaly, abdominal pain, reluctance to move
Pale mucous membranes and occasionally petechial and ecchymotic haemorrhages (Figure 11.7)
Lymphadenopathy, tonsillitis, pharyngitis
Corneal oedema during the convalescent period
Neurological signs (varied) associated with vasculitis
Bloody diarrhoea with or without vomiting associated with intestinal tract involvement
Coughing due to bronchitis/bronchiolitis
Collapse

Figure 11.6: Clinical features associated with canine adenovirus-1 infection.

Diagnosis

Non-specific abnormalities include:

- A neutropenia and leucopenia early in the disease
- A leucocytosis during the recovery period
- Thrombocytopenia in most cases
- Prolonged bleeding times and coagulation disorders resulting from liver and vascular endothelial damage (Figure 11.7)
- Increased concentrations of liver enzymes, reflecting hepatocellular damage.

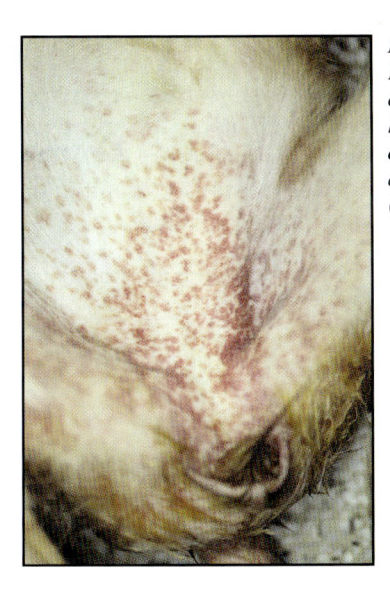

Figure 11.7: Petechiation and ecchymotic haemorrhages in a dog with canine adenovirus infection. (© Dr Bryn Tennant.)

Ante-mortem confirmation of CAV-1 infection relies on isolating the virus from faecal samples or oropharyngeal swabs taken into virus transport media, and/or demonstrating a rise in antibody titres to CAV-1 in paired serum samples taken 14–21 days apart. The presence of a high antibody titre in an unvaccinated puppy with compatible clinical signs would be highly suggestive but not definitive evidence of CAV-1 infection.

Post-mortem examination reveals enlargement and mottling of the liver often with fibrinous exudates attached to the liver capsule. The gall bladder may be oedematous and haemorrhagic. The diagnosis may be confirmed after histological examination of the liver.

Treatment and prevention

No specific therapy is available for CAV-1 infection. Symptomatic supportive therapy for acute liver failure is required for more severely affected dogs. Immunization with CAV-1 or CAV-2 vaccines is highly efficient in protecting against disease. Modified live CAV-1 vaccines are associated with adverse effects, primarily the development of corneal oedema. All dog vaccines currently contain modified live CAV-2, and protection may persist for as long as 6 years (Ford and Schultz, 2000).

Canine herpesvirus

Canine herpesvirus is one agent responsible for fading puppy syndrome. It is an acute and rapidly fatal multisystemic disease. Hepatocellular necrosis is one feature of this condition. Canine herpesvirus is discussed further in Chapter 12.

Feline coronavirus

Feline infectious peritonitis (FIP) commonly involves the liver, resulting in a granulomatous hepatopathy (Figure 11.8) and severe liver dysfunction. See Chapter 9 for a detailed discussion of FIP.

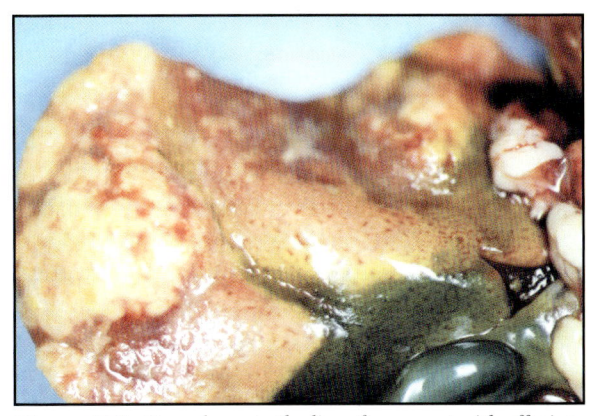

Figure 11.8: Granuloma in the liver from a cat with effusive feline infectious peritonitis. (© Dr Bryn Tennant.)

Acidophil cell hepatitis

Canine acidophil cell hepatitis is a rare hepatic disease, associated with acute or chronic hepatitis, cirrhosis and liver failure. Little has been reported on this disorder. A transmissible agent, possibly a virus, may be the cause, but it has not been characterized. The clinical features of the disease are vague and non-specific and relate to hepatic damage. Diagnosis is based on histology.

Toxoplasmosis

Toxoplasmosis is caused by an obligate intracellular coccidian parasite, *Toxoplasma gondii*. The liver is one of several organs that may be infected by *T. gondii*. This protozoan causes multifocal hepatic necrosis and hepatic failure, resulting in jaundice, abdominal pain and pyrexia. Concomitant infection of other organs results in other signs, e.g. dyspnoea, uveitis and CNS abnormalities. Serum biochemical changes relating to liver involvement include increased ALT, ALP and bilirubin concentrations. For further discussion on the pathophysiology, diagnosis and treatment of toxoplasmosis, see Chapter 15.

Miscellaneous infections

Systemic mycoses, such as histoplasmosis and coccidioidomycosis, may involve the liver, resulting in granulomatous lesions, hepatomegaly, ascites and jaundice. Involvement of other organ systems, e.g. intestinal tract (histoplasmosis), respiratory tract and lymphoid tissue, give rise to other clinical signs. These infectious agents do not occur in the UK.

Other infectious agents that cause multisystemic disease and can involve the liver, although not always causing clinically significant hepatic damage, are listed in Figure 11.1. *Rhodococcus equi* has been associated with a case of necrotizing pyogranulomatous hepatitis, osteomyelitis and myositis (Cantor *et al.*, 1998).

Blue green algae may cause hepatotoxicity as several contain toxins. Consumption of water containing these algae may cause convulsions and death in a few minutes or hepatocellular necrosis over days. The diagnosis may be suspected with an appropriate history and histology. Confirmation requires demonstration of the toxin or algae in the gastrointestinal tract.

Aflatoxins produced by the fungus *Aspergillus* are very rare causes of fulminant liver necrosis. Aflatoxicosis may develop following consumption of contaminated food.

Opisthorchis felineus is a liver fluke that infests cats, dogs and foxes. It is common in eastern Europe and Siberia but sparse in other areas. Light infestations may be asymptomatic. Heavy infestations may cause cholangiohepatitis and pancreatitis. *Metorchis conjunctus* is the common liver fluke in dogs and cats in North America and may cause cholangiohepatitis and pancreatitis. It may be seen in the UK in imported animals. Fluke infestations may be diagnosed by demonstrating eggs in faeces.

Capillaria hepatica is a nematode that lives in the liver. Infections are sporadic; prevalence in the UK is unknown. The adult worm may provoke a mild traumatic hepatitis and its eggs may induce granuloma formation. Rodents are the usual definitive hosts. Diagnosis is by histology. Eggs are not seen in faeces.

Some strains of canine parvovirus (see Chapter 8) have been demonstrated in the liver after natural infection, but the clinical importance of this is unclear.

Neospora caninum (see Chapter 15) may occasionally infect the liver, causing hepatic damage.

PANCREATITIS

Infectious diseases of the pancreas are uncommon. Infectious agents can spread to the healthy and inflamed pancreas:

- By reflux into the pancreatic duct (from intestinal lumen or bile duct)
- Haematogenously
- Via lymphatics or transcoelomically from extrapancreatic septic foci
- By direct implantation after abdominal trauma
- Following transmural migration from the colon.

The risk of bacterial colonization is proportional to the extent of pancreatic damage. In the cat bacteria frequently colonize the healthy pancreas, but the clinical importance of this is unclear. Most cases of pancreatitis are found to be sterile when examined at laparotomy or post mortem examination. The importance of bacterial reflux as a trigger factor in the early pathogenesis of pancreatitis is unknown.

Aetiology

There are many potential inciting causes of pancreatitis (Figure 11.9), most of which do not involve infectious agents. Once inflammation and pancreatic damage are established, bacteria may have a secondary role; all animals with pancreatitis should be considered at risk of developing secondary opportunistic bacterial infection. Pancreatitis may be seen alone, in association with cholangiohepatitis and inflammatory bowel disease in the cat or cholangiohepatitis in the dog or, rarely, as part of a multisystemic infection.

Nutrition: high-fat diets
Hyperlipoproteinaemia
Drugs: suspect drugs include thiazide diuretics, frusemide, sulphonamides, azathioprine, tetracycline and corticosteroids
Toxins: cholinesterase inhibiting insecticides
Pancreatic duct obstruction
Duodenal reflux
Hypercalcaemia
Trauma
Ischaemia/reperfusion
Infections

Figure 11.9: Potential causes of pancreatitis.

Systemic fungal (e.g. *Aspergillus* spp.) and yeast (e.g. *Candida albicans*) infections may involve the pancreas, resulting in major damage, although these are rare. Viral, mycoplasmal and parasitic infections have been cited as infecting the pancreas, although their clinical importance is unclear. Pancreatic abscessation is a rare disorder, the aetiology of which is unclear in most cases. The abscesses are often sterile and may reflect a complication of or sequel to pancreatitis.

Clinical and historical findings

The clinical features of pancreatitis relate to activation of digestive enzymes within the pancreas and subsequent autodigestion. Pancreatic abscessation presents similarly to pancreatitis. Clinical signs vary from mild abdominal pain with or without vomiting to severe signs of an abdominal catastrophe, with shock and collapse. Bacterial involvement tends to result in more severe clinical signs. Dehydration, cranial abdominal pain and occasionally an abdominal mass and ascites are reported. Involvement of the biliary tract can result in jaundice, and bleeding disorders and respiratory distress may develop.

Diagnosis

Confirmation of pancreatic inflammation is difficult. Radiography is useful in ruling out other causes of abdominal pain, but on its own cannot confirm the diagnosis. There may be loss of radiographic detail in the cranial abdomen, displacement of the stomach and duodenum, thickening and corrugation of the duodenal wall, ileus in the duodenum and colon (static gas shadows) and gastric distension due to outflow obstruction. Ultrasonography is likely to be more useful than radiography in demonstrating pancreatic disease with loss of echodensity and identification of cysts, abscesses and non-homogenous masses expected.

Clinical pathology findings are non-specific. Haematology may show a neutrophilia with a left shift and an increased packed cell volume. Azotaemia is often present, which is either prerenal in origin or may reflect the development of acute renal failure. Increased concentrations of liver enzymes and bilirubin indicate hepatocellular and biliary tract involvement. Hyperglycaemia associated with increased concentrations of glucagon, cortisol and catecholamines and/or decreased insulin secretion may develop in the dog and cat. Hypoglycaemia has been reported in the cat and is probably caused by a combination of anorexia and sepsis. Increased concentrations of pancreatic enzymes may be helpful in the dog but not in the cat. Any increase in amylase and lipase concentrations may, however, relate as much to reduced renal function as it does to pancreatic damage. Increased serum trypsin-like immune activity suggests pancreatic damage but it is cleared rapidly, and normal values are often seen.

Treatment

Treatment is generally supportive. Fluid and electrolyte balance should be maintained, food withheld to minimize pancreatic secretions, analgesia (pethidine) provided and any complications such as respiratory distress and disseminated intravascular coagulation managed. As bacteria may colonize the inflamed pancreas and exacerbate any damage, prophylactic antibacterial therapy with trimethoprim–sulphonamide, fluoroquinolone or cefotaxime is indicated.

SPLENITIS

Infectious conditions that target reticuloendothelial organs (e.g. FIP, fungal infection) are causes of splenic disease but only usually as part of a multisystemic disorder. Infectious agents that specifically target the spleen are rare. They gain access to the spleen via haematogenous and lymphatic routes or following penetration of the abdominal wall. The spleen's highly efficient phagocytic function removes bacteria from blood, thereby providing some protection against bacterial infections.

Aetiology

Figure 11.10 lists the categories and causes of infectious splenitis.

Clinical and historical features

Suppurative splenitis usually presents acutely or subacutely although chronic disease may be found. It can be difficult to distinguish splenomegaly due to infection from other causes of splenomegaly such as splenic torsion, non-infectious inflammatory splenomegaly, infiltrative disorders, hyperplasia or congestion. Clinical features of splenitis are often vague and non-specific and include anorexia, weight loss, depression, pyrexia, splenomegaly and cranial abdominal pain. Where splenitis accompanies a multisystemic disease process, clinical signs reflect damage to other organs; these infections are covered elsewhere in this manual (see Figure 11.10).

Suppurative splenitis
Penetrating abdominal wounds
Migrating foreign bodies
Haematogenous bacterial spread from a primary focus, e.g. bacterial endocarditis, septicaemia, tuberculosis
Toxoplasmosis (see Chapter 15)
Canine adenovirus-1 (see section on liver)

Necrotizing splenitis
Salmonellosis (see Chapter 8)
Canine adenovirus-1 (see section on liver)

Lymphoplasmacytic splenitis
Ehrlichiosis (see Chapter 5)
Pyometra (see Chapter 12)
Brucellosis (see Chapter 12)
Haemobartonellosis (see Chapter 5)

Granulomatous splenitis
Histoplasmosis
Mycobacteriosis (see Chapter 6)
Leishmaniasis (see Chapter 5)

Pyogranulomatous splenitis
Feline infectious peritonitis (see Chapter 9)
Blastomycosis
Sporotrichosis

Figure 11.10: Categories of infectious disorders that involve the spleen of the dog and cat.

Diagnosis

Clinical pathology

Routine serum biochemistry is rarely of any value other than in documenting the involvement of other organ systems in a multisystemic problem. Haematological changes associated with splenitis depend on the inciting cause. Suppurative splenitis would be expected to result in a neutrophilia. Where the infectious agent also involves bone marrow, haematological changes reflect marrow damage. Urinalysis is of no value in the investigation of splenic disease except that splenic torsion often results in haemoglobinuria.

Serology
Serology is of value in assessing multisystemic viral conditions that affect the spleen (e.g. feline coronavirus, toxoplasmosis, CAV-1).

Imaging
Ultrasonography may demonstrate:

- Focal parenchymal abnormalities, including cysts, abscesses, haematoma and neoplasia
- Diffuse increase in echogenicity with gas-forming bacteria
- Normal or decreased echogenicity without parenchymal lesions in congestive and infiltrative disorders.

Histopathology and cytology
Cytological examination of transabdominal fine-needle aspirates of the spleen can provide a diagnosis and should be considered in all cases of splenomegaly. If a definitive diagnosis cannot be made, histopathological examination of splenic tissue after splenectomy is indicated. If a bacterial cause is suspected, tissue should also be submitted for culture.

Treatment
Splenectomy is indicated for suppurative splenitis, particularly if gas-forming bacteria are evident. Bacterial splenitis secondary to trauma or a migrating foreign body may respond to antibacterial therapy. Most other causes of splenitis involve other organ systems, and the management of these infectious agents is discussed in the relevant chapters (see Figure 11.10).

REFERENCES AND FURTHER READING

Adamus C *et al.* (1997) Chronic hepatitis associated with leptospiral infection in vaccinated beagles. *Journal of Comparative Pathology* **117**, 311-328

Cantor *et al.* (1998) VapA-negative *Rhodococcus equi* in a dog with necrotizing pyogranulomatous hepatitis, osteomyelitis and myositis. *Journal of Veterinary Diagnostic Investigation* **10**, 297-300

Carmichael LE (1999) Canine viral vaccines at a turning point - a personal persepective. *Advances in Veterinary Medicine* **41**, 289-307

Ford and Schultz (2000) Vaccines and vaccinations: issues for the 21st century. In: *Current Veterinary Therapy XIII*, ed. RW Kirk, pp. 250-253. WB Saunders, London

Grad *et al.* (1990) Localization of inflammation and virions in canine adenovirus type 2 bronchiolitis. *American Review of Respiratory Disease* **142**, 691-699

Hall E (1998) Hepatobiliary system. In: *Manual of Small Animal Clinical Pathology*, ed. Davidson *et al.*, pp. 161-186. BSAVA, Cheltenham

Kelly WR (1993) Inflammation of the liver and biliary tract. In: *Pathology of Domestic Animals*, ed. Jubb *et al.*, pp. 359-381. Academic Press, San Diego

Rutgers HC and Haywood S (1998) Chronic hepatitis in the dog. *Journal of Small Animal Practice* **29**, 679-690

Steger-Lieb A *et al.* (1999) An old disease with a new face: canine leptospirosis does not lose its relevance. *Schweizer Archiv für Tierheilkunde* **141**, 499-507

CHAPTER TWELVE

The Reproductive Tract and Neonate

Gary England

CHAPTER PLAN

Introduction
Female reproductive tract
  Normal bacterial flora
  Juvenile vaginitis
  Vaginitis
  Atrophic (post-spay) vaginitis
  Cystic endometrial hyperplasia/pyometra
  Resorption/abortion
  Metritis
  Mastitis
Male reproductive tract
  Normal preputial discharge
  Posthitis
  Canine herpesvirus
  Orchitis
  Epididymitis
  Bacterial prostatitis
  Prostatic abscessation
The neonate
  Septicaemia
  Viral infections
Further reading

INTRODUCTION

In humans, infections of the reproductive tract do not seem to play a major part in reproductive tract disease when compared with the high rate of embryo loss associated with genetic defects. In animals, however, a wide variety of infectious agents produce disease of the pregnant and non-pregnant female, the male and the neonate.

FEMALE REPRODUCTIVE TRACT

Various bacteria and viruses may affect the reproductive tract of the female. They are not always venereal pathogens; indeed, many clinical conditions are caused by the opportunistic proliferation of commensal organisms. The collection of a relevant history may help to construct a list of differential diagnoses. The most important factors to consider are:

- Previous parity
- Litter size
- Onset of puberty
- Present cyclicity
- General medical history.

A clinical examination should help to rule out systemic disease:

- The appearance of the vulva and any associated discharge should be noted. A mucoid discharge is common during both early pregnancy and the early luteal phase; in the queen, vulval swelling and discharge are rarely observed in any physiological state
- Digital examination of the vestibule and caudal vagina may detect pathology
- Enlargement of the mammary glands occurs during the luteal phase
- The uterus may be palpated in the caudal abdomen dorsal to the bladder; enlargement occurs in pregnancy, during oestrus and in cases of uterine pathology
- Examination of exfoliative vaginal cytology helps to determine the stage of the oestrous cycle
- Vaginal endoscopy can determine the stage of the oestrus cycle, document the nature of vaginal pathology and detect the origin of a vulval discharge (cervical or urethral)
- Ultrasonography is especially useful for the detection of physiological and pathological changes of the reproductive tract (England, 1995)
- Laparoscopy and laparotomy may detect pathological and cyclical changes within the reproductive tract.

One of the commonest clinical presentations of reproductive tract disease is vulval discharge; this results from physiological and pathological conditions (Figure 12.1). Bacteria cultured from the vestibule or vagina should be interpreted with care because of the

186 Manual of Canine and Feline Infectious Diseases

Nature of discharge	Condition	History	Appearance of vulva	Cytological findings	Comments
Clear or straw coloured	Oestrus	Expected in 'heat'	Swollen or slightly soft	LEC, AEC, RBC, no WBC	Attractive to males
Mucoid	Normal luteal phase	Recent oestrus	Large but soft	PBC, SEC, WBC	No malaise
	Normal pregnancy	Pregnant/recent oestrus	Large but soft	PBC, SEC, WBC	No malaise, does not threaten pregnancy
Purulent	Juvenile vaginitis	Before first 'heat'	Normal	PBC, SEC, WBC	May respond to antimicrobials. Recovery after puberty
	Vaginitis	Variable but often excessive licking, attractive to males	Depends on stage of cycle	Depends on stage of cycle	Specific causes include certain bacterial or viral infections, chemical irritation (urine), mechanical irritation (FB), neoplasia and anatomical abnormalities
	Atrophic vaginitis	Several years after surgical neutering	Normal	PBC, SEC, WBC	May respond to antimicrobial and parenteral or topical oestrogen
Purulent/haemorrhagic	Pyometra	Oestrus 2–8 weeks previously	Slightly swollen	WBC, SEC, LEC, RBC, bacteria, debris	Diagnosis by using ultrasonography or radiography. Often malaise
	Metritis	Recent parturition	Large	Multinucleated cells, LEC, uterine cells	Severe malaise
Haemorrhagic	Pro-oestrus	Expected in 'heat'	Swollen	SEC, LEC, RBC, WBC	Attractive to males
	Oestrus	Expected in 'heat'	Swollen or large but soft	LEC, AEC, RBC, no WBC	Attractive to males
	Follicular cysts	Prolonged oestrus	Swollen	LEC, AEC, RBC	Attractive to males, may be unwell if persistent high oestrogen causes bone marrow suppression
	Vaginal ulceration	Recent mating	Depends on stage of cycle	RBC, depends on the stage of cycle	Rare, usually immediately after mating, but signs may develop up to 2 weeks later
	Placental separation	Pregnant	Normal or swollen	RBC, mucus	Diagnosis of pregnancy essential. Confirmation of fetal stress may be made by detection of lowered heart rate by using ultrasonography
	Subinvolution of placental sites	Persistent discharge after parturition	Slightly swollen	RBC, polynucleated often vacuolated cells present	No malaise. Ultrasonography may show areas of non-involution
	Transmissible venereal tumour	Only within certain countries	Depends on stage of cycle	RBC, tumour cells on impression smear	Clinical appearance usually confirms diagnosis
	Cystitis	Frequent urination	Depends on stage of cycle	RBC, mucus	Haematuria
Haemorrhagic/brown	Resorption abortion	Pregnant	Slightly enlarged	RBC, mucus, debris	May detect absence of embryonic heart beat. Ultimately uterus has similar appearance to one post-partum
Green/brown	Parturition	Pregnant	Slightly swollen	RBC, SEC, uterine cells	Mammary enlargement and signs of first- and second-stage parturition
	Dystocia/placental separation	Pregnant with subsequent non-productive straining	Slightly swollen	RBC, SEC, uterine cells	Ultrasonography may be useful for confirming fetal viability

Figure 12.1: Differential diagnoses of vulval discharge in the bitch.
AEC = anuclear epithelial cells; FB = foreign body; LEC = large epithelial cells; PBC = parabasal cells; RBC = red blood cells; SEC = small epithelial cells; WBC = polymorphonuclear leucocytes. Adapted from England (1996).

wide range of species in normal bacterial flora (see below). Although neutrophils (polymorphonuclear leucocytes) are common within the discharge of bitches with inflammation, they are also normally present in the vaginal smear of any non-oestral bitch. Dogs are frequently attracted to a bitch with a vulval discharge, regardless of its cause.

Normal bacterial flora

Despite popular misconceptions, many bacterial species are present in the vagina of clinically normal bitches. Aerobic commensals, including *Escherichia coli*, *Staphylococcus* spp., *Proteus* spp., *Pseudomonas* spp. and β-haemolytic streptococci (e.g. *Streptococcus canis*), probably originate from skin and the gastrointestinal tract. Although the bacterial flora changes after mating, these changes are not permanent.

In some countries (particularly Central and South America and areas in the USA) *Brucella canis* is a cause of clinical disease; this organism is not present in the UK. Before mating their bitches, some owners request bacteriology of the vagina. This practice is pointless in countries where *B. canis* is absent. It is irrational to exclude animals from mating on the basis of positive culture results for commensal bacteria such as β-haemolytic streptococci. The use of antibacterials against commensal bacteria is irresponsible and ineffective. Bacteria commonly isolated from animals with vaginitis are commensal organisms, which proliferate because of alterations to local environmental factors. Such organisms are not primary pathogens (van Duijkeren, 1992).

Juvenile vaginitis

Prepubertal or juvenile vaginitis may occur in bitches as young as 8 weeks. There is frequently a creamy vulval discharge and sticky material on the hairs around the vulva. The discharge contains epithelial cells, neutrophils and normal commensal bacteria. There is usually no systemic illness. The condition may result from poor mucosal immunity and usually disappears after priming of the reproductive tract with oestrogen when the bitch enters her first oestrus. Bitches respond temporarily to parenteral antimicrobials; however, treatment is usually not warranted, and the condition resolves after the first oestrus. The condition is rare in the queen.

Vaginitis

Bitches and queens with a mucoid, mucopurulent or purulent vulval discharge are frequently diagnosed with vaginitis; however, other conditions, many physiological, may result in such a clinical picture (see Figure 12.1). A diagnosis of true vaginitis should be made on the basis of:

- A persistence of a discharge of purulent material
- Clinical signs of vaginal or vestibular inflammation, including increased vascularity of the vaginal wall and the presence of neutrophils within the discharge
- Discomfort of the bitch – often manifest as excessive licking.

The bitch is often attractive to dogs. In most cases there is a specific underlying cause such as:

- Chemical irritation (urine)
- Mechanical irritation (foreign body)
- Neoplasia
- Anatomical abnormalities of the vagina (stricture).

In each case, vaginal bacteriology shows large numbers of commensal organisms. Diagnosis of the specific cause requires digital, endoscopic and contrast radiographic examination of the caudal genitourinary tract. Removal of the underlying cause rapidly results in a cure. Rarely, primary bacterial or viral infections result in vaginitis (see below). In some animals no causal factor is identified – these are often older animals that respond to parenteral or topical oestrogen therapy; a condition now considered to be atrophic vaginitis (see below).

Brucella canis is the only specific bacterial cause of infertility. It is not found in the UK. Occasionally heavy pure growths of other bacterial species in association with clinical signs are considered important, although pure growths may be isolated from normal dogs.

Canine herpesvirus may cause genital lesions; bitches may develop vesicular vaginal or vestibular lesions, and severe vaginitis has been reported after experimental infection. Calicivirus has been isolated from bitches with vaginal vesicles. Its importance as a major pathogen is unclear.

Vaginitis should be differentiated from perivulval dermatitis, which develops in the skin folds around the vulva.

Atrophic (post-spay) vaginitis

Some bitches show signs of being attractive to dogs several years after surgical neutering. In such cases, there is usually a small volume of vulval discharge containing neutrophils and commensal bacteria, similar to that found in juvenile vaginitis. The condition may result from an absence of oestrogen in the reproductive tract epithelium causing decreased local immunity. The administration of low-dose parenteral oestrogen or the topical application of creams containing oestrogen may control the clinical signs.

Cystic endometrial hyperplasia/pyometra

In the normal bitch or queen, oestradiol causes an increase in the size of endometrial glands and alters epithelial cell morphology from cuboidal to columnar. Under the influence of progesterone, the glands become hyperplastic and hypertrophic. Cystic endometrial hyperplasia (CEH) develops when the response to progesterone is exaggerated and prolonged, which may result in hydrometra or mucometra; abdominal enlargement may be the only clinical sign. Pyometra develops when bacterial colonization of the uterus occurs concurrently with CEH.

Bacteria may enter the uterus during oestrus when the cervix is open and persist into the luteal phase, when they proliferate in the environment of increased endometrial gland secretion, resulting in the development of a pyometra. The bacteria commonly isolated from animals with pyometra are commensal species normally found in the vagina (see above). Pyometra is less common in the queen because, in general, ovulation is induced by coitus, and a large number of queens are surgically neutered. Pyometra may also be induced by the therapeutic administration of progestogens and oestrogens (e.g. for the treatment of unwanted mating). In general, pyometra commonly affects middle-aged and elderly females. There is no relation to parity or a history of reproductive disease. When a complete history is available it is usually found that the female was in oestrus a few weeks before the illness. In the bitch, the owner may consider the vulval discharge to be a continuation of oestrus (see Figure 12.1).

Clinical signs include vulval discharge (a chocolate brown colour with a characteristic odour; Figure 12.2), lethargy, inappetence, polydipsia and polyuria, vomiting, nocturia, diarrhoea and abdominal enlargement. In about one third of cases there is no discharge, and fluid is retained within the uterus (closed-cervix pyometra).

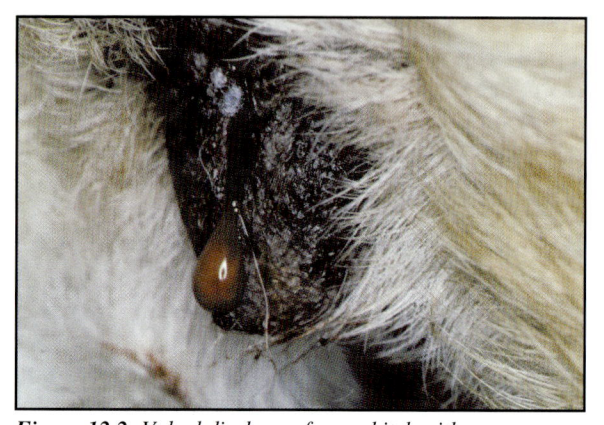

Figure 12.2: Vulval discharge from a bitch with pyometra. (© Dr Ian Ramsey.)

Diagnosis can be made on the basis of clinical findings together with the identification of an enlarged fluid-filled uterus by using transabdominal palpation, radiography or ultrasound examination (Figure 12.3). Animals with closed-cervix pyometra generally have an absolute neutrophilia, which is not necessarily present in those with open-cervix pyometra. The polydipsia is due to reduced permeability for water in the distal convoluted tubule of the kidney, probably caused by the formation of immune complexes.

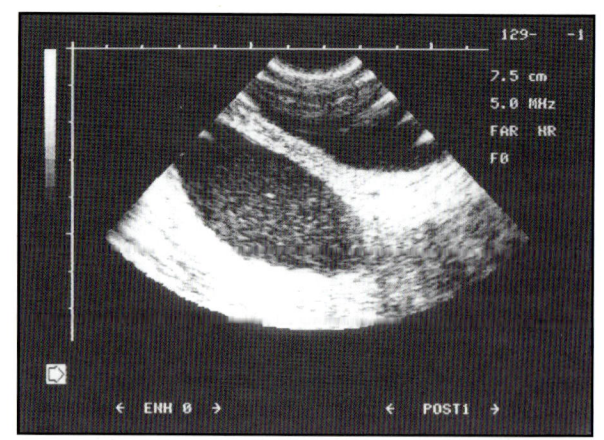

Figure 12.3: Ultrasound image of pyometra in a bitch, showing the large fluid-filled uterus adjacent to the bladder. The uterus contains echogenic material. (5.0 MHz transducer, scale in centimetres.)

Ovariohysterectomy is the treatment of choice for pyometra. Intravenous fluid therapy is essential to maintain renal perfusion if the animal is toxaemic. Attention should be paid to plasma electrolytes and acid–base status because complications associated with endotoxaemia, septicaemia, bacteraemia and uraemia are common.

Medical therapy may be attempted in valuable breeding animals. Several regimens have been reported, including oestrogens (presumably to relax the cervix) and drugs to induce uterine contraction (including ergometrine, quinine and etamiphylline). Because pyometra is a disease of the luteal phase stimulated by progesterone, there has been considerable interest in prostaglandins to lyse the corpora lutea and to promote uterine contractions. Prostaglandins have been used successfully in animals with open-cervix pyometra but are not recommended when the cervix is closed.

A protocol of 0.25 mg/kg dinoprost daily by subcutaneous injection has been recommended, although 0.125 mg/kg twice daily may result in fewer adverse effects. These, which include restlessness, pacing, hypersalivation, tachypnoea, vomiting, diarrhoea, pyrexia and abdominal pain, may be severe and can persist for up to 60 minutes. Admission to hospital and careful observation of the patient is necessary during such treatment. Prostaglandin therapy should be combined with appropriate broad-spectrum antimicrobial agents and intravenous fluids. The success of treatment is variable, with around 40% of animals subsequently achieving pregnancy.

Other treatment options include repeated administration of the prolactin inhibitor cabergoline (terminates the luteal phase) with a prostaglandin such as cloprostenol or dinoprost. These regimens are anecdotally successful but there are no scientific studies that confirm their efficacy. Recently, the progesterone receptor antagonist, aglepristone, has been reported to be effective for the treatment of pyometra, although it is not widely available (Galac *et al.*, 2000).

Resorption and abortion

There are many causes of embryonic resorption or fetal abortion in the bitch and queen, including embryonic abnormalities, an abnormal maternal environment and infectious agents. Embryonic resorption may result in the loss of all the embryos or a reduced litter size; ultrasonography can show resorption of one or two conceptuses in up to 10% of pregnancies (Figure 12.4). In most cases of embryonic resorption there is a serosanguineous vulval discharge (Figure 12.5), and the dam may be systemically unwell when the cause is an infectious organism. Expulsion is the commonest sequel to fetal death, and usually there is a dark-red vulval discharge; the aborted material may be eaten by the female and thus be unavailable for inspection.

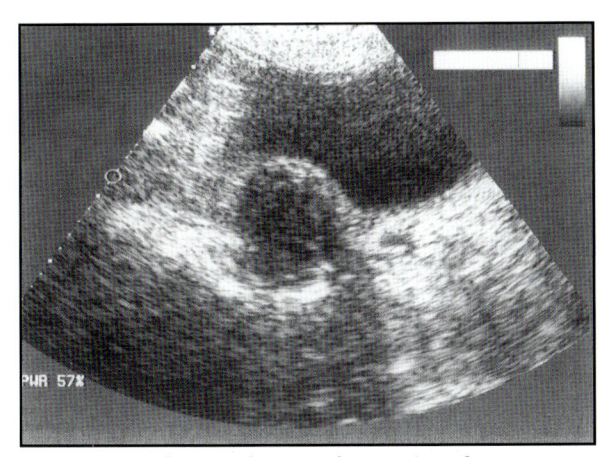

Figure 12.4: Ultrasound image of resorption of an embryonic vesicle in a bitch. There is collapse of the vesicle and loss of the normal anechoic fluid region. (7.5 MHz transducer, scale in centimetres.)

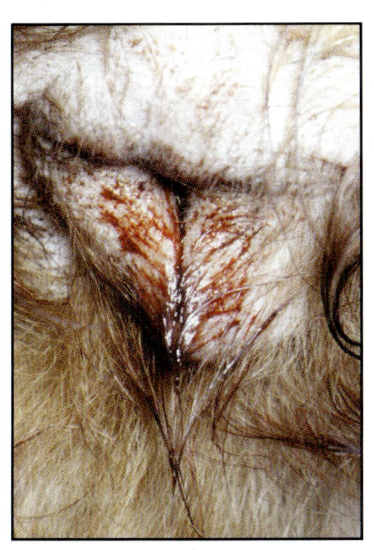

Figure 12.5: Haemorrhagic vulval discharge from a bitch with embryonic resorption.

In most cases, treatment at the time of a resorption is not warranted unless the female becomes systemically unwell. The most important aim is to establish a diagnosis. Treatment to prevent an ongoing abortion is inappropriate, and it is best to encourage expulsion with ecbolic agents such as oxytocin, combined with parental fluid therapy and antimicrobials. Progesterone should not be administered during an abortion since it encourages closure of the cervix and may therefore result in endotoxaemia.

The cause of resorption/abortion may be established by serological examination of the dam and the isolation of bacteria from the fetal membranes and stomach. In many cases, non-specific bacteria, including *Escherichia coli*, *Streptococcus* spp., *Proteus* spp. and *Pseudomonas* spp. are also identified.

Resorption and abortion in bitches

Brucella canis: Abortion caused by *B. canis* occurs most commonly between days 45 and 55 of pregnancy, although early fetal resorption or the birth of stillborn or, rarely, weak puppies may occur. *B. canis* can be transmitted in several ways, including contact both with aborted fetal or placental tissue and with the vaginal discharge of infected bitches, venereal transmission and congenital infection. The most common means of infection is venereal.

Between 1.5% and 6.6% of dogs in the USA have antibodies to *B. canis*, but the organism is not present in the UK. The isolation of the bacterium from blood or aborted tissue is diagnostic of the disease; however, there may be prolonged periods when the bitch is not bacteraemic, so that a negative blood culture result does not rule out infection. Diagnosis by using a plate agglutination test for screening and tube agglutination for confirmation is not difficult; titres of 1:200 or greater are diagnostic of infection.

Toxoplasma gondii: Infection with *T. gondii* is an uncommon cause of abortion in the bitch. The public health consequences of *Toxoplasma* should be considered whenever it is diagnosed. *T. gondii* may also cause premature birth, stillbirth and neonatal deaths. Surviving puppies may carry the infection (see Chapter 15).

Canine herpesvirus: The outcome after exposure to canine herpesvirus (CHV) depends largely on the time of infection. Abortion generally follows infection in mid-pregnancy, whereas infection during early pregnancy may result in fetal death and mummification, and infection during late pregnancy results in premature birth. It seems that infection of the pregnant bitch results in the production of placental lesions and direct transmission to the fetus. Infected placentae are macroscopically underdeveloped and possess small greyish-white foci, which are characterized by focal necrosis and the presence of eosinophilic intranuclear inclusion bodies.

Canine herpesvirus has also been recovered from vesicular lesions on the genitalia of bitches. Frequently these lesions develop during pro-oestrus, suggesting that venereal transmission is important in adult bitches. Recrudescent canine herpes with virus shedding may be stimulated by the stress of pregnancy and parturition.

Diagnosis of herpesvirus infection is difficult. In adults the virus is excreted intermittently and is difficult to isolate. Virus is shed for 2-3 weeks following primary infection and may also be shed intermittently following times of immunosuppression or stress. Serology is of little value as antibody levels are often low or undetectable. Culture and serological testing are not accurate or effective in screening dogs or bitches for infection. No vaccine is available.

Canine distemper virus: Experimental exposure of pregnant bitches to canine distemper virus produces either clinical illness in the bitch with subsequent abortion or subclinical infection of the bitch and the birth of clinically affected puppies. This provides evidence for transplacental transmission, although the frequency of this under natural conditions is unknown. See Chapter 6 for more information on distemper.

Canine adenovirus: Infection with canine adenovirus during pregnancy can result in the birth of dead puppies or weak puppies that die a few days after parturition. In most cases the virus is ingested by the neonate and causes subsequent mortality. Carrier bitches occur and may act as a source of infection for puppies. See Chapter 11 for more information on this infection.

Resorption and abortion in queens

Feline leukaemia virus: Feline leukaemia virus (FeLV) may cause a variety of conditions of the reproductive tract, including embryonic resorption. Fetal abortion and the birth of permanently infected kittens also occur. The virus seems to cross the placenta, although abortion may result from secondary bacterial infection after FeLV-induced immunosuppression.

Owners should be encouraged to test queens before mating and discouraged from breeding from affected ones because their offspring will be persistently infected. Infected kittens usually develop an FeLV-related disease soon after birth. See Chapter 5 for further discussion on the diagnosis and management of FeLV.

Feline herpesvirus: Abortion during the fifth or sixth week of pregnancy may follow infection with feline herpesvirus (FHV). In experimental studies both uterine and placental lesions have been shown, although in the clinical situation abortion may result from a non-specific reaction to the infection, such as pyrexia. Abortion due to herpesvirus is normally diagnosed on the basis of the clinical signs and isolation of the virus. All breeding animals should be vaccinated as this provides immunity against infection. See Chapter 6 for further information on FHV.

Feline panleucopenia virus: Abortion is a common complication of feline panleucopenia virus infection. In many cases the clinical signs are stillbirth, neonatal death and the birth of kittens with cerebellar hypoplasia. The virus passes across the placenta and the outcome depends on the time of infection; infection in early pregnancy results in fetal abortion, whereas infection later in pregnancy results in cerebellar hypoplasia and stillbirths. The virus is transmitted by direct contact with saliva, faeces and urine, and diagnosis is made on the basis of the clinical signs, histopathological findings, virus isolation and a rising antibody titre. All breeding animals should be vaccinated. See Chapter 8 for more information on this infection.

Feline coronavirus: Abortion during the last 2 weeks of pregnancy is not uncommon after infection with feline coronavirus (FCoV). The virus may also cause endometritis, stillbirths, chronic upper respiratory tract disease and fading kitten syndrome. Diagnosis is made by serological and pathological investigation (see Chapter 9 for more information on this infection).

Toxoplasmosis: Abortion may rarely result from infection with *Toxoplasma gondii*; some kittens are born with congenital infection. The role of this organism in abortion can be shown by serological screening. See Chapter 15 for more information on toxoplasmosis.

Chlamydophilosis: Formerly known as *Chlamydia psittaci* var. *felis*, the organism *Chlamydophila felis* may cause abortion in the queen. The aetiology of the abortion and the mode of transmission has not been elucidated, although the organism may be isolated from the reproductive tract of aborting queens. Direct isolation of the organism and the demonstration of high antibody titres suggests infection, although these findings should be interpreted with care as the organism may be opportunistic.

Metritis

Metritis is associated with bacterial infection of the uterus after abortion, parturition, fetal and/or placental retention and obstetric manipulation. Clinical signs of depression, pyrexia, anorexia and purulent vaginal discharge are usually noted 2 to 3 days after parturition. A neutrophilia with a left shift is common, and enlargement of the uterus may be identified by radiography, palpation or ultrasonography. As metritis is a bacterial disorder without the underlying hormonal component found in pyometra, conservative medical management is feasible. Broad-spectrum antimicrobial therapy is required, and both oxytocin and ergometrine have been used to stimulate myometrial activity and to induce uterine drainage.

Mastitis

Mastitis is uncommon in dogs and cats. Its most important manifestation is acute mastitis during early lactation. The commonest agents involved are *Escherichia coli*, *Staphylococcus* spp. and *Streptococcus* spp. The microbes gain access from the skin. In the mammary gland they tend to develop localized abscesses, although gangrene has been reported. Affected glands are firm, warm and painful. A greyish, often bloody fluid, which may contain pus, may be expressed. The diagnosis can be confirmed by cytological examination and culture of the expressed material. Treatment involves appropriate antibacterial therapy based on sensitivity testing. Ampicillin, amoxycillin and cephalosporins achieve high concentrations in milk and should be considered prior to culture results being known. Application of warm compresses to affected glands several times a day will ease pain and swelling. Mammary abscesses require surgical drainage. Analgesics, such as non-steroidal anti-inflammatory drugs, are indicated.

MALE REPRODUCTIVE TRACT

Several bacteria affect the reproductive tract of the male. With the exception of *Brucella canis*, these are not venereal pathogens, but as with the female are commensal organisms that have an opportunistic role in disease. When obtaining a history, particular attention should be paid to the:

- Owner's observations of the clinical signs
- Breeding history
- Administration of any pharmaceutical compounds
- General medical history.

As in the female, a full clinical examination is mandatory. In the tom, physical examination of the reproductive tract is limited to inspection and palpation of the external genitalia, whereas in the dog rectal palpation of the prostate gland is also possible. Testes should be examined and compared for their size and consistency. The epididymis should be palpated and the epididymal tail, which is usually pea sized in the dog, should be noted. The prostate gland should be symmetrical, with a dorsal median furrow. The position of the prostate gland is variable, although it is usually intrapelvic. An increase in size occurs normally with advancing age. The prepuce should be examined for abnormal discharges and the penis exposed for inspection of abnormalities.

The collection of a semen sample by manual stimulation of the penis in the presence of a bitch in oestrus may provide diagnostic information on diseases of the testes, epididymides and prostate. Biopsy samples of the testes may be obtained by incision or needle aspiration, although this is not advisable in breeding animals as the procedure is followed by a marked inflammatory response and subsequent fibrosis. Ultrasonography is especially useful for imaging the prostate and testes. Further evaluation of the prostate gland in the dog may be achieved by needle aspiration or biopsy of the gland and cytological assessment of material obtained after per rectal massage of the prostate gland and the immediate lavage and re-aspiration of the prostatic urethra with 5 ml of sterile saline given via a urinary catheter.

One of the commonest clinical presentations of reproductive tract disease is a preputial discharge (Figure 12.6). There are many causes of preputial discharge and these are not always associated with primary infectious diseases.

Normal preputial discharge

A small volume of mucopurulent preputial discharge is normal in the dog. Many aerobic bacteria may be isolated, including *Staphylococcus* spp., *Escherichia coli*, *Streptococcus* spp., *Proteus* spp. and *Pseudomonas* spp. As in the vagina of the bitch, these organisms are commensals. Parenteral or topical antimicrobial agents result in a temporary reduction in the discharge but are not warranted.

Posthitis

Excessive preputial discharge may be associated with posthitis (inflammation of the prepuce). Preputial trauma, foreign bodies and tumours must be eliminated as primary causes. In many cases the aetiology remains unknown; mycoplasmas were implicated but they have been found in normal dogs. In these cases, when the prepuce appears normal, the prostate, epididymides and testes should also be carefully examined to eliminate them as sources of the discharge.

Treatment involves removal of the predisposing cause and flushing of the preputial cavity and penis with an antimicrobial ointment/solution (e.g. amoxycillin–clavulanate intramammary tubes) or weak antiseptic solutions. Parenteral drugs are usually of little value. Some traumatic lesions may necessitate surgical debridement.

Canine genital herpes

Genital lesions associated with CHV infection include: hyperaemia; petechiation; development of lymphoid nodules, especially over the base of the penis; and preputial reflection. An associated serous discharge from the preputial orifice may be evident. The lesions, which appear 3 days after infection, are self-limiting and regress 4–5 days later. Concurrent conjunctivitis has been reported (see Chapter 16). Pustule formation and ulceration do not appear to be features of genital herpesvirus infection in the male dog. For diagnosis, see above, under Female reproductive tract.

192 Manual of Canine and Feline Infectious Diseases

Nature of discharge	Condition	History	Appearance of external genitalia	Cytological findings	Comments
Mucoid–mucopurulent	Normal	Unremarkable	Normal	LEC, WBC	Often presented because of owner concern but no clinical signs. Can be large volume
	Lymphoid hyperplasia	Unremarkable	Small raised nodular lesions on penis	LEC, WBC	Common and 'normal' finding in many dogs
	Phimosis	May be excessive licking. Pain at attempted coitus	Small preputial orifice and inability to protrude penis	LEC, WBC	May urinate into sheath producing secondary inflammation. May require surgical enlargement
Mucopurulent	Bacterial prostatitis	Young adult. Acute stage may show vomiting and malaise. Chronic may show wasting and faecal tenesmus	Normal	LEC, WBC, bacteria	Clinical presentation depends on whether disease is acute or chronic or if abcessation has developed. Gland is often painful when palpated
Purulent	Posthitis	Frequent and excessive licking. Inflammation of the preputial lining	Swollen sheath	LEC, WBC, bacteria	Commonly an underlying cause such as FB, trauma or neoplasia. Primary bacterial infections are rare
(Purulent) or none	Orchitis/epididymitis	Swelling of the testes/epididymides. Frequent licking and self-trauma	Swelling of scrotum	WBC, bacteria	May have no discharge. Common clinical signs are related to the testes and epididymides
Haemorrhagic	Benign prostatic hyperplasia	Older dog. Faecal tenesmus is common	Normal	LEC, WBC	Prostatomegaly detected on palpation. May also have haemospermia
	Prostatic neoplasia	Older dog. Poor condition. Faecal tenesmus	Normal	Tumour cells, LEC, RBC	Palpation and ultrasonography useful but may require biopsy for accurate diagnosis
	Urethral prolapse	Rare. Masturbation	Normal — may be trauma to prepuce	RBC	Small 'button-like' prolapse easily visible on extrusion of penis
	Penile neoplasia	Rare. May be history of coitus in the case of transmissible venereal tumour	Cauliflower-like lesions on surface of penis	Tumour cells, RBC	Surgical resection and penile amputation may be necessary

Figure 12.6: Differential diagnoses of preputial discharge in the dog.
FB = foreign body; LEC = large epithelial cells; RBC = erythrocytes; WBC = polymorphonuclear leucocytes.

Orchitis

Inflammation of the testis may be infectious or non-infectious in origin. The former is rare in the UK but not uncommon in countries where *Brucella canis* is endemic. Infected dogs have acute swelling of the testes and epididymides, resulting in spermatozoal abnormalities and infertility. The organism may be found in semen or detected serologically. After the culture of bacteria from an animal with orchitis, antimicrobial sensitivity should be established to allow effective treatment. Infective orchitis may also occur after retrograde passage of urine and result in suppurative inflammation and abscess formation, often necessitating castration. Traumatic orchitis is most common in the tom and may be complicated by infection and haemorrhage. Conservative therapy involving broad-spectrum antimicrobial preparations may be successful, although surgical debridement or castration may be necessary.

Epididymitis

Infectious agents may enter the epididymis via the vas deferens or seminiferous tubules, through the vaginal tunic (traumatic) or haematogenously. A specific syndrome of epididymitis, orchitis and scrotal oedema, in association with pyrexia, depression and swelling of one or more limbs, has been associated with *Pseudomonas pseudomallei* infection. Outside the UK, *Brucella suis* may cause a granulomatous epididymitis and prostatitis. The epididymis becomes enlarged and painful and the resulting inflammation may cause fibrosis and obstruction. Culture of the second fraction of the ejaculate may help to isolate bacterial causes. Appropriate antimicrobial therapy may then be helpful, although castration may be necessary. Serology for brucellosis should be undertaken in dogs that have been imported to the UK or in areas where *Brucella canis* is endemic.

Bacterial prostatitis

Bacterial prostatitis is not uncommon in young adult dogs. It is not reported in toms. Dogs generally show signs of systemic illness, with vomiting and pain in the caudal abdomen. There is usually a neutrophilia, and the prostate gland is painful and has an irregular contour on palpation. Collection of the third fraction of the ejaculate, urethral washings after massage of the prostate or urine culture may help with diagnosis. Commonly *Escherichia coli*, *Proteus* spp., *Staphylococcus* spp., *Streptococcus* spp., *Klebsiella* spp. and *Pseudomonas* spp. are identified, and there are usually large numbers of neutrophils within the prostatic fluid.

The ultrasonographic appearance (Figure 12.7) may be similar to that of benign prostatic hyperplasia, such that these conditions cannot be differentiated by ultrasonography. Most commonly the gland is diffusely affected and has a heterogeneous appearance, with poorly marginated regions of hyper- and

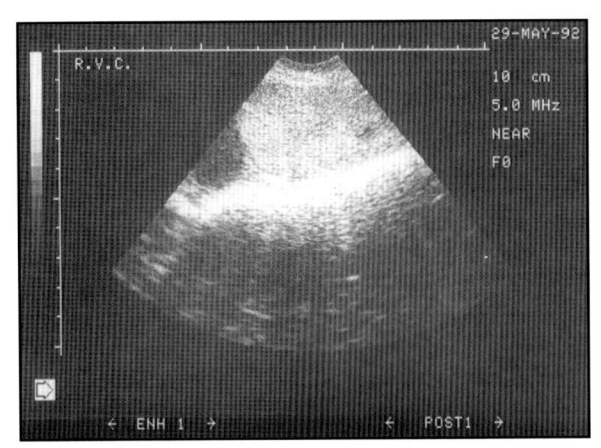

Figure 12.7: Ultrasound image of bacterial prostatitis in a dog. The prostate gland is enlarged and generally is heterogenously echogenic, with poorly defined zones of hypoechogenicity. (5.0 MHz transducer, scale in centimetres.)

hypoechogenicity. Various sized hypoechoic zones may be present, probably representing focal accumulations of pus.

Antimicrobial agents (based on culture and sensitivity) should be given for at least 21 days. The blood-prostate barrier is not intact during acute inflammation, so many antibacterial agents are efficacious.

Chronic prostatitis may follow inadequate treatment of an acute episode, although in some cases it may be secondary to a chronic urinary tract infection or similar. In this case there may be further enlargement of the gland, detected ultrasonographically, with greater distortion of the prostatic architecture. Treatment is difficult because the blood–prostatic barrier is normally intact. Factors such as lipid solubility, ionization and protein binding affect the ability of agents to cross the blood–prostate barrier.

Culture of the prostatic fluid, with Gram staining and sensitivity testing to antibacterials, is advisable in all cases. If the organism is Gram-positive then erythromycin, clindamycin, chloramphenicol or trimethoprim are likely to be useful. For Gram-negative organisms, chloramphenicol, trimethoprim or enrofloxacin are preferred. Therapy should be continued for at least 6 weeks, after which re-culture should be performed to establish a clinical cure.

Prostatic abscessation

Chronic prostatitis may progress to form large pockets of purulent exudate (abscessation). Dogs may have various signs attributed to prostatic enlargement, and there is frequently a haemorrhagic or purulent urethral discharge, which may be constant or intermittent. Some dogs may present with septic shock after rupture of an abscess. There is frequently, but not always, a leucocytosis, and dogs commonly have clinical signs of a recurrent cystitis. Prostatic abscesses can be readily detected by ultrasonography. The central fluid-filled regions are often asymmetrical, and the entire gland has a distorted appearance (Figure 12.8a). *Escherichia coli* is the predominant organism cultured from these cases. Surgical drainage is the treatment of choice. The abscess cavities should be opened and care taken to avoid damage to the urethra (Figure 12.8b). The gland should be flushed with sterile saline and then the cavities should be omentalized (Figure 12.8c). After surgery, antimicrobial therapy is required for several months.

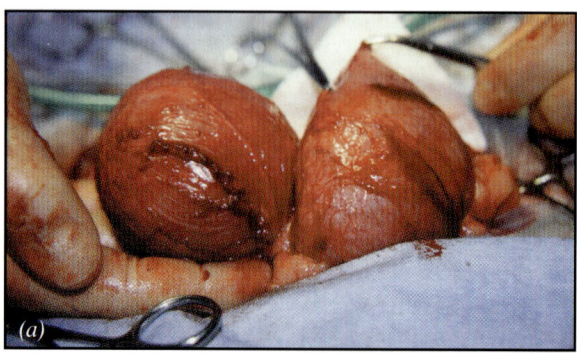

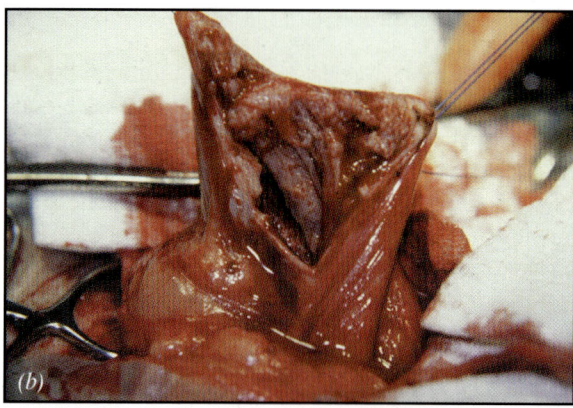

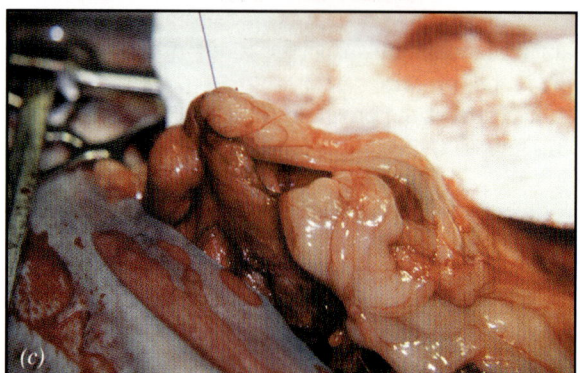

Figure 12.8: (a) Gross appearance of prostatic abscess. The abscess is positioned to the right of the bladder. (b) The abscess has been opened and the cavity drained. (c) The abscess has been omentalized. (Courtesy of Mr R. N. White.)

THE NEONATE

The most common problem within the neonatal period is fading puppies or kittens. Fading neonates usually die when less than 1 week old. There is a multitude of factors associated with this loss, but the inherent susceptibility of being newborn contributes to the animal's ultimate demise. Neonates have poor mechanisms of both thermoregulation and fluid and energy balance, are immunologically incompetent, and may have abnormal lung surfactant composition. When combined with poor management regimens and poor mothering behaviour of the dam, the risk of neonatal mortality may be high. About 50% of neonatal deaths can be attributed to the following four groups.

- Infection
- Maternal and management-related deficiencies
- Low birthweight
- Congenital abnormalities.

Septicaemia

The inherent vulnerability of the neonate puts it at risk of colonization by several bacterial agents. Infection with organisms such as *Staphylococcus* spp., *Escherichia coli*, *Klebsiella* spp., *Enterobacter faecalis*, *Streptococcus* spp., *Enterococcus* spp., *Pseudomonas* spp., *Bacteroides* spp., *Salmonella* spp. and *Bordetella bronchiseptica* may result in clinical illness. In each case death may occur rapidly with few initial clinical signs. In some circumstances, ill health results in frequent crying, restlessness and hypothermia, and this progresses to clinical signs of diarrhoea and/or dyspnoea, with resultant dehydration or cyanosis and ultimately death. In certain circumstances some neonates are more chronically affected and fail to grow as expected before the onset of obvious clinical disease.

Most passive immunity follows from the intake of colostrum, and gut transfer occurs only during the first 48 hours of life. It is vital, therefore, to ensure that a neonate has an adequate intake of colostrum to protect against infectious organisms.

In most cases diagnosis is made on the basis of the clinical history and signs. Blood cultures may be useful but usually neonates have either recovered or died before the results are available. In the case of bordetellosis, oropharyngeal swabs may be useful for diagnosis. Regardless of the cause, rapid and aggressive treatment with intravenous fluid therapy, oral electrolytes, broad-spectrum antimicrobial agents and oxygen is essential. Despite such treatment, mortality can be high.

Viral infections

Viral infections are not common in the neonate, especially when vaccination programmes are practised in the adult. Maternally derived antibody frequently provides protection for several weeks.

Canine herpesvirus (CHV)

Puppies can become infected with CHV *in utero*, during birth or in the early neonatal period. Infectious virus may be excreted by the bitch from lesions of genital herpes and in bodily secretions, including saliva, following primary infection or after recrudescence of latent infection. Infection may result in the birth of congenitally infected puppies that are weak and die soon after birth.

Puppies infected at birth or postnatally up to 2 weeks of age may develop generalized systemic disease that is often fatal, often without any premonitory signs. Resistance to systemic disease is sharply age-related: pups exposed after 2 weeks of age will not develop systemic illness. The disease has an incubation period of 3–7 days. Clinical signs include vomiting, refusal to eat, shallow and rapid breathing, abdominal pain, widespread petechial and ecchymotic haemorrhages, nasal discharge and CNS signs. In adults or older puppies, CHV may produce mild upper respiratory tract infection (see Chapter 6), although most infections are inapparent. Following infection, the virus may become latent.

Some bitches may produce several affected litters, whereas with others only the first litter is affected, presumably owing to subsequent protection in the puppies against disease (although not infection) by maternally derived antibody over the risk period.

Diagnosis of neonatal CHV infection is made following post-mortem examination and histological assessment of systemic organs, including kidney, liver and lungs. Virus isolation is difficult and usually unrewarding. For information on CHV infection in adults, see earlier in this chapter.

Others

Other viral causes of fading puppies include canine adenovirus and canine distemper virus infection, although these are rare.

In cats, feline immunodeficiency virus (FIV) and FeLV can both infect kittens transplacentally as well as perinatally and result in neonatal death after a few weeks of age. Neonatal deaths and the birth of kittens with cerebellar hypoplasia are not uncommon after infection with feline panleucopenia virus during pregnancy. Feline coronavirus has also been implicated in cases of upper respiratory tract disease and fading kitten syndrome. In each of these cases, clinical evaluation and information from serology and post-mortem examination may be combined to make a diagnosis. This may be useful for future preventive medicine regimens but may offer little help in the treatment of an ongoing infection. Treatment of such cases is usually empirical, as described above.

FURTHER READING

Allen WE and Dagnall GRJ (1982) Some observations on the aerobic bacterial flora of the genital tract of the dog and bitch. *Journal of Small Animal Practice* **23**, 325–336

Brownlie J and England GCW (1999) Viral infections with pathological consequences for reproduction in veterinary species. In: *Viral Infections on Obstetrics and Gynaecology*, ed. DJ Jeffries and CN Hudson, pp. 289–333. Arnold, London

England GCW (1995) Small animal reproductive ultrasonography. In: *Veterinary Ultrasonography*, ed. PJ Goddard, pp. 55–85. CAB International, London

England GCW (1996) Infertility in the bitch and queen. In: *Veterinary Reproduction and Obstetrics*, 7th edn, ed. GH Arthur et al., pp. 497–515. WB Saunders, London

Galac S, Koostra HS, Butinar J, Bevers MM, Dielman SJ, Voorhout G and Okkers AC (2000) Termination of mid-gestation pregnancy in bitches with aglepristone, a progesterone receptor antagonist. *Theriogenology* **53**, 941–950

Simpson GM, England GCW and Harvey MJ (1998) *Manual of Small Animal Reproduction and Neonatology*. BSAVA, Cheltenham

van Duijkeren E (1992) Significance of the vaginal bacterial flora in the bitch: a review. *Veterinary Record* **131**, 367–370

CHAPTER THIRTEEN

The Skin

Ian Mason, Ross Bond, Danièlle A. Gunn-Moore and Andrew Sparkes

CHAPTER PLAN

Introduction
Approach to infectious dermatopathies
Parasitic skin disease
    Ctenocephalidiasis (fleas)
    Pediculosis (lice)
    Mange (mites)
        Sarcoptes
        Cheyletiella
        Demodex
        Otodectes
        Trombicula
    Helminthiasis
        Hookworm and *Pelodera* dermatitis
Bacterial skin disease
    Pyoderma
    Cat bite abscesses
    Cutaneous mycobacterial disease
    Others
Fungal skin disease
    Dermatophytosis
    Malassezia pachydermatis
    Others
Protozoal skin disease
    Leishmaniasis
Viral skin disease
Algal skin disease
Otitis
    Bacterial/fungal otitis
    Otodectes cynotis
References and Further Reading

INTRODUCTION

This chapter is concerned with infections that primarily affect the skin and with systemic infections that may manifest with signs of skin disease. The first two sections describe skin defence mechanisms and the approach to a dermatological problem. Subsequent sections provide details on individual organisms.

THE SKIN'S DEFENCE MECHANISMS

For an organism to establish an infection in the skin it must first overcome the skin's immune and non-immune defence mechanisms. These include:

- Secretory immunoglobulin A (SIgA)
- Cell-mediated immunity
- The physical barrier provided by epithelial cells
- Desquamation, which constantly rids the skin of microbes
- Inhibition of microbial growth due to skin dryness and low surface pH.

Secretory immunoglobulin A (SIgA) is found in sweat glands and on the skin surface, and inhibits the adherence of bacteria and viruses, thereby preventing colonization/infection. It also neutralizes toxins. It has been suggested that a deficiency of SIgA predisposes to local infections, allowing the development of such diseases as anal furunculosis, atopy, chronic/recurrent dermatitis and otitis externa. This remains unproven.

Non-immune defence mechanisms are affected by many factors. Alterations to the local environment (e.g. persistently wet skin), physical integrity (e.g. trauma, burns) and the presence of underlying disease (e.g. neoplasia, systemic disease) predispose to skin infection.

APPROACH TO INFECTIOUS DERMATOPATHIES

Diagnosis of infectious dermatological disease should be on the basis of history, physical examination and laboratory results; infectious and non-infectious dermatopathies often present similarly, and detailed information is required to distinguish between them.

History
In addition to general historical information regarding the health of the animal, specific information relating to the presence of pruritus, alopecia, papules or other dermatological signs must be recorded. The chronological order in which these signs develop can be useful. Knowledge of the management of the animal, previous treatment and the coexistence of skin disease in other animals or humans in the household is invaluable (Figure 13.1).

Patient profile	
Breed - Note the following predilections:	
Boxer, Dobermann Pinscher, Great Dane, Persian cat	Acne (superficial folliculitis)
Boxer, Bull Terriers, Shar Pei, West Highland Terrier	Demodicosis
Jack Russell Terrier, Yorkshire Terrier, Persian cat	Dermatophytosis
Bulldog, Pug, Shar Pei, Persian cat	Intertrigo
Basset Hound, Miniature Poodle, spaniels, West Highland Terrier	*Malassezia* dermatitis
Spaniels, poodles, German Shepherd Dog	Otitis externa
German Shepherd Dog	Perianal fistulae
Age - Note the following:	
Before 1 year	Impetigo Demodicosis Dermatophytosis
1-3 years	Primary idiopathic pyoderma
General and dermatological history questions:	
Has the animal been abroad? Was the animal acquired from a breeder, pet shop, puppy farm or a rescue society? Did the animal arrive with the problem or develop skin disease soon after? Are in-contact animals or humans affected? Any exposure to potential source of infection - foxes, grooming parlour, boarding kennels, shows etc? First sign noticed? Which body regions first affected, which regions affected now? Sudden or gradual onset of disease? Flea control (if any)? Housing - indoors, outdoors?	

Figure 13.1: Case history information of value in assessing skin cases.

Clinical examination

A full clinical examination may identify underlying systemic disorders or other unrelated problems that can influence subsequent management decisions and priorities for investigation. The entire skin, including mucous membranes and ear canals, should be carefully examined under good illumination and the nature of lesions (e.g. papules, pustules, macules, nodules, alopecia) noted and recorded, preferably on a two-dimensional lesion map. The distribution of lesions may indicate specific diagnoses; a good example of this is flea allergy dermatitis where the lesions occur in the dorsal rear quadrant of the skin. Skin infections and infestations lead to a range of clinical features (Figure 13.2); knowledge of these is helpful in the formulation of a list of differential diagnoses.

Clinical feature	Dermatosis
Pruritus	Ectoparasites, pyoderma
Alopecia	Demodicosis, dermatophytosis
Scaling/crusting	Ectoparasites, pyoderma, *Malassezia* dermatitis, Leishmaniasis
Papules/pustules	Pyoderma, ectoparasites
Malodour	*Malassezia* dermatitis, pyoderma
Pododermatitis	Demodicosis, hookworm, *Pelodera* dermatitis, harvest mites

Figure 13.2: Clinical features of infectious dermatoses.

Differential diagnosis and laboratory investigations

In almost all instances, a short list of differential diagnoses can be generated using historical and clinical information. This enables the selection of focused confirmatory diagnostic tests. Figure 13.3 lists the infectious agents that may be associated with skin disease. Figure 13.4 lists differential diagnoses for miliary dermatitis. Differential diagnoses for infectious causes of other dermatopathies are given in relevant sections.

PARASITES		BACTERIA	
Dogs	*Cats*	*Dogs*	*Cats*
Ctenocephalides felis – cat flea *Ctenocephalides canis* – dog flea *Linognathus setosus* – sucking louse *Trichodectes canis* – biting louse *Sarcoptes scabiei* *Cheyletiella* sp. *Demodex canis* *Neotrombicula autumnalis*	*Ctenocephalides felis* – cat flea *Ctenocephalides canis* – dog flea *Felicola subrostratus* – biting louse *Cheyletiella* sp. *Otodectes cynotis* *Neotrombicula autumnalis*	*Staphylococcus intermedius* *Staphylococcus aureus* *Staphylococcus felis* *Proteus* sp. *Pseudomonas* sp. *Mycobacteria* sp. *Nocardia asteroides* *Borrelia burgdorferi* *Dermatophilus congolensis* *Rickettsia rickettsii** *Brucella canis**	*Staphylococcus intermedius* *Staphylococcus aureus* *Proteus* sp. *Pseudomonas* sp. *Mycobacterium* sp. *Nocardia asteroides* *Dermatophilus congolensis*
NEMATODES		**FUNGI/YEASTS**	
Dogs	*Cats*	*Dogs*	*Cats*
Pelodera strongyloides *Ancylostoma* sp. *Uncinaria* sp.		*Microsporum* spp. *Trichophyton* spp. *Malassezia* spp. *Candida* spp. *Sporothrix schenkii*	*Microsporum* spp. *Trichophyton* spp. *Malassezia* spp. *Sporothrix schenkii*
PROTOZOA		**VIRUSES**	
Dogs	*Cats*	*Dogs*	*Cats*
Leishmania sp. *Caryospora* sp. *Neospora caninum* *Sarcocystis*-like coccidia	*Toxoplasma gondii*	Distemper virus Papilloma virus	Poxvirus Feline parapoxvirus Contagious pustular dermatitis Feline sarcoma virus Feline leukaemia virus

*Figure 13.3: Infectious agents of the skin. * Do not occur in the UK.*

Hypersensitivity	Ectoparasites	Microbial
Flea bite	Notoedric mange (extinct in UK?) Pediculosis Cheyletiellosis Otodectic mange	Bacterial pyoderma Dermatophytosis

Figure 13.4: Infectious causes of feline 'miliary dermatitis'.

Various techniques are used to collect and analyse laboratory samples from animals with skin disease:

- Direct observation of lice and fleas
- Tape-stripping – this is a rapid and simple method (Figure 13.5) used to detect fungi and superficial pathogens that do not burrow into skin, e.g. *Cheyletiella* spp. Occasionally ear mites (*Otodectes cynotis*), flea faeces or *Trombicula* mites may be identified.
- Coat brushings (Figure 13.5) – these are used to identify flea faeces and *Cheyletiella* spp. Brushings collected on a new or sterilized toothbrush may be cultured for dermatophytes; the dermatophyte culture medium is inoculated directly by the toothbrush
- Smears from pustules in pyoderma – these may also be used in the diagnosis of demodicosis
- Microscopy of skin scrapings (Figure 13.5) – this is the method of choice for detecting burrowing mites such as *Sarcoptes scabiei* and *Notoedres cati*. Skin scrapes should be performed on several carefully selected areas, as multiple specimens are more likely to yield a positive test result, particularly for sarcoptic mange. These sites should be at the periphery of large lesions, avoiding areas of hyperkeratinization or exudation

Microscopy of skin scrapings
1. Clip hair (if present) carefully with scissors
2. Moisten skin surface with mineral oil
3. Scrape surface with No. 10 scalpel blade (if near eyes, a scraping spatula may be used)
4. Scrape until slight bleeding is seen
5. Smear material collected on blade on to a microscope slide
6. Add a small amount of mineral oil (liquid paraffin) and a cover slip
7. Examine under microscope using lowest power objective lens
Examination of coat brushings
1. Hold the animal in standing or sitting position over a large sheet of white paper towelling
2. Comb or brush the coat. Remove hair and debris trapped between teeth of comb and place this material on the paper towelling (in addition to this, scale, hair and other material will drop from the coat directly on to the paper)
3. Examine the material with a hand-held magnifying lens for evidence of flea faeces
4. Add water to any material suspected to be flea faeces – these will disolve and stain the paper rust-red
5. Examine any other material under the microscope for evidence of parasites other than fleas
Tape-stripping
1. Apply clear adhesive tape to the areas with most scale
2. Press firmly down
3. a) Mount the strip of adhesive tape on a glass slide and view immediately
b) If yeast infection is suspected, stain with a Romanowsky-type stain (e.g. Diff-Quik) and examine under a X100 objective
Choose an adhesive tape that resists the staining process; some tapes curl and disintegrate when stained, making examination and interpretation difficult
Smears from pustules
1. Clip the hair
2. Extrude the mites from hair follicles by gently pinching the skin. If this procedure is done properly it is only mildly painful to the animal
3. Scrape the extruded material on to a glass slide for processing

Figure 13.5: Techniques for finding ectoparasites.

- Smears from needle aspirates of fluid-containing lesions or solid lesions, or impression smears from ulcers. These allow bacterial, yeast and fungal infections to be detected. Gram or modified Wright's staining of a slide provides some indication as to the predominant type of bacteria present. The presence of inflammatory cells containing phagocytosed bacteria or fungal hyphae is consistent with infection. Extracellular bacteria only suggest colonization. The presence of eosinophils, basophils or mast cells raises the suspicion of ectoparasitism. Unusual infectious agents may be identified (e.g. actinomycetes, mycobacteria, *Leishmania*)
- Histopathology – this may be useful in the diagnosis of some infectious agents. It allows the dermatosis to be confirmed as an infectious disorder and may indicate specific infectious agents (e.g. *Demodex*, fungi)
- Serology for *Sarcoptes* and flea saliva antibody.

PARASITIC SKIN DISEASE

Ctenocephalidiasis (fleas)

Flea-induced skin disease is the commonest problem in veterinary dermatology practice. Dermatitis arises after fleas have bitten the animal; although there is some uncertainty about the precise pathogenesis of the skin disease, it is clear that a complex series of immunological mechanisms, including hypersensitivity, is involved. *Ctenocephalides felis felis* (abbreviated to *C. felis*) is the species of flea most commonly associated with pet dogs and cats in the UK, whereas the dog flea *C. canis* is more common in Eire.

Disease can occur in virtually any adult dog or cat at any time of the year, although many cases start in late summer or early autumn. Intermittent exposure to fleas may predispose to the development of flea-bite hypersensitivity. Fleas are the intermediate host of the tapeworm *Dipylidium caninum*, and affected animals may have a history of infestation with this endoparasite. Fleas may also be responsible for the transmission of *Haemobartonella felis* and other blood-borne infections. The life cycle of *C. felis* is shown in Figure 13.6.

Clinical features

Flea infestation results in a wide range of clinical signs, from subclinical to severe dermatitis. The spectrum of disease reflects the flea burden and the immunological status of the host. Classically, moderate to severe pruritus, self-induced alopecia and excoriation are present. In dogs, hyperpigmentation, scale formation, pyoderma and other secondary changes may be observed. In the cat, miliary

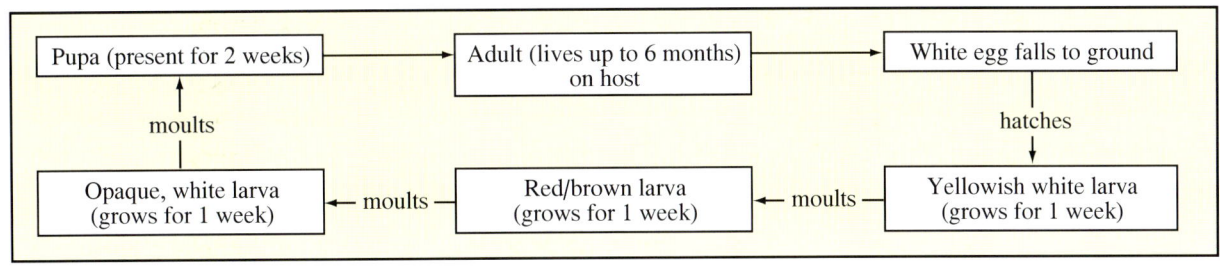

```
Pupa (present for 2 weeks) ──→ Adult (lives up to 6 months) on host ──→ White egg falls to ground
         ↑                                                                       │
       moults                                                                  hatches
         │                                                                       ↓
Opaque, white larva  ←─ moults ─ Red/brown larva  ←─ moults ─ Yellowish white larva
(grows for 1 week)              (grows for 1 week)            (grows for 1 week)
```

Figure 13.6: Flea life cycle.

dermatitis, symmetrical alopecia (self-induced) and eosinophilic skin diseases may be present. Lesions predominantly affect the dorsal rear quadrant of the trunk (i.e. rump, dorsolumbar sacral area and lateral, caudal thighs).

Differential diagnosis
The differential diagnoses for flea infestation are shown in Figure 13.7.

Hypersensitivity (atopy, dietary, contact, insects other than fleas)

Other ectoparasites (mites, lice)

Pyoderma and/or *Malassezia* dermatitis – should be considered in dogs, although they usually occur as secondary complications of other diseases

Dermatophytosis (in cats)

Figure 13.7: Differential diagnoses for flea infestation.

Diagnosis
Presence of fleas or flea faeces within the coat is often indicative of a flea-related skin disease, although this may be an incidental finding as many animals carry fleas asymptomatically. Immunological tests measure flea saliva antigen-specific antibodies in serum or assess the skin reaction after an intradermal injection of flea extract. Currently, neither is regarded as being completely reliable. In many instances, the diagnosis is based on the resolution of skin lesions after appropriate insecticidal therapy. This can be misleading as some cases that respond to such therapy are caused by other parasites, such as mites.

Treatment and prognosis
Fleas are susceptible to various ectoparasiticides (see Chapter 2). It is essential that environmental control is carried out concomitantly with treatment of the animal. All animals in a household must be treated. Regular preventive treatment is recommended. Environmental control includes washing the pet's bedding, regular use of a vacuum cleaner and, in some cases, application of insecticides (e.g. permethrin) and insect growth regulators.

Prognosis is excellent, although the problem may recur if flea control is allowed to lapse. Furthermore, in some multi-pet households in hot humid weather, flea control may be impossible to implement effectively.

Pediculosis (lice)
Lice infestation may develop in various situations, ranging from overcrowded, dirty and badly managed kennels to those with good management systems. Dogs and cats that are young, old or debilitated may be more susceptible. Lice are host-specific and only survive for a few days in the environment. They are classified as either sucking (suborder Mallophaga) or biting (suborder Anoplura) lice. In the UK, only one type of louse is found on cats, *Felicola subrostratus* (biting), whereas dogs may be infested with sucking lice (*Linognathus setosus*) and biting lice (*Trichodectes canis*). The life cycle of a louse is shown in Figure 13.8.

Clinical features
Clinical signs are variable, and some animals may be unaffected carriers. Pruritus, excoriation, crusting and scaling may be present to a variable degree. Miliary dermatitis may be present in cats. In severe infestations with sucking lice, anaemia and debility may be seen.

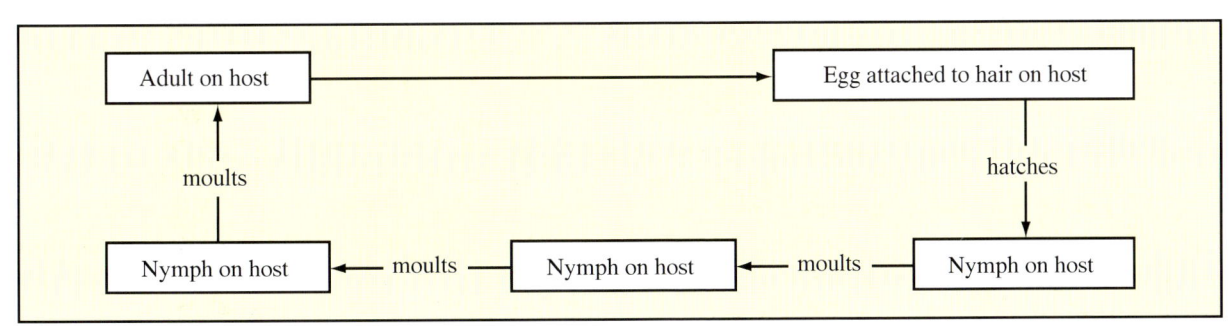

```
Adult on host ─────────────────────────→ Egg attached to hair on host
     ↑                                              │
   moults                                        hatches
     │                                              ↓
Nymph on host ←─ moults ─ Nymph on host ←─ moults ─ Nymph on host
```

Figure 13.8: Louse life cycle (14–21 days).

Hypersensitivity (atopy, dietary, contact, insects other than lice)

Other ectoparasites (mites or fleas)

Pyoderma and/or *Malassezia* dermatitis – should be considered in dogs, although they usually occur as secondary complications of other diseases

Dermatophytosis (in cats)

Figure 13.9: Differential diagnoses for pediculosis.

Differential diagnosis
The differential diagnoses for pediculosis are listed in Figure 13.9.

Diagnosis
Adult parasites and eggs attached to hairs may readily be seen with the naked eye or with the aid of a magnifying lens.

Treatment and prognosis
Lice are susceptible to most insecticides (see Chapter 2). Insecticidal shampoos (e.g. those containing selenium sulphide or carbaryl), fipronil spray or imidacloprid spot-on may be effective. Poor management practices should be addressed to prevent reinfestation. Environmental treatment is not necessary as the parasites do not survive long in the environment and are host-specific. The prognosis is excellent.

Mange (mites)

Sarcoptes scabiei
Sarcoptes scabiei (the cause of scabies or sarcoptic mange) infests dogs and other Canidae such as foxes. Cats may be affected, but this is rare and usually associated with concurrent immunodeficiency. Infestation usually follows direct contact with affected dogs, although there is anecdotal evidence that indirect contact with affected wild foxes may lead to disease. Humans in contact with affected dogs may develop a pruritic papular urticarial rash.

Clinical features: The disease is characterized by severe self-trauma and pruritus of the pinnae (Figure 13.10), elbows, brisket and limbs. Anti-inflammatory, or even immunosuppressive, doses of glucocorticoids may fail to control pruritus, and this is a significant diagnostic pointer.

Differential diagnosis: The differential diagnoses for scabies are listed in Figure 13.11.

Diagnosis: Microscopical examination of skin scrapings (see Figure 13.5) reveals evidence of parasites in most instances (Figure 13.12), provided that a meticulous search of the collected material is made. In some cases it is impossible to confirm the diagnosis, and trial therapy is required; this is acceptable practice

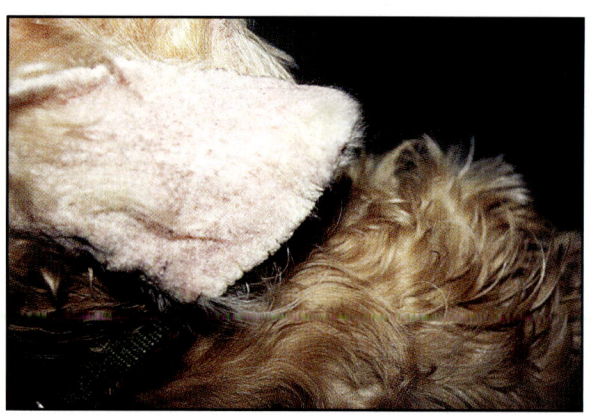

Figure 13.10: Concave aspect of pinna of Cocker Spaniel with sarcoptic mange. There is alopecia with scale and thick crusting at the pinnal margins.

Hypersensitivity (atopy, dietary, contact, insects)

Other ectoparasites

Pyoderma and/or *Malassezia* dermatitis – should be considered in dogs, although they usually occur as secondary complications of other diseases

Dermatophytosis (in cats)

Figure 13.11: Differential diagnoses for scabies.

provided that clinical signs and history are compatible with this diagnosis. Serological assays are available. Investigation of possible immunosuppressive disease should be undertaken in cats.

Treatment and prognosis: In the UK, products licensed for the treatment of canine scabies include amitraz (note that the Chihuahua is reported to be susceptible to toxic effects and that this agent is unlicensed for use in cats), phosmet and selamectin (spot-on treatment). The dips should be sponged on to the skin surface and allowed to dry without rinsing. Treatment should be repeated at least twice at weekly to 2-weekly intervals, and all animals in the household should be treated. Long-haired dogs should be clipped before treatment. A short course of glucocorticoid therapy may be necessary on welfare grounds; however, this may lead to the erroneous impression that the tentative diagnosis of sarcoptic mange was correct in cases where the diagnosis was not confirmed microscopically. The prognosis is excellent provided that reinfestation does not occur.

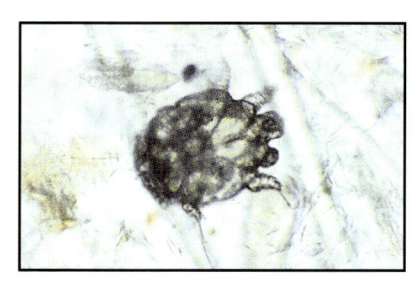

Figure 13.12: Sarcoptes scabiei var. canis.

***Cheyletiella* spp.**
The mites of the genus *Cheyletiella* infest dogs, cats and rabbits, and may cause skin disease in humans. There are three species of veterinary significance:

- *C. yasguri* (usually associated with dogs)
- *C. blakei* (the feline parasite)
- *C. parasitivorax* (principally found on rabbits).

The parasites are not host-specific, and it is not uncommon to find *C. parasitivorax* on cats. Although animals of any age are susceptible to infestation, cheyletiellosis is most common in puppies from pet shops and breeding establishments.

Clinical features: The clinical signs of cheyletiellosis are variable degrees of pruritus (leading to self-trauma and alopecia), scale and papules. In some cases, large quantities of scale are present.

Differential diagnosis: The differential diagnoses for cheyletiellosis are listed in Figure 13.13.

> Hypersensitivity (atopy, dietary, contact, insects (including fleas))
>
> Other ectoparasites (other mites, lice)
>
> Pyoderma and/or *Malassezia* dermatitis – should be considered in dogs, although they usually occur as secondary complications of other diseases
>
> Dermatophytosis (in cats)
>
> Keratinization disorders such as sebaceous adenitis and primary idiopathic seborrhoea

Figure 13.13: Differential diagnoses for cheyletiellosis.

Diagnosis: Microscopy of material from the skin and coat (skin scrapings, coat brushings and adhesive tape specimens; Figure 13.5) is indicated in cases where cheyletiellosis is suspected (Figure 13.14). Cats are adept at grooming and may remove most of the parasites, making it difficult to find the organism. Microscopy of adhesive tape specimens may reveal the presence of eggs attached to hairs.

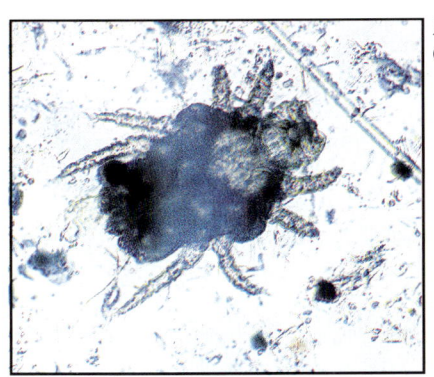

Figure 13.14: Cheyletiella.

Treatment and prognosis: Although there is no product licensed for the treatment of *Cheyletiella* in the UK, dichlorvos, selamectin, selenium sulphide and fipronil are effective therapies. The prognosis is excellent.

***Demodex* spp.**
Demodex mites are commensal inhabitants of normal mammalian skin, and disease most often occurs when immunity is compromised. Demodicosis is rare in the cat but more common in the dog. *Demodex* mites live in the hair follicles, and infestation occurs when mites are transferred from dam to offspring during suckling.

Clinical features: Several clinical presentations of demodicosis are recognized in dogs, although there may be overlap between these syndromes.
  Localized demodicosis is characterized by:

- Focal or multifocal hair loss combined with erythema and scale
- Lesions affecting the face, particularly around the eyes and the lip commissures
- Onset at a few months of age
- Spontaneous resolution
- A proportion of cases becoming generalized.

In generalized demodicosis:

- Onset is usually in dogs less than 18 months old
- Lesions are widespread
- Alopecia, superficial and deep pyoderma, malodour and pruritus are usually evident
- Marked peripheral lymphadenopathy, crusting, oedema and exudation may be present
- Secondary superficial pyoderma (see below) may be a complicating factor and may induce pruritus
- A proportion of cases may resolve spontaneously.

Adult-onset demodicosis:

- Is seen in dogs aged 4 years or older
- May develop secondary to immunosuppressive therapy and systemic diseases such as hyperadrenocorticism, hypothyroidism or neoplasia
- Has similar features to those seen in juvenile-onset generalized demodicosis, although there may also be concurrent clinical signs of the primary systemic disease.

Demodectic pododermatitis:

- Is a variant of demodicosis, with a somewhat unfavourable prognosis
- May occur in isolation or associated with the generalized form

- Is characterized by severe foot swelling, lameness, crusting, erythema and alopecia (Figure 13.15)
- Is invariably associated with severe secondary pyoderma
- May be associated with extremely severe popliteal and prescapular lymphadenopathy.

Differential diagnosis: The differential diagnoses for demodicosis are listed in Figure 13.16.

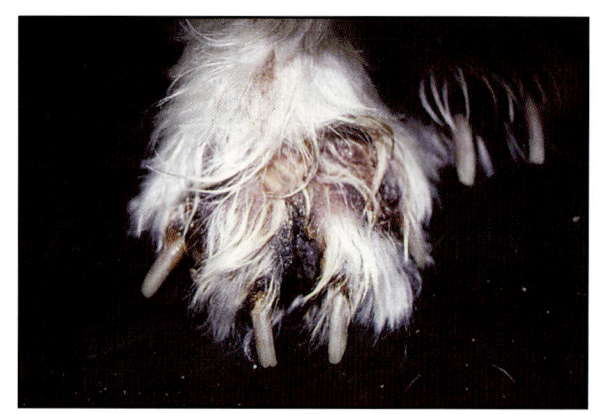

Figure 13.15: Demodectic pododermatitis in a West Highland Terrier. There is alopecia, hyperpigmentation, erythema and exudation.

- Hookworm and *Pelodera* dermatitis
- Deep and superficial pyoderma associated with other primary diseases
- Dermatophytosis in puppies (may be mistaken for localized demodicosis)
- Rare disorders such as pemphigus foliaceus, lupus erythematosus and dermatomyositis
- Cutaneous neoplasia.

Figure 13.16: Differential diagnoses for demodicosis.

Diagnosis: Follicular or pustular smears, skin scrapings or plucked hairs can be examined microscopically mounted in liquid paraffin or following clarification with 10% potassium hydroxide. *Demodex* mites (Figure 13.17) are easily damaged and identification may be harder following potassium hydroxide treatment. Diagnosis requires the demonstration of several mites and, preferably, several life cycle stages. Finding one mite may not necessarily prove the presence of demodicosis as *Demodex* may be present in small numbers in normal skin. Further pustule smears, skin scrapings or plucked hairs should be obtained in this instance.

Treatment and prognosis: Localized demodicosis is regarded as a mild disease that usually heals spontaneously. Many dermatologists do not treat this condition. However, it is argued that as a proportion of cases may become generalized, treatment of early localized cases

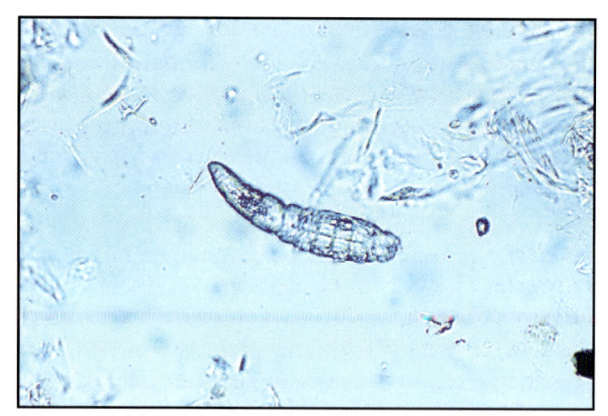

Figure 13.17: Demodex canis.

may prevent this from occurring. Amitraz mixed with propylene glycol (1:50) applied every 48 hours may be effective. Alternatively, benzoyl peroxide gel should be gently applied to the lesions daily.

Generalized forms of demodicosis (especially adult-onset cases) and demodectic pododermatitis require rigorous treatment. These forms of demodicosis have a poor prognosis and may be life-threatening. The cost and difficulty of treatment in older dogs, along with the likelihood that the disease will recur, should be discussed with the owner before treatment is undertaken.

Amitraz is the only product licensed for the treatment of demodicosis. It should be applied to the entire skin surface weekly, according to the manufacturer's instructions. Cost-saving measures such as using small volumes of dip or local treatment are futile. Long-haired dogs should be clipped before treatment. The use of an antibacterial shampoo a few hours before dipping may be beneficial. Secondary pyoderma should always be assumed to be present and treated accordingly. In adult-onset cases, once the patient's condition is stable, investigations of likely primary causes should be undertaken. However, in many instances, the primary cause remains obscure.

In some cases it is impossible to resolve the lesions, or, once in remission, the problem recurs swiftly. In such instances, the use of ivermectin (an unlicensed treatment) has been recommended. This is a somewhat hazardous procedure as idiosyncratic and breed-associated adverse fatal neurological reactions have been reported after the use of this drug. Ideally, such treatment should be under the guidance of a specialist in veterinary dermatology. Milbemycin oxime is available in the USA and parts of Europe to treat demodicosis.

For demodectic pododermatitis, in addition to the use of generalized amitraz treatment, amitraz mixed with propylene glycol at twice the standard concentration of active ingredient may be applied daily to the feet. This is an unlicensed treatment, and the advice of a dermatology specialist should be sought before embarking on such therapy.

The prognosis for demodicosis depends on the form of disease present. Juvenile-onset and localized forms of the disease have a favourable prognosis and may resolve spontaneously. Generalized and adult-onset forms have a much poorer prognosis; such cases may be impossible to resolve. Some apparently cured cases may recur months or years later. Demodectic pododermatitis has a very poor prognosis.

Otodectes cynotis

Otodectes cynotis is generally found in the ear canal; however, all stages of the life cycle have been found on the general skin surface in cats and therefore this mite should be considered as a possible, albeit rare, cause of dermatitis. Typically, *Otodectes* mites are associated with otitis externa in dogs and cats (see below).

Clinical features: Clinical signs are usually restricted to the ear. Ectopic lesions may be found on the rump, neck and tail. The presentation may be similar to flea-bite hypersensitivity or miliary dermatitis.

Diagnosis and treatment: The diagnosis is made by demonstration of the mite on microscopy of coat brushings. Selamectin has been licensed for use against this parasite in cats (and dogs in some other countries). Treatment of aural infections is covered later in this chapter.

Trombiculidiasis (harvest mites)

The larvae of the trombiculid mites are parasitic, resemble minute red or yellow spiders, have six legs (adults have eight) and are just visible to the naked eye. *Neotrombicula autumnalis* is the European harvest mite. It attaches to skin and ingests tissue fluids. There is intense pruritus at the site of attachment as a result of an allergic reaction to the salivary secretions. Infestation shows a seasonal incidence, occurring in late summer and autumn. Lesions are most often found in the feet of dogs and on the paws, head and ears of cats. Gross lesions are small erythematous papules on which are gathered the mites. Self-trauma may be seen. Diagnosis is through demonstration of the presence of the mite. Treatment with fipronil spray has been reported as being successful.

Helminthiasis

Hookworm and *Pelodera* dermatitis

Pelodera strongyloides is a free-living nematode that lives in damp conditions or decaying organic matter. The hookworms *Ancyclostoma* spp. and *Uncinaria* spp. are primary gastrointestinal pathogens. Larvae of *P. strongyloides* and of the hookworms may invade the skin of dogs kennelled in an unclean environment and bedded on plant-derived material such as wood shavings or straw.

Clinical features: Dogs with *Pelodera* dermatitis present with intense pruritus and erythematous papular eruptions affecting those parts of the body that contact the ground. Papules later develop crusts and scale and become secondarily infected. Hookworm dermatitis is less pruritic, with alopecia and erythema on the feet and other parts of the skin in contact with the ground.

Differential diagnosis: The following causes of pedal dermatitis should be considered in the differential diagnosis:

- Demodectic pododermatitis
- Irritant contact dermatitis
- Hypersensitivity (atopic dermatitis, adverse reactions to foods, contact).

Diagnosis: History and clinical signs may be suggestive of these infestations. *Pelodera strongyloides* can be detected on microscopy of skin scrapings (small, 625–650 µm long, motile nematode larvae) and histologically in biopsy specimens. Hookworms are rarely found on histopathology, but eggs may be found on examination of the faeces of affected dogs.

Treatment and prognosis: *Pelodera* dermatitis is treated by destroying all contaminated bedding or moving the animal into clean accommodation. The environment should be sprayed with an appropriate chemical such as malathion or diazinon, and the animal should be treated with a parasiticidal dip at least twice on a weekly basis. Environmental treatment of hookworm dermatitis is similar to that described for *Pelodera*, and an anthelmintic with activity against intestinal hookworm infestation should be prescribed.

The prognosis is good if the condition is diagnosed early.

BACTERIAL SKIN DISEASE

Normal mammalian skin is very resistant to microbial disease, due to the presence of well developed defence mechanisms. Disease occurs when the virulence of the pathogen overwhelms cutaneous immunity. In some instances infection is due to a virulent pathogen such as a dermatophyte. However, it is not uncommon for disease to be associated with proliferation and invasion of normally harmless commensal organisms such as *Staphylococcus intermedius* or *Malassezia pachydermatis*. Such infections usually have a primary cause such as hypersensitivity or systemic disease that appears to compromise skin immunity. This situation is most commonly seen in dogs, where it has been shown that epidermal anatomical barriers against infection are less well developed than in other mammals.

Pyoderma

Pyoderma is commonly encountered in canine practice and has recently been recognized as a somewhat under-diagnosed skin disease in cats. In dogs, the bacterium most commonly involved is *Staphylococcus intermedius*, and this may be the most common pathogen in cats; however, other genera of bacteria (and other staphylococci such as *S. felis* or *S. aureus*) are occasionally associated with this disorder.

Clinical features: Pustules are regarded as one of the principal features of pyoderma yet, paradoxically, are rarely seen in dogs and cats. The epidermis of canine and feline skin is thin and therefore pustules are fragile and short lived. Instead of pustules, a range of lesions may be present such as scale, crust, hyperpigmentation and epidermal collarettes that occur subsequent to the rupture of pustules (Figure 13.18).

The clinical features of pyoderma vary depending on the primary cause, the anatomical location and the depth of infection (Figure 13.19). Pruritus is a variable feature as the primary disease may or may not be pruritic. The production of inflammatory mediators and enzymes by bacteria may lead to pruritus.

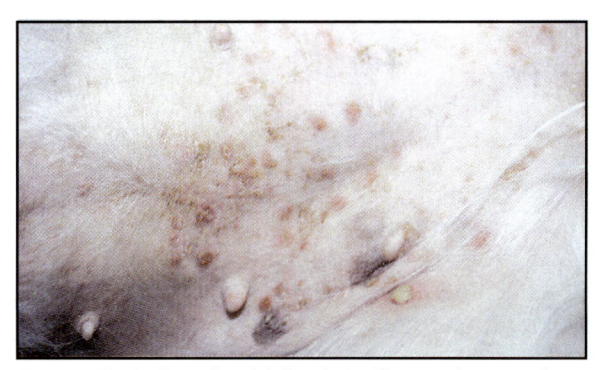

Figure 13.18: Superficial folliculitis affecting the ventral abdomen of a dog showing a pustule and many crusted papules.

Depth of infection	Underlying causes
Surface pyoderma	
Acute moist dermatitis	Flea allergy, otitis externa, anal sacculitis, inadequate grooming, poor coat ventilation, painful musculoskeletal conditions
Intertrigo	Anatomical defects (facial, lip, tail, vulvar, body folds)
Superficial pyoderma	
Impetigo	Often idiopathic; may be associated with poor husbandry
Folliculitis	
Deep pyoderma	Demodicosis, hypothyroidism, hypersensitivity, foreign body, idiopathic

Figure 13.19: Clinical features of pyoderma.

Differential diagnosis: Pustules may occur in diseases other than pyoderma; such disorders are usually immune-mediated (Figure 13.20). Hyperpigmentation is a non-specific finding associated with chronic inflammatory and endocrine dermatoses and some developmental and neoplastic disorders.

Pyoderma – superficial, impetigo, folliculitis, canine acne, interdigital pyoderma
Immune-mediated disease – pemphigus group, bullous pemphigoid and other diseases of the dermal–epidermal junction
Subcorneal pustular dermatosis
Bullous impetigo
Sterile eosinophilic pustular dermatitis

Figure 13.20: Differential diagnoses for pustules in canine skin.

Diagnosis: Pyoderma is usually diagnosed on the grounds of clinical examination and response to appropriate antimicrobial therapy. Although many cases may be recognized readily by the clinician, there are instances where the disease is difficult to identify. This is particularly so in cases of canine superficial folliculitis and feline pyoderma.

Diagnostic tests that may assist in establishing that bacterial infection is present include cytology of pustule contents, culture for identification of the bacteria and antibacterial sensitivity testing.

In recurrent or refractory cases it is of pivotal importance that the primary cause of the disease be identified. The patient should be assessed for fungal infection, ectoparasite infestation, systemic metabolic or endocrine diseases and hypersensitivity. There are numerous primary causes of pyoderma and the reader is referred to the Further Reading list for sources of information on their detailed investigation.

Treatment and prognosis: All patients with pyoderma should receive antimicrobial therapy for at least 2 weeks beyond remission of clinical signs. In cases of deep pyoderma, treatment should be extended until at least a month after clinical recovery. In most instances, the dose of systemic antimicrobial agents should be double the standard recommended dose for infections of other organ systems. The habitual use of glucocorticoids in the management of pyoderma is contraindicated as the disease may recur once glucocorticoid therapy ceases. Such recurrences are usually more severe than the previous episode of disease and far more difficult to bring into remission.

The prognosis for pyoderma is variable. For example, a trivial case of acute moist dermatitis associated with flea infestation may be cured by the appropriate use of insecticidal and antibacterial agents. Conversely, severe deep pyoderma associated with serious systemic disease may be impossible to manage.

Cat bite abscesses

Cat bite abscesses are amongst the commonest bacterial infections encountered in small animal practice. The rapid healing of puncture wounds such as bites and scratches in feline skin favours the formation of large subcutaneous pockets of purulent exudate.

Clinical signs and diagnosis

Clinical signs depend on the site of the abscess. Typically, however, a soft painful mass is readily identified on clinical examination. Common sites of cat bite abscesses include the head, limbs and sacral area. Pyrexia is common and may result in inappetance and depression. Other clinical signs may result from extension of the abscess to include deeper structures such as bone, muscle and central nervous tissue. Bacterial osteomyelitis, arthritis, and myositis will all produce lameness. Seizures and pronounced head pain may result from meningitis. Occasionally the abscess may not be apparent on clinical examination and in these cases the signs are non-specific. A neutrophilia, with or without a left shift, is often found.

Cat bite abscesses classically contain a creamy white exudate, but anaerobic infections tend to be associated with an exudate that is more malodourous and haemorrhagic. The most common organisms isolated from cat bite abscesses are, unsurprisingly, those that are normally found in the oral cavity. Anaerobes are more common than aerobes (see Figure 13.21). Routine bacterial culture is not often performed and it is acceptable to reserve this procedure for recurring abscesses. Cats that are bitten may also become infected with feline immunodeficiency virus (see Chapter 5).

Anaerobes
Porphyromonas spp. (*Bacteroides*)
Fusobacterium spp.
Peptostreptococcus spp.
Clostridium spp.
Aerobes
Pasteurella spp.
Actinomyces spp.
Nocardia spp.
Staphylococcus spp.
Rhodococcus spp.
Enterobacteriaceae (including *Escherichia*)
Streptococcus spp.

Figure 13.21: Main bacterial isolated from cat bite abscesses (adapted from Greene, 1998).

Treatment

Surgical drainage is essential for mature abscesses. Flushing of the abscess cavity with hydrogen peroxide or any one of several bactericidal solutions has not been demonstrated to improve the prognosis. Maintaining adequate drainage after surgery is important to prevent the abscess recurring.

Immature abscesses or cases involving a more diffuse cellulitis may be responsive to treatment with antibacterials alone. Drug choice is often empirical, but the high prevalence of anaerobic organisms limits the choice to clindamycin, cephalosporins and penicillins. Fluoroquinolones (such as enrofloxacin, marbofloxacin and difloxacin) are less effective against obligate anaerobes and their use should be restricted to those cases that have been shown to be sensitive to them.

Consideration should be given to castrating entire male cats to prevent future fight wounds. Elective castration should not be performed at the same time as abscess drainage.

Cutaneous mycobacterial disease

Cutaneous tuberculosis

Cutaneous tuberculosis may be caused by *Mycobacterium tuberculosis*, *M. bovis*, *M. microti*, a newly recognized *M. microti*-like variant or *M. avium*. Most cases in the UK appear to be caused by the *M. microti*-like variant or by *M. bovis*. The organisms act either as primary or secondary pathogens. The disease is rare, and cats are affected more often than are dogs. Adult cats with a hunting or fighting lifestyle are most frequently affected. Co-infection with FIV or FeLV does not appear to play a role.

Cutaneous lesions usually consist of firm raised dermal nodules (Figure 13.22) but ulceration, non-healing wounds and draining sinus tracts, as well as depigmentation of hair (Figure 13.23), may also be seen. Granulomatous tissue may extend into the subcutaneous structures, muscle or bone. Lesions often involve the face, neck, paws, tail base or perineum, i.e. 'fight and bite' sites.

If the disease becomes disseminated, a range of clinical signs may be seen, including abdominal enlargement, dyspnoea, right-sided heart failure, generalized lymphadenopathy, weight loss and fever. Granulomatous uveitis and CNS signs have been seen

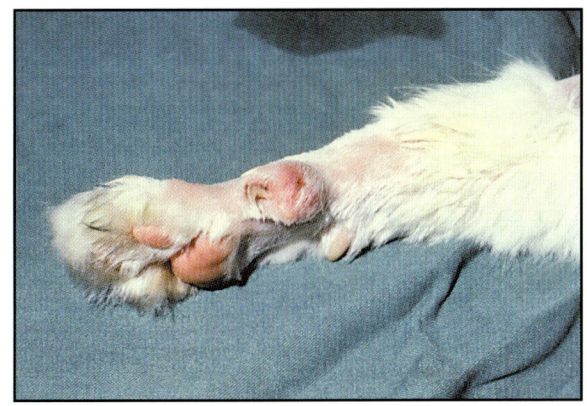

Figure 13.22: Nodule and swelling of the accessory carpal in a cat with tuberculosis caused by Mycobacterium microti-*like variant. Reproduced from Gunn-Moore and Shaw (1997) with the kind permission of* In Practice.

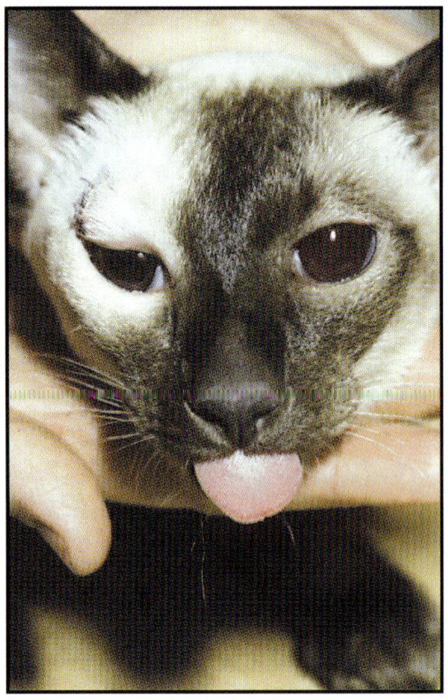

Figure 13.23: Depigmentation of hair and swelling of the right upper eyelid in a cat with tuberculosis caused by Mycobacterium microti-*like variant. A biopsy site can be seen at the right lateral canthus. Reproduced from Gunn-Moore and Shaw (1997) with the kind permission of* In Practice.

in cats. Feline leprosy, deep bacterial and fungal granulomata, eosinophilic granuloma and neoplasia may be confused with cutaneous tuberculosis.

Mycobacterial infection is diagnosed by a positive result from Ziehl-Neelsen staining of organisms within aspirates and/or biopsy samples (see Chapter 1). Intradermal tuberculin testing and specific antibody assays are generally unhelpful. Once the mycobacterial species has been identified, it is possible to evaluate zoonotic risk, treatment options and prognosis. Until the organism has been cultured it must be considered to be a potential human pathogen.

When only cutaneous lesions and/or regional lymphadenopathy are evident, treatment may be considered; however, it is important first to consider several points:

- Given the potential zoonotic risk, all members of the affected cat's household must be involved in decision making
- In households inhabited by people with HIV infection or undergoing chemotherapy, it is *strongly advised* that treatment not be considered as an option and that euthanasia of the affected animal be carried out
- If the affected animal has generalized disease, productive pulmonary involvement or extensive draining cutaneous lesions, the potential risk of human infection is such that euthanasia of the animal is the only option
- Treatment is long term and can be difficult to maintain given the fact that some animals are difficult to medicate, the inherent toxicity of some of the drugs, and the financial costs involved.

Antimycobacterial treatment is initiated once a presumptive diagnosis is made and ideally consists of an initial and a continuation phase:

- Initial phase – at least three drugs used for at least 2 months increases the chance of control and minimizes the development of resistant mycobacteria. The combination of rifampicin, isoniazid and ethambutol, which may be used to treat tuberculosis in humans, is markedly hepatotoxic to dogs and cats. Mycobacteria are susceptible to fluoroquinolones and variably susceptible to some macrolides (clarithromycin and azithromycin). The use of clarithromycin, rifampicin and enrofloxacin in this phase is the safest combination
- Continuation phase – two drugs are used for at least a further 4–6 months, depending on the extent of disease. Rifampicin and either enrofloxacin or clarithromycin are suggested. In cases where resistance develops, the rifampicin–isoniazid–ethambutol combination may be considered. If necessary, ethambutol can be substituted by dihydrostreptomycin or pyrazinamide. Rifampicin and isoniazid are more effective and less toxic than ethambutol and dihydrostreptomycin and are consequently more appropriate choices if only two drugs are required (Gunn-Moore and Shaw, 1997)
- In cats where triple therapy is not feasible, treatment should involve two drugs given for 6–9 months.

Surgical excision of small cutaneous lesions may be considered but is successful in few cases without concurrent antimicrobial therapy. Debulking larger lesions risks wound dehiscence and local recurrence.

For cutaneous mycobacteriosis the prognosis is guarded, though long-term remission has been achieved in many cats. If a cat is not to be treated, euthanasia should be performed to remove the potential zoonotic risk. The animal should then be cremated rather than buried.

Feline leprosy
Feline leprosy, a granulomatous condition, is associated with acid-fast bacteria that cannot be cultured by standard techniques. *Mycobacterium lepraemurium* has been suggested as the cause of feline leprosy, although this has not been confirmed. Infection is believed to occur via rodent bite wounds or soil contamination of cutaneous wounds. Feline leprosy is not considered to be a zoonotic disease. It is seen most often in cats living in areas with a temperate maritime climate, such as the UK. Young adult cats are more often affected, with no sex or breed predisposition.

Single or multiple non-painful and freely mobile haired, alopecic or ulcerated nodules develop on the head, limbs (Figure 13.24) and occasionally the trunk. An animal may present with abscesses and fistulae that fail to heal. Regional lymphadenopathy may be present, but systemic disease is rare. The main differential diagnoses are cutaneous tuberculosis, deep bacterial and fungal granulomata, eosinophilic granuloma, and neoplasia.

Cytology/histopathology and Ziehl-Neelsen staining are required for diagnosis; typically large numbers of acid-fast organisms are seen within macrophages. Culture is unrewarding, but should be performed in all cases as the clinical signs and histopathology can mimic those of feline tuberculosis.

Surgical removal of small nodules is recommended. Enrofloxacin should be prescribed once the diagnosis is confirmed. Clofazamine has been used in a limited number of cases where surgical removal proved difficult. Dapsone is considered too toxic for use in cats. Prognosis is good, and spontaneous resolution may occur.

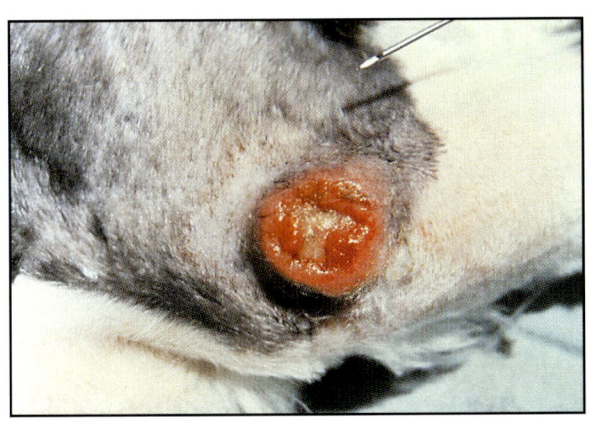

Figure 13.24: Ulcerated nodule on forelimb of a cat with feline leprosy, showing classic 'rolled edge' appearance (surrounding hair clipped). Reproduced from Gunn-Moore and Shaw (1997) with the kind permission of In Practice.

Opportunistic mycobacterial disease
Opportunistic mycobacterial disease is caused by saprophytic mycobacteria including *Mycobacterium chelonae, M. fortuitum, M. smegmatis* and *M. phlei* that are found in soil, water and decaying vegetation. Disease usually follows contamination of cutaneous wounds. Because the organisms are lipophilic they are particularly pathogenic when inoculated into adipose tissue. Gastrointestinal or respiratory infections are rarely seen. Cats are more susceptible to opportunistic mycobacterial infections than are dogs. Adult cats who hunt or fight are most often affected. Infection with feline immunodeficiency virus or feline leukaemia virus does not appear to play a role.

Infection is usually seen as panniculitis, with multiple punctate draining tracts and associated subcutaneous nodules, giving a 'salt and pepper shaker' appearance. Coalescence produces large areas of ulcerated non-healing tissues that are extremely painful. Disease may be exacerbated by surgery; dehiscence is common. Feline leprosy, nocardiosis, deep mycotic infections, bacterial furunculosis and panniculitis should be differentiated from opportunistic mycobacterial infections.

Histopathology from lesions caused by opportunistic mycobacteria reveals pyogranulomatous panniculitis. Mycobacteria can be difficult to identify, even when special stains are used, but culture is the diagnostic test of choice because the organisms are relatively easy to grow.

Treatment should be based on culture and antibacterial agent sensitivity. Generally, *M. fortuitum* and *M. smegmatis* are sensitive to the fluoroquinolones, whereas *M. chelonae* is sensitive to clarithromycin. In severely affected cases double or triple therapy – as used to treat cutaneous tuberculosis – may be considered, using a combination of enrofloxacin, clarithromycin and/or rifampicin. Antibacterial therapy should be continued for 6-12 weeks. If performed, surgical intervention should be radical and combined with antibacterial therapy. Prognosis is poor to guarded and deteriorates further when previous attempts at surgery have proved unsuccessful.

Nocardiosis
Nocardia spp. are Gram-positive, partially acid-fast, branching filamentous aerobes. Skin infection is rare and occurs most commonly through penetrating wounds, especially if a foreign body such as a grass seed is present. In debilitated hosts, cutaneous nocardiosis may develop secondary to pulmonary nocardiosis. Working dogs may be predisposed to this disease. The incubation period is long and varies from week to months.

Clinical signs are variable:

- Cutaneous lesions begin as granulomata that may develop into subcutaneous abscesses, cellulitis, ulcerated nodules and draining tracts. Fine granular material may be present in the exudate, which is brownish-red
- Systemic signs (pyrexia, lethargy, pyothorax and dyspnoea) may be present
- Neurological signs are present in some cases.

The main differential diagnoses include:

- Cutaneous tuberculosis
- Feline leprosy
- Atypical mycobacterial infections
- Foreign body (or cat bite) abscesses
- Demodicosis
- Panniculitis
- Subcutaneous and deep mycoses
- Deep pyoderma.

Cytological examination of exudate, bacterial culture and/or skin histopathology may be diagnostic. It is essential to find and remove any penetrating foreign body. After surgical debridement and drainage, the animal should receive antibacterials for several months on the basis of culture and sensitivity testing. The prognosis is guarded. See Chapter 6 for more information on nocardiosis.

Borreliosis

Borreliosis or Lyme disease is caused by the spirochaete *Borrelia burgdorferi* and transmitted by ticks of the genus *Ixodes*; infection is thus most common where tick exposure is likely to occur. Subclinical infection is common in the dog. Skin lesions reported in dogs infected with *B. burgdorferi* include urticaria, erythema and moist dermatitis, although the role of this organism in causing the lesions is not clear. There are few diseases that produce both joint lesions and cutaneous abnormalities. Leishmaniasis, systemic lupus erythematosus and drug eruptions should be considered as possible differential diagnoses. See Chapter 14 for more information on Lyme disease.

Dermatophilosis

Dermatophilosis, caused by *Dermatophilus congolensis*, is a very rare disease in dogs and cats. The lesions are multiple oval-shaped plaques composed of matted hair and exudate. Lesions are non-pruritic but may be painful. In the cat, deep pyogranulomatous fistulous lesions, particularly in the region of the popliteal lymph node, have been described. Diagnosis is made following culture of the organism.

Management of dermatophilosis requires the elimination of predisposing factors such as moisture, arthropod bites and skin trauma. Topical povidone-iodine soaks can be used to improve skin hygiene. Systemic antibacterials are usually required. *Dermatophilus* is usually susceptible to ampicillin, cephalosporins, cloxacillin, lincomycin and tetracyclines. It is resistant to erythromycin and sulphonamides.

Miscellaneous bacterial infections

Septicaemia may result in septic thrombosis of cutaneous vessels, with resultant deep necrotizing skin lesions. Rocky Mountain spotted fever caused by *Rickettsia rickettsii* (not present in the UK) is associated with vasculitis that can result in oedema and dermatitis of the scrotum, deep dermal necrosis of ear tips, nasal planum, nipples and digits (see Chapter 5). *Brucella canis* has been isolated from chronic, ulcerative nodular plaque-like lesions (nodular to diffuse pyogranulomatous dermatitis) in a dog (see Chapter 12).

FUNGAL SKIN DISEASE

Dermatophytosis

Dermatophytosis (ringworm) is caused by infection of the keratinized layers and appendages (hair and nails) of the skin by a group of specialized filamentous fungi (dermatophytes). Around 40 individual dermatophyte species are recognized and are classified in one of three genera:

- *Epidermophyton*
- *Microsporum*
- *Trichophyton*.

Geophilic
Microsporum gypseum
M. fulvum
Trichophyton terrestre
Zoophilic
M. canis
M. equinum
M. persicolor
T. verrucosum
T. equinum
T. mentagrophytes var *mentagrophytes*
T. mentagrophytes var *erinacei*
Anthropophilic
Epidermophyton floccosum
M. audouinii
T. rubrum
T. tonsurans
T. mentagrophytes var *interdigitale*

Figure 13.25: *Ecological classification of some common dermatophytes.*

Individual dermatophytes are also classified on the basis of their major reservoir in nature, as either anthropophilic (humans), zoophilic (animals) or geophilic (soil) (Figure 13.25).

Dermatophytosis is a common fungal skin infection of dogs and cats, with the prevalence varying between countries, being highest in warm and humid climates. The disease is about three times more common in cats than it is in dogs, and it is one of the commonest zoonotic infections.

Epidemiology

The most common cause of feline and canine dermatophytosis is *Microsporum canis*. Despite its name, cats are considered to be the natural reservoir for this organism. In a large UK study (Sparkes, 1993; Figure 13.26) *M. canis* was responsible for 92% of feline and 65% of canine dermatophyte cases. Most other dermatophytes isolated from cats and dogs are thought to be acquired from rodents during hunting (e.g. *Trichophyton mentagrophytes*, *M. persicolor*, *T. erinacei*) or, less commonly, from the soil (e.g. *M. gypseum*, *M. fulvum*, *T. terrestre*). There is a marked age predisposition, with young animals (particularly those less than a year of age) being the highest risk group. In cats, *M. canis* is more common in multi-cat households, where the organism can spread rapidly. There is good evidence that long-haired cats are predisposed to disease.

Most dermatophytes infect both the stratum corneum and hairs, producing a sheath of arthrospores around infected hairs. Vast numbers of these resistant spores are produced during infection, and they are the main infectious particles of dermatophytes. Direct contact between animals is probably the most efficient

Dermatophyte species	No. Cats (%)	No. Dogs (%)
Microsporum canis	827 (92)	309 (65)
Trichophyton mentagrophytes	50 (6)	114 (24)
T. erinacei	0	15 (3)
M. persicolor	4 (0.5)	12 (3)
T. terrestre	8 (1)	9 (3)
M. fulvum	1	3
M. gypseum	1	3
Others	4	10

Figure 13.26: Species isolated from 895 cats and 475 dogs with dermatophytosis in the UK. Data from Sparkes (1993).

means of transmission. However, widespread dissemination of infected material and prolonged survival of arthrospores in the environment (up to 18 months or more for *M. canis*) means that infected hair and keratinous debris shed into the environment are also important sources of infection.

Clinical features
The incubation period for dermatophytosis is typically several days to 3 weeks. The duration of infection varies considerably from short-lived self-limiting infections to those lasting many months or years. The commonest clinical sign is one or more discrete areas of alopecia that develop as a consequence of the increased fragility of infected hairs. Typically there will be an irregular or circular alopecic patch of varying size, accompanied by variable scaling, crusting, thickening and erythema (Figure 13.27). Central healing of lesions can be observed, with growth of new hair surrounded by an area of alopecia. Dermatophytosis may also present with other clinical manifestations, including widespread disease where most or all of the body is affected, causing generalized alopecia and scaling, folliculitis, granuloma (pseudomycetoma), miliary dermatitis in cats (Figure 13.28) and paronychia. In some cats with *M. canis* infection, a chronic focal disease may develop with few or no observable clinical signs ('asymptomatic carriers').

The lesions produced by dermatophyte infections are variable and clinically indistinguishable from those that may be observed in many other cutaneous diseases.

Differential diagnosis
In cats many diseases mimic dermatophytosis, as the appearance of dermatophytosis may be very pleomorphic. Key differential diagnoses in the dog include demodicosis, localized superficial pyoderma, sebaceous adenitis and pemphigus foliaceus.

Diagnosis
The three tests most widely used to confirm dermatophytosis are:

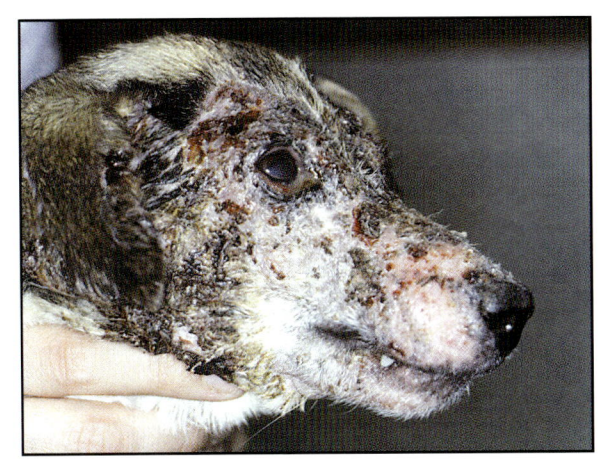

Figure 13.27: Trichophyton mentagrophytes infection in a Jack Russell Terrier. Note the severe crusting and erosions.

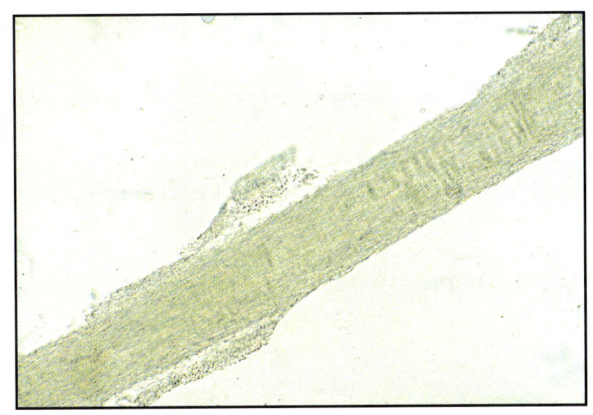

Figure 13.28: Plucked hair preparation from a cat infected with Microsporum canis. The photomicrograph shows arthrospores on the hair.

- Examination of hairs under ultraviolet light (Wood's lamp illumination)
- Direct microscopic examination of hairs, nails or scale
- Fungal culture.

These are discussed in more detail in Chapter 1.

Treatment and prognosis
Although many infections are self-limiting, treatment of dermatophytosis in animals is recommended to prevent spread of the disease and reduce the zoonotic risk. Treatment may involve topical therapy (creams, shampoos, dips), systemic therapy, or a combination (see Chapter 2 for antifungal drugs). Some may be recalcitrant to therapy.

Treatment for individual dogs or cats: The only systemic agent currently licensed for use in animals is griseofulvin. This drug should be given with a fatty meal. **Pregnant women should not handle griseofulvin.** Duration of treatment varies according to response (which should be monitored clinically and by culture) but is typically 6–12 weeks. As in humans, infections recalcitrant to griseofulvin are encountered, and treatment during pregnancy is contraindicated owing to the teratogenic nature of the drug. Side effects occasionally reported with griseofulvin include ataxia, anaemia, neutropenia, bone marrow hypoplasia and hepatopathy.

Itraconazole is clinically efficacious in the treatment of feline dermatophytosis, and few side effects have been reported. Based on the experience in human medicine, it is likely that itraconazole may be intrinsically more effective than griseofulvin in the treatment of dermatophytosis. Terbinafine has excellent activity against dermatophytes. A recent study suggested lufenuron may be an effective systemic agent for dermatophytes in dogs and cats.

Topical therapy with azoles (e.g. ketoconazole enilconazole), may speed resolution of disease. As topical creams are unable to penetrate to the infected hair within the hair follicle, systemic therapy is also recommended unless specifically contraindicated.

While creams may be applied to focal lesions, more extensive disease requires the use of dips or shampoos. There is little critical information available on the most appropriate preparations for small animal dermatophytoses. Enilconazole is licensed as a topical agent (dip) for use in dogs but not in cats. A shampoo combining 2% chlorhexidine and 2% miconazole used twice weekly as an adjunct to systemic (griseofulvin) therapy enhances resolution of disease in infected cats and significantly reduces environmental contamination.

Clipping lesions aids penetration of topical agents and reduces environmental contamination with arthrospores. Total body clipping of hair as has been advocated for long- or medium-haired animals, may traumatize the skin and facilitate spread of the disease. For focal lesions, careful clipping of the hair (with scissors) 2 or 3 cm beyond the visible extent of the lesion is recommended. Clipping should be repeated 2–4 weeks after starting systemic therapy, as infected hair shafts previously within the hair follicles should be exposed. Clipped hair should be disposed of carefully (ideally burned).

Treatment of animal colonies: Special consideration needs to be given to multi-cat households where dermatophytosis is identified. In addition to careful environmental decontamination, infected cats should be separated from uninfected cats, with topical prophylactic treatment (shampoos/dips) for the uninfected group and additional systemic treatment for the infected group. In practice, separation is often difficult to achieve, and it is usually better to treat the entire colony with both systemic and topical therapy. Systemic therapy provides excellent prophylaxis for uninfected cats, and this regimen is the most likely to eradicate infection from a colony. Careful monitoring of response (brush cultures from animals – ideally two negative culture results should be obtained 4 weeks apart) is necessary prior to cessation of therapy to ensure therapy is not stopped too early.

Disinfectants and antifungals recommended for fomite and environmental decontamination include 5% lime sulphur, 0.5–5% sodium hypochlorite, 2% glutaraldehyde, 1–2% chlorhexidine and 0.2% enilconazole. There have been few or no controlled studies to confirm the efficacy of many of these agents. Where widespread environmental contamination is present – and in particular within a house – effective disinfection may be difficult to achieve. Wherever feasible, the environment and fomites should be treated and thorough and regular vacuum cleaning of carpets and furnishings undertaken to reduce the burden of infection.

The prognosis is excellent in most cases, although occasionally the disease may be difficult to manage in dogs with *Trichophyton* infection and long-haired cats (especially those kept in groups).

Malassezia

Malassezia yeasts are principally isolated from skin and mucous membranes of a variety of mammals and birds. *M. pachydermatis* is a normal inhabitant of healthy canine skin and mucosae. It is most often found in sites such as the external ear canal, interdigital skin, the haired skin of the lip region and the anal mucosa. It is of importance as it is a common opportunistic pathogen of dogs and, to a lesser extent, cats. Other species, such as *M. sympodialis* and *M. globosa*, can be isolated from the skin of healthy cats; their significance as pathogens is not yet clear.

M. pachydermatis can be associated with otitis externa and generalized canine skin disease. Quantitative studies of *M. pachydermatis* show that population densities in lesional skin in dogs with *Malassezia* dermatitis often exceed those of healthy dogs by 100- to 10 000-fold. Skin populations in healthy Basset Hounds, a breed predisposed to *Malassezia* dermatitis, exceed those of healthy dogs of other breeds, reflecting the susceptibility of this breed to the disease. Some atopic dogs have abnormally high *M. pachydermatis* populations in affected and unaffected areas. Concurrent increases in cutaneous bacterial populations, particularly of *Staphylococcus intermedius*, are often observed in dogs with *Malassezia* dermatitis.

The factors that allow the transition from commensal carriage to opportunistic infection are not well understood. In some cases, other skin diseases such as hypersensitivity disorders and keratinization defects are diagnosed; however, the specific physical, chemical or immunological defects that allow yeast proliferation have not been identified.

Clinical features

Breeds predisposed to *Malassezia* dermatitis include Basset Hounds, Dachshunds, Cocker Spaniels and West Highland White Terriers, although there are geographical differences. Males and females are equally at risk. Hot humid weather seems to favour the development of infection in some parts of the world. The clinical characteristics associated with *M. pachydermatis* include:

- Localized or generalized lesions
- Erythema, alopecia and varying degrees of scaling or greasy exudation (Figure 13.29)
- Hyperpigmentation and lichenification often develop in chronic cases
- Mild to extremely severe pruritus
- Affected areas include the external ear canal, face, ventral neck, axillae, groin, interdigital skin or other intertriginous areas
- Frenzied facial pruritus
- Clinical signs that may mimic or coexist with lesions caused by allergic skin diseases (especially atopic disease) ectoparasitic infestations or keratinization defects.

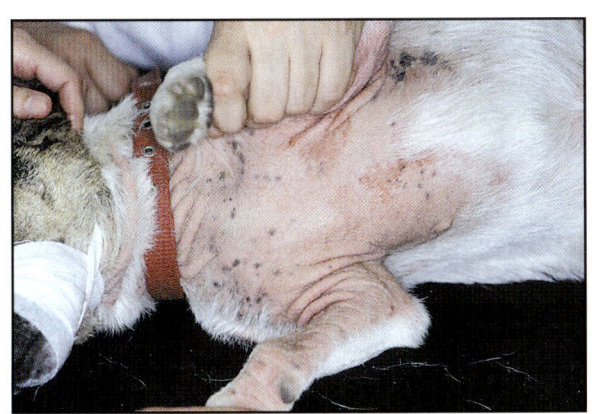

Figure 13.29: Alopecia and inflammation associated with chronic Malassezia *infection.*

Differential diagnosis
Malassezia dermatitis should be suspected when dogs present with greasy, malodorous and inflammatory skin disease. Clinical signs may either mimic or complicate allergic skin disease and keratinization defects. Predisposing causes of the yeast infection (e.g. hypersensitivity, endocrinopathy) and concurrent bacterial pyoderma will also have to be considered and appropriate diagnostic tests undertaken to identify and correct these complicating factors.

Diagnosis
The principal diagnostic criteria for *Malassezia* dermatitis are consistent clinical signs, increased *M. pachydermatis* populations on lesional skin and a good clinical and mycological response to appropriate antifungal therapy. The yeast can be demonstrated readily in most cases through cytological techniques (Figure 13.30), although culture and biopsy can also be helpful.

Tape-stripping is a rapid and simple method (see Figure 13.5). The yeast has a characteristic 'peanut'-shape and populations should be considered to be elevated if the yeast is readily identified. It is important to choose an adhesive tape which resists the staining process; some tapes curl and disintegrate when stained making examination and interpretation difficult.

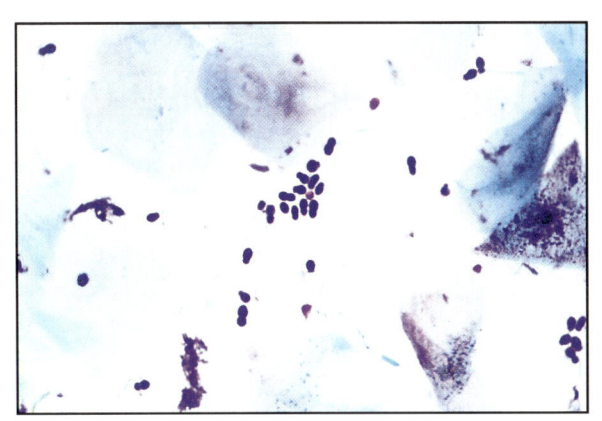

Figure 13.30: Photomicrograph of Malassezia *yeasts.*

The yeast can be isolated from skin using standard swabbing techniques, although quantitative methods provide more information. The contact plate technique is most applicable in clinical practice; small agar plates are directly applied to affected skin for 10 seconds, removed, incubated at 32–37°C for 3–7 days, and the colonies counted (Bond *et al.*, 1994). Sabouraud's dextrose agar can be used, although lipid-containing media such as modified Dixon's agar support the growth of the occasional more lipid-dependent variants of *M. pachydermatis* and enable the isolation of the lipid-dependent *Malassezia* spp. found on cats. In most healthy dogs, populations in the axillae and groin are typically present at less than 1 colony-forming unit (cfu) per square centimetre, but large populations can be found on lip folds and interdigital skin. There are also breed differences in 'normal' populations; population densities in the axillae of some healthy Basset Hounds exceed 10 cfu/cm^2. These findings emphasize the importance of response to therapy as a diagnostic criterion.

The yeast may be demonstrated histopathologically in the epidermal stratum corneum; however, this technique is not as sensitive as cytological and cultural methods, probably owing to disruption of the epidermal stratum corneum that occurs during routine processing. Identification of the yeast in biopsy material should prompt trial therapy, but failure to find the yeast does not exclude its presence and potential significance.

Treatment and prognosis
The aim of treatment is to reduce yeast and bacterial skin populations and to correct any underlying diseases that favour the development of infection. The yeast occupies a superficial location within the stratum corneum and is therefore susceptible to topical therapy. A 2% miconazole plus 2% chlorhexidine shampoo is very effective, with excellent degreasing,

anti-*Malassezia* and antibacterial properties when used every 3 days. Alternative treatments include shampoos containing selenium sulphide, chlorhexidine and benzoyl peroxide. Azole-containing creams, ointments and lotions are suitable for the treatment of focal lesions.

Systemic therapy with azole antifungal drugs may be used in cases where topical therapy is impractical or where signs are severe. Ketoconazole is usually effective, although it is not licensed for this use in dogs in most countries, and occasional adverse effects, including severe hepatotoxic reactions after high doses, have been reported. Itraconazole is effective and may be better tolerated. If the response to therapy is incomplete despite anti-yeast therapy, or if clinical signs relapse, then the patient should be evaluated for concurrent disease. In many cases the reason for the relapse is unclear, and lifelong maintenance treatment to control clinical signs is required.

Topical therapy is often sufficient to maintain dogs in clinical remission; the frequency of bathing should be adjusted according to the needs of the patient. Animals will go into permanent remission if the primary cause of the disease is determined and corrected. If this is not achieved, lifelong antimicrobial therapy is needed.

Candidiasis

Candidiasis is a rare disease of dogs caused by yeasts of the genus *Candida*. These commensal organisms of the gastrointestinal and genital mucosae act as opportunistic pathogens in animals debilitated by systemic disease or those undergoing treatment with immunosuppressive drugs.

Clinical features

Mucocutaneous erosion or ulcerated exudative and erythematous lesions with thick crusts and associated malodour may develop at any mucosal or mucocutaneous site, e.g. nail beds, nares, scrotum, external ear, perineal skin. Secondary bacterial infection is usually a feature. Lesions seem to be painful, and signs of systemic illness are sometimes evident. Candidiasis may complicate other diseases of the mucocutaneous areas such as some of the immune-mediated disorders. Localized infections with *Candida* spp. may affect bitches around the vulvar area; this is more likely to occur if poorly ventilated skin folds are present.

Differential diagnosis

Immune-mediated diseases such as bullous pemphigoid and similar clefting disorders of the basement membrane zone should be considered as possible causes of mucocutaneous ulceration. Other differential diagnoses include pemphigus vulgaris, erythema multiforme, hepatocutaneous syndrome (superficial necrolytic dermatitis) and drug eruptions.

Diagnosis

Histopathology of biopsy material may indicate the presence of an underlying immune-mediated or drug-induced disease. In some instances fungi will be found on histology, although false negatives may occur. Cytology from lesions reveals evidence of the yeast (budding cells and pseudohyphae). The yeast is readily isolated.

Treatment and prognosis

Severe cases in which several sites are affected should be investigated to determine the primary immunosuppressive illness. Use of systemic antifungal drugs such as itraconazole, fluconazole or ketoconazole for up to 2 weeks after resolution of lesions is recommended. None of these drugs, however, is licensed for this use in domestic animals in the UK. Furthermore, hepatotoxicity has been reported in some dogs after treatment with ketoconazole. Localized lesions may be treated with topical antifungal agents such as miconazole or clotrimazole. In some instances, surgical correction of infected skin folds is required

The prognosis for localized cases is good, especially if the underlying anatomical defect is corrected surgically. In generalized cases the prognosis is guarded to poor as any underlying disease is often life-threatening.

Subcutaneous and systemic mycoses

Several fungi other than dermatophytes and yeasts have been rarely associated with skin disease in dogs and cats. Subcutaneous mycotic infections occur at the site of inoculation after a bite or other trauma. An example of a subcutaneous mycosis occasionally encountered in the UK is sporotrichosis associated with *Sporothrix schenkii*. Systemic mycoses may affect the skin, although there is usually concurrent internal disease; examples include cryptococcosis and aspergillosis. Many of these diseases are potentially zoonotic and therefore specimens should be handled carefully and suitable protective clothing worn. Diagnosis is based on cytological examination of exudate, fungal culture and histopathology. Treatment may be difficult and should be based on knowledge of the fungus present. See Chapter 6 for further information.

PROTOZOAL SKIN DISEASE

Leishmaniasis

Infection with *Leishmania* spp. leads to multisystemic disease (see Chapter 5) with cutaneous manifestations. The disease is rare in the UK but cases may be seen in dogs that have visited Mediterranean areas of France and Spain. Leishmaniasis can affect humans.

Clinical features
Most commonly there is a non-pruritic exfoliative dermatosis. Nodules (which may become ulcerated) are present in advanced cases. The disease is characterized by the presence of periorbital rings of alopecia, depigmentation of the planum nasale and lymphadenopathy. Systemic signs of infection include fever, depression, weight loss, muscle weakness, polyarthritis, blood coagulation disorders and renal failure.

Differential diagnosis
Several rare disorders should be considered in the differential diagnosis including zinc-responsive dermatosis, pemphigus foliaceus, sebaceous adenitis, systemic and subcutaneous mycoses, systemic and malignant histiocytosis and neoplasia (epitheliotropic lymphoma).

Diagnosis, treatment and prognosis
See Chapter 5 for a discussion of these areas.

Miscellaneous protozoal infections
Toxoplasma gondii has been associated, rarely, with nodular skin lesions in the cat. *Caryospora* is a rare cause of pyogranulomatous dermatitis in puppies. Immunosuppression may be required for disease to develop. The primary hosts for this coccidian parasite are reptiles and raptors. There are no reports of its occurring in the UK. *Neospora caninum* has been reported to cause multifocal ulcerated cutaneous lesions in a dog. A *Sarcocystis*-like coccidian parasite has been associated with diffuse necrotizing, haemorrhagic and suppurative skin lesions.

VIRAL SKIN DISEASE

Feline cowpox
Infection with feline cowpox virus is seen occasionally and is probably acquired from hunting small mammals such as rodents and insectivores.

Clinical features
The primary lesion seems to be a bite wound on an extremity or the head. Viral replication and a period of viraemia then ensues, during which some animals develop mild pyrexia, inappetence and depression. About 10–14 days after infection, generalized secondary lesions start as macules but become crusted, ulcerated and nodular (Figure 13.31). Pruritus is variable. A small proportion of affected cats develop oral vesiculation or ulceration. There is usually a slow spontaneous recovery, although residual scarring may be seen. Immunosuppression with glucocorticoids or co-infection with FIV may lead to systemic poxvirus infections characterized by severe skin lesions and pneumonia.

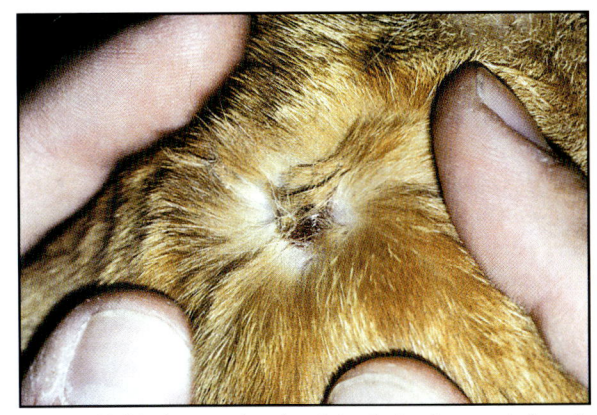

Figure 13.31: A crusted and nodular lesion in a cat infected with feline cowpox. (Courtesy of Hilary O'Dair.)

Differential diagnosis
Fungal and bacterial nodular and ulcerated disease, eosinophilic granuloma, mast cell tumour and other neoplasms should be considered in the differential diagnosis.

Diagnosis
Histopathology of biopsy material (including immunocytochemistry), serological testing and electron microscopy or viral isolation from crusts or biopsy specimens are diagnostic. Serology is unable to differentiate feline cowpox from other orthopox viruses. It is recommended that the advice of a specialist laboratory is sought before harvesting samples for diagnosis.

Treatment and prognosis
There is no specific treatment for feline cowpox. Glucocorticoids are strongly contraindicated; it is imperative that these lesions are not confused with glucocorticoid-responsive lesions such as eosinophilic plaques. Supportive antimicrobial therapy may be necessary in some cases.

The prognosis is excellent. Most cases resolve spontaneously. The disease is a potential zoonosis, and there is a risk of fatal human infection of immunocompromised people (e.g. those with HIV or undergoing chemotherapy) if they are in contact with a viraemic cat.

Other viral infections

- Parapoxvirus infections may be seen rarely in cats and even more rarely in dogs. Clinical signs include multiple crusting lesions with scab formation around the head, that may take several weeks to heal. The lesions resemble contagious pustular dermatitis (CPD) of sheep and goats. Canine and feline parapoxviruses may be related to, or identical to, the viruses that cause CPD but this has not been demonstrated. As CPD is infectious to humans, where it is known as orf, it is sensible to wear gloves when handling animals suspected of having parapoxvirus or material

from them. Diagnosis relies on demonstration of the virus by electron microscopy of scab material. Treatment is conservative. Glucocorticoids are contraindicated
- Distemper virus causes hyperkeratosis, particularly of the footpads (see Chapter 6 for details on canine distemper)
- Papilloma virus causes cutaneous and mucosal papillomas (warts) (see Chapter 8)
- Feline sarcoma virus has been associated with cutaneous fibrosarcomas in young cats (see Chapter 5)
- Feline leukaemia virus has been associated with the development of various skin neoplasms, including lymphoma, and may predispose to pyoderma through its immunosuppressive effects (see Chapter 5)
- There are a couple of reported cowpox infections in dogs.

ALGAL SKIN DISEASE

Prototheca

Prototheca spp. are opportunistic pathogens that are very rarely associated with systemic infections. Cutaneous protothecosis has been described in the dog in the UK and in cats elsewhere. The condition is characterized by multiple small grey-white or tan ill-defined nodules. Histopathology may be helpful but diagnosis is confirmed by culture or immunofluorescence.

OTITIS

Infectious organisms (bacteria, yeasts and *Otodectes* mites) are often associated with cases of otitis externa in dogs and cats. Bacteria and yeasts are not considered to be primary causes of disease of the external ear but instead may act as perpetuating factors in the pathogenesis of otitis externa. The bacteria and yeasts involved are commensal organisms and may be found in the normal ear canal of a large proportion of dogs and cats. Many factors influence the development of otitis. They are categorized as either:

- Primary causes of aural inflammation – foreign bodies, hypersensitivities (e.g. atopy), sebaceous gland disorders (e.g. seborrhoea, hypothyroidism), immune-mediated skin disease and ectoparasite infestation
- Predisposing factors – conformation (e.g. drooping pinna, excess hair in ear canal, narrow canal), excess moisture in ear, administration of cleansing agents into the ear canal, obstruction to normal air flow by polyps or neoplasms
- Perpetuating factors – overgrowth of commensal bacteria/fungi, mucosal hyperplasia, otitis media, errors in treatment.

Bacterial/fungal otitis

The bacteria involved in otitis include *Staphylococcus intermedius,* coagulase-negative staphylococci, α- and β-haemolytic streptococci, *Pseudomonas aeruginosa, Proteus mirabilis, Escherichia coli* and *Klebsiella* spp. The usual yeast isolated from cases of otitis externa is *Malassezia pachydermatis,* although other species including *M. sympodialis* and *M. furfur* have been isolated.

Clinical signs

Clinical features vary from mild irritation and a slight discharge to severe pain and a heavy purulent discharge. Infection may be localized to the external ear or may involve the middle ear and rarely the inner ear.

Diagnosis

Prolonged inflammation associated with microbial infections often leads to irreversible changes within the ear canal. Therefore otitis externa should always be investigated thoroughly and promptly:

- Physical examination should highlight any predisposing factors that may need to be addressed to allow long-term management
- Cytology allows a semi-quantitative assessment of microbial numbers. Repeated cytology can provide an indication of any response to treatment. Normal aural mucosal smears should contain few bacteria or yeasts per oil immersion field
- Bacterial and fungal culture and sensitivity testing may be indicated to document the specific organisms present and to guide the appropriate therapy; they are essential if otitis media is present
- Radiography of the middle ear is indicated where rupture of the ear drum occurs or when relapsing infections are encountered. However, many cases of otitis media do not show radiographic changes. Culture of samples from the middle ear should be considered if there is radiological evidence of otitis media or if relapsing infections with tympanic membrane rupture are encountered.

Treatment and prognosis

Successful treatment of otitis can be difficult. Any underlying primary or predisposing factor must be identified and corrected if possible. Topical antibacterial therapy is valid for simple uncomplicated infections where secondary changes have not developed. When mucosal hyperplasia, otitis media or multiresistant organisms such as *Pseudomonas aeruginosa* are present, aggressive therapy is indicated. One or more of the following may be required:

- Lavage of the external ear canal and, if the ear drum is ruptured, the middle ear with sterile saline/water, using a Spreull's needle to remove debris, on one or more occasions. Beware of penetrating into the inner ear; ensure the Spreull's needle is directed ventrally when passed into the bulla
- Lavage of the external ear canal and, if the ear drum is ruptured, the middle ear with povidone-iodine (1% solution) or chlorhexidine (1% solution), which is effective in managing multiresistant bacterial infections. These agents are potentially ototoxic, but deafness does not seem to be common. The middle ear must be thoroughly rinsed with sterile saline after use of these chemicals and a pharyngeal pack inserted to prevent inhalation of any material that passes down the auditory tube during the lavage procedure. Lavage of the ear with diluted acetic acid is recommended by some authors to treat *Pseudomonas* spp; however, it is rather irritant and should only be used in cases that cannot be managed by other means
- Ceruminolytics such as squalene, dioctyl sulphosuccinate, carbamide peroxide and glycerin are indicated to soften waxy debris. They should be applied to the ear 10–15 minutes prior to lavage. They are potentially ototoxic
- Topical antimicrobial therapy has only a limited part to play. Aqueous products are preferred, but even they are unlikely to penetrate the whole of the external ear canal. They can be administered into the outer and middle ear through a Spreull's needle if lavage is being performed. Although many are potentially ototoxic, further compromise of hearing does not appear to be clinically significant. Sensitivity testing should guide antimicrobial choice in such cases
- Oral antimicrobial therapy is often helpful in managing bacterial otitis and is essential when resistant organisms or otitis media are present or where alterations to the ear canal prevent effective administration of topical drugs
- Topical corticosteroids ameliorate inflammation and reduce ceruminous secretions
- Oral corticosteroids at anti-inflammatory doses are beneficial in the management of severe or chronic otitis. They not only reduce inflammation but also inhibit proliferation of the mucosa
- Lateral wall resection/vertical canal ablation are indicated to remove diseased mucosa that harbour bacteria and to provide drainage for the horizontal canal. In some cases complete resection of the external ear and bulla osteotomy are required. Readers are advised to consult surgical texts for information on case selection and operative procedures.

The prognosis depends on the extent of any secondary changes and whether the underlying causes can be addressed.

Otodectes cynotis

Clinical signs
Animals infested with *Otodectes cynotis* may be virtually free of disease and act as asymptomatic carriers of the mite or show severe signs of otic discomfort and pruritus. Typically, owners complain that their cat or dog has aural exudate, pruritus, self-trauma, head shaking and apparent discomfort and pain. The pinnae may be carried low against the head, and head tilting may be present. In severe cases there is usually a thick dark brown to black crumbly waxy aural exudate.

Diagnosis
Auroscopy of the ear canal may reveal the parasites as small pearly white mobile organisms in the ear canal. In some cases only small numbers of mites are present, and they may be difficult to detect. In such cases, samples of aural wax should be carefully taken from the ear canal using a cotton-tipped swab. The wax is then suspended in mineral oil and examined microscopically.

Treatment and prognosis
Topical preparations containing an acaricidal, antimicrobial, anti-inflammatory and other active ingredients for installation into the ear canal have traditionally been used to control ear mites. These polypharmacy products control inflammation and secondary bacterial infection as well as having acaricidal effects. Some products that lack a specific acaricidal agent are also effective in the management of ear mite infestations; the mechanisms by which this occurs are incompletely understood. All animals within the household should be treated to prevent reinfestation from apparently unaffected carrier animals. Treatment should be continued for at least 3 weeks as it is likely that most medicaments used are not ovicidal. The systemic drug selamectin is also effective.

If cases of otitis externa associated with ear mites are identified promptly and treated appropriately, then the prognosis is good; however, neglected or misdiagnosed animals swiftly develop secondary infections and other changes, which may be difficult to resolve.

DRUG DOSAGES

See Appendix 3.

REFERENCES AND FURTHER READING

Ben-Ziony Y and Arzi B (2000) Use of lufenuron for treating fungal infections of dogs and cats: 297 cases (1997-1999). *Journal of the American Veterinary Medical Association* **217**, 1510-1513

Bond R, Collin NS and Lloyd DH (1994) Use of contact plates for the quantitative culture of *Malassezia pachydermatis* from canine skin. *Journal of Small Animal Practice* **35**, 68-72

Bond R, Rose JF, Ellis JW and Lloyd DH (1995) Comparison of two shampoos for treatment of *Malassezia pachydermatis*-associated seborrhoeic dermatitis in Basset Hounds. *Journal of Small Animal Practice* **36**, 99-104

Crespo MJ, Abarca ML and Cabanes FJ (2000) Otitis externa associated with *Malassezia sympodialis* in two cats. *Journal of Clinical Microbiology* **38**, 1263-1266

Greene CE (1998) Feline abscesses. In: *Infectious Diseases of the Dog and Cat*, 3rd edn, ed. Greene CE, pp.328-330. WB Saunders, Philadelphia

Gunn-Moore DA, Jenkins PA and Lucke VM (1996) Feline tuberculosis: a literature review and discussion of 19 cases caused by an unusual mycobacterial variant. *Veterinary Record* **138**, 53-58

Gunn-Moore DA and Shaw S (1997) Mycobacterial disease in the cat. *In Practice* **19**, 493-501

Mason IS (1995) Approach to the animal with skin disease. In: *Handbook of Small Animal Dermatology*, ed. KA Moriello and IS Mason. Pergamon Press, Oxford

Mason KV and Evans AG (1991) Dermatitis associated with *Malassezia pachydermatis* in 11 dogs. *Journal of the American Animal Hospital Association* **27**, 13-20

Paterson S (1999) Miconazole/chlorhexidine shampoo as an adjunct to systemic therapy in controlling dermatophytosis. *Journal of Small Animal Practice* **40**, 163-166

Raake P, Mayser P and Wein R (1998) Demonstration of *Malassezia furfur* and *M. sympodialis* together with *M. pachydermatis* in veterinary specimens. *Mycoses* **41**, 493-500

Shearer D (1993) The discharging sinus. In: *Manual of Small Animal Dermatology*, ed. PH Locke, RG Harvey and IS Mason, pp.74-82. BSAVA, Cheltenham

Sparkes AH, Gruffydd-Jones TJ, Shaw SE, Wright AI and Stokes CR (1993) Epidemiological and diagnostic features of canine and feline dermatophytosis in the United Kingdom from 1956-1991. *Veterinary Record* **133**, 57-61

CHAPTER FOURTEEN

The Musculoskeletal System

Chris May

CHAPTER PLAN

Introduction
Infective arthritis
   Bacterial arthritides
      Lyme disease
      Mycoplasmal arthritis
      Bacterial L-forms and arthritis
      Tubercular arthritis
   Other arthritides
Osteomyelitis
   Bacterial osteomyelitis
   Fungal osteomyelitis
   Protozoal osteomyelitis
   Viral osteomyelitis
Discospondylitis
   Bacterial discospondylitis
   Fungal discospondylitis
Infective myopathies
   Focal bacterial myopathies
   Protozoal myopathies
References and further reading

INTRODUCTION

Musculoskeletal infections are uncommon when compared with skin, urogenital or gastrointestinal infections, and they do not often constitute life-threatening events. Musculoskeletal infections can, however, cause irreversible debilitating secondary changes and should always be given prompt and appropriate treatment. Musculoskeletal infections are best considered in the following sections:

- Infective arthritis (infection of synovial joints)
- Osteomyelitis (infection of bones)
- Discospondylitis (infection of intervertebral discs)
- Infective myopathies (infection of muscles).

The most common musculoskeletal infections are bacterial, either from haematogenous spread, which is more common than is often appreciated, or from penetrating wound injury. Possible primary sources of haematogenous bacterial infections include:

- Tooth root abscesses
- Urinary tract infections
- Anal sac infections
- Pyodermas
- Bacterial endocarditis
- Omphalophlebitis (in very young puppies and kittens).

The most common causes of penetrating wounds are:

- Iatrogenic (e.g. surgery)
- Road traffic accidents
- Bite wounds (especially in cats).

In addition to bacterial infections, some consideration must be given to viral, protozoal and fungal infections in the musculoskeletal system, although these are generally rare in the UK.

INFECTIVE ARTHRITIS

Infective arthritis is an inflammatory arthropathy caused by an infective agent, which can be cultured from the affected joint or joints. Bacteria are the most common cause of infective arthritis in dogs and cats, but several other infective agents can cause an arthropathy.

Bacterial arthritides

Bacterial infection may be introduced to a joint by penetration or haematogenous spread (see above). Most infections of joints in cats are probably associated with bite wounds resulting from fights. However, many dogs present with bacterial infective arthritis without a history of penetrating injury, suggesting a haematogenous infection. The nature of the ensuing joint disease varies with the infecting bacterium. The clinical presentation may vary from a mild non-erosive condition to a severe rapidly progressive destructive disease.

Most cases of bacterial arthritis concern a single joint; involvement of more than two joints is most often secondary to severe systemic bacterial infections, such as bacterial endocarditis, or omphalophlebitis, in which there is a major bacteraemic component.

Figure 14.1 shows the bacteria commonly isolated from infected joints.

220 Manual of Canine and Feline Infectious Diseases

Bacterial genus	Comments
Common*	
Staphylococcus	Most common in infective arthritis and osteomyelitis Particularly *S. intermedius* Usually β-lactamase positive
Streptococcus	Usually Lancefield group G
Escherichia	Usually haemolytic
Pasteurella	
Proteus	
Actinomyces	Anaerobe
Bacteroides	Anaerobe
Fusobacterium	Anaerobe
Clostridium	Anaerobe: particularly associated with myositis
Peptostreptococcus	Anaerobe
Less common	
Pseudomonas	
Erysipelothrix	Found in a few cases of infective arthritis
Klebsiella	
Nocardia	
Corynebacterium	
Salmonella	Very uncommon
Brucella	Particularly found in infective arthritis and discospondylitis Not found in UK Uncommon elsewhere

*Figure 14.1: Bacteria associated with musculoskeletal infections. *In the majority of original case series, have been isolated on at least one occasion.*
NB. In some cases there may be mixed infections, including both aerobic and anaerobic bacteria. Culture of anaerobic bacteria is difficult and their presence in infected tissues may remain unconfirmed.

History and clinical findings

Bacterial infective arthritis affects all breeds of dog and all ages. The larger breeds are most often affected, and there is a male to female ratio of 2:1. In most cases the history is of an acute onset of lameness in a single limb. Sometimes the lameness is chronic, with an insidious onset, reflecting less severe pathology. Pre-existing joint disease, such as osteoarthritis, or joint trauma may predispose a joint to secondary bacterial infection by the haematogenous route. Most traumatic injuries, other than fractures or luxations, improve within 48 hours whereas infected joints do not. Care should be taken in monitoring patients after minor joint trauma in case of conversion to infection. If there is any doubt, the joint should be examined under anaesthesia, radiographed and synovial fluid analysis performed to confirm the diagnosis (see below).

Clinical examination may demonstrate:

- A warm swollen joint that elicits pain when touched or manipulated
- Erythema or other discoloration of the overlying skin
- Fluid distension of the joint due to excessive synovial fluid production
- Local lymphadenopathy
- Muscle atrophy of the affected limb (often occurs rapidly).

Systemic signs, such as inappetence, pyrexia and lethargy, only occur in around one third of all cases.

Diagnostic plan

Bacterial arthritis can resemble many other inflammatory arthropathies. The diagnosis of bacterial arthritis is confirmed by culture of the organism from synovial fluid and/or synovial membrane. Sensitivity testing to antibacterial agents is an important prelude to therapy in bacterial infective arthritis. The diagnostic plan for suspected bacterial joint infections is:

- Radiograph affected or suspected joints
- Laboratory investigations – obtain synovial fluid samples for cytology and bacterial culture and sensitivity before any antibacterials are given
- Consider synovial membrane biopsy
- Consider making a search for a primary infective source if haematogenous infection is suspected.

Radiography: Radiological features vary with the type of infection and its duration. In the early stages there may only be soft tissue swelling around the joint, due to inflammation and oedema, and these radiographic changes cannot be differentiated from similar changes in acute traumatic arthritis. Later there is often a marked periarticular periosteal bone reaction and sometimes calcification of the periarticular soft tissues. A reduction in the joint space may be seen because of the loss of articular cartilage. Subchondral bone erosions and irregular areas of sclerosis may be found (Figure 14.2).

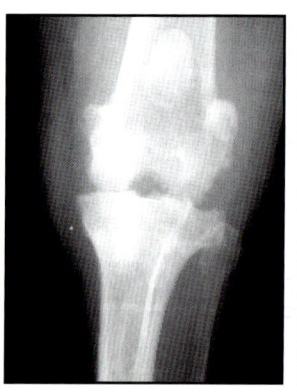

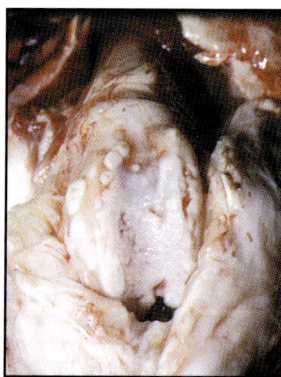

Figure 14.2: Radiograph and gross pathological specimen of the stifle of a dog with chronic destructive bacterial arthritis. Infection occurred as a complication of stifle surgery with inadequate aseptic technique, and despite antibacterial therapy at the time of surgery. There is periarticular new bone proliferation and severe erosion of the articular cartilage. The subchondral bone shows a mixed pattern of destruction and sclerosis. Treatment was by amputation.

In chronic cases, secondary osteoarthritic changes and subluxation resulting from ligament damage may be seen. Fibrous or bony ankylosis is occasionally found in end-stage cases.

Haematology: Routine haematology is not a reliable indicator of septic arthritis because leucocytosis, as a result of neutrophilia and a left shift, is an inconsistent finding.

Synovial fluid analysis: Synovial fluid analysis is probably the single most useful laboratory investigation for suspected bacterial infective arthritis. Synovial fluid is obtained by fine needle aspiration (Figure 14.3). Gross changes in synovial fluid may include:

- Increased volume
- Turbid or blood-tinged fluid
- Poor viscosity
- The high levels of fibrinogen in an inflammatory synovial fluid may cause it to clot on exposure to air (unlike normal synovial fluid).

Cytological changes in synovial fluid are particularly helpful in distinguishing bacterial infective arthritis from other arthropathies, such as immune-mediated joint disease and traumatic arthritis (Figure 14.4). Although such changes can be identified on smears made in the practice, this technique is relatively insensitive and depends on the skills of the observer (Gibson *et al.*, 1999). Samples should routinely be submitted for formal cytological analysis. Changes characteristic of bacterial infective arthritis include:

- Markedly increased numbers of white cells, mostly neutrophils
- Toxic neutrophils with pyknotic nuclei, or ruptured or degranulated neutrophils: large numbers of neutrophils (>5-10 per high powered field) on a smear is highly suggestive of bacterial infective arthritis (Figure 14.5).

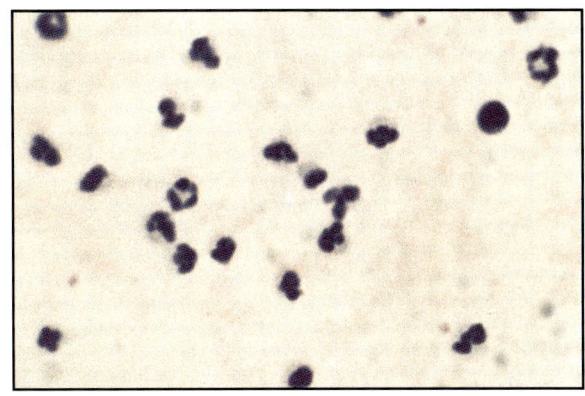

Figure 14.5: Cytological smear of synovial fluid from a joint with bacterial arthritis. The neutrophils are mildly degenerate with ragged nuclear margins. In some cases neutrophils show no evidence of degenerative change. No bacteria are seen; this is quite common in bacterial arthritis. (Courtesy of Elizabeth Villiers.)

Direct culture of infected synovial fluid may only yield a positive result in 50% of cases. The success rate can be increased by collecting the synovial fluid into blood culture medium for transport to the laboratory for aerobic and anaerobic culture (see Chapter 1). Prior use of antibacterial agents seriously reduces the chance of a successful culture.

When antibacterials have already been given, it may be necessary to withdraw all antibacterial therapy for 5-7 days before attempting cultures. Failure to respond to antibacterial therapy is, however, usually

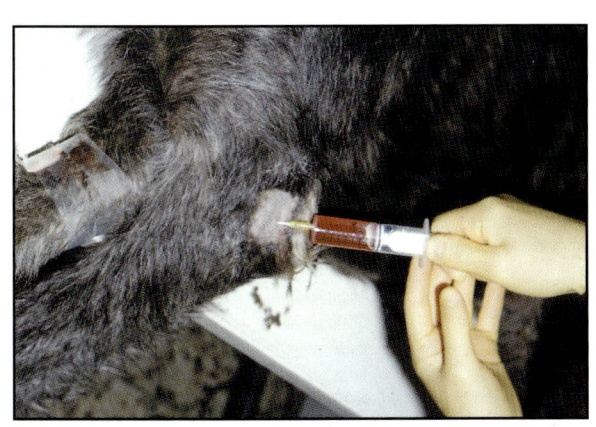

Figure 14.3: Synovial fluid being aspirated from an infected elbow joint. A small area of fur is clipped and aseptically prepared as for surgery. Drapes are unnecessary. Maps of approaches for synoviocentesis are provided by Houlton (1994).

	Normal joint	Degenerative joint disease	Immune-mediated arthritis	Bacterial arthritis
Colour	Clear/pale yellow	Yellow	Yellow (may be blood tinged)	Yellow (may be blood tinged)
Clarity	Transparent	Transparent	Transparent or opaque	Opaque
Viscosity	Very high	High	Low/very low	Very low
Protein (g/dl)	2.0-2.5	2.0-3.0	2.5-5.0	>4.0
White cells (× 10^6/l)	<1	1-5	>5	>5
Neutrophils	<5%	<10%	10-95%	>90%
Mononuclear cells	>95%	>90%	5-90%	<10%

Figure 14.4: Synovial fluid analysis in dogs and cats.

because of inappropriate treatment, particularly lack of surgical drainage or inappropriate choice of agent.

If there has been prior antibacterial therapy, it may be preferable to establish only a presumptive diagnosis on the basis of synovial fluid cytology and radiological features. Appropriate therapy (see below) is then instigated and the patient monitored carefully for a response to treatment. If a satisfactory response is not obtained, all therapy must be withdrawn for a 7-day period, and synovial membrane biopsies obtained for culture and histopathology.

Synovial membrane cultures: There is some debate about the relative merits of attempted cultures from synovial membrane rather than from synovial fluid. It is less invasive to obtain synovial fluid, but synovial membrane biopsies may offer more reliable culture results. Synovial membrane biopsies are used for culture whenever an open approach is made to a suspected infected joint (e.g. for surgical drainage) or when synovial fluid cultures are negative in the face of other indicators of joint infection. Culture from synovial membrane biopsies is also often convenient when the diagnosis is in such doubt that there is an indication for synovial biopsy for other purposes, such as histopathology.

Treatment

The mainstay of therapy is a prolonged course of systemic antibacterials. Antibacterial therapy should be initiated with a broad-spectrum β-lactamase-resistant bactericidal preparation while laboratory confirmation of the diagnosis is pending. The author's preference is for clavulanate-potentiated amoxycillin or a cephalosporin combined with metronidazole (see Appendix 3).

The antibacterial agent should only be changed if indicated by subsequent sensitivity tests. In particular, bacteriostatic drugs such as the lincosamides (lincomycin and clindamycin) and tetracyclines should be avoided unless specifically indicated by culture and sensitivity test results. Systemic antibacterial therapy is continued for at least 4-6 weeks, or for 2 weeks after the complete resolution of clinical signs. Gentamicin-impregnated polymethylmethacrylate beads may be used in refractory cases provided the organism is sensitive to gentamicin (Brown and Bennett, 1989).

Joint lavage (Figure 14.6) and drainage (Figure 14.7) are indicated if the clinical signs are severe, if there is rapid joint destruction, or in immature animals where increased intra-articular pressure can have deleterious effects on neighbouring physes.

Method 1: Needle aspiration
In most cases, particularly in early disease, drainage and lavage is adequately achieved by needle aspiration Sterile saline is the most appropriate solution for lavage The use of antibacterial solutions is unnecessary and may cause further harm. Penetration of systemic antibacterials to the inflamed synovial membrane is very good.
Method 2: Open drainage
In chronic cases, or if attempts at needle aspiration prove inadequate, open surgical drainage is required: 1. The joint is opened and drained of fluid and fibrin 2. The joint is lavaged thoroughly with copious quantities (2-10 litres) of sterile saline at body temperature 3. The joint is closed, with Penrose drains left in place for 3-5 days   Suction drainage may be applied if available Physical restraints are almost always needed to prevent the animal chewing the drains Analgesia with non-steroidal anti-inflammatory drugs (NSAIDs) is almost always required.
Method 3: Distension irrigation
This is a useful way of continuously removing debris and damaging enzymes from the articular cavity The procedure is painful and requires repeated sedation or anaesthesia in all but the most amenable of animals 1. Sterile saline is infused into the joint under aseptic precautions via preplaced irrigation tubes, with the outlet blocked 2. The infusion is continued to distend the joint, so that the lavage solution penetrates all corners of the articular cavity before draining the joint completely The technique may be repeated several times over a 2-3-day period Physical restraints are almost always needed to prevent the animal chewing the drains Analgesia with NSAIDs is almost always required.
All methods
During, and immediately following, drainage the joint must be rested by using strict confinement and support bandaging Later, in the recovery phase, controlled exercise, such as passive flexion/extension, short lead walks and swimming are helpful for maintaining range of movement in the joint Exercise is gradually increased after the first 4 weeks.

Figure 14.6: Joint lavage.

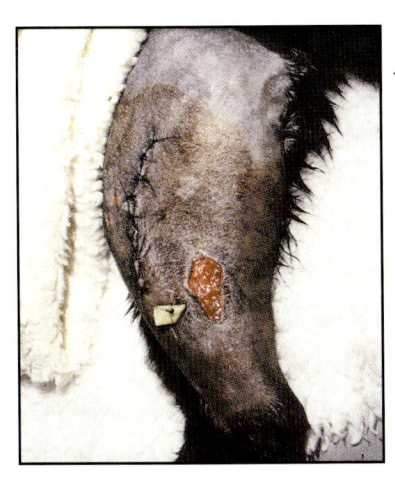

Figure 14.7: Stifle joint of a cat with open wounds and bacterial infective arthritis after a bite injury. Penrose drains have been placed in the joint.

In rare cases, a degree of inflammation persists in the joint after elimination of the offending organism as a result of ongoing immune responses to persisting microbial antigens. Such lameness quickly responds to low-dose prednisolone therapy (0.1–0.2 mg/kg orally every 24 hours), but this should only be given after repeated synovial membrane or fluid culture results are negative and when there is only mild chronic inflammatory change on synovial membrane histology or synovial fluid cytology.

Prognosis
Prognosis depends on several factors:

- Prompt diagnosis and appropriate treatment is critical to a good prognosis
- Chronic infection, rapidly destructive infections or any infection with severe joint destruction all merit a guarded to poor prognosis
- Multiple joint infections are more difficult to treat
- Systemic infections are more difficult to treat, and some, such as bacterial endocarditis, carry a very poor prognosis when there is joint involvement
- A guarded prognosis is justified in immature animals because of the additional risk of secondary physeal damage.

Of 57 dogs with bacterial infective arthritis in one survey, 56% made a complete recovery, 32% had a mild residual lameness and 12% responded poorly and had severe persistent lameness (Bennett and Taylor, 1988).

Lyme disease
Lyme disease is a non-erosive inflammatory arthropathy caused by the tick-borne spirochaete *Borrelia burgdorferi*. Serious morbidity associated with *B. burgdorferi* seems to be rare in dogs in the UK. Lyme disease has not been diagnosed in cats in the UK.

Diagnosis in dogs usually depends on a history of previous tick infestation, often 2–3 months before the onset of clinical signs. The typical presenting signs are a migratory monoarthritis or pauciarthritis (inflammation of up to five joints, symmetrical or asymmetrical). True polyarthritis is rare. Episodes of lameness typically last only a few days, although repeat episodes may occur. There may be fever and lymphadenopathy. Rare manifestations include neurological signs and myocarditis. The cytological changes in synovial fluids from dogs with Lyme disease are often more typical of a low-grade immune-mediated joint disease than of a bacterial infection (see Figure 14.4).

The diagnosis is difficult to confirm. Serological testing is helpful, but subclinical infections can occur, and the antibodies to *B. burgdorferi* may cross-react with other spirochaetes. A positive serological test does not equate to a diagnosis of Lyme disease, but animals with clinical Lyme disease are unlikely to be negative for anti-*Borrelia* antibodies. Up to 28% of dogs exposed to ticks in the UK have a positive antibody titre to *B. burgdorferi* without having clinical Lyme disease (May *et al.*, 1991). Evidence of a rising titre is sometimes helpful, but it is generally of most importance to correlate all the clinical, cytological and serological findings in order to establish sufficient evidence for the diagnosis. To this end a set of diagnostic criteria has been suggested (Figure 14.8). Even in low numbers, the organism can be detected by sensitive molecular biology techniques such as the polymerase chain reaction (PCR) or *in situ* hybridization, but these are not in common use for routine diagnosis at the present time.

A	A history of potential exposure to *Borrelia burgdorferi*. Usually preceding onset of arthropathy by several weeks
B	Seasonal incidence: associated with peaks in tick activity, particularly the nymph or adult stages, which are more likely to transmit *B. burgdorferi*
C	Appropriate clinical signs: including fever, malaise, lethargy, inappetence, lymphadenopathy, lameness, carditis (heart block), neurological signs and, possibly, glomerulonephritis
D	Laboratory support for the diagnosis: in cases of Lyme arthritis this should include radiographic evidence of a synovial effusion and synovial fluid analysis consistent with synovitis
E	Positive serological test for *B. burgdorferi*. Some asymptomatic animals are positive for anti-*Borrelia* antibodies
F	Response to antibacterial therapy
G	Identification of *B. burgdorferi* in blood, urine, synovial fluid, cerebrospinal fluid (CSF) or tissues
H	Culture of *B. burgdorferi* from blood, urine, synovial fluid, CSF or tissues
I	Exclusion of other possible causes of similar clinical signs: including traumatic arthritis, osteoarthritis and the immune-mediated polyarthritides.

A diagnosis of Lyme disease in dogs should satisfy criteria A, C, D, E and I. Criterion F should subsequently be satisfied in almost all cases. Ideally, criteria G and H should also be satisfied, but this may be difficult as the organism is difficult to culture and may only be present in very low numbers.

Figure 14.8: Criteria for diagnosis of Lyme disease in dogs. Adapted from Bennett and May, 1995.

A response to treatment with tetracyclines or penicillin derivatives is normally found within 7 days of starting therapy, but it is advisable to continue antibacterial treatment for at least 2 weeks after the resolution of all clinical signs. Most cases have an excellent prognosis, particularly if diagnosed and treated promptly.

Mycoplasmal arthritis

Mycoplasmal infection of joints may arise as a result of the spread of organisms from localized sites of active or latent infection in the mucous membranes of the airways, conjunctivae or urogenital tract. This is most likely to occur in debilitated or immunosuppressed animals. In cats the possibility of coinfection with retroviruses should always be considered. *Mycoplasma spumans* infection has been associated with a polyarthritis syndrome of young Greyhounds (Barton *et al.*, 1985), but this has not been seen in the UK. The articular surfaces are markedly eroded, with loss of cartilage, making this an important differential diagnosis for canine rheumatoid arthritis and multiple bacterial joint infections. Mycoplasmal arthritis can be treated with tylosin, gentamicin or erythromycin.

Bacterial L-forms and arthritis

L-forms are bacteria deficient in cell walls, which are differentiated from *Mycoplasma* because they may revert to the parent state in culture. Bacterial L-forms have been associated with longstanding antibacterial-unresponsive polyarthritis in a dog and a progressive erosive fistulating purulent arthropathy in cats. Extensive case reports are lacking. It is uncertain whether the L-forms are true pathogens or merely represent coincidental pathology. Treatment is the same as for mycoplasmal arthritis.

Tubercular arthritis

Arthritis is one manifestation of tuberculosis associated with the human type of *Mycobacterium tuberculosis* in dogs. Tuberculosis in dogs has become rare in parallel with the human disease, and it is now of most importance only because of the potential public health implications. Mycobacteria have also been identified in the joints of cats. See Chapter 6 and 13 for more information on mycobacteriosis.

Other arthritides

Fungal arthritis

Fungal infections of joints have been described with a range of organisms, including *Coccidioides*, *Blastomyces*, *Filobasickiella* (*Cryptococcus*), *Sporotrichum* and *Aspergillus*. However, fungal arthritis is infrequent in dogs and cats and it has not yet been described in the UK. Treatment with antifungal drugs has been variably successful.

Rickettsial arthritis

Polyarthritis is being increasingly recognized in association with rickettsial infections (in particular ehrlichiosis and Rocky Mountain spotted fever). None of these infections is endemic in the UK. See Chapter 5 for further details.

Protozoal arthritis

Leishmaniasis is often associated with a polyarthritis. Synovial fluid analysis demonstrates large numbers of macrophages filled with *Leishmania* organisms. See Chapter 5 for further details on leishmaniasis.

Viral arthritis

Certain wild and vaccine strains of feline calicivirus (FCV) are joint pathogens in cats and can cause lameness in kittens. The arthritis might be a direct pathogenic effect of the virus or a result of immune-complex hypersensitivity. The arthritis is usually self-limiting and is of less clinical importance than the other lesions produced by the virus. Small doses of corticosteroids (0.1–0.2 mg/kg orally every 24 hours) may be of help in cats with arthritis during convalescence from infection.

Specific viral infections of joints are unknown in dogs. A transient arthropathy of dogs may be associated with either natural infection or vaccination with viruses such as canine distemper virus (CDV) or parvovirus.

OSTEOMYELITIS

Osteomyelitis literally means 'inflammation of bone', including the marrow and cortex, however the term is most commonly applied to infections of bone. Bacteria are the most common agents infecting bone in dogs and cats, but osteomyelitis has also been associated with fungal and viral infections.

Bacterial osteomyelitis

Bacterial invasion of bone may occur by any of three routes:

- Post-traumatic osteomyelitis
  - By direct penetration of the bone (usually iatrogenic or as a result of an open fracture)
  - Invasion from local soft tissue infection
- Haematogenous osteomyelitis
  - Spread from a site of infection elsewhere in the body; the primary site often remaining occult.

Undoubtedly, the vast majority of cases of bacterial osteomyelitis occur because of poor aseptic technique at the time of open reduction of fractures (nosocomial infection). Open reduction of fractures should always be performed under strict aseptic precautions: perioperative antibacterial therapy is not an effective substitute for good aseptic technique.

Bacterial osteomyelitis is also usually classified as 'acute' or 'chronic'. There is no accurate means of distinguishing these definitions, but broad guidelines can be applied in the history and clinical signs and radiographic and laboratory features. Acute bone inflammation resulting from bacterial infection is characterized by a leucocytic infiltration, phagocytosis of the infecting organisms and the release of proteolytic enzymes, which result in the classic signs of heat, pain, swelling and disuse.

Localized ischaemia is an important contributory factor in the establishment of many, if not all, cases of bacterial osteomyelitis. Ischaemia may also occur as a secondary event owing to intraosseous vascular thrombosis. Severe localized ischaemia leads to bone death, sequestration and the development of draining sinuses in chronic lesions.

History and clinical findings
Bacterial osteomyelitis usually presents with an obvious lameness and a localized painful and swollen bone lesion. There is usually a history of fracture repair or other bone trauma, such as a bite wound.

Systemic signs of infection, including local lymphadenopathy, pyrexia, depression and inappetence, are not consistently present and are rare in chronic osteomyelitis.

Some cases of haematogenous osteomyelitis present with multiple bone involvement, and the metaphyses of juveniles are especially at risk from this form of the disease (Dunn *et al.*, 1992). Such cases of metaphyseal osteomyelitis require careful differentiation from metaphyseal osteopathy (hypertrophic osteodystrophy) (Figure 14.9). See Viral osteomyelitis (below) for more information. Typically, the radiographic features of metaphyseal osteomyelitis are far more diffuse and aggressive than those in metaphyseal osteopathy. Bone biopsy or a good response to prolonged appropriate antibacterial therapy may be the only means of confirming the diagnosis in some cases.

In chronic cases of osteomyelitis heat, pain and swelling are less obvious but are still present. There may be weight loss and the development of discharging sinus tracts, muscle atrophy, fibrosis and contracture. Joint infection can occur in association with infection of a neighbouring bone, and it may be difficult to determine whether infection of the joint or bone was the primary event, particularly in the case of discospondylitis (see below). It is rare for bacterial osteomyelitis to spread from one bone to another across a synovial joint, but bone infection either side of the joint commonly occurs in discospondylitis.

Diagnostic plan
The diagnostic plan for suspected bacterial osteomyelitis is:

- Radiograph affected or suspected bones
- Laboratory investigations
  - Consider haematological analyses
  - Obtain biopsy specimens for bacterial culture and sensitivity testing before any antibacterials are given if possible
  - Consider histopathological analysis of bone biopsy specimens.

Radiography: The radiographic appearance of bacterial osteomyelitis varies with the stage in the disease process. In the acute stages there is often only soft tissue swelling with no apparent osseous abnormality. There may be gas lucencies in neighbouring soft tissues.

As the lesion becomes more chronic, osseous changes typical of an aggressive bone lesion develop (Figure 14.10). These include extensive periosteal new bone proliferation and irregular bone lysis and sclerosis. Focal lysis is often especially apparent adjacent to metal implants.

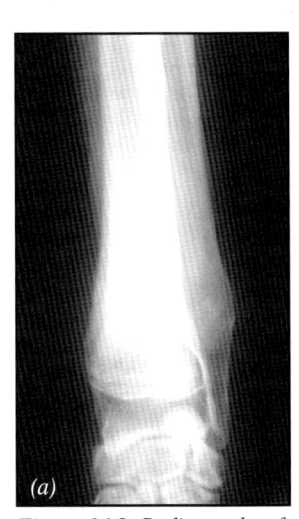

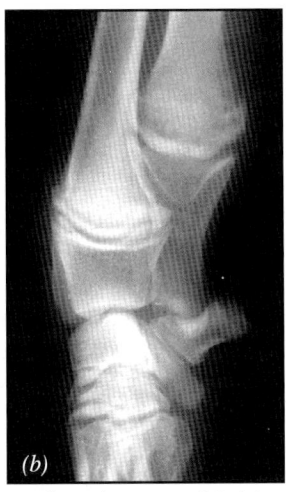

Figure 14.9: Radiographs of metaphyseal osteomyelitis (a) and metaphyseal osteopathy (b). Both conditions occur in young dogs and usually involve several limb bones. Metaphyseal osteomyelitis arises as a result of haematogenous spread of infection to the metaphyses of the long bones of a juvenile dog. The radiographic changes are superficially similar to those seen in metaphyseal osteopathy, but the lucencies within the bone do not form the distinct radiolucent line ('double growth plate') typical of metaphyseal osteopathy. The cause of metaphyseal osteopathy is unknown but an association with canine distemper virus has been suggested. (© Martin Sullivan, University of Glasgow.)

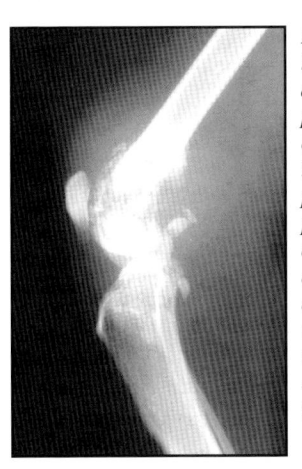

Figure 14.10: Radiograph of bacterial osteomyelitis in the distal femur of a cat. Note the presence of characteristic changes of an aggressive bone lesion (i.e. a mixed pattern of destruction and proliferation of the bone with a poorly defined margin demarcating normal from abnormal bone). On the basis of the radiographs alone, these changes do not reliably differentiate between infection and malignancy.

When infection complicates a fracture there may be sequestration and involucrum formation and/or a delayed union or non-union, which is usually hypertrophic.

Aggressive bone lesions associated with infection cannot be reliably differentiated from bone malignancy on the basis of radiological features alone. Other factors may assist in the differentiation, e.g. the presence of pulmonary metastases or spontaneous fracture indicates a neoplastic process. Furthermore, a radiologically aggressive bone lesion at a site of predisposition for bone malignancy in the older, large breed dog without a history of bone trauma is unlikely to be osteomyelitis. However, a radiologically aggressive bone lesion at a site of recent internal fixation of a fracture is most likely to be infection. Malignancies and infections occasionally arise at the site of longstanding fractures or repairs, and in these cases one must be more circumspect in the absence of a bone biopsy.

Routine blood screens: Haematological and serum biochemical analyses are often of little help in confirming a suspected diagnosis of bacterial osteomyelitis. Leucocytosis, as a result of neutrophilia and a left shift, is an inconsistent finding.

Culture of bone biopsies: A bone biopsy or implants taken directly and aseptically from the infected bone at the time of surgery should be submitted for aerobic and anaerobic bacteriological culture and antimicrobial sensitivity testing. Alternatively, biopsies from soft tissues neighbouring the bone may be used. Anaerobic culture is essential as around 60% of all cases of osteomyelitis have an anaerobic component (Muir and Johnson, 1992). Prior administration of antibacterials reduces the chance of a successful culture result. Swabs from draining sinus tracts are not satisfactory because the tracts are commonly invaded by secondary bacteria.

If there is any uncertainty about the diagnosis, particularly with regard to the possibility of malignancy, a further biopsy specimen should be fixed in formalin and submitted for histopathological examination.

Treatment

Treatment of osteomyelitis often depends on a combination of surgical and medical therapies:

- Sequestra and necrotic soft tissues are surgically debrided to leave only healthy vascularized bone. Surgical implants, which may act as a continuing focus for infection, are removed
- Drainage is established to eliminate dead space. Consider reaming the medullary cavity to drain the bone. Drainage may be maintained by open-wound management or by the insertion of drainage tubes (Daly, 1985)
- Persistent fracture instability is often a major factor in osteomyelitis secondary to fracture repair. Achieving absolute rigidity at the fracture site can be an important adjunct to controlling the infection
- Antibacterial therapy is directed by the results of antimicrobial sensitivity testing. While awaiting laboratory test results, therapy should be instigated with a broad-spectrum β-lactamase resistant bactericidal agent. Consider using clavulanate-potentiated amoxycillin or cephalosporin derivatives in this intervening period. Metronidazole may be included for its action against anaerobes
- Change the initial choice of antibacterial only if indicated by subsequent sensitivity tests. Avoid bacteriostatic drugs such as the lincosamides (lincomycin and clindamycin) and tetracyclines unless specifically indicated by culture and sensitivity test results
- Poor blood supply is important in the pathogenesis of osteomyelitis and can limit the ability of the immune system to clear infections only controlled by bacteriostatic drugs. High doses of antibacterials are necessary to facilitate penetration of areas with poor blood perfusion
- Administration of systemic antibacterial agents should continue for a minimum of 6 weeks or for 2 weeks after the complete resolution of clinical signs
- Surgical implantation of gentamicin-impregnated polymethylmethacrylate beads may be helpful in selected cases with multiple resistant infections (Brown and Bennett, 1989)
- Nursing adjuncts to therapy include regular attention to dressings and drains. Movement should be restricted in the early stages of treatment, but prolonged exercise restriction is inadvisable as this may encourage the formation of adhesions.

Prognosis

The prognosis varies with the stage of the disease. Haematogenous osteomyelitis often has a good response to a prolonged course of antibacterials, provided the primary source of infection can also be eliminated. Post-traumatic osteomyelitis normally has a good prognosis provided appropriate treatment is instigated promptly. This can be expensive. The prognosis becomes more guarded with chronic osteomyelitis as therapy can be prolonged and expensive, with relapses sometimes occurring months or even years later, and there may be irreversible soft tissue changes.

Fungal osteomyelitis

With the exception of aspergillosis, fungal osteomyelitis is rare. Most cases have a restricted geographical distribution and some have never been diagnosed in the UK. Osteomyelitis associated with *Cryptococcus neoformans* has been reported in one dog in the UK (Brearley and Jeffery, 1992).

Aspergillosis usually causes bone infection as an extension of mycotic rhinitis or sinusitis. Treatment hinges on the administration of antifungal agents (Sharp *et al.*, 1991). *Aspergillus* spp. occasionally disseminate to other body systems, including the skeleton, and may present as a discospondylitis (see Fungal discospondylitis, below) (Day and Penhale, 1988).

Protozoal osteomyelitis
Protozoal osteomyelitis is rare. It has been found in association with leishmaniasis and may, in some instances, be the only clinical manifestation of the disease (Figure 14.11). See Chapter 5 for further details on leishmaniasis.

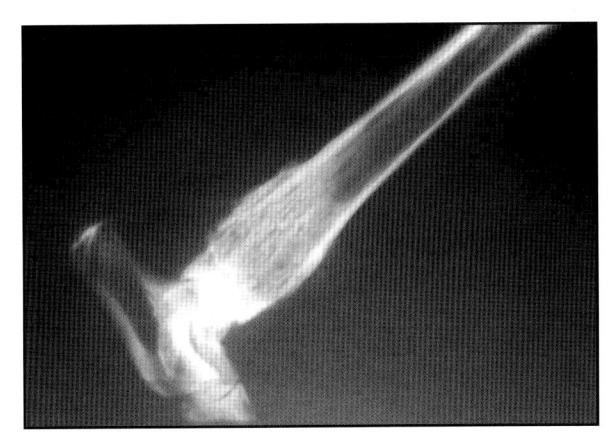

Figure 14.11: Radiograph showing osteomyelitis that was found to be caused by leishmaniasis. (Courtesy of Artur Font.)

Viral osteomyelitis
It is well established that viruses can infect bone in dogs and cats. In experimental situations, viruses can occasionally cause identifiable bone lesions, such as necrosis (Mee *et al.*, 1992). However, a confirmed role for viruses in clinical infections of bone remains elusive.

Metaphyseal osteopathy (MO; hypertrophic osteodystrophy) is a polyostotic inflammatory disease of immature dogs. Most recent evidence suggests an infective aetiology for MO. Metaphyseal lesions have been recognized in dogs with clinical CDV infection (Baumgartner *et al.*, 1995), and blood taken from dogs with MO caused clinical CDV infection when infused into unvaccinated recipients. Mee *et al.* (1992, 1993) demonstrated RNA and mRNA of CDV in osteoblasts and bone marrow cells of CDV-infected dogs and in the affected metaphyses of dogs with MO. Nevertheless, CDV has yet to be confirmed as an aetiological agent in the pathogenesis of MO, and it is possible that MO is a syndrome associated with individuals, who are genetically at risk, meeting any one of several inflammatory agents.

DISCOSPONDYLITIS

Discospondylitis is the term applied to infection of the intervertebral discs and adjacent vertebral bodies. It occurs when bacteria or fungi are implanted by:

- Haematogenous spread of infection
- Migrating foreign bodies, such as plant awns
- Iatrogenic contamination at the time of spinal surgery
- Extension from paravertebral infections or penetrating wounds.

Of these, haematogenous spread of infection is probably the most common, although discospondylitis is more common in dogs in areas where grass awn infections are a problem. Most cases of discospondylitis are bacterial. The lumbosacral disc space and the discs of the thoracolumbar junction are most commonly affected.

Bacterial discospondylitis
The spectrum of organisms isolated from cases of bacterial discospondylitis is similar to that of bacterial osteomyelitis (see above). Although not endemic in the UK, *Brucella canis* can produce a discospondylitis. In endemic areas *B. canis* titres should be examined from all dogs with discospondylitis because it is a major zoonosis.

History and clinical findings
Any age or breed of dog may be affected by bacterial discospondylitis, but young adults of the larger breeds seem to be predisposed. It has been reported in cats, but is rare. Predominant clinical signs include:

- Spinal pain – common and may be severe
- Persistent or recurring pyrexia – common
- Neurological deficits – including ataxia, weakness, hyperaesthesia, hyperreflexia, hyporeflexia, paralysis and urinary incontinence
- Dramatic weight loss
- Severe wastage of paraspinal muscles.

Diagnosis may be difficult as clinical signs can be non-specific. Discospondylitis should always be considered as a differential diagnosis for pyrexia of unknown origin (see Chapter 7).

Diagnostic plan
The diagnostic plan for suspected bacterial discospondylitis is:

- Spinal radiography
- Consider myelography if neurological deficits present
- Consider haematological analyses
- Consider lumbar puncture and cerebrospinal fluid (CSF) analysis (if neurological deficits present)

- Obtain specimens (disc aspirate, CSF, blood or urine) for bacterial culture and sensitivity before any antibacterials are given
- Consider surgical biopsy specimens.

Radiography and myelography: Good quality spinal radiographs are essential to the diagnosis of discospondylitis although clinical signs occasionally precede radiographic signs. The earliest radiographic finding is narrowing of the intervertebral space. More frequently, advanced changes are found at the time of radiography (Figure 14.12):

- Destruction of vertebral bone either side of the disc space giving it an irregular appearance
- An apparently increased width to the disc space as a result of end-plate destruction
- There is often sclerosis of the vertebral bodies either side of the lytic area and shortening of the affected vertebral bodies by end-plate destruction
- Ventral spondylosis is often prolific but is not, in itself, a diagnostic indicator of disc infection
- Multiple discs may be affected, but care must be taken to differentiate such cases from fungal discospondylitis (see below).

Myelography should be considered in patients with neurological deficits that may be candidates for decompressive surgery. Referral to a specialist centre may be advisable.

Laboratory investigations: As with other bacterial infections of the skeletal system, haematological and biochemical variables in the peripheral blood are not changed consistently, although they may provide supportive evidence for a systemic inflammatory process in cases of fever of unknown origin.

CSF from affected animals may be normal or may have an increased protein content and/or increased white blood cell numbers, with a predominance of neutrophils, particularly if the infection has extended to the spinal canal and is causing a meningitis or myelitis (see Chapter 15).

The single most useful test to confirm a suspected case of bacterial discospondylitis is the submission of samples for bacterial culture and sensitivity testing. With lumbosacral infections, a fine needle aspirate can be obtained directly from the disc by lumbar puncture. This is, however, technically difficult to achieve without experience and is not feasible at other spinal sites. Alternatives include:

- Blood cultures
- CSF cultures, particularly if there are neurological deficits or evidence of extension of infection into the spinal canal on CSF analysis
- Urine cultures. It has long been suggested that urinary tract infections might be a source of microorganisms that spread haematogenously and localize to the intervertebral discs. Recent evidence, however, suggests that concurrent urinary tract and disc infections are coincidental. Affected dogs may also have other concurrent infections, e.g. of the skin and peripheral synovial joints.

Treatment

Most cases of discospondylitis are treated with long-term systemic antibacterials and with confinement. The criteria for drug management are similar to those for bacterial osteomyelitis (see above). Culture results may be negative in some cases, and if sensitivities are not available a broad-spectrum β-lactamase-resistant bactericidal agent should be used.

Prognosis

The prognosis depends on the ability to eliminate the causative organism and on the degree of neurological deficits. Generally, the prognosis is good for animals with only spinal pain but becomes guarded to poor as neurological signs progress.

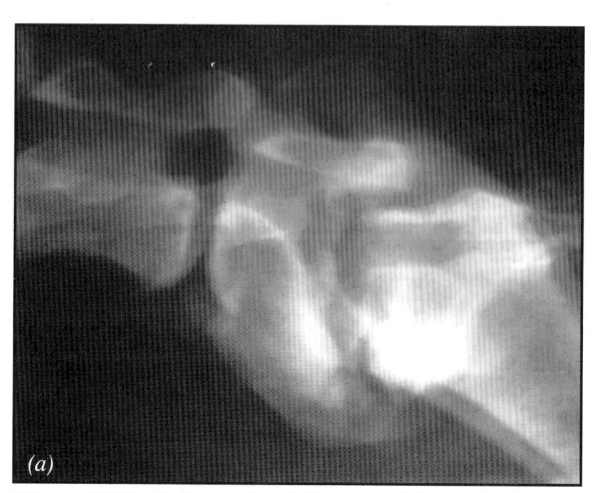

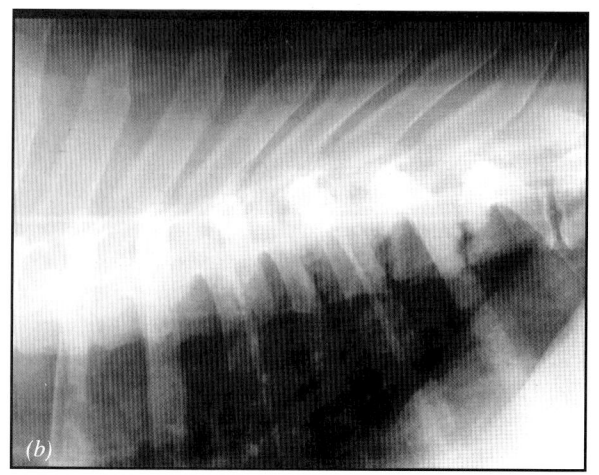

Figure 14.12: Radiographs of discospondylitis in (a) lumbosacral and (b) thoracic intervertebral joints. Note the new bone formation and destruction of the end-plates in both radiographs. ((b) courtesy of Dr Ian Ramsey, University of Glasgow.)

Surgical decompression or stabilization is indicated in cases with obvious neurological deficits. Stabilization is also indicated in the management of chronic, recurrent or non-responsive discospondylitis. Surgical management can be combined with curettage, which facilitates collection of material for bacterial cultures and allows thorough debridement of necrotic material. The surgical management of discospondylitis is both technically demanding and expensive. Referral to a specialist centre should be considered.

Fungal discospondylitis

Among other skeletal sites, disseminated *Aspergillus* spp. infections occasionally present as a discospondylitis. In particular in this context, *Aspergillus* spp. have been associated with a syndrome of multiple discospondylitis to which German Shepherd bitches are particularly predisposed. Often, affected dogs do not have serum antibodies to the organism. Treatment is with prolonged, or permanent, systemic antifungal drugs, but the prognosis is poor.

INFECTIVE MYOPATHIES

Infectious agents involving muscle in dogs and cats include:

- Focal bacterial myopathies
- Protozoal myopathies (toxoplasmosis, neosporosis)
- Parasitic myopathies (Craig, 1989)
- Generalized bacterial myopathies, e.g. associated with leptospirosis.

Of these, only focal bacterial myopathies and protozoal myopathies are of great clinical importance.

Focal bacterial myopathies

Focal bacterial myopathies are relatively uncommon in dogs and cats. They typically result from trauma such as bite wounds, road traffic accidents or contaminated surgery. Clinical signs are typical of local inflammation, with lameness and heat, pain, swelling and disuse localized to the affected muscle group. Common organisms include *Staphylococcus intermedius* and *Clostridium perfringens*.

Radiography usually only demonstrates soft tissue swelling. However, there may be a reactive periostitis on neighbouring bones, and gas shadows are seen when gas-forming organisms such as *C. perfringens* are present (Figure 14.13).

Tissue biopsies should be obtained for bacterial culture and sensitivity testing. The mainstay of treatment is antibacterial therapy, and the criteria for selection are similar to those for bacterial osteomyelitis. *Clostridium* spp. infection is best treated with metronidazole or clindamycin. Surgical debridement of necrotic tissue and surgical drainage may be indicated.

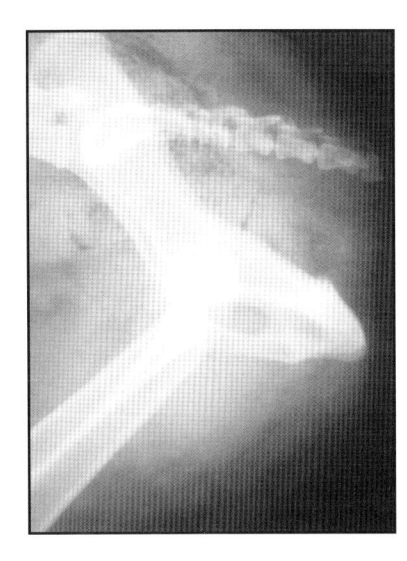

Figure 14.13: Radiograph of clostridial myositis. Note the gas densities within the soft tissues. (© Dr Bryn Tennant.)

Rarely, *C. tetani* infection of muscles may occur. Typically affected animals present within 5 days of sustaining a wound.

Protozoal myopathies

Polymyositis has been recorded in dogs and cats in association with both *Toxoplasma gondii* and *Neospora caninum* infections (see Chapter 15). The classic presentation of protozoal myopathy in dogs is pelvic limb extensor rigidity. Most affected animals are under 4 months of age, although cases are documented in adults. Typically there is muscle atrophy and hyporeflexia. The extensor rigidity may be so severe that it induces physeal fractures in young dogs.

Muscle hyperaesthesia has been documented in association with feline toxoplasmosis (Lappin *et al.*, 1989) Protozoal infection should be considered as a differential diagnosis in hyperaesthetic cats.

Hepatozoon canis and related species are found in Africa, southern Europe, Asia and America. The infection is transmitted by the tick *Rhipicephalus sanguineus*. American isolates have been associated with polymyositis and show signs of severe muscle wastage, pyrexia and depression, with purulent ocular and nasal discharges. Unusually, despite these signs, many dogs retain a good appetite. The disease has a prolonged course and there may be periods of apparent remission. Haematology usually demonstrates a leucocytosis, due to a neutrophilia with a left shift, and a mild non-regenerative anaemia. Radiography may demonstrate a widespread periosteal reaction. Isolates from the other geographical regions seem to be less pathogenic and cases are presented with a mild systemic illness without polymyositis. The organism can be seen in peripheral neutrophils (non-American isolates) or muscle biopsies (American isolates). There is no well established protocol for treatment, although various antiprotozoal drugs have been tried. Providing analgesia with non-steroidal drugs during episodes is helpful. Relapses after apparently successful therapy are common and most dogs eventually die from the disease.

DRUG DOSAGES

See Appendix 3.

REFERENCES AND FURTHER READING

Barton MD, Ireland L, Kirschner JL and Forbes C (1985) Isolation of *Mycoplasma spumans* from polyarthritis in a greyhound. *Australian Veterinary Journal* **62,** 206

Baumgartner W, Boyce RW and Alldinger S (1995) Metaphyseal bone lesions in young dogs with systemic canine distemper virus infection. *Veterinary Microbiology* **44,** 201-209

Bennett D and May C (1995) Joint diseases of dogs and cats. In: *Textbook of Veterinary Internal Medicine, 4th edn*, ed. SJ Ettinger and EC Feldman, pp. 2032-2076 WB Saunders, Philadelphia

Bennett D and Taylor DJ (1988) Bacterial infective arthritis in the dog. *Journal of Small Animal Practice* **29,** 207-230

Brearley MJ and Jeffery N (1992) Cryptococcal osteomyelitis in a dog. *Journal of Small Animal Practice* **33,** 601-604

Brown A and Bennett D (1989) The use of gentamycin impregnated methylmethacrylate beads for the treatment of bacterial infective arthritis. *Veterinary Record* **123,** 625-626

Craig TM (1989) Parasitic myositis of dogs and cats. *Seminars in Veterinary Medicine and Surgery (Small Animal)* **4,** 161-167

Daly WR (1985) Orthopaedic infections. In: *Textbook of Small Animal Surgery, 1st edn*, ed. DH Slatter, pp. 2020-2034 WB Saunders, Philadelphia

Day MJ and Penhale WJ (1988) Humoral immunity in dogs with disseminated *Aspergillus terreus* infection in the dog. *Veterinary Microbiology* **16,** 283-287

Dunn JK, Dennis R and Houlton JEF (1992) Successful treatment of two cases of metaphyseal osteomyelitis in the dog. *Journal of Small Animal Practice* **33,** 85-89

Gibson NR, Carmichael S, Li A, Reid WJ, Normand EH, Owen MR and Bennett D (1999) Value of direct smears of synovial fluid in the diagnosis of canine joint disease. *Veterinary Record* **144,** 463-465

Houlton JEF (1994) Ancillary aids to diagnosis. In: *Manual of Small Animal Arthrology*, ed. JEF Houlton and R Collinson, pp. 22-38 BSAVA Publications, Cheltenham

Lappin MR, Greene CE, Winston S, Toll SL and Epstein ME (1989) Clinical feline toxoplasmosis. Serologic diagnosis and therapeutic management of 15 cases. *Journal of Veterinary Internal Medicine* **3,** 139-143

May C, Bennett D and Carter SD (1991) Serodiagnosis of Lyme disease in UK dogs. *Journal of Small Animal Practice* **32,** 170-174

Mee AP, Gordon MT, May C, Bennett D, Anderson DC and Sharpe PT (1993) Canine distemper viral transcripts detected in the bone cells of a dog with metaphyseal osteopathy. *Bone* **14,** 59-67

Mee AP, Webber DM, May C, Bennett D, Sharpe PT and Anderson DC (1992) Detection of canine distemper virus in bone cells in the metaphyses of distemper-infected dogs. *Journal of Bone and Mineral Research* **7,** 829-833

Muir P and Johnson KA (1992) Anaerobic bacteria isolated from osteomyelitis in dogs and cats. *Veterinary Surgery* **21,** 463-466

Sharp NJ, Harvey CE and O'Brien JA (1991) Treatment of canine nasal aspergillosis/penicillosis with fluconazole (UR-49,858). *Journal of Small Animal Practice* **32,** 513-516

Thomas WB (2000) Diskospondylitis and other vertebral infections. *Veterinary Clinics of North America* **30,** 169-182

CHAPTER FIFTEEN

The Nervous System

Clare Rusbridge

CHAPTER PLAN

Introduction
Diagnosis of nervous system infections
    Lesion localization
    Clinical pathology
    Cerebrospinal fluid analysis
    Diagnostic imaging
Infections resulting in cranial or spinal pain
    Bacterial meningitis/meningoencephalitis
    Viral meningoencephalitis
Infections resulting in multifocal neurological signs
    Toxoplasmosis
    Neosporosis
    Cryptococcosis
    Other fungal infections
    Distemper
    Feline infectious peritonitis
    Feline leukaemia virus
Infections resulting in altered behaviour
    Rabies
    Borna disease and feline staggering disease
    Feline immunodeficiency virus
    Feline spongiform encephalopathy
    Feline parvovirus
Infections resulting in muscle spasm
    Tetanus
Infections resulting in tetraparesis
    Botulism
References and further reading

INTRODUCTION

Compared with other organs, infection of the nervous system is rare. To establish itself within the nervous system the infectious agent must overcome the normal defence mechanisms such as the blood–brain/nerve barrier, astrocytes and the phagocytic microglia. Host factors such as compromise of the blood–brain barrier or immunodeficiency contribute to the likelihood of infection. The nervous system has no secondary lymphoid tissue and has low concentrations of humoral defence mechanisms such as complement. Once an infection has become established it usually progresses rapidly. Prompt diagnosis and treatment are essential. Inflammatory mediators are neurotoxic, and other consequences of inflammation, e.g. increased blood flow or oedema, are equally undesirable in the confined space of the nervous system. Most of the clinical signs of nervous system infection are due to inflammation, and the clinician must distinguish infection from more common causes of inflammation such as primary immune-mediated disease. In addition to the lack of specific signs, diagnosis of nervous system infections is made more difficult by the problems of demonstrating the organism and the limited availability of some diagnostic aids, e.g. magnetic resonance imaging (MRI) and computed tomography (CT).

DIAGNOSIS OF INFECTION

Lesion localization

Neurological diagnosis requires the affected parts of the nervous system to be identified. Figure 15.1 provides a useful summary of the clinical signs that are seen with diseases of parts of the nervous system. Neurological texts, such as the BSAVA's *Manual of Small Animal Neurology*, should be consulted for further assistance in localizing lesions within the nervous system.

Clinical pathology

Haematology is useful but generally non-specific. White blood cell counts can often be normal even when there is significant CNS inflammation. Serum biochemistry may help eliminate metabolic disorders, e.g. hepatic encephalopathy. It is useful to assess creatine kinase (CK) and aspartate aminotransferase (AST) concentrations for an indication of muscle involvement.

Cerebrospinal fluid analysis

Cerebrospinal fluid (CSF) analysis is the most important diagnostic test in the evaluation of CNS inflammation. CSF can be collected from either the cerebellomedullary cistern or the caudal lumbar subarachnoid space. CSF generally flows in a cranial

Manual of Canine and Feline Infectious Diseases

Clinical signs	Forebrain	Brain stem	Cerebellum	C1-C5 spinal cord	C5-T2 spinal cord	T3-L3 spinal cord	L4-S3 spinal cord	Peripheral nervous system	Neuromuscular junction	Muscle
Seizures	✓ or ✗	✗	✗	✗	✗	✗	✗	✗	✗	✗
Behavioural change	✓ or ✗	✗	✗	✗	✗	✗	✗	✗	✗	✗
Mental status	Depressed Stuporous Comatose	Depressed Stuporous Comatose	N	N	N	N	N	N	N	N
Tremor	✗#	✗	Intention	✗	✗	✗	✗	Muscle	Muscle	Muscle
Ataxia	✓ or ✗	✓	✓	✓	✓	✓PL	✓PL	✗	✗	✗
Circling	✓ or ✗	✓ or ✗	✗	✗	✗	✗	✗	✗	✗	✗
Paresis	✓	✓	✗	✓	✓	✓PL	✓PL	✓	✓	✓
Proprioceptive deficits	Contralateral	Ipsilateral	✗	Ipsilateral	Ipsilateral	Ipsilateral	Ipsilateral	✓ or ✗	✗	✗
Deficit menace response	✓ Contralateral ✓ or ✗	CNVII	✓ or ✗ normal vision	✗	✗	✗	✗	CNVII	CNVII	✗
Cranial nerve (III-XII) deficits	✗	✓ or ✗	✗	✗	✗	✗	✗	✓ or ✗	✓ or ✗*	✓ or ✗*
Limb muscle tone	N	N or ↑	N or ↑ or ↓	↑	↓TL ↑PL	↑PL	↓PL	↓	↓	↓ or ↑
Limb muscle atrophy	✗	✗	✗	✗	✓TL	✗	✓PL	✓ or ✗	✓ or ✗	✓
Spinal reflexes	N or ↑	N or ↑	N	N or ↑	↓TL ↑PL	↑PL	↓PL	↓	N or ↓	N or ↓
Pain	✓ or ✗ (head/cranial cervical)	✓ or ✗	✗	✓ or ✗	✓ or ✗	✓ or ✗	✓ or ✗	✓ or ✗	✗	✓ or ✗

Figure 15.1: Clinical signs associated with dysfunction of each functional area of the nervous system. Involvement of more than one section suggests multifocal disease, which is the hallmark of CNS infection/inflammation.
✓, present; ✗, not present; N, normal; PL, pelvic limbs only; TL, thoracic limbs only; ↓, decreased, ↑, increased; CNVII, may have facial nerve deficits; *, no actual cranial nerve deficits but may have dysphagia, dysphonia, regurgitation, poor gag; C, cervical spinal cord segment; T, thoracic spinal cord segment; L, lumbar spinal cord segment; S, sacral spinal cord segment; #, rarely action or resting tremor may be seen.

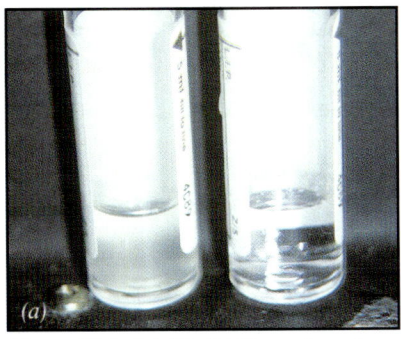

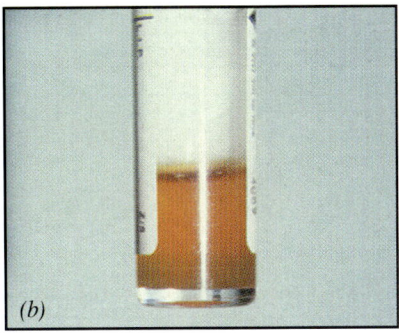

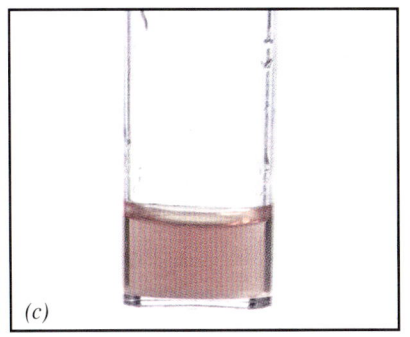

Figure 15.2: *(a) (Right) Normal cerebrospinal fluid (CSF) sample. (Left) Sample with marked turbidity; the cell count was 4600 cells/ml. A change in turbidity is not detected until the cell count is >100 cells/ml; therefore, gross examination of CSF is not sufficient for detecting inflammatory disease. Reproduced from* In Practice *(1997)* **19***, 324 with permission. (b) Xanthochromia, a yellow discoloration associated with degradation of old haemorrhage or an increased protein concentration (e.g. in feline infectious peritonitis); occasionally it is seen in icteric patients. (c) CSF with a pink discoloration is most commonly due to iatrogenic blood contamination. In this instance centrifugation produces a clear supernatant.*

to caudal direction, and it is preferable to collect from a site caudal to the suspected lesion. Collection methods are described in the BSAVA's *Manual of Small Animal Neurology* (Wheeler, 1995) and in several textbooks. Some nervous system infections are associated with an increased risk of brain herniation after CSF collection. MRI or CT may be of value in the preoperative assessment and are essential for the diagnosis of this complication. Collecting CSF from the caudal lumbar subarachnoid space does not decrease the risk of herniation.

The collected sample should be examined for colour and turbidity (Figure 15.2) and a cell count, differential and total protein determined. Ideally the sample should be handled by a dedicated laboratory; however, it is often advantageous for the clinician to perform some tests in their own practice laboratory to identify the disease process while laboratory results are awaited. Cell counts can be obtained using a haemocytometer, and a differential count can be obtained after sedimentation of the sample (Figure 15.3). Autoanalysers are unable to count the low numbers of cells that are present in normal and abnormal CSF accurately and so should not be used. Before obtaining the CSF, it is important to determine from the commercial laboratory how they wish the sample to be handled.

Normal CSF is a clear fluid with a low cell count and protein concentration (Figure 15.4). Increases in cell numbers or protein concentration suggest an inflammatory response. The fluid can be submitted for measurement of specific antibody titres. Immunoglobulins do not pass an intact blood–brain barrier, so a positive titre suggests that the infectious agent is present in the CNS. Figure 15.5 outlines the approach to interpretation of CSF cytology, and Figure 15.6 shows some examples of such investigations.

CSF should be cultured anaerobically and aerobically. For optimal results it should be innoculated into liquid broth in a similar manner to that used for culturing blood (see Chapter 7). Sensitivity testing should be performed using antibacterials that are known to cross

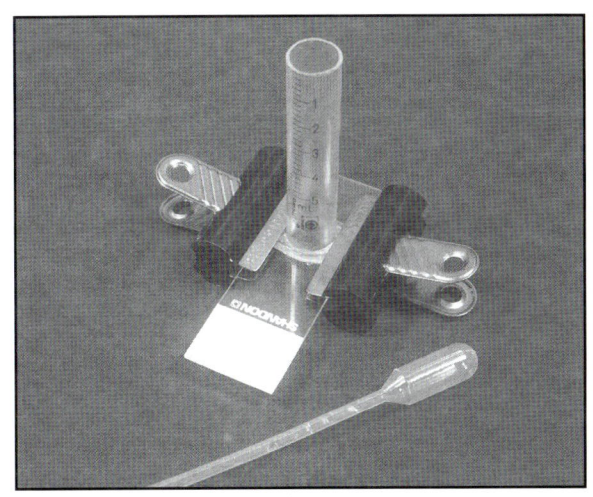

Figure 15.3: *Sedimentation chamber for practice laboratory preparation of cerebrospinal fluid (CSF) for cytological evaluation. The top has been cut off a 5 ml syringe and a small quantity of silicone grease applied to the base to create a waterproof seal. Care must be taken to ensure that the 'hole' in the centre is free of grease. The chamber is then clamped to a glass microscope slide using bulldog clips. Collected CSF is added to the chamber and left to stand in a refrigerator for 25 minutes. The supernatant is then pipetted off, the cylinder removed, and the slide allowed to air dry before being stained and examined. Reproduced from* In Practice *(1997)* **19***, 327 with permission.*

Variable	Normal finding
Colour	Colourless
Turbidity	Clear
Total white blood cell count	<6 cells/µl
Total red blood cell count	0
Cytology	Few monocytes and lymphocytes (rarely neutrophils)
Total protein Cisternal Lumbar	<0.3 g/l <0.45 g/l

Figure 15.4: *Normal values for routine cerebrospinal fluid analysis.*

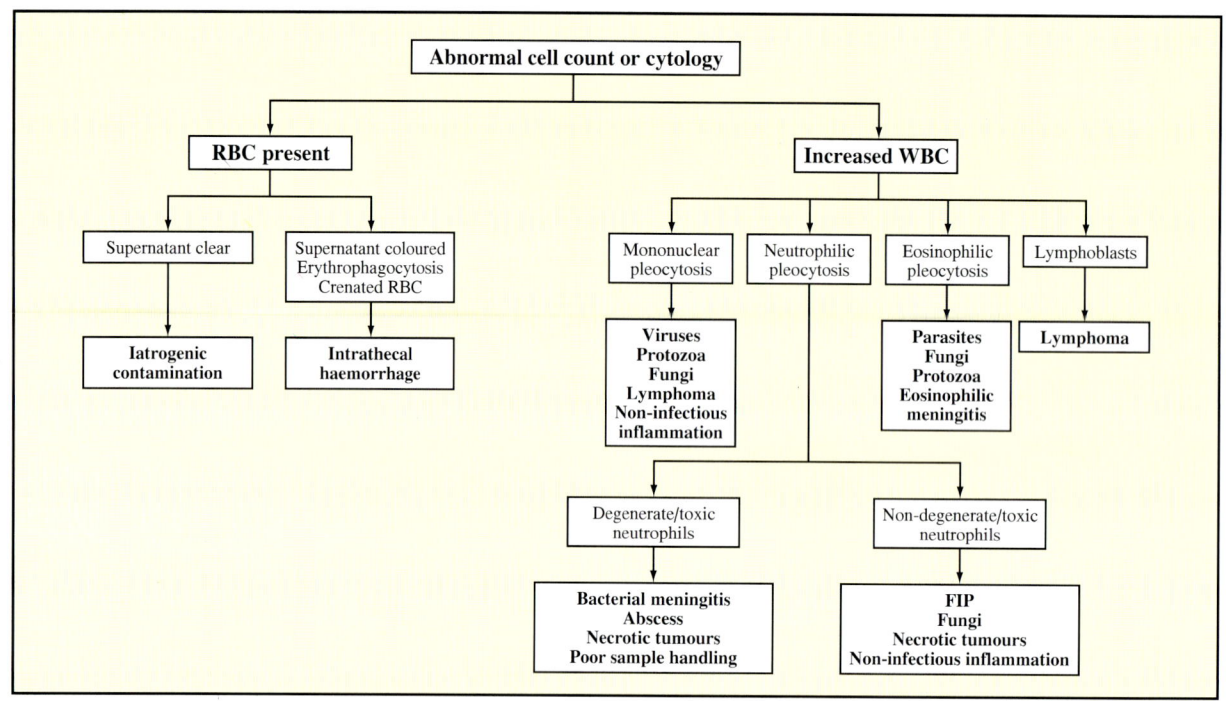

234 Manual of Canine and Feline Infectious Diseases

Figure 15.5: Flow chart showing approach to interpretation of cerebrospinal fluid cytology. RBC, red blood cells; WBC, white blood cells.

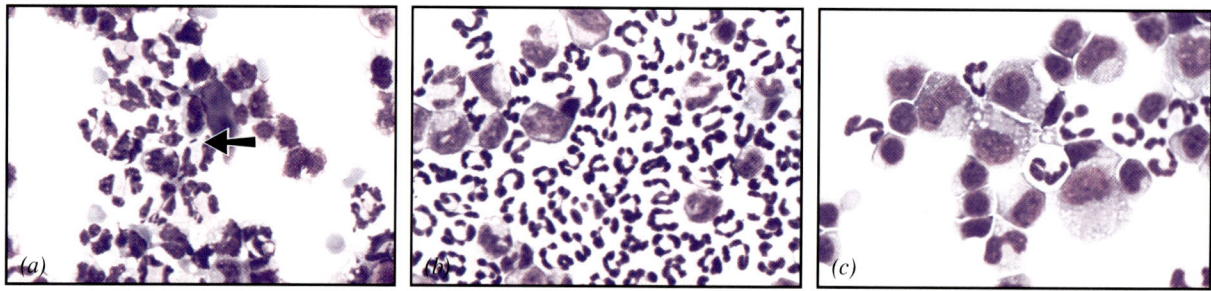

Figure 15.6: Examples of cerebrospinal fluid cytology. (a) Bacterial meningitis: there is a neutrophilic pleocytosis; many of the cells are dead or dying and there are intracellular bacteria (arrowed). (b) Steroid-responsive meningoencephalomyelitis; unlike in bacterial meningitis the neutrophils are healthy and there are no intracellular bacteria. (c) Granulomatous meningoencephalomyelitis: a mononuclear and neutrophilic pleocytosis is evident with a predominance of macrophages with abundant lacy cytoplasm (reticulum cells).

the normal blood–brain barrier (such as potentiated sulphonamides, metronidazole and fluoroquinolones). Sensitivity to other antibacterials may still be clinically useful in animals with abnormal blood–brain barriers.

A crude method of determining protein concentration is to put a few drops of CSF on a urinary reagent strip. The normal value is trace to 0.3 g/l (+1). This method is unreliable for mild increases and should be reinforced by laboratory determination. Refractometers are not sufficiently sensitive to detect the low protein concentrations that are present in CSF.

Normal CSF protein contains about 75% albumin; an increase in the globulin component suggests immune-mediated disease. Although it is possible for practitioners to make a quantitative assessment of globulin concentration by the Pandy test, determination of total protein, albumin and globulin concentrations in a commercial laboratory is preferred. The Pandy test is performed by adding a few drops of CSF to 1 ml of phenol solution (10 mg of carbolic acid crystals made up to a volume of 100 ml in distilled water) and then shaken. Appropriate safety measures should be taken when handling phenol solutions. Normal CSF develops a slight turbidity. CSF containing increased globulin concentrations develops a white turbidity, which is graded on a scale of +1 to +4.

Diagnostic imaging

Plain radiography and ultrasonography are almost always unhelpful in the assessment of suspected cases of nervous system infection. Myelography may be useful in excluding some differential diagnoses. The value of MRI and CT is restricted by their limited availability but, if they are available, then they are important tools in determining the nature and likely aetiology of CNS inflammation. They are also important for eliminating other more common differential diagnoses such as neoplasia.

INFECTIONS RESULTING IN CRANIAL OR SPINAL PAIN

Meningeal irritation causes spinal pain and may develop secondary to inflammation or spinal cord compression. The most common clinical manifestation is cranial cervical pain, i.e. the animal may have a low head carriage and pain on ventroflexion of the neck. Multifocal spinal pain may be seen in some inflammatory conditions. With the exception of discospondylitis (see Chapter 14), infectious causes of spinal pain are rare and other differential diagnoses should be considered (Figure 15.7). The main infectious causes of spinal pain are summarized in Figure 15.8.

Bacterial meningitis/meningoencephalitis

With the exception of a few neurotropic species, e.g. *Listeria*, bacteria are opportunistic invaders of the CNS. There are three potential routes of infection:

- Direct extension, e.g. from otitis interna or sinusitis
- Bacterial embolization within the brain, e.g. from a bacterial endocarditis
- Bacterial penetration of the blood–brain barrier, e.g. systemic infection from an infected umbilical cord in a neonate.

Penetration of the blood–brain barrier only occurs if there is a sustained bacteraemia and a compromised immune system. Bacterial meningitis is very rare in

Disease	Relative frequency
Infectious	
Bacterial meningitis	Very rare
Viral meningitis/ meningoencephalomyelitis	Rare
Discospondylitis	Occasional
Feline infectious peritonitis	Common
Lymphoma (feline leukaemia virus (FeLV) induced)	Common
Non-infectious	
Degenerative intervertebral disc disease	Very common
Steroid-responsive meningoencephalomyelitis/ polyarteritis	Common in the dog
Granulomatous meningoencephalomyelitis	Common in the dog
Pug/Maltese Terrier/Yorkshire Terrier encephalitis	Uncommon
Eosinophilic meningoencephalomyelitis	Occasional
Atlantoaxial subluxation	Occasional
Brain tumour, e.g. meningioma	Occasional
Spinal neoplasia (including FeLV-negative lymphomas)	Common
Other space-occupying lesions	Rare
Spinal trauma	Common

Figure 15.7: Differential diagnosis of spinal pain.

Infectious disease	Other clinical signs	CSF cell count	CSF protein	CSF cytology	Other diagnostic tests
Bacterial meningitis	Severely depressed, pyrexia +/- other neurological deficits	Moderately to markedly increased	Moderately to markedly increased	Toxic neutrophils Intracellular bacteria	CSF culture (in blood culture bottle) ?CSF glucose <60% serum glucose†
Viral meningitis/ meningoencephalomyelitis	Depressed, pyrexia +/- other neurological deficits	Normal to moderately increased	Normal to moderately increased	Mononuclear cells occasionally mixed	CSF anti-distemper antibody titre Fundic examination
Discospondylitis (see Chapter 14)	One or more focuses of pain especially cervical and lumbosacral areas Pyrexia, depression	Normal to mildly increased	Normal to mildly increased	Mononuclear cells +/- neutrophils	Radiography MRI Blood and urine culture
Feline infectious peritonitis (see Chapter 9)	Multifocal signs especially vestibular disease and seizures	Moderately to markedly increased	Moderately to markedly increased	Neutrophils Unproductive tap common	CSF Feline coronavirus antibody titre
Lymphoma (FeLV-induced) (see Chapter 5)	Multifocal signs especially cranial nerve deficits, Horner's syndrome and cauda equina signs	Normal to mildly increased	Normal to mildly increased	Mature lymphocytes Neoplastic lymphoblasts may be seen	FeLV and FIV titres WBC differential Bone marrow cytology MRI Thoracic/abdominal radiography

Figure 15.8: Infectious causes of spinal pain.
FeLV, feline leukaemia virus; FIV, feline immunodeficiency virus; MRI, magnetic resonance imaging; mildly increased (cerebrospinal fluid (CSF) 5–50 cells/ml, total protein <1 g/l); moderately increased (CSF >50 cells/ml, total protein >1g/l); markedly increased (CSF >500 cells/ml, total protein >2g/l), †, not quantified in domestic animals. Note that steroid therapy may result in normal cell counts and protein; WBC, white blood cell count.

small animals and there should be evidence of a source of infection and predisposition, e.g. cranial trauma or immunosuppression.

The most common isolates from bacterial meningitis in the dog and cat are *Staphylococcus* spp. Infection with *Pasteurella, Actinomyces, Nocardia, Flavobacterium, Streptococcus* and anaerobes including *Peptostreptococcus, Bacteroides, Fusobacterium* and *Eubacterium* have also been reported.

Clinical signs
The clinical signs of bacterial meningitis/meningoencephalitis include:

- Depression
- Pyrexia
- Cervical pain
- Hyperaesthesia
- Photophobia
- Generalized rigidity
- Seizures
- Papilloedema
- Evidence of ophthalmic inflammation on fundic examination
- Systemic signs, e.g. septic shock and bradycardia; these are common. Limb weakness is uncommon unless there is spinal cord involvement.

Diagnosis
Bacterial meningitis is confirmed by CSF analysis and culture but there is considerable risk of brain herniation after cisternal or lumbar puncture in such cases. Cell counts are typically markedly increased, with toxic neutrophils and intracellular bacteria (see Figure 15.6a). If intracellular bacteria are not present then the diagnosis should be reconsidered. Haematology and biochemical changes are usually non-specific, e.g. a neutrophilia with left shift. The absence of a leucocytosis does not exclude bacterial meningitis.

MRI or CT may be useful to determine the extent of disease and to exclude some differential diagnoses. MRI or CT is also invaluable for detecting bacterial cerebritis and abscessation (Thomas, 1999).

Treatment
Antibacterial therapy should be initiated as soon as possible. It is important to select a bactericidal drug that penetrates the blood-brain barrier and achieves a high CSF concentration (see Chapter 2). The author's preferences are potentiated sulphonamides until culture/Gram stain results are obtained, as these drugs also have significant antiprotozoal activity (see later). Treatment should be continued for 2 weeks after resolution of clinical signs. Restriction of fluid intake increases mortality so intake must be monitored and supplemented to at least maintenance requirements if necessary.

Dead and dying bacteria (bacterial cell walls and lipopolysaccharides) trigger the inflammatory cascade, and initiation of antibacterial therapy can make the disease worse. Short-term steroid therapy has been used in some cases of human meningitis (Knockaert, 1994) and may be beneficial in canine bacterial meningitis. Steroid therapy does not seem to affect the time to achieve CSF sterility; if used, steroids should be given 10-20 minutes before antibacterials. No benefit is seen if steroids are given more than 12 hours after the onset of clinical signs. It is essential that a CSF sample be obtained before steroids are administered. Steroid therapy in bacterial meningitis is still controversial as glucocorticoids may potentiate ischaemic injury to neurons, reduce penetration of the antibacterial into the CSF and prevent adequate clinical assessment of the response to therapy.

Viral meningoencephalitis
CNS viral infections are often suspected on the basis of clinical signs, a CSF lymphocytic pleocytosis and/or a suggestive MRI or histological appearance (Figure 15.9). For example, a feline polioencephalomyelitis and a non-suppurative encephalomyelitis have been described and are suspected to be of viral origin. Some cases will make a spontaneous recovery without treatment; some seem to be immune-mediated and respond to immunosuppressive therapy. It is likely that new techniques such as PCR will allow new viral diseases to be identified (see also Borna disease, below).

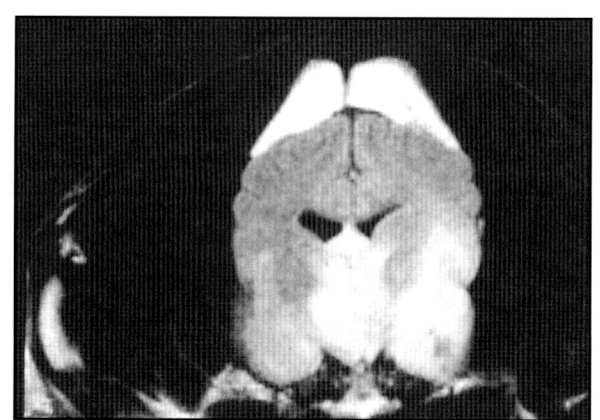

Figure 15.9: Magnetic resonance image from a 4-year-old Boxer, which presented after status epilepticus. A FLAIR transverse brain image is shown. There is increased signal (i.e. white) within the limbic system, indicative of oedema. The multifocal nature suggests an inflammatory aetiology and the grey matter localization a viral cause. A similar appearance has been seen in humans with herpesvirus encephalitis. Cerebrospinal fluid analysis revealed a mild lymphocytic/ neutrophilic pleocytosis; virus isolation and serology for canine herpesvirus and distemper virus were negative.

INFECTIONS RESULTING IN MULTIFOCAL NEUROLOGICAL SIGNS

Infections that are associated with multifocal neurological signs in dogs and cats are summarized in Figures 15.10 and 15.11, respectively.

Disease	Common clinical signs	CSF cell count	CSF protein	CSF cytology	Other useful diagnostic tests	Frequency
Neosporosis	PNS/muscle and hepatic involvement typical	Normal to mildly increased	Normal to mildly increased	Neutrophils Eosinophils	Antibody titres Serum biochemistry Electrophysiology Radiography	Occasional
Distemper	Seizures Caudal fossa disease Optic neuritis Spinal cord signs Spinal pain	Normal to moderately increased	Normal to moderately increased	Mononuclear cells occasionally mixed	CSF antibody titre MRI Indirect immunofluorescence antigen test	Occasional
Cryptococcosis	Seizures and caudal fossa disease +/- systemic signs	Normal to moderately increased	Mildly to markedly increased	Mixed (mononuclear and PMN cells)	Demonstration of organisms by India ink stain CRAG titre (serum/CSF) MRI/CT	Rare
Toxoplasmosis	Altered mental state, seizures Systemic signs	Normal to moderately increased	Normal to mildly increased	Mixed (mononuclear and PMN cells)	Serum biochemistry Radiography Antibody titres Electrophysiology	Rare
Rabies	Behavioural changes Paralysis, CN signs	Unknown	Unknown	Mononuclear cells	Antibody for viral antigen	Rare
Tick-borne encephalitis	Pyrexia, PNS signs, altered mental state, seizures, vestibular signs	Mildly to markedly increased	Mildly to markedly increased	Mononuclear cells, predominantly lymphocytes	Serum/CSF antibody titre	Seasonal in endemic areas only (central Northern Europe)
Neuroborreliosis	PNS signs (especially facial nerve) and pain	Unknown	Unknown	Unknown	Serum/CSF antibody titre Erythematous skin lesion about 7 weeks previously	Endemic areas only
Pseudorabies (Aujeszky's disease)	Peracute usually rapidly fatal disease Ptyalism, pruritus, depression, restlessness, aimless wandering	Unknown	Unknown	Unknown	History of contact with pigs or cattle Ingestion of contaminated meat or offal	Rare

Figure 15.10: Infections resulting in multifocal CNS signs in the dog. CN, cranial nerve; CT, computed tomography; MRI, magnetic resonance imaging; mildly increased (cerebrospinal fluid (CSF) 5–50 cells/ml, total protein <1 g/l); moderately increased (CSF >50 cells/ml, total protein >1g/l); markedly increased (CSF >500 cells/ml, total protein >2g/l); PMN, polymorphonuclear cells. PNS, peripheral nervous system.

238 Manual of Canine and Feline Infectious Diseases

Disease	Common clinical signs	CSF cell count	CSF protein	CSF cytology	Other useful diagnostic tests	Frequency
Neosporosis	PNS/muscle and hepatic involvement typical	Normal to mildly increased	Normal to mildly increased	Neutrophils Eosinophils	Antibody titres Serum biochemistry Electrophysiology Radiography	Occasional
Distemper	Seizures Caudal fossa disease Optic neuritis Spinal cord signs Spinal pain	Normal to moderately increased	Normal to moderately increased	Mononuclear cells occasionally mixed	CSF antibody titre MRI Indirect immunofluorescence antigen test	Occasional
Cryptococcosis	Seizures and caudal fossa disease +/− systemic signs	Normal to moderately increased	Mildly to markedly increased	Mixed (mononuclear and PMN cells)	Demonstration of organisms by India ink stain CRAG titre (serum/CSF) MRI/CT	Rare
Toxoplasmosis	Altered mental state, seizures Systemic signs	Normal to moderately increased	Normal to mildly increased	Mixed (mononuclear and PMN cells)	Serum biochemistry Radiography Antibody titres Electrophysiology	Rare
Rabies	Behavioural changes Paralysis, CN signs	Unknown	Unknown	Mononuclear cells	Antibody for viral antigen	Rare
Tick-borne encephalitis	Pyrexia, PNS signs, altered mental state, seizures, vestibular signs	Mildly to markedly increased	Mildly to markedly increased	Mononuclear cells, predominantly lymphocytes	Serum/CSF antibody titre	Seasonal in endemic areas only (central Northern Europe)
Neuroborreliosis	PNS signs (especially facial nerve) and pain	Unknown	Unknown	Unknown	Serum/CSF antibody titre Erythematous skin lesion about 7 weeks previously	Endemic areas only
Pseudorabies (Aujeszky's disease)	Peracute usually rapidly fatal disease Ptyalism, pruritus, depression, restlessness, aimless wandering	Unknown	Unknown	Unknown	History of contact with pigs or cattle Ingestion of contaminated meat or offal	Rare

Figure 15.10: Infections resulting in multifocal CNS signs in the dog.
CN, cranial nerve; CT, computed tomography; MRI, magnetic resonance imaging; mildly increased (cerebrospinal fluid (CSF) 5–50 cells/ml, total protein <1 g/l); moderately increased (CSF >50 cells/ml, total protein >1g/l); markedly increased (CSF >500 cells/ml, total protein >2g/l); PMN, polymorphonuclear cells. PNS, peripheral nervous system.

Toxoplasmosis

Toxoplasma gondii is an apicomplexan protozoan with an intestinal sexual stage in the cat and an asexual tissue stage in mammals or birds (Figure 15.12). Clinical disease is always related to the extraintestinal stage, which rapidly multiplies and is dispersed to other tissues via lymph and blood. Intracellular multiplication results in cell death, and, in the event of a heavy infection, widespread tissue necrosis may be present. In most instances the host's antibody response limits the invasion and induces the parasite to encyst in the brain, skeletal and cardiac muscles or liver (Dubey, 1994). These tissue cysts survive for the life of the organism, and clinical disease only occurs if they are reactivated.

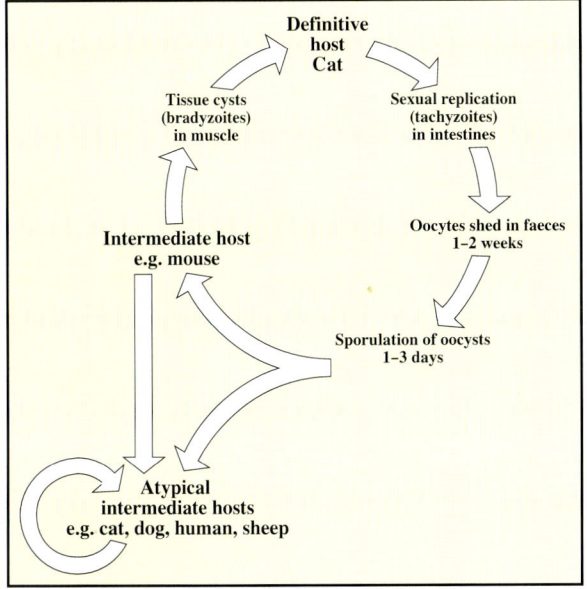

Figure 15.12: Life cycle of Toxoplasma gondii.

Animals can be infected by *T. gondii* after ingestion of infective tissues or by ingestion of food or water contaminated with infective faeces; most infections are subclinical. If infection of a naive animal occurs during pregnancy, *T. gondii* can multiply in the placenta and spread to the fetus.

Clinical signs

Toxoplasmosis is often included in the differential diagnoses of neurological diseases, but it is rare. It is a multisystemic infection; neurological signs are seen in about 10% of affected animals, are multifocal in nature and may include derangement of consciousness, seizures, visual loss, poor coordination, circling, torticollis, anisocoria and spinal cord dysfunction. It is highly unlikely that the animal will only have neurological signs. Systemic signs, in approximate order of prevalence, include:

- Pyrexia
- Anorexia
- Ophthalmitis (especially uveitis)
- Pneumonia
- Hepatitis
- Myositis
- Pancreatitis
- Myocarditis
- Cutaneous lesions (rare).

Descriptions of many of these signs are provided in the appropriate chapters in this manual. Although immunosuppression is thought to play a part in the development of toxoplasmosis, comparatively few animals have concurrent infections or illnesses. Feline immunodeficiency virus (FIV) infection does not predispose towards toxoplasmosis, unlike HIV in humans; however, severe immunosuppression caused by canine distemper virus (CDV) can activate latent protozoal infections (Tipold *et al.*, 1992).

Diagnosis

Haematological changes, if present, are non-specific. Abnormal liver enzyme and bile acid concentrations are common. Animals with pancreatitis may have increased concentrations of amylase and/or lipase. Myositis may be indicated by an increased CK concentration. Thoracic radiographs may reveal a diffuse interstitial and alveolar pneumonia and compensatory emphysema.

It is difficult to diagnose toxoplasmosis confidently. The only dependable method is to demonstrate tachyzoites in a biopsy or aspirate from an animal with appropriate clinical signs (Figure 15.13). Alternatively a presumptive diagnosis can be made using serology, clinical signs of disease, exclusion of other causes and response to antiprotozoal drugs. Tests for IgG antibodies are unreliable as many animals have a low or negative titre in acute toxoplasmosis. In addition most cats are exposed to *T. gondii* and many normal cats will have a high titre and remain positive for months to years post infection. A fourfold increase in an IgG titre is indicative of recent or active infection, but this necessitates two samples 2-4 weeks apart and not all animals show such an increase.

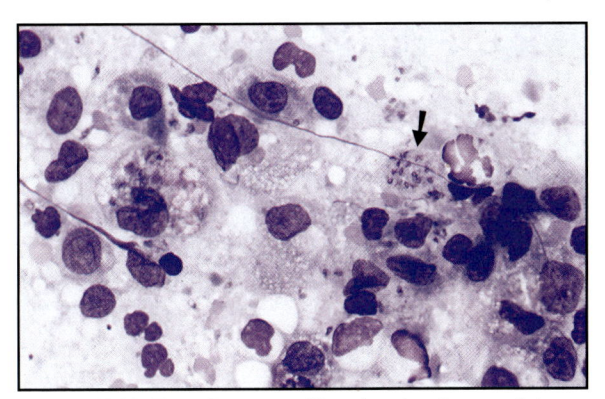

Figure 15.13: Toxoplasma gondii *tachyzoites (arrowed) in an imprint of consolidated lung tissue. When such pyogranulomatous lesions exudate into the airways it may be possible to identify macrophages and tachyzoites on a bronchoalveolar lavage (BAL) preparation. BAL is preferable to tracheal wash because it retrieves cells from the small airways. (Picture kindly donated by Dr Glade Weiser, HESKA Corporation.)*

A positive IgM titre is a more reliable indication of a recent or active infection. Experimentally, positive titres develop within 2-3 weeks post inoculation and are generally negative by 16 weeks post inoculation. CSF antibody titres may be useful; however, normal cats can be positive.

The accuracy of the diagnostic testing depends on the methodology. The modified agglutination test (using acetone-fixed tachyzoites) is superior to the Sabin-Feldman dye test, and IgM and IgG ELISAs. The commercially available latex agglutination and indirect haemagglutination tests, which use soluble *T. gondii* antigens, have a low sensitivity (Dubey *et al.*, 1995a,b).

Treatment
T. gondii is sensitive to clindamycin and combinations of sulphonamide with dihydrofolate reductase and thymidylate inhibitors (e.g. trimethoprim and pyrimethamine). A combination of trimethoprim, a sulphonamide and pyrimethamine is believed to be superior; however, haematological variables should be monitored, and folic acid supplementation is advisable. Corticosteroid therapy is contraindicated.

Control
Toxoplasmosis is a major cause of death in HIV-infected humans, and congenital infection can result in mental retardation and blindness. It is also an important cause of abortion and neonatal mortality in sheep and goats. Cats that have shed *T. gondii* cysts are immune to reshedding of oocysts for many months. FIV- and FeLV-infected cats do not shed more oocysts. The main sources of infection to humans are soil or litter trays contaminated with infected faeces or eating undercooked meat, especially lamb and pork. There are no drugs that will kill tissue cysts; however, they are killed in meat that is frozen to -12°C, cooked to an internal temperature of 67°C or gamma irradiated. The possibility of infection after touching cats is minimal due to their fastidious grooming and because their hard faeces do not stick to their fur.

Toxoplasma-like protozoans
Toxoplasma-like cysts have been reported as incidental findings in cats' brains and as a cause of myelitis. They are morphologically distinct from *T. gondii* and about twice the size. Disease seems to be associated with bradyzoites rather than tachyzoites.

Neospora caninum
Neospora caninum is structurally similar to *T. gondii* but immunologically distinct; until 1988 infections were misdiagnosed as toxoplasmosis. Like *T. gondii*, *Neospora* has a sexual phase in the definitive host and an asexual phase in the intermediate host. Unlike *T. gondii*, *N. caninum* tissue cysts are only found in the CNS and the dog is the definitive host (McAllister *et al.*, 1998). Clinical disease in dogs is only associated with the asexual phase (Figure 15.14). There is no evidence of natural feline infection. *Neospora* infection is one of the most important causes of bovine abortion and can cause clinical disease in sheep, goats and horses.

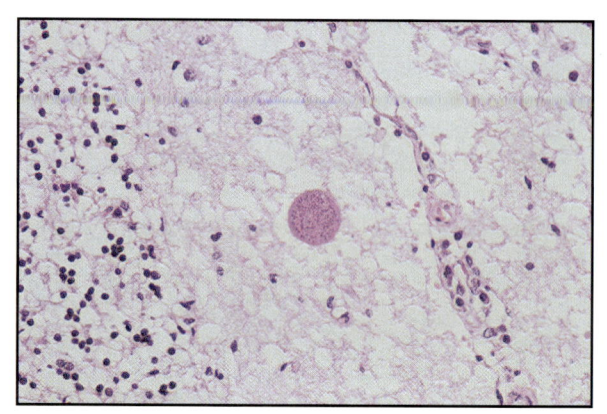

Figure 15.14: Neospora *bradyzoite cyst within the brain of an 18-month-old Boxer euthanased after a 6-month progressive history of paraparesis with urinary and faecal incontinence. Unlike toxoplasmosis, bradyzoite cysts are found only within the CNS in neosporosis. Dogs are both intermediate and definitive hosts for* Neospora caninum.

Clinical signs
Disease in the dog is characterized by two clinical syndromes dependent on the age of the dog. Transplacental infection of puppies results in a rapidly progressive and ascending paraplegia with faecal and urinary incontinence. The combination of polyradiculoneuritis, myositis and upper motor neuron paralysis commonly results in rigid pelvic limb extension (Figure 15.15). Such infections are acquired from dams who are carriers and do not develop clinical signs of disease (Dubey, 1992). In older dogs the clinical syndrome can be subtler and is characterized by multifocal nervous system disease. There is almost always disease of the peripheral nerves and muscle. Like toxoplasmosis, neosporosis can be a multisystemic infection; however, evidence of pneumonia, hepatitis, pancreatitis, myocarditis or dermatitis is less common than in toxoplasmosis. Pyrexia and anorexia are unusual in the early stages of disease (Barber and Trees, 1996). Older dogs may have been infected transplacentally; however, the role of other sources of infection is not known.

Diagnosis
Haematological changes, if present, are often non-specific; occasionally there is an eosinophilia. Increased concentrations of creatine kinase, alanine aminotransferase and bile acids are common. Radiographs may demonstrate hepatomegaly and pulmonary involvement. Hepatic changes may be seen with ultrasonography. Electromyography may reveal spontaneous muscle activity - a consequence of denervation or myositis. Nerve conduction velocities

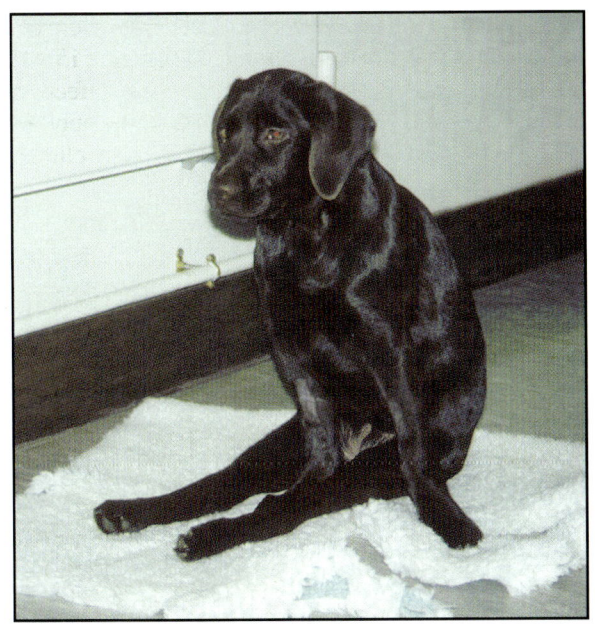

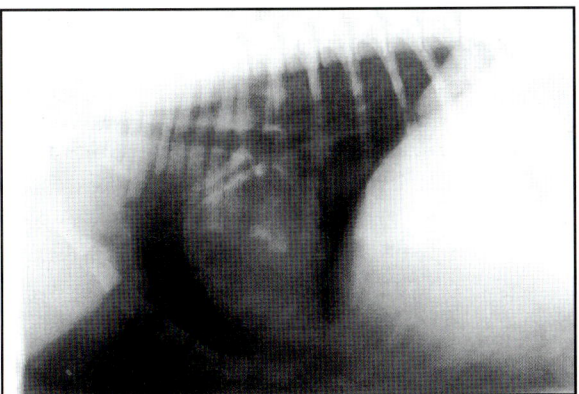

Figure 15.15: A 15-week-old puppy with neonatal neosporosis. The puppy had a 7-day history of pelvic limb proprioceptive deficits, progressing to areflexic paraplegia with faecal and urinary incontinence. Note the rigid pelvic limb hyperextension. (Reproduced from Journal of Small Animal Practice *(1995)* **36***, 172–177 with permission.) The thoracic radiograph shows an interstitial pattern of the dorsal lung fields and hepatomegaly.*

may be normal or reduced. CSF may be normal or may show a neutrophilic or eosinophilic pleocytosis and increased protein concentration.

A positive antibody titre in addition to appropriate clinical signs is a reliable indication of infection. Dogs with clinical neosporosis have titres of 1:800 or higher (Barber and Trees, 1996). Titres often remain persistently increased despite successful therapy. Dams of affected puppies usually have titres of 1:200 or higher. Subsequent litters from these dams may be affected: the parasite may be reactivated and antibody titres can rise during pregnancy.

Treatment
A similar treatment regimen to that described above for toxoplasmosis is recommended. The prognosis is fair for adult-onset disease if the clinical signs are not severe and treatment is instigated promptly. The time course in puppies is rapid and dogs with pelvic limb hyperextension are unlikely to have a good outcome. As a precaution any puppy demonstrating neurological signs should be treated until titre results are obtained. If an infected puppy is identified inquiries should be made as to the health of the siblings as littermates are often also affected although not always simultaneously. Antibacterial treatment of the dam prior to or during pregnancy does not protect subsequent litters from being infected.

Cryptococcosis
Cryptococcus neoformans is a saprophytic fungus that rarely infects small animals. Pigeons are thought to be important in transmission; however, cases can occur in indoor cats. The organism is protected by a hypoantigenic capsule, and as a result infection stimulates very little inflammatory response. The usual route of infection is inhalation of the aerosolized organism, and concurrent immunosuppression is thought to be important in the pathogenesis. The animal should be investigated for concurrent disease, e.g. FIV/FeLV infection or neoplasia. Spread to the CNS is haematogenous or a result of direct extension through the cribriform plate.

Clinical signs
The signs of CNS involvement are of a space-occupying lesion or are secondary to obstruction of CSF flow (e.g. hydrocephalus, raised intracranial pressure and papilloedema). Onset is very variable but signs are typically slowly progressive. Although the organism is found in the meninges, the animal does not display signs commonly attributed to meningitis because there is a minimal inflammatory reaction. Neurological signs are typically multifocal; seizures, altered mental status and caudal fossa signs (e.g. ataxia, vestibular syndrome, cranial nerve deficits, cerebellar disease) are the most common. Solitary brain or epidural spinal masses can also occur. The CNS may be the only system involved or may be part of a more generalized disease. Other common clinical signs include anorexia, lethargy, weight loss, ocular disease (especially chorioretinitis), nasal/respiratory signs, gastrointestinal signs and cutaneous lesions. Pyrexia is not a common sign (Berthelin *et al.*, 1994a; Gerds-Grogan and Dayrell-Hart, 1997).

Diagnosis
Haematology is usually unremarkable but there may be a monocytosis (Gerds-Grogan and Dayrell-Hart, 1997). CSF analysis may demonstrate a neutrophilic, eosinophilic, mononuclear or mixed pleocytosis with an increased protein concentration (Berthelin *et al.*, 1994b). There is a high risk of brain herniation after CSF sampling. Changes may be seen on MR and CT images.

The diagnosis can be confirmed by demonstration of the organism or by a latex agglutination test for capsule antigen (CRAG titre). Antibody titres are not useful because of the lack of a host immune response. The easiest way to demonstrate the organism is in cytological specimens (e.g. nasal exudate, urine, CSF, pleural effusion; Figure 15.16). Biopsy of lesions or culture (and sensitivity) on Sabouraud's dextrose is also possible. A positive CRAG titre is a fairly reliable indication of disease; however, false positives do occur. If a positive CRAG titre result is the only indication of disease then a presumptive diagnosis can based on response to treatment (Berthelin *et al.*, 1994b).

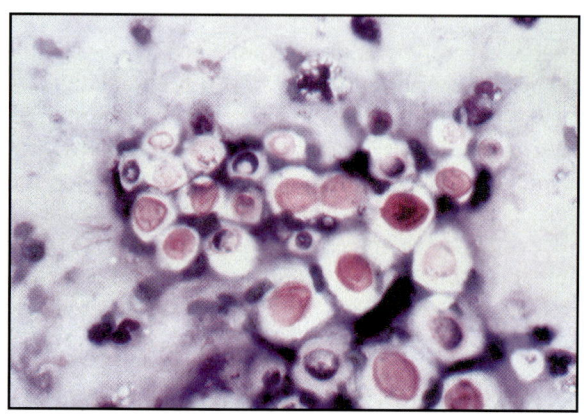

Figure 15.16: Cryptococcus neoformans *stained with Wright's Giemsa. Most stains (including Diff-Quik®) will not affect the capsule so that the organism itself appears in a clear halo, sharply demarcated from the background. Mayer's mucicarmin stains the capsule red, and India ink stains it black. (Picture kindly donated by Dr Glade Weiser, HESKA Corporation.)*

Treatment
Fluconazole or itraconazole are the agents of choice for CNS cryptococcosis. Flucytosine and ketoconazole are cheaper, but less effective, alternatives. Two to three weeks of therapy may be required before visible improvement. There is a danger of withdrawing therapy too early, and it is recommended to continue treatment until there are two negative CRAG titre results 1 month apart. If titres are still positive after 2 years then treatment should be discontinued if the titre is not rising. In the event of fulminating life-threatening disease, treatment should be initiated with amphotericin B and then switched to one of the above drugs as soon as the animal is stable.

The clinician may also need to manage the increased intracranial pressure. Corticosteroids may not adversely affect the outcome but should not continue after antifungal treatment is started. Ventricular shunt placement has been advocated for management of hydrocephalus, and surgical removal of large brain or spinal masses is also recommended. These procedures require referral to a specialist neurosurgical service.

Other fungal diseases
Other fungi that cause disseminated disease fall into two groups:

- Primary pathogens, e.g. *Histoplasma* and *Blastomyces*
- Opportunistic invaders, e.g. *Aspergillus* and *Penicillium*.

The primary pathogens do not occur in the UK. Neurological involvement due to infection with *Aspergillus* or *Penicillium* tends to be seen as a rare consequence of discospondylitis or osteomyelitis. Extension of nasal aspergillosis through the cribriform plate has also been seen.

Distemper
Neurological signs of distemper virus infection may occur 2 weeks to many years after systemic signs. In some instances systemic signs may have been mild or not present at all. Neurological signs may be seen in vaccinated dogs, presumably because there is infection with a wild strain to which the dog is not fully protected. Virus replication in the acute form of the disease induces a non-inflammatory demyelination, which may be fatal if the host is unable to mount an immune response. If the immune response is suboptimal, the virus may persist and stimulate an inflammatory demyelination owing to the release of toxic substances (Tipold *et al.*, 1992).

Clinical signs
Clinical signs may be focal or multifocal and are acute in onset and progressive. Common features include:

- Seizures
- Depression
- Caudal fossa signs (e.g. vestibular syndrome, cranial nerve deficits, cerebellar disease)
- Optic neuritis
- Behavioural changes
- Spinal cord signs.

Myoclonus is said to be a classic sign but actually occurs in less than 50% of cases. Distemper virus infection may predispose towards protozoal infections (Tipold *et al.*, 1992). It has also been suggested that distemper virus may be involved in the pathogenesis of subacute diffuse sclerosing encephalitis (so-called 'old dog encephalitis'). This rare disease is characterized by central blindness, personality change, dementia and compulsive pacing/circling, depressed postural responses and exaggerated spinal reflexes (Vandevelde *et al.*, 1980). Other more common causes of cortical dysfunction, e.g. neoplasia, hepatic encephalopathy or granulomatous meningoencephalomyelitis, should be excluded before diffuse sclerosing encephalitis can be diagnosed.

The diagnosis and treatment of canine distemper are covered in Chapter 6.

Feline infectious peritonitis

Feline infectious peritonitis (FIP) is the most common infectious meningoencephalomyelitis in cats, and neurological signs are generally associated with the dry form of the disease. The most common neurological signs are:

- Altered mental state
- Central vestibular disease
- Proprioceptive deficits
- Tetraparesis/plegia
- Seizures
- Cerebellar signs
- Spinal pain
- Cranial nerve deficits.

Signs are usually multifocal but may be focal; involvement of the caudal fossa (brain stem and cerebellum) is very common. About two thirds of cases have systemic signs in association with neurological signs (Kline *et al.*, 1994). CSF analysis can be helpful for diagnosis (Baroni and Heinold, 1995). In comparison to other feline viral diseases which generally have low cell counts and protein levels, CSF white blood cell counts are usually >100 cells/µl and consist predominantly of neutrophils. CSF protein concentration is typically >2 g/l (Rand *et al.*, 1994). A positive result for CSF anti-FCoV antibody titre is very suggestive of disease (provided the sample is uncontaminated with blood); serum antibody measurements are variable and assays may, rarely, give negative results. Non-productive CSF taps are common as CSF pathways become obstructed by inflammatory cells. Further diagnostic imaging such as MRI and CT may be useful; obstructive hydrocephalus and hydromyelia with contrast enhancement of the choroid plexus (choroiditis), meninges (meningitis) and ependyma (ependymitis) have been described (Kline *et al.*, 1994; Thomas 1999). FIP is discussed in detail in Chapter 9.

Feline leukaemia virus

Feline leukaemia virus (FeLV) does not seem to directly infect the nervous system; however, it may cause neurological signs by oncogenic or immunosuppressive mechanisms. Besides lymphoma (the most common CNS tumour in the cat), FeLV has also been implicated in the development of olfactory neuroblastoma (Schrenzel *et al.*, 1990). FeLV may also predispose animals to other diseases such as cryptococcidiosis. FeLV is discussed in detail in Chapter 5.

INFECTIONS RESULTING IN ALTERED BEHAVIOUR

Rabies

Rabies is a disease of worldwide importance (Figure 15.17). In 1994 there were 34,110 human deaths recorded from the disease and almost all were from dog bites. The virus is inoculated by the bite into muscle from where it migrates towards the CNS via the peripheral nerves. Once in the CNS replication initially occurs in grey matter and then the virus disseminates rapidly via the white matter tracts. Subsequently the virus spreads centrifugally along neural pathways to salivary glands, serous glands, heart and skin.

Any mammal may be infected with rabies and in most rabies-infected parts of the world the disease is maintained in a wildlife reservoir. In most of Europe rabies is found principally in foxes, with dogs, cattle, horses and humans being regarded as aberrant, end hosts. Oral vaccination has resulted in a 65% decrease in cases of fox rabies over the 12 years to 1997 (Müller, 1997). In other parts of the world, notably the Indian subcontinent, Asia, Africa and Central and South America, the dog is a major reservoir of rabies. Turkey is the only European country with a rabies reservoir in dogs. A 10-year survey of British bats failed to demonstrate any evidence of rabies (Whitby *et al.*, 1996).

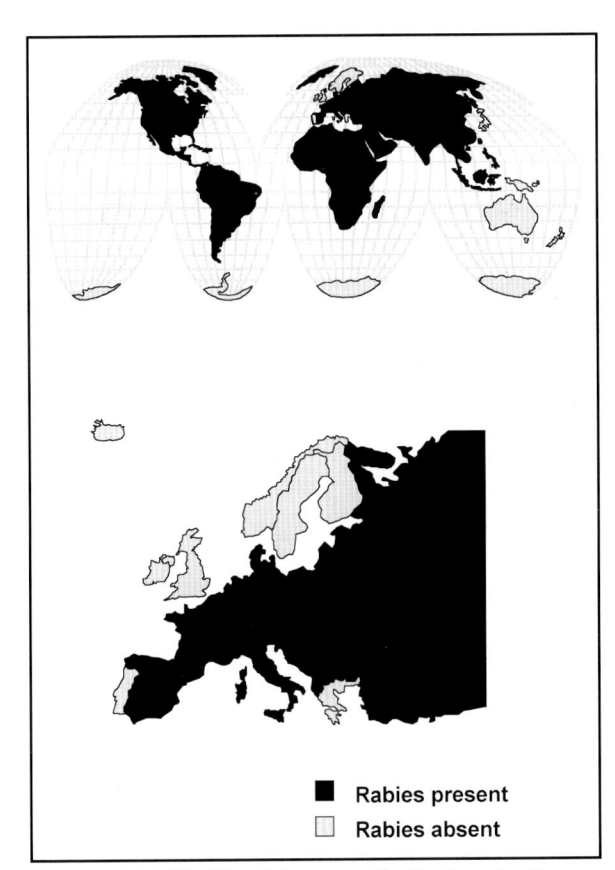

Figure 15.17: World and European distribution of rabies.

Clinical signs

The incubation period is very variable (12 days to 1 year) but the average is 4–6 weeks. The incubation period is shorter when a larger initial dose of virus is given or when the bite is on the head or neck. Clinical signs are traditionally divided into furious (Figure 15.18a), encephalitic and paralytic dumb forms (Figure 15.18b); however, the distinction is often not clear and both presentations progress towards paralysis, coma, circulatory insufficiency and death. Animals mounting an immune response seem to get the furious form and die more quickly. The dumb form is very uncommon in cats. Pyrexia, excitability and nervousness are early signs. Other behavioural changes include hypersensitivity, abnormal vocalization, abnormal sexual behaviour and attacking/eating inanimate objects. In the dumb form the animal is more lethargic although it may still bite. Cranial nerve signs may be observed such as dysphonia and dysphagia (resulting in drooling of saliva). Paralytic weakness may initially start in the bitten limb and progress to involve all limbs and pharyngeal and respiratory muscles; seizures rarely occur (Wandeler, 1995). Rabies can resemble several other conditions (Figure 15.19).

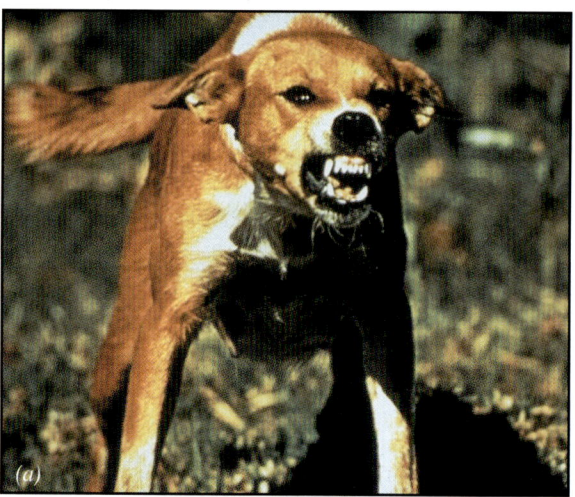

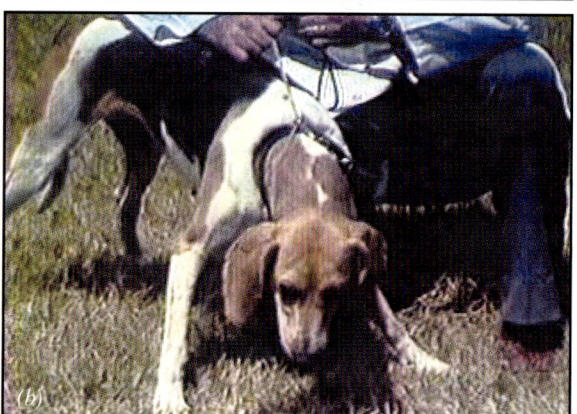

Figure 15.18: Rabies. (a) The 'furious' form of the disease is only seen in some cases. (Photograph courtesy of Mérial.) Animals with the paralytic or dumb form (b, courtesy of Dr Stephen Simpson) may still display unprovoked aggression.

Behavioural changes
Brain neoplasia
Bacterial, viral, protozoal or fungal infections, granulomatous meningoencephalomyelitis or other inflammations (see Figures 15.7, 15.10 and 15.11)
Acquired hydrocephalus
Cerebral infarct
Toxicity, e.g. lead
Thiamine deficiency
Degenerative CNS disorders, e.g. lysosomal storage diseases
Metabolic disease, e.g. hepatic or uraemic encephalopathy, hypoglycaemia
Pica as a consequence of systemic disorders, e.g. anaemia
Dysphonia/dysphagia/drooling saliva
Neuromuscular disease, e.g. myasthenia gravis, polyneuropathies, trigeminal neuritis, facial nerve paralysis and myopathies
Brain stem lesions, e.g. neoplasia
Oesophageal foreign body
Pharyngeal disease
Idiopathic phenobarbitone-responsive hypersalivation
Tetanus
Paresis
Neuromuscular disease, e.g. myasthenia gravis, polyneuropathies
Disc disease
Spinal neoplasia
Bacterial, viral, protozoal or fungal infections, granulomatous meningoencephalomyelitis or other inflammatory conditions (see Figures 15.7, 15.10 and 15.11)

Figure 15.19: Differential diagnoses for rabies.

Public health considerations

With the exception of an outbreak after the First World War (due to soldiers smuggling dogs into Britain), rabies has been absent from Britain since the introduction of quarantine in 1901 apart from a few isolated cases in quarantined animals.

Rabies is a notifiable disease in the UK. Anyone who knows or suspects that an animal has rabies in the UK must report it immediately to the police or their local divisional veterinary office. Detailed plans have been established under the Rabies (Control) Order 1974 for the handling of such cases. The animal should be kept in a cage and euthanasia should not be performed while awaiting further instructions from the relevant authorities (who are called Consultants in Communicable Disease Control in England and Wales and Consultants in Public Health Medicine for Communicable Disease and Environmental Health in

Scotland). About 25 cases of suspected rabies are investigated each year. Since 1970 none has proven positive, but eternal vigilance is the price of safety.

If a human is bitten by an animal that is suspected to have rabies then the wound should be washed immediately and aggressively with a 20% soap solution or a quaternary ammonium compound. Ethanol solution (43% or stronger) can also be applied to wounds. Deep puncture wounds can be effectively cleaned by irrigation using a 20 ml syringe. Medical help should be sought while this washing is in progress. Immediate vaccination is most successful when combined with local and systemic human rabies immune globulin although passive immunization is not always necessary. Humans that are accidentally injected with animal rabies vaccines do not require post-exposure prophylaxis.

Diagnosis
Fluorescent antibody testing for viral antigen in fresh refrigerated brain is the preferred technique at post mortem examination. Ante-mortem testing is also possible, but rather unreliable, on CSF, saliva, serum, cytological smears from nasal mucosa, and corneal and skin biopsies.

Treatment
There is no treatment for rabies, which is always fatal.

Control
Vaccination is effective at preventing rabies and should be used in all dogs and cats in countries where the disease is endemic. Inactivated vaccines are available in the UK for use in dogs and cats as part of the Pet Travel Scheme (see Appendix 2). Two injections, 2 to 4 weeks apart, are given as a primary course after the animal is 3 months old, and booster vaccinations should be given every 2 years (dogs) or 1 year (cats). A modified live virus vaccine is available in some other countries.

Vaccine-induced rabies
The modified live virus vaccine (not available in the UK) may result in clinical disease in dogs and cats 10–21 days after vaccination. A flaccid paralysis of the inoculated limb develops first, then the contralateral limb becomes involved and the disease progresses over a few days to rigidity in all four limbs and dementia. The prognosis is guarded; clinical recovery has been reported in dogs after 1–3 months. In dogs a polyradiculoneuritis can develop characterized by flaccid tetraparesis and depressed spinal reflexes. This carries a reasonable prognosis, and regeneration of peripheral nerves occurs in 1–2 months (Chrisman, 1991).

Borna disease and feline staggering disease
Borna disease virus (BDV) is endemic in eastern and southern Germany, eastern Switzerland and western Austria where it infects several large animal species. There has been a single case report in a dog, which displayed anorexia, lethargy and non-specified CNS signs. There is some evidence of its presence in the UK (Reeves *et al.*, 1998). Cats can become infected with a virus that is related to, but distinct from, Borna virus (Lundgren *et al.*, 1995). The disease produced is referred to as 'feline staggering disease'.

Clinical signs
Feline staggering disease initially presents as a behavioural change characterized by an initial hyperactivity, aggression or excitability followed by lethargy and withdrawal. Other signs may include pyrexia, hypersensitivity to sound and touch, skin tremors (especially of eyelids and whiskers), an altered voice and pelvic limb ataxia progressing to hindlimb paresis. In experimental disease the cats recovered from the acute phase, but some neurological deficits were permanent. It has been suggested that feline staggering disease and feline polioencephalomyelitis are the same disease as both are characterized by a non-suppurative meningo-encephalomyelitis (Lundgren *et al.*, 1995, 1997).

Diagnosis
Feline staggering disease is difficult to diagnose in the living animal. The virus is a commensal, and many healthy animals may express antibodies. Therefore demonstrating anti-Borna virus antibody is not useful. Experimentally infected and ill animals often do not develop circulating antibodies or develop them late in the disease course. To diagnose Borna virus infection definitively requires either a reverse transcriptase-polymerase chain reaction (RT-PCR) or immunohistochemistry. CSF analysis may reveal a mild mononuclear pleocytosis. MRI and CT should be performed to eliminate brain neoplasia, which is the most common pathological cause of behavioural change in the cat.

Treatment
Effective treatment has not been established. Immunosuppressive therapy may be effective as Borna disease is an immune-mediated disease and immunosuppressed animals are unaffected.

Feline immunodeficiency virus encephalopathy
Feline immunodeficiency virus (FIV) is a neurotropic virus that infects microglia and astrocytes resulting in neuronal damage and cortical atrophy. The virus enters the brain early in the disease process and may cause neurological abnormalities at any time; however, signs of an encephalopathy usually develop after clinical signs of immune system failure (Podell *et al.*, 1997). Neurological disease is only reported in 1–5% of naturally occurring cases of FIV, possibly because euthanasia is performed once clinical signs of immunological dysfunction develop. Secondary opportunistic infections, e.g. FIP and cryptococcosis, may result in neurological signs in FIV-infected cats.

Clinical signs

An early and persistent sign is abnormal stereotypical motor behaviour characterized by repetitive compulsive roaming. Other changes include aggression, reclusiveness, disorientation, polyphagia, excessive lip licking, changes in sleep patterns and stereotypical paddling of the limbs. Other neurological deficits include anisocoria with delayed pupillary light responses, ataxia with pelvic limb paresis and proprioceptive deficits, visual deficits and seizures.

Diagnosis

FIV encephalopathy may be suspected on the basis of appropriate clinical signs in an FIV-infected cat. Other causes of CNS disease, e.g. opportunistic infections and lymphoma, should be ruled out. CSF analysis may reveal a mild mononuclear pleocytosis and increased protein concentration. MRI may demonstrate cortical atrophy, mild ventricular enlargement owing to cortical atrophy and discrete white matter lesions. Electrophysiological abnormalities are common and include increased frontal cortex slow wave activity, abnormal spindle activity in slow wave sleep, delayed visual and auditory evoked responses, and decreased spinal and peripheral nerve conduction velocities.

Treatment

AZT has been shown to have an ameliorating affect on HIV encephalopathy, which seems to be a similar disease to FIV encephalopathy. See Chapter 5 for further details on FIV.

Feline spongiform encephalopathy

Feline spongiform encephalopathy (FSE) results from infection with an unclassified agent that is either an unconventional virus or an altered form of naturally occurring protein - the prion protein. The disease is characterized by fibril accumulation and neuronal disease or death. The agent is thought to be the same as that causing BSE in cattle and variant Creutzfeldt-Jakob disease in humans. FSE was first reported in 1990 and since specified bovine offal has been excluded from pet food, the incidence of FSE has been decreasing. FSE has been confined to Great Britain with the exception of single cases in Norway, Ireland and Liechtenstein.

Clinical signs

The disease has a long incubation period. It has not been seen in animals under 14 months old; the average age of affected cats is 7 years. Initial behavioural changes are characterized by nervousness or aggression and may precede more obvious neurological signs by several months or even years. Other reported changes include:

- Polyphagia
- Polydipsia
- Cessation of, or excessive, grooming
- Aberrant defecation or urination
- Drooling/excessive salivation
- Inability to retract claws
- Impaired vision
- Weight loss or gain (as in cattle)
- Muscle fasciculation
- Bruxism.

Affected cats develop a characteristic gait often described as staggering or crouching. It is similar to the gait seen with cerebellar disease but probably reflects disease of the extrapyramidal system. They often have a resting head tremor and are hyperaesthetic to sound and touch. Seizures and nystagmus are rarely seen. Once gait abnormalities develop, the progression is often rapid over 1-3 months.

Diagnosis

At present the diagnosis can only be confirmed by histopathology, although the clinical signs may be very suggestive of the condition. Post mortem examination should be carried out by a veterinary pathologist, and the disease is notifiable after a histological diagnosis. There is no effective treatment.

Feline parvovirus

Infection of queens with feline parvovirus in late pregnancy may result in a variety of defects in their kittens. The most common of these is cerebellar hypoplasia. Affected kittens may have a wide based crouching gait with an intention tremor. Affected kittens may seem normal at rest. Not all kittens in a litter are affected to the same extent. Other defects include forebrain lesions, which result in seizures and behavioural changes and retinal damage. These may occur independently of cerebellar hypoplasia. Affected kittens may learn to compensate and so may make suitable indoor pets. Kittens infected *in utero* with feline parvovirus may excrete the virus for the first 6 weeks of life and so may be a source of environmental contamination. See Chapter 8 for further information on the diagnosis and management of feline parvovirus.

INFECTIONS RESULTING IN MUSCLE SPASM

Tetanus

Tetanus is a consequence of contamination of wounds with spores of the anaerobic bacterium *Clostridium tetani*. The spores convert to the vegetative form, multiply and produce two exotoxins, which bind to axons of peripheral nerves and ascend to the spinal cord within a few hours. The toxins then bind to the neuronal cell bodies of inhibitory interneurons, preventing the release of the inhibitory neurotransmitter glycine and resulting in overactivity of motor neurons. Blood and CSF distribution of the toxin also occurs.

Clinical signs

Clinical signs develop 2–20 days after the initial wounding. The classic signs of a rocking-horse stance, lock jaw and risus sardonicus are easy to recognize (Figure 15.20); however, it is preferable to recognize early signs of muscle spasm before the animal becomes critically ill. Clinical signs are often most pronounced in the area where the toxin has first gained access to the nervous system. Cats are more resistant than dogs and may develop localized tetanus (Figure 15.21). In severe cases respiratory distress can result from spasm of the larynx or respiratory muscles and there may be sympathetic signs such as arrhythmias, elevated blood pressure, hyperthermia and vasoconstriction.

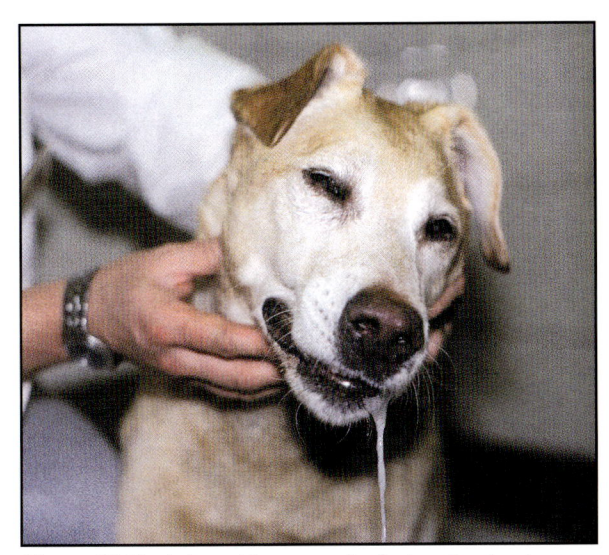

Figure 15.20: A dog with tetanus displaying the classic risus sardonicus (sneering expression) owing to released inhibition of the facial nerve. The ears are pulled erect and the forehead is wrinkled. There is a torticollis due to unequal involvement of the neck muscles. Saliva is falling from the mouth due to swallowing difficulties. The dog's first signs were difficulty opening the jaw and inability to close the left eye 2 weeks after dental treatment. Full signs of generalized tetanus were apparent 5 days later.

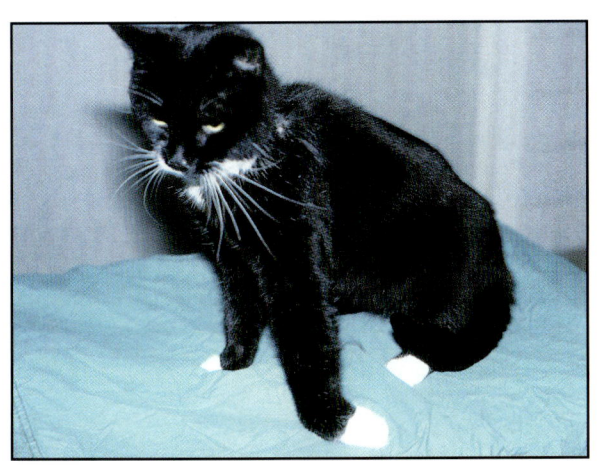

Figure 15.21: Localized tetanus in a cat. The spread of the toxin has been restricted to neurons innervating local muscle groups close to the site of injury, and the signs of muscle stiffness are confined to one limb only. (Courtesy of Malcolm McKee.)

Diagnosis

There are very few diseases that result in acute onset muscle stiffness, and the clinical signs of generalized tetanus are highly suggestive of the condition. Localized tetanus can be more confusing depending on the muscle groups involved. Muscle enzyme concentrations may be increased and electromyography demonstrates non-specific changes. Bacterial culture from wounds is nearly always unrewarding. The main differential diagnosis of both forms of tetanus is a polymyositis. The distinction between tetanus and a polymyositis is usually made on clinical grounds. Muscle pain, less resistance to limb flexion (especially on repeated stimulation) and very high concentrations of creatine kinase are more prominent in cases of polymyositis. The possibility of strychnine poisoning should also be eliminated.

Treatment

The aims of treatment are: to stop further toxin production; to prevent further toxin binding; and to provide supportive care. It is important to search for and debride wounds; the most common sites are the digits.

The most appropriate antibacterials are penicillin (amoxycillin and ampicillin are less effective) or metronidazole and these should initially be given intravenously.

Tetanus antitoxin at a dose of 30 000–100 000 IU for dogs and 5000 IU for cats is given intravenously. A test dose of 0.1 ml subcutaneously should be given 30 minutes beforehand to ensure there are no adverse reactions. The antitoxin may be repeated on a daily basis; however, it is questionable whether this is beneficial. The author has found that outcome in severe cases is improved if antitoxin is also given intrathecally (500–3000 IU diluted 1 in 10 in sterile water), thus preventing spread of the toxin by CSF pathways. This should only be attempted by veterinary surgeons who are experienced at performing myelography. The antitoxin has no effect on bound toxin, which remains attached for 3 weeks or more. As a result clinical signs will take at least this long to resolve, and typically it is 2–3 months before the animal is normal.

Handling and stress aggravates the condition and the animal should be kennelled in a quiet darkened area. Management of hyperthermia (secondary to muscle contraction and sympathetic effects) can be difficult. Sedation with benzodiazepines, acepromazine or barbiturates can reduce muscle spasm. Other supportive care such as fluid therapy, turning every 4 hours and prevention of decubital ulcers is often necessary.

Affected animals may have eating difficulties due to trismus, spasm of the pharyngeal muscles, megaoesophagus or hiatal hernia. Feeding liquidized food is helpful, and in severe cases pharyngostomy or gastrostomy feeding may be necessary.

INFECTIONS RESULTING IN TETRAPARESIS

Botulism

Clostridium botulinum spores are normal inhabitants of the alimentary canal of herbivores and survive for long periods in the environment. Under anaerobic conditions the bacteria produce several types of neurotoxin. Dogs and cats seem to be most susceptible to type C neurotoxin.

The clinical syndrome of botulism can occur in three different ways:

- Ingestion of the preformed toxin in food or carrion
- Wound botulism after contamination of wound with spores
- Infant botulism (toxicoinfectious botulism) where bacteria succeed in germinating from spores in the intestine when they would otherwise be prevented from doing so by a normal gut flora.

The toxin initially binds to the exterior of somatic and autonomic nerve terminals (it is still susceptible to neutralization at this stage). Once acetylcholine release occurs the toxin passes into the nerve terminals and interferes with the further release of acetylcholine. The toxin binds irreversibly. Recovery is by axonal sprouting and reinnervation.

Clinical signs

Signs occur 1–2 days after consumption of food and 1–2 weeks after wound contamination and may be preceded by gastrointestinal signs. The speed of onset is proportional to the amount of toxin ingested and is characterized by an ascending flaccid paralysis with hyporeflexia. Cranial nerves are usually affected, resulting in dysphonia, dysphagia, facial paralysis and poor gag reflex and tongue movement with megaoesophagus. There may be parasympathetic signs such as decreased salivation and lacrimation, mydriasis with sluggish pupillary light reflexes, constipation and urinary retention. Sensation is preserved. Severe cases may die from cardiac arrest or respiratory failure. Even mild cases can die from aspiration pneumonia.

Diagnosis

There are very few infections that result in neuromuscular disease and other differentials should be considered (Figure 15.22). Serum biochemistry (including creatine kinase and aspartate aminotransferase) is useful to eliminate metabolic causes of weakness and inflammatory myopathies. Thoracic radiographs are advisable to assess for megaoesophagus, aspiration pneumonia and thymoma (associated with paraneoplastic diseases such as myasthenia gravis). In one study of canine botulism slow motor and sensory nerve conduction velocities were reported (Van Nes *et al.*, 1986). As the disease progresses, electromyography may demonstrate fibrillation potentials, prolonged insertional activity and spontaneous high voltage complexes (Scully *et al.*, 1997). Demonstration of the toxin is not practical (as it requires innoculation into mice). Culture of *C. botulinum* from faeces is difficult and the significance of isolating the organism is controversial. A nerve or muscle biopsy may be appropriate to exclude some non-infectious differential diagnoses. A laboratory should be contacted before the biopsy is obtained to ensure the sample is handled according to their specifications.

Botulism
Acute polyradiculoneuritis
Distal denervating disease
Myasthenia gravis
Neospora/Toxoplasma
Ionophore toxicity, e.g. lasalocid, monensin
Organophosphate and carbamate toxicity
Antibacterials associated neurotransmission disorder
Tick paralysis

Figure 15.22: *Differential diagnosis for acute onset flaccid paralysis.*

Treatment

Most cases survive with appropriate supportive care; the speed of recovery is inversely proportional to severity of intoxication and varies between 14 and 24 days. Laxatives or an enema are advisable to remove unabsorbed toxin. Polyvalent antitoxin is of questionable efficacy in dogs and cats and must be given before the toxin binds, i.e. before clinical signs become apparent. Drugs that enhance acetylcholine release, such as 3,4-diaminopyridine, should only be used in acute cases if antitoxins are also given to block further uptake of toxin (Critchley, 1991). If the animal has a megaoesophagus then feeding the animal from a height and raising the head, neck and chest for 30 minutes after feeding is advisable. If the animal is unable to lift its head and has a megaoesophagus then gastrostomy tube feeding is indicated. Thoracic radiographs should be obtained every few days to check for aspiration pneumonia and if present broad-spectrum antibacterials (against anaerobes and aerobes) should be given. Corticosteroids are contraindicated.

DRUG DOSAGES

See Appendix 3.

REFERENCES AND FURTHER READING

Barber JS and Trees AJ (1996) Clinical aspects of 27 cases of neosporosis in dogs. *Veterinary Record* **139**, 439-443

Baroni M and Heinold Y (1995) A review of the clinical diagnosis of feline infectious peritonitis viral meningoencephalomyelitis. *Progress in Veterinary Neurology* **6**, 88-93

Berthelin CF, Bailey CS, Kass PH, Legendre AM and Wolf AH (1994a) Cryptococcosis of the nervous system in dogs, Part 1: epidemiologic, clinical and neuropathological features *Progress in Veterinary Neurology* **5**, 88-97

Berthelin CF, Legendre AM, Bailey CS, Kass PH and Wolf AH (1994b) Cryptococcosis of the nervous system in dogs, Part 2: Diagnosis, treatment, monitoring, and prognosis *Progress in Veterinary Neurology* **5**, 136-146

BSAVA Scientific Committee (1996) Feline spongiform encephalopathy. *Journal of Small Animal Practice* **37**, 198-199

Chrisman CL (1991) Rabies. In: *Problems in Small Animal Neurology*, ed. CL Chrisman, pp. 151-153. Lea and Febiger, Philadelphia

Critchley EMR (1991) A comparison of human and animal botulism: a review. *Journal of the Royal Society of Medicine* **84**, 295-298

Dubey JP (1992) *Neospora caninum* infections. In: *Current Veterinary Therapy XI*, ed. RW Kirk, pp. 263-266. WB Saunders, Philadelphia

Dubey JP (1994) Toxoplasmosis. *Journal of the American Veterinary Medical Association* **205**, 1593-1598

Dubey JP, Lappin MR and Thulliez P (1995a) Diagnosis of induced toxoplasmosis in neonatal cats. *Journal of the American Veterinary Medical Association* **207**, 179

Dubey JP, Lappin MR and Thulliez P (1995b) Long term antibody responses of cats fed *Toxoplasma gondii* tissue cysts. *Journal of Parasitology* **81**, 887-893

Gerds-Grogan S and Dayrell-Hart B (1997) Feline cryptococcosis: a retrospective evaluation. *Journal of the American Animal Hospital Association* **33**, 118-122

Hemachudha T and Phuapradit P (1997) Rabies. *Current Opinion in Neurology* **10**, 260-267

Kline KL, Joseph RJ and Averill DR (1994) Feline infectious peritonitis with neurological involvement: clinical and pathological findings in 24 cats. *Journal of the American Animal Hospital Association* **30**, 111-118

Knockaert DC (1994) Bacterial meningitis: diagnostic and therapeutic considerations. *European Journal of Emergency Medicine* **1**, 92-103

Lundgren AL, Johannisson A, Zimmermann W, Bode L, Rozell B, Muluneh A, Lindberg R and Ludwig H (1997) Neurological disease and encephalitis in cats experimentally infected with Borna disease virus. *Acta Neuropathologica* **93**, 391-401

Lundgren AL, Zimmermann W, Bode L, Czech G, Gosztonyi G, Lindberg R and Ludwig H (1995) Staggering disease in cats: isolation and characterization of the feline Borna disease virus. *Journal of General Virology* **76**, 2215-2222

McAllister MM, Dubey JP, Lindsay DS, Jolley WR, Wills RA and McGuire AM (1998) Dogs are definitive hosts of *Neospora caninum*. *International Journal for Parasitology* **28**, 1473-1478

Podell M, Hayes K, Oglesbee M and Mathes L (1997) Progressive encephalopathy associated with CD4/CD8 inversion in adult FIV-infected cats. *Journal of Acquired Immune Deficiency Syndromes and Human Retrovirology* **15**, 332-340

Rand JS, Parent J, Percy D and Jacobs R (1994) Clinical, cerebrospinal fluid, and histological data from twenty-seven cats with primary inflammatory disease of the central nervous system. *Canadian Veterinary Journal* **35**, 103-110

Reeves NA, Helps CR, Gunn-Moore DA, Blundell C, Finnemore PL, Pearson GR and Harbour DA (1998) Natural Borna disease virus infection in cats in the United Kingdom. *Veterinary Record* **143**, 523

Schrenzel MD, Higgins RJ, Hinrichs SH, Smith MO and Torten M (1990) Type C retroviral expression in spontaneous feline olfactory neuroblastomas. *Acta Neuropathologica Berlin* **80**, 547-553

Scully RE, Mark EJ, McNeeley WF, Ebeling SH and Phillips LD (1997) Case records of the Massachusetts General Hospital. *New England Journal of Medicine* **337**, 184-190

Thomas WB (1999) Nonneoplastic disorders of the brain. *Clinical Techniques in Small Animal Practice* **14**, 125-147

Tipold A, Vandevelde A and Jaggy A (1992) Neurological manifestations of canine distemper virus infection. *Journal of Small Animal Practice* **33**, 466-470

Van Nes JJ, van der Most and van Spijk D (1986) Electrophysiological evidence of peripheral nerve dysfunction in six dogs with botulism Type C. *Research in Veterinary Science* **40**, 372-376

Vandevelde M, Kristensen B, Braund KG, Green CE, Swango LJ and Hoerlein BF (1980) Chronic canine distemper virus encephalitis in mature dogs. *Veterinary Pathology* **17**, 17-29

Wandeler AI (1995) The clinical disease in animals In: *Rabies in a changing world*, ed. PH Beynon and ATB Edney, pp. 8-12. BSAVA Publications, Cheltenham

Wheeler SJ (1995) *Manual of Small Animal Neurology*, 2nd edn. BSAVA Publications, Cheltenham

Whitby JE, Johnstone P, Parsons G, King AA and Hutson AM (1996) Ten-year survey of British bats for the existence of rabies. *Veterinary Record* **139**, 491-493

CHAPTER SIXTEEN

The Eye

David Gould

> **CHAPTER PLAN**
>
> **Introduction**
> **The ophthalmic examination**
>   Distinguishing conjunctivitis from uveitis
>   Approach to the 'red eye'
> **Conjunctivitis and keratitis**
>   Diagnostic plan for conjunctivitis and keratitis
>   Infectious conjunctivitis and keratitis in dogs
>   Infectious conjunctivitis and keratitis in cats
>   Feline herpesvirus and feline calicivirus
>   *Chlamydophila*
>   *Mycoplasma*
> **Dacryocystitis**
> **Uveitis and retinitis**
>   Differentiating active from inactive chorioretinitis
>   Diagnostic plan for uveitis and chorioretinitis
>   Infectious uveitis in dogs
>   Infectious uveitis in cats
> **Optic neuritis**
> **Further reading**

INTRODUCTION

The ocular surface is protected by mucosal surface immunity, mediated by lacrimal and conjunctival tissues. IgA, produced by plasma cells within the conjunctiva, coats its surface and is secreted into the tears. To a lesser extent, other antibody subtypes and immune cells are also present within the tear film. In addition, lacrimation has a flushing action to aid removal of surface contaminants. The conjunctiva has an extensive vascular supply and a large lymphoid cell population that reacts quickly and aggressively to pathogens. Mast cells allow an almost instantaneous immune response, by the release of cytokines upon antigen stimulation. Dendritic cells and macrophages constantly survey the conjunctival surface for antigens, which are processed and presented to helper T lymphocytes in the local lymph nodes. With chronic antigenic stimulation, lymphocyte expansion occurs locally within the conjunctiva itself, and lymphoid follicles may become grossly visible across the conjunctiva.

Because of this powerful mucosal immunity, primary bacterial infections of the ocular surface are uncommon in the dog. Most develop secondary to traumatic injury, eyelid abnormalities or tear film deficits. Primary bacterial infection is more common in the cat.

Intraocular infections can develop from penetrating wounds or haematogenous spread. An ophthalmic examination should always be included as part of a general physical examination where a systemic infectious disease is suspected, because it can give important clues to the aetiology and severity of the condition.

THE OPHTHALMIC EXAMINATION

A logical approach to the examination minimizes the risk of missing abnormalities. Figure 16.1 gives a suggested examination protocol.

Referral should be offered in all cases of uncertain diagnosis, as failure to provide prompt and accurate treatment can be deleterious to many eye conditions.

Distinguishing conjunctivitis from uveitis

Approach to the 'red eye'
Depending on their location within the eye, ocular infections may cause conjunctivitis, keratitis or uveitis. All these may present as painful reddened eyes and therefore when assessing such cases it is vital to identify the condition involved. It is not acceptable to prescribe a topical antibacterial and plan to assess the animal's response in a few days; conditions such as anterior uveitis need immediate treatment or extensive intraocular pathology can ensue, such as secondary glaucoma.

| 1 | **Distant examination before restraining animal for closer inspection** |

Subtle signs of ocular discomfort such as increased blink rate may disappear when the animal is faced with the stress of a hands-on examination.

| 2 | **Close examination** |

First in normal lighting conditions and then in a darkened room with focal illumination, with a transilluminator or a pen torch to examine the external globe, eyelids and periorbita.

| 3 | **Schirmer tear test** |

This should be performed in all cases of ocular discharge, conjunctivitis or lacklustre cornea, and must be performed before topical drops are applied.

| 4 | **Cranial nerve tests** |

These are performed in normal lighting conditions (menace and tracking responses, palpebral blink, corneal blink, oculocephalic reflex) and in the dark with focal illumination (direct and consensual pupillary light reflexes, dazzle reflex).

| 5 | **Swabs or scrapes (if required)** |

If an infectious conjunctivitis is suspected, a swab from the conjunctival fornix should be taken. Topical anaesthesia is not usually required for this (topical anaesthesia is always necessary before taking corneal swabs or conjunctival or corneal scrapes). All swabs must be taken before the application of fluorescein dye, since this can interfere with some laboratory tests. To improve sensitivity, the swab should be moistened with sterile saline or water before use and transported quickly to the diagnostic laboratory.

| 6 | **Topical fluorescein** |

This should be applied in cases of reddened and painful eyes to identify corneal ulceration. It is wise to flush the surface of the eye with water or saline after application, since the dye can pool at sites of previously healed deep ulcers. The remainder of the examination is best performed in a darkened room.

| 7 | **Assessment of the anterior segment** |

Focal illumination can be used to look at the depth of the anterior chamber (shallow in uveitis, deep in glaucoma and posterior lens luxation), for the presence of inflammatory material in the anterior chamber and for iris abnormalities (swollen muddy appearance in active anterior uveitis, increased pigmentation in chronic uveitis).

| 8 | **Distant direct ophthalmoscopy** |

The ophthalmoscope is held close to the observer's eye in the normal way, but the patient is examined at arm's length. This is useful to compare pupil sizes and to identify opacities in the visual axis, such as cataracts.

| 9 | **Examination of the fundus** |

Since this can be difficult through a constricted pupil, it is advisable to dilate the pupil with a topical mydriatic such as 1% tropicamide. A low intensity of illumination maximizes patient comfort and cooperation. Indirect ophthalmoscopy with a lens and a pen torch in a darkened room is ideal for examining larger areas of the fundus; although the technique takes a little practice, it is not difficult to master. The optic disc, superficial retinal blood vessels and tapetal and non-tapetal fundus should be examined for abnormalities. Close direct ophthalmoscopy with an ophthalmoscope can then be used to examine discrete areas of the fundus.

Figure 16.1: Suggested protocol for an ophthalmic examination.

Figure 16.2 lists the differential diagnoses for inflamed and painful eyes. By following a basic examination protocol, it is usually not difficult to differentiate conjunctivitis from anterior uveitis or glaucoma (Figure 16.3). Once the extent of inflammation has been determined, a more specific differential diagnosis should be considered.

Conjunctivitis	Retrobulbar disease
Keratitis	Episcleritis
Anterior uveitis	Scleritis
Glaucoma	

Figure 16.2: Differential diagnoses for the inflamed and painful eye.

> **1** **Identify the layer of vascular engorgement**
>
> Conjunctival redness may mask episcleral hyperaemia or congestion, which is a sign of a deeper inflammation such as uveitis or glaucoma.
>
> - *Conjunctival hyperaemia*
>   Long straight vessels, perpendicular to the limbus, move within the conjunctiva as the lids are moved; rapidly constrict with topical 10% phenylephrine.
>
> - *Episcleral hyperaemia*
>   Short vessels, perpendicular and close to the limbus, deeper red in colour, do not move with conjunctiva; take longer to constrict with topical 10% phenylephrine.
>
> - *Scleral hyperaemia*
>   Deep red or purple vessels, run parallel to the limbus.
>
> **2** **Look for signs of intraocular disease**
>
> - *Visual deficits*
>   Conjunctivitis does not affect vision. Anterior uveitis is not usually blinding unless severe. Acute glaucoma causes severe visual deficits or blindness.
>
> - *Corneal oedema*
>   Glaucoma and uveitis cause diffuse corneal oedema, giving a cloudy stippled effect to the cornea. Localized corneal oedema may surround corneal ulcers. Corneal oedema is not found with conjunctivitis.
>
> - *Abnormal iris position and appearance*
>   The anterior chamber may appear deep in glaucoma, shallow in anterior uveitis. If the condition is unilateral, it helps to compare the eyes. In acute anterior uveitis, the iris is swollen, with loss of stromal detail, or may be hyperaemic.
>
> - *Abnormal pupil size and light response*
>   Anterior uveitis causes a constricted pupil. Glaucoma creates a dilated pupil.
>   The direct pupillary light response is poor or absent in glaucoma and poor in anterior uveitis.
>
> - *Abnormal dazzle response*
>   The dazzle response may also help to distinguish between anterior uveitis and glaucoma. Shining a strong light into the eye (preferably in a darkened room) initiates a blink response and shows that retinal and optic nerve function is present. The dazzle response is usually absent in acute glaucoma but present in anterior uveitis.
>
> - *Specialized investigations*
>   More specialized diagnostic investigations, such as tonometry and slit-lamp assessment, may be available in some practices; if not, referral should be considered.

Figure 16.3: Diagnostic plan for the inflamed and painful eye.

CONJUNCTIVITIS AND KERATITIS

Diagnostic plan for conjunctivitis and keratitis

Figure 16.4 lists the differential diagnoses for conjunctivitis and keratitis, and a diagnostic plan is outlined in Figure 16.5. It is necessary to rule out non-infectious causes of conjunctivitis before assuming an infectious cause. In dogs, common non-infectious causes of conjunctivitis include keratoconjunctivitis sicca, eyelid defects (e.g. entropion, distichiasis), allergy or environmental irritant, traumatic injury and foreign bodies. In cats, keratoconjunctivitis sicca and eyelid defects are uncommon, and the major cause of non-infectious conjunctivitis is traumatic injury.

Swabs

If infectious conjunctivitis is suspected, a conjunctival swab is indicated. Although it may be impractical to do this in every case, it is advisable if there is a poor response to treatment or if the diagnosis is uncertain. In dogs, swabs should be sent for bacterial culture and sensitivity testing. In cats, if *Chlamydophila* or feline herpesvirus infection is suspected, conjunctival and oropharyngeal swabs are advised and must be placed in appropriate transport media before transport to the laboratory.

Smears

Conjunctival smears are useful in many cases of conjunctivitis. The smears may be submitted unstained to

254 Manual of Canine and Feline Infectious Diseases

PRIMARY CONJUNCTIVITIS
Infectious
Dogs
Bacteria (mostly *Staphylococcus* spp.)
Canine distemper virus
Canine adenovirus-1
Rickettsia spp.
Cats
Chlamydophila felis (formerly *Chlamydia psittaci*)
Mycoplasma spp.
Feline herpesvirus-1
Feline calicivirus
Allergic/irritant
Retained foreign body
Dust, wind, smoke
Acid or alkali burns
Topical medications
SECONDARY CONJUNCTIVITIS
Tear film abnormalities
Eyelid defects
Corneal ulceration
Retrobulbar or periorbital disease
Neoplastic infiltration

Figure 16.4: Differential diagnoses for conjunctivitis and keratitis.

---

1 Take history
Onset, duration, previous ocular problems, systemic signs, trauma, allergy, other pets (with or without signs).

2 Perform a Schirmer tear test
To rule out keratoconjunctivitis sicca.

3 Examine eyelids
Conformation, hair defects, normal blinking, palpebral blink reflex.

4 Take conjunctival swab/smear
Fairly vigorous swabbing techniques are required to obtain sufficient conjunctival cells (in cats an orophayngeal swab is often required as well).
- *Romanowsky or rapid cytological (e.g. Diff-Quik®) with or without Gram stains of smear*
  Viral inclusion bodies
  Chlamydophila inclusion bodies
  General type of bacterium
- *Laboratory analysis of swab*
  Virus and chlamydial isolation (cats)
  Culture and sensitivity (dogs and cats)

5 Apply topical anaesthesia
To evert nictitating membrane and to look for foreign bodies or take a conjunctival scrape if cytology is required.

6 Apply fluorescein stain
To identify corneal ulceration and tear drainage problems.

Figure 16.5: Diagnostic plan for conjunctivitis and keratitis.

---

a commercial laboratory or stained in a practice laboratory for immediate examination. The Romanowsky-type stains are preferred by most cytologists, although the rapid stains are usually satisfactory. If large numbers of bacteria are present, a Gram stain (see Chapter 1) of a smear may give a useful indication as to the organism while awaiting laboratory test results. Gram-positive solitary cocci or those in clusters are consistent with *Staphylococcus* spp. and those in chains to be *Streptococcus* spp. Gram-negative rods are consistent with *Pseudomonas* spp.

Some caution is required when interpreting laboratory results as bacteria can be isolated from the conjunctiva of up to 90% of normal dogs and 50% of normal cats. Scanty growths of Gram-positive aerobes (most commonly *Staphylococcus* spp.) are likely to be incidental, but heavy growths of Gram-positive bacteria and any culture of Gram-negative bacteria are more likely to be clinically significant.

Infectious conjunctivitis and keratitis in dogs

Viral disease

Canine distemper virus: Many ocular manifestations of canine distemper have been reported, including acute and chronic conjunctivitis, keratoconjunctivitis sicca, anterior uveitis, retinochoroiditis, optic neuritis and cortical blindness. The respiratory disease is discussed in more detail in Chapter 6.

Acute conjunctivitis is found in the early stages of distemper in conjunction with systemic signs. Initially the ocular discharge is serous, and conjunctival scrapes show a mononuclear cell response and occasionally viral inclusion bodies within epithelial cells. Over 7-10 days the discharge becomes mucopurulent as secondary bacterial conjunctivitis develops, and this is concomitant with a neutrophil response.

Acute and chronic keratoconjunctivitis sicca have been reported with canine distemper. The virus is thought to target the lacrimal glandular tissue directly, causing a dacryoadenitis. In most dogs, spontaneous resolution of tear production has been reported to occur over 4-8 weeks, but chronic keratoconjunctivitis may result, presumably depending on the degree of lacrimal gland damage during infection. Symptomatic treatment includes topical tear replacements and topical broad-spectrum antibacterials. If tear production does not return in 2 or 3 months, parotid duct transposition may be necessary.

Canine adenovirus: A conjunctivitis may accompany anterior uveitis in canine adenovirus infections (see Chapter 11 for details of canine adenovirus).

Bacterial disease

A wide range of bacterial species has been implicated in conjunctivitis, but Gram-positive organisms predominate, most notably *Staphylococcus* and *Streptococcus* spp. Fusidic acid, chloramphenicol and neomycin are active against these species and are a suitable first-line treatment for canine bacterial conjunctivitis.

Pseudomonas aeruginosa is a Gram-negative bacterium that may cause conjunctivitis. It may also infect the cornea if there is overlying epithelial damage, and the subsequent release of proteases may cause melting corneal ulceration (Figure 16.6). Gentamicin or tobramycin are active against *Pseudomonas* spp. If melting corneal ulceration is present, specialist advice should be sought urgently.

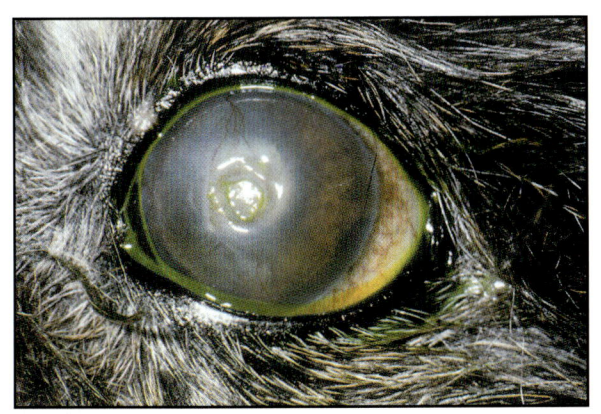

Figure 16.6: A melting corneal ulcer in a crossbreed dog. Corneal stromal necrosis and superficial neovascularization are present. Pseudomonas aeruginosa *was isolated from the lesion. (Courtesy of Dr Sheila Crispin.)*

Secondary bacterial conjunctivitis is common in keratoconjunctivitis sicca. Typically, this presents as a bilateral tenacious mucopurulent discharge that is partly responsive to topical antibacterial treatment (Figure 16.7). *Staphylococcus* spp. and *Streptococcus* spp. are the most common isolates.

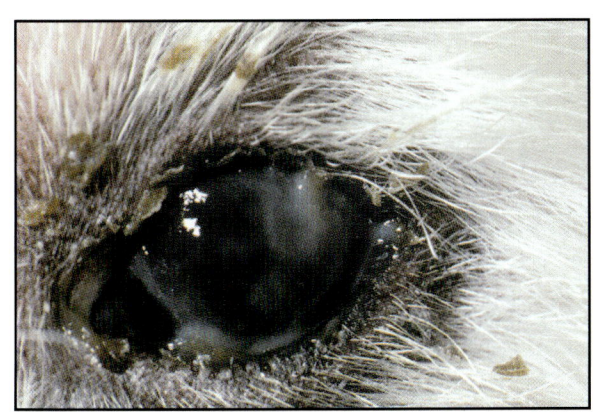

Figure 16.7: Keratoconjunctivitis sicca and secondary bacterial conjunctivitis in a West Highland White Terrier. (Courtesy of Dr Sheila Crispin.)

Rickettsial disease

Rickettsias such as *Ehrlichia canis* and *Rickettsia rickettsii* cause conjunctivitis in the acute stages of disease, but these diseases are not endemic in the UK. The chronic stage of *E. canis* infection is occasionally found in imported dogs, but uveitis and bleeding disorders rather than conjunctivitis are a feature of chronic disease. See Chapter 5 for further details on *E. canis*.

A different *Ehrlichia* species, related or identical to *E. phagocytophilia* (the cause of tick-borne fever in cattle and sheep), has been reported in working dogs in Scotland, where it causes acute conjunctivitis in association with rhinotracheitis, pyrexia, lethargy and neurological signs. These signs must be distinguished from canine distemper.

Infectious conjunctivitis and keratitis in cats

Feline herpesvirus (FHV), feline calicivirus, *Chlamydophila felis* and *Mycoplasma* spp. are possible causes of infectious feline conjunctivitis. Of these, FHV and *C. felis* are by far the most important. In many cases, the history and clinical signs indicate the pathogen involved. For example, conjunctivitis alone is most likely to be due to *C. felis*, whereas conjunctivitis with upper respiratory tract disease is more likely to be due to FHV. Feline herpesvirus is also the only pathogen to cause a primary keratitis.

Despite sometimes convincing clinical appearances, laboratory confirmation of the pathogen is often difficult. This may be due to poor collection technique, delays in transport to the laboratory and limited sensitivity of some tests. With the development of molecular biological diagnostics, the laboratory diagnosis rate can be expected to improve.

Feline herpesvirus and feline calicivirus

Clinical features: FHV and feline calicivirus cause acute conjunctivitis in association with upper respiratory tract disease, primarily in young adult cats. In contrast to *Chlamydophila* infections, nasal discharge and sneezing are usually present. The clinical signs of conjunctivitis are non-specific. The acute phase of infection usually resolves within 2–3 weeks, but persistent infection may occur. FHV is the commonest cause of chronic conjunctivitis in cats. Conjunctival adhesions may occur after severe infection in young kittens, and this may cause chronic problems such as tear overflow (owing to adhesions across the nasolacrimal punctae), keratitis (owing to restricted eyelid and third eyelid movement) and keratoconjunctivitis sicca (owing to occlusion of the lacrimal gland ducts).

FHV also causes acute and chronic keratitis. In acute infections, corneal ulceration is found in addition to conjunctivitis. Although the ulcer resolves spontaneously, latency is established in 80% of cases. A variety of clinical presentations have been described in chronic FHV keratitis, including multiple punctate keratitis, dendritic keratitis (Figure 16.8), stromal keratitis (Figure 16.9), corneal sequestrum (Figure 16.10), eosinophilic keratitis and keratoconjunctivitis sicca.

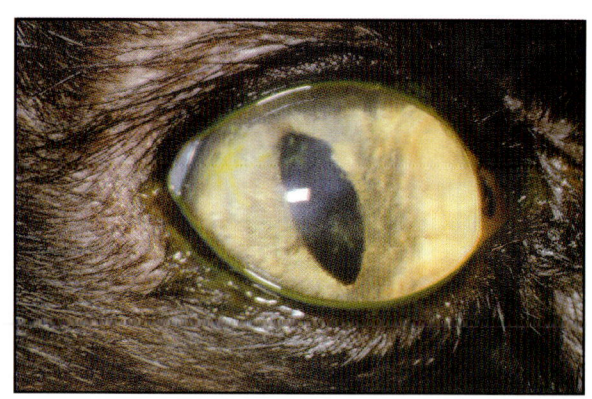

Figure 16.8: Multiple dendritic corneal ulcers, stained with fluorescein, in feline herpesvirus infection. (Courtesy of Dr Sheila Crispin.)

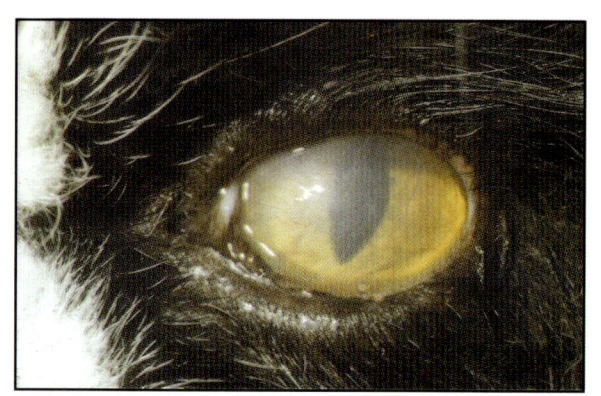

Figure 16.9: Chronic stromal keratitis in feline herpesvirus infection. Symblepharon formation and chronic eyelid thickening were also present.

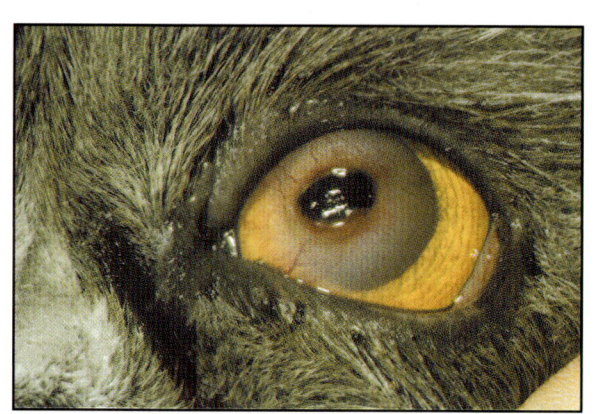

Figure 16.10: Feline herpesvirus infection. Corneal sequestrum with corneal oedema and superficial corneal neovascularization. (Courtesy of Dr Sheila Crispin.)

Diagnosis: Diagnosis is by immunofluorescent staining of conjunctival scrapes or by isolation of the virus from conjunctival or oropharyngeal swabs. Both require special transport medium, obtained from the laboratory offering the service. As with *Chlamydophila* isolation, a vigorous swab technique and rapid transport to the laboratory are required. In the USA, the polymerase chain reaction (PCR) is used to identify FHV DNA from ocular samples, and this is likely to become available in the UK.

Treatment: The viral causes of feline conjunctivitis are difficult to treat, and effective topical antiviral agents are not widely available in the UK. Trifluorothymidine, idoxuridine, vidarabine, bromovinyldeoxuridine and acyclovir (in order of decreasing efficacy) have all been shown to have some activity against FHV in vitro.

Trifluorothymidine may be obtained in the UK from selected medical suppliers. The frequency of application can make treatment difficult; the drug should be applied hourly for the first day then five times daily.

Acyclovir (the only topical antiviral agent widely available in the UK) has very limited efficacy against FHV in vitro although it may have some effect if used in conjunction with human α-interferon.

Topical and systemic human α-interferon have been used in acute FHV infections, although controlled clinical trials are awaited. Because the drug is supplied in high concentrations (e.g. 5 million IU/ml), serial dilutions are required to obtain suitable concentrations for dosing.

Recently, oral L-lysine has become popular as a treatment for chronic FHV-1 infection, based on the in vitro observation that it inhibits viral replication (but only in the presence of low arginine levels, so whether it will work in vivo is unknown). L-Lysine can be obtained from health food shops, but the preparation should not contain propylene glycol, which may be toxic in cats. Clinical trials are still under way to determine the validity of using this amino acid (see Figure 16.28 for an anecdotal dose). Results were equivocal in clinical trials in humans. None of the above treatments is licensed for use in cats.

Chlamydophila

Chlamydophila felis (formerly known as *Chlamydia psittaci* var. *felis*) is the commonest cause of acute conjunctivitis in cats in the UK, isolated from up to 30% of cases. It is also an important cause of chronic conjunctivitis, accounting for 18% of cases in one study. It causes a primary conjunctivitis that can persist for weeks or longer in multicat households, where cats can pass the infection between each other.

Epidemiology and clinical features: Most commonly the disease causes conjunctivitis in young cats (from 5 weeks to 9 months of age), although it can also infect adult cats. The causal agent, *Chlamydophila felis*, is an intracellular bacterium that replicates in the cytoplasm of conjunctival epithelial cells. In experimental infections, clinical signs develop from around 3 days after challenge. Although ultimately a bilateral conjunctivitis develops, initially the disease tends to be unilateral, with a serous ocular discharge, blepharospasm (Figure 16.11), conjunctival hyperaemia and chemosis. Corneal ulceration is not a feature. Over time, the discharge may change from serous to mucopurulent.

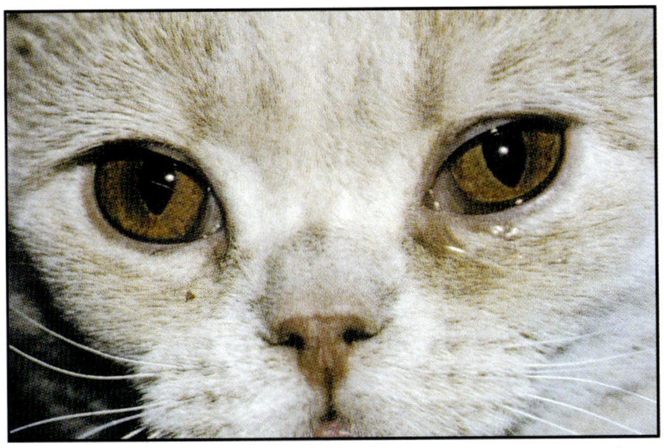

Figure 16.11: Acute chlamydophilosis in a young cat. Left blepharospasm and serous ocular discharge are present. (Courtesy of Dr Andrew Sparkes.)

Often the cat displays no systemic signs of disease, although in some cases mild upper respiratory tract signs (sneezing and nasal discharge) may develop. The cat usually remains bright and responsive.

It is known that conjunctival challenge leads to excretion of the organism from the urogenital and gastrointestinal tracts. Although this usually causes no signs of clinical disease, chronic intermittent vomiting and diarrhoea have been documented. The urogenital and gastrointestinal routes may be a source of infection for other cats, especially if litter trays are shared.

The ocular signs are self-resolving in most cases, although some cats become persistent symptomless carriers and are capable of passing the disease to other cats. Treatment is aimed at reducing the severity and length of the clinical signs.

Diagnosis: A conjunctival scrape obtained under topical anaesthesia and stained with Giemsa may identify intracellular inclusion bodies and allow a quick diagnosis. However, this needs to be performed early in infection (days 4–7), and interpretation may be difficult if the clinician is not used to such analysis.

Immunofluorescent staining to identify chlamydial antigen is a sensitive test, capable of picking up one infected cell from a sample. However, a reasonably vigorous swab technique is needed to ensure conjunctival cells are collected, and the swab must be sent quickly in chlamydial transport medium, which can be obtained from laboratories offering the test. It is important to take the conjunctival swab before applying topical fluorescein solution, which may interfere with the laboratory test.

Serology to identify anti-chlamydial antibodies is possible, but because 9% of healthy cats have such antibodies, an accurate diagnosis relies on rising titres over a 4-week period, which limits the usefulness of such a test.

Identification of chlamydophilial DNA from a conjunctival swab, using PCR, is now available in the UK and is likely to become the predominant diagnostic test for the disease. Theoretically it is by far the most sensitive test available for chlamydophilosis. Also, since DNA is extremely stable, the transport problems associated with other techniques should not occur. However, because it is not known how long chlamydial DNA might remain within conjunctival tissue after active infection has been cleared, and because the test identifies DNA rather than actively infected cells, this might lead to false-positive test results.

Treatment: The antibacterials of choice for chlamydial infections are the tetracyclines. Topical and systemic treatments are available and both are effective if used for sufficient periods of time, although clinical trials have shown that treatment with systemic tetracycline is more effective than topical treatment in eliminating the agent and achieving resolution of clinical disease. Also, frequent application of topical ointments for a prolonged period is often poorly tolerated by cats, and owner compliance is important. Systemic doxycycline is the treatment of choice. It is vital to treat all cats in the household, whether clinical disease is apparent or not, to prevent disease cycling. In addition to systemic treatment, topical chlortetracycline ointment (three times daily) may be used concurrently, although it is not essential.

In pregnant queens and young kittens, long courses of topical tetracycline ointment are often recommended to reduce the risk of incorporation of systemic tetracyclines into developing bones and teeth. However, this adverse effect has never been reported in animals. The bacterium is labile and survives less than 24 hours outside host cells.

Vaccination: Cell culture-derived vaccines give major protection against the clinical signs of disease although they will not necessarily stop infection and shedding or development of carriers. The protection lasts around 1 year.

Zoonosis: The zoonotic risk from feline chlamydophilosis is low, although there have been a few isolated reports of suspected zoonosis. For this reason it is wise to recommend simple hygiene precautions, such as hand washing after dosing, handling and litter removal. The risk of zoonotic transmission is presumably greater for immunocompromised individuals.

Mycoplasma

The *Mycoplasma* species *M. felis* and *M. gatae* are normal conjunctival inhabitants of cats, and there is debate as to whether they are primary pathogens. Experimental conjunctival inoculation with *M. felis* has been reported to induce disease in young cats, but other experimental studies with a variety of mycoplasmal strains have failed to do so. It is likely that they are rare primary pathogens but may cause disease in conjunction with *Chlamydophila* or FHV, or in immunocompromised cats. Mycoplasmosis is not thought to be a major cause of chronic conjunctivitis.

DACRYOCYSTITIS

Inflammation of the nasolacrimal system is most commonly due to a retained foreign body, with or without secondary bacterial infection. The typical presentation is a profuse unilateral mucopurulent ocular discharge, which is only mildly painful and is non-responsive to topical antibacterial treatment. Nasolacrimal cannulation and flushing usually allows the foreign body to be expelled from the opposing punctum.

UVEITIS AND RETINITIS

Inflammation of the uveal tract is usually classified into anterior uveitis (involving the iris and ciliary body), intermediate uveitis (involving the pars plana of the ciliary body) and posterior uveitis (involving the choroid). This is a useful clinical classification, as these conditions present with different signs. However, since these structures are contiguous, infections or inflammation may involve them all, to varying degrees.

Anterior uveitis

Anterior uveitis presents as a painful red eye but, unlike conjunctivitis, signs of intraocular disease are always present (see Figure 16.3). Vision may be impaired although the animal is rarely rendered blind, in contrast to glaucoma. Episcleral hyperaemia, corneal oedema, miosis and a swollen or hyperaemic iris are present. Aqueous flare is always present but is difficult to visualize without a slit-beam. The anterior chamber is often shallow and the intraocular pressure is low, although this may be hard to determine without a tonometer. Hyphaema or hypopyon may be present.

As the disease becomes chronic, the iris becomes darkened and signs of pain lessen. Inflammatory deposits may adhere to the corneal endothelium where they are visible with direct illumination as keratic precipitates. Anterior or posterior synechiae (adhesions of the iris to the cornea or lens, respectively) and secondary cataracts may develop.

Intermediate uveitis

Intermediate uveitis may release inflammatory material into the adjacent anterior vitreous where it may be visible behind and at the edges of the pupil, giving what has been described as a 'snowbanking' appearance (see Figure 16.25).

Posterior uveitis (chorioretinitis)

Posterior uveitis almost always extends to involve the adjacent retina, therefore chorioretinitis is a more accurate description of the disease. Because there are no pain fibres in this region, inflammation is painless and therefore may go unnoticed in veterinary practice; often only when the disease is severe enough to affect vision or if anterior segment structures become involved are acute inflammations identified. For this reason it is important to examine the fundus if systemic signs of disease are present.

Differentiating active from inactive chorioretinitis

Active and inactive chorioretinitis can be differentiated relatively easily. In active chorioretinitis, inflammatory cells accumulate and appear as grey focal opacities across the fundus. In more severe inflammation, subretinal oedema may develop, creating localized areas of retinal detachment. These are visible as circumscribed lesions, over which the superficial retinal blood vessels may be seen to change direction as they follow the path of the elevated retina. The underlying tapetum appears hyporeflective. If the inflammation progresses, the detachment may progress to involve larger areas of the retina. Haemorrhage may also occur with acute inflammation. It may be subretinal, intraretinal, preretinal or intravitreal in location.

Inflammatory material may also accumulate within the vitreous, giving the effect of a local or generalized haziness to the fundus (see Figure 16.16a). This may make areas of the fundus difficult to visualize during ophthalmoscopy.

In inactive chorioretinitis, hyperreflective lesions are seen across the fundus (see Figure 16.16b). The tapetum appears hyperreflective in these areas because the overlying retina degenerates after inflammation. Unlike the inherited generalized progressive retinal atrophies, the affected regions are focal and bilaterally non-symmetrical. The underlying retinal pigment epithelium may hypertrophy and produce pigment within the lesions. Across the non-tapetal fundus, the retinal pigment epithelium (which is usually pigmented in this region) may become hypopigmented or hyperpigmented.

It is common during routine ocular examinations to identify inactive fundic lesions that are indicative of a previous chorioretinitis or retinochoroiditis. In such cases it is usually impossible to identify an aetiology.

Diagnostic plan for uveitis and chorioretinitis

The differential diagnoses for uveitis are extensive (Figure 16.12). In practice, only a limited number of these conditions are likely to be encountered. The history, other ocular findings and systemic signs may also point towards the aetiology. Because similar aetiological agents are implicated in anterior uveitis and chorioretinitis, the diagnostic plan is similar (Figure 16.13).

A large component of anterior uveitis is immune mediated, with an aggressive host immune response responsible for much of the intraocular pathology. Therefore symptomatic treatment with topical corticosteroids and topical atropine is indicated in addition to treatment specific for the aetiological agent. It is important to

The Eye

INFECTIOUS
Dogs

Viral
    Canine adenovirus
    Canine distemper virus
    Canine herpesvirus
    (Rabies)
Protozoal
    Toxoplasma gondii
    Neospora caninum
    (*Leishmania donovani*)
Bacterial
    Penetrating corneal inoculation
    Bacterial sepsis
    Leptospira spp.
    ?*Borrelia burgdorferi*
    (*Brucella canis*)
Rickettsial
    (*Ehrlichia canis*)
    (*Ehrlichia platys*)
Mycotic/algal
    Cryptococcus neoformans
    (*Histoplasma capsulatum*)
    (*Blastomyces dermatiditis*)
    (*Coccidioides immitis*)
    (*Prototheca* spp.)

Cats

Viral
    Feline coronavirus
    Feline immunodeficiency virus
    Feline leukaemia virus
Protozoal
    Toxoplasma gondii
Bacterial
    Penetrating corneal inoculation
    Bacterial sepsis
    (Mycotic)

Parasitic
Angiostrongylus vasorum *Toxocara canis* *Diptera* spp. (*Dirofilaria*)
NON-INFECTIOUS
Traumatic
Blunt or penetrating injury
Reflex uveitis
Immune-mediated
Lens-induced Phacolytic (rapidly growing or hypermature cataracts) Phacoclastic (lens capsule rupture) Vaccine reaction Autoimmune disease
Systemic disease
Toxaemia Bleeding disorders Granulomatous meningoencephalitis Systemic histiocytosis Diabetes mellitus Hyperlipidaemia Hypertension
Neoplasia
Intraocular tumour Local invasion from extraocular tissues Metastatic disease

Figure 16.12: Differential diagnoses for uveitis. (Agents in parentheses are not endemic in the UK.)

---

1 **Take history**

Age, breed, vaccination status, history of travel abroad, environment, other pets, history of trauma, other clinical signs

2 **Perform clinical examination**

Ophthalmic examination
Acute or chronic uveitis, anterior or posterior, unilateral or bilateral. Any other ophthalmic signs (e.g. corneal penetration)

General examination
Signs of systemic disease, traumatic injury

3 **Perform serology/virology**

If an infectious agent is suspected

Dogs: *Toxoplasma*, *Neospora*, others if suspected from history or clinical signs

Cats: feline immunodeficiency virus, feline leukaemia virus, feline coronavirus, *Toxoplasma*

4 **Perform haematology/serum biochemistry**

If an infectious agent or systemic disease is suspected

Serum protein electrophoresis may be useful in many cases:

- Monoclonal globulinaemia in multiple myeloma, ehrlichiosis, leishmaniasis
- Polyclonal globulinaemia in other chronic infections or inflammations, e.g. ehrlichiosis, leishmaniasis, neoplasia in dogs and FIP, feline immunodeficiency virus, toxoplasmosis, lymphocytic cholangitis, neoplasia in cats
- Increased $\alpha 2$-globulin concentrations in FIP

5 **Perform ultrasonography**

If any suspicion of intraocular neoplasia, intraocular haemorrhage, retinal detachment

6 **Perform radiography**

Chest and abdominal radiographs to look for effusions if FIP is suspected or to look for metastatic disease

Figure 16.13: Diagnostic plan for uveitis.

select a topical corticosteroid that has good intraocular penetration, such as prednisolone acetate drops (applied 3–6 times daily until the uveitis is controlled, then at a gradually reducing dose). However, if corneal ulceration or penetration is present, then topical (and systemic) corticosteroids should be avoided. In such cases, a topical non-steroidal anti-inflammatory drug such as ketorolac (applied topically 3–6 times daily) may be used instead. Alternatively, a systemic non-steroidal drug such as carprofen can be used.

260 Manual of Canine and Feline Infectious Diseases

Infectious uveitis in dogs

Viral disease

Canine adenovirus-1: CAV-1 causes acute anterior uveitis with corneal oedema (Figure 16.14), which is usually self-resolving over a period of weeks. CAV-1 is now uncommon owing to widespread vaccination. Live attenuated CAV-1 vaccines caused acute uveitis in some cases therefore live CAV-2 vaccines (which confer protection against both species) are now used. See Chapter 11 for further details on CAV-1.

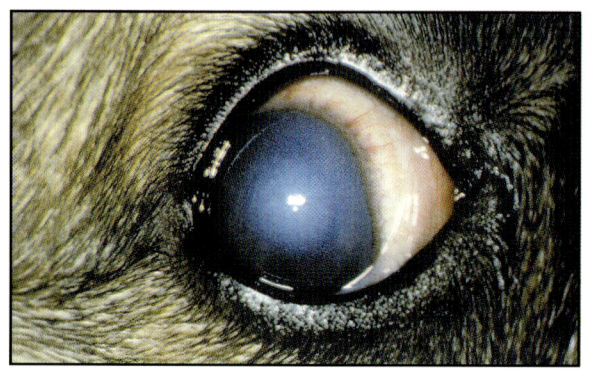

Figure 16.14: Acute anterior uveitis with corneal oedema and episcleral hyperaemia caused by canine adenovirus-1 infection. (Courtesy of Dr Sheila Crispin.)

Canine herpesvirus: Canine herpesvirus causes a fatal neonatal disease in litters of puppies, with severe anterior uveitis and chorioretinitis in addition to systemic signs. It is not a clinical problem in adult dogs. See Chapter 12 for further details on CHV.

Canine distemper virus: Retinochoroiditis may occur in canine distemper, with focal areas of active inflammation visible across the tapetal and non-tapetal fundus. The lesions are not usually severe enough to cause blindness. The virus may also directly target the optic nerve, causing optic neuritis, which presents as sudden onset blindness. This may be unilateral or bilateral. See Chapter 6 for further details on canine distemper.

Bacterial disease

A wide range of bacterial species can cause anterior uveitis if they gain access to the anterior segment. The most common site of entry is through the cornea after a penetrating injury. Cat scratch injuries most commonly inoculate *Pasteurella* spp. Treatment consists of topical antibacterials, with symptomatic treatment for anterior uveitis. A broad-spectrum topical agent that is able to penetrate the cornea and reach therapeutic levels in the anterior chamber is needed, such as chloramphenicol solution. Systemic antibacterials may also be used.

Any septicaemic bacterial disease may localize to the eye, where it may cause anterior uveitis or chorioretinitis. Systemic antibacterial treatment is indicated in addition to symptomatic treatment for anterior uveitis. Several specific bacterial infections have been associated with anterior uveitis.

Brucellosis: *Brucella canis* is most commonly associated with epididymitis in dogs and abortion/stillbirth in bitches. However, it can infect other tissues, including the eye, where it may cause recurrent anterior uveitis. It is not currently found in the UK. See Chapter 12 for further details on brucellosis.

Borreliosis: *Borrelia burgdorferi* is a spirochaete that causes Lyme disease in humans and dogs (although it is rare in the UK). It has been associated with canine uveitis. See Chapter 14 for further details on borreliosis.

Leptospirosis: *Leptospira interrogans* is a spirochaete that causes leptospirosis in humans and dogs but rarely affects cats. Several serovars are known. Clinical effects vary from peracute infection, which may be fatal, to chronic or subclinical disease. All forms of the disease may show uveitis. See Chapter 11 for further details on leptospirosis.

Rickettsial disease

Ehrlichiosis: *Ehrlichia canis* and *E. platys* have been implicated in ophthalmological disease, in conjunction with systemic signs. Acute *E. canis* infection may be accompanied by acute conjunctivitis, subconjunctival haemorrhage, anterior uveitis and retinal haemorrhage. *E. canis* can also cause chronic disease, which may be encountered in the UK, even in imported dogs that have undergone quarantine. In addition to systemic signs, a monoclonal hypergammaglobulinaemia can cause hyperviscosity syndrome, with resultant conjunctival and episcleral congestion (Figure 16.15), hyphaema, anterior uveitis, intraocular or retinal haemorrhage, retinal blood vessel thickening and tortuosity and retinal detachment. See Chapter 5 for further details on *E. canis*.

E. platys has been reported to cause a mild canine uveitis but is not likely to be found in the UK.

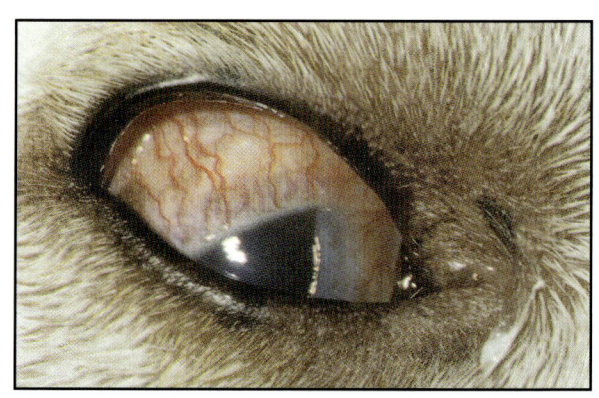

Figure 16.15: Chronic ehrlichiosis in a Labrador Retriever. The dog was from Sardinia but had lived in the UK for 2 years before presentation. Conjunctival and episcleral congestion, third eyelid protrusion and corneal oedema are evident, due to hyperglobulinaemia and anterior uveitis.

Other rickettsias: Rocky Mountain spotted fever (caused by *Rickettsia rickettsii*) occurs in the USA and South America. A similar disease, Mediterranean spotted fever (*R. conorii*), is endemic in much of Africa and the Mediterranean. Signs in acute disease are similar to those in acute *Ehrlichia canis* infection. Unlike ehrlichiosis, chronic disease does not occur, so these diseases are unlikely to be found in the UK.

Salmon poisoning disease (caused by *Neorickettsia helminthoeca*) occurs on the western coast of the USA. It is an acute disease characterized by pyrexia, depression, anorexia, mucopurulent ocular discharge and serous nasal discharge. It is responsive to tetracyclines. See Chapter 8 for further details on salmon poisoning disease.

Mycotic and algal diseases

Mycotic and algal infections are a cause of anterior or posterior uveitis in some parts of the world but are only likely to be encountered in the UK in imported animals. Cryptococcosis, histoplasmosis, blastomycosis, candidiasis and protothecosis have been reported.

Protozoal diseases

Toxoplasmosis and neosporosis: Toxoplasmosis can occur in intermediate or definitive hosts, when tachyzoites invade tissues and organs. In the dog, toxoplasmosis can cause either a generalized multisystemic disease or present primarily as a neurological disease. Ophthalmological manifestations may include anterior uveitis, chorioretinitis and optic neuritis (Figure 16.16). See Chapter 15 for further details on toxoplasmosis.

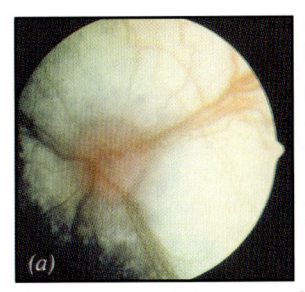

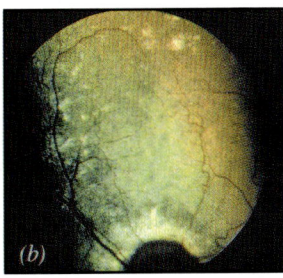

Figure 16.16: (a) Acute toxoplasmosis in a crossbreed dog that presented with sudden onset blindness. Retinochoroiditis and optic neuritis are present, with a swollen optic disc and overlying vitreal inflammatory debris in the acute phase. (b) The same dog after treatment. Focal areas of hyperreflectivity are present across the tapetal fundus, where the overlying retina has thinned. A hyperreflective peripapillary halo surrounds the optic disc, at the site of the previous optic neuritis. (Courtesy of Dr Sheila Crispin.)

Neospora caninum causes similar clinical signs, including neurological disease, polymyositis, myocarditis, hepatitis and dermatitis. Ophthalmological changes include chorioretinitis and extraocular myositis. See Chapter 15 for further details on neosporosis.

Leishmaniasis: Ocular lesions in leishmaniasis include conjunctivitis, keratitis, anterior uveitis and panophthalmitis, as well as periorbital alopecia and scaling (Figure 16.17). Chronic leishmaniasis may cause a polyclonal hyperglobulinaemia, with resultant ocular signs of hyperviscosity (see Chapter 5 for more details on leishmaniasis).

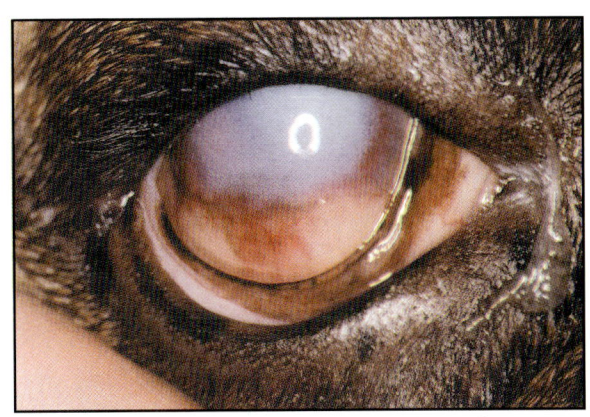

Figure 16.17: Leishmaniasis in a Boxer. Chronic keratitis and anterior uveitis are present. Superficial and deep corneal neovascularization, corneal pigmentation, cellular infiltration and corneal oedema are visible. (Courtesy of Dr Sheila Crispin.)

Parasitic disease

Migrating parasites may gain access to the anterior or posterior segment of the eye and induce uveitis. *Toxocara canis* (Figure 16.18) and *Angiostrongylus vasorum* (Figure 16.19) are possible causes in the UK. Abnormal migration of nasal bot fly larvae (*Oestrus ovis*) and warble fly larvae (*Hypoderma* spp.) may also cause uveitis. *Dirofilaria immitis* may be encountered in imported dogs.

If the parasite is in the anterior chamber it may be directly visible. Focal granulomatous chorioretinitis may be found in the posterior segment (Figure 16.19). Since a dead larva within the anterior segment of the eye often provokes a more severe inflammatory response than a living one, management relies on surgical removal of the parasite rather than the use of antiparasiticides.

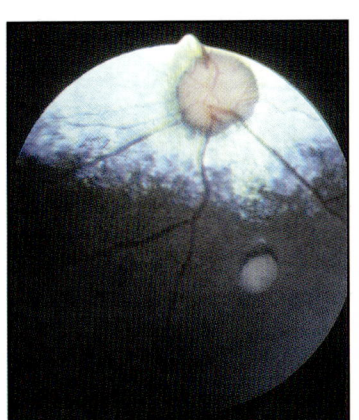

Figure 16.18: Parasitic cyst within the non-tapetal fundus of a Whippet. This was presumed to be caused by Toxocara canis. (Courtesy of Dr Sheila Crispin.)

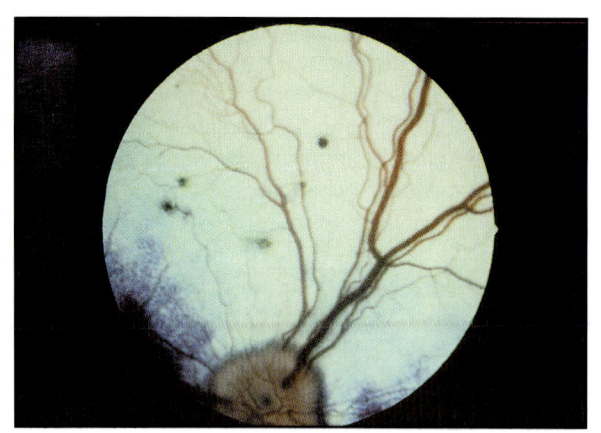

262 Manual of Canine and Feline Infectious Diseases

Figure 16.19: Granulomatous lesions across the tapetal fundus of a Staffordshire Bull Terrier with active Angiostrongylus vasorum *infestation. Presumed to be associated with encysted larvae.*

Infectious uveitis in cats

Viral disease
Viral infections are important causes of anterior and posterior uveitis in the cat.

Feline infectious peritonitis: Feline coronavirus is a common cause of uveitis in the cat (see Chapter 9). Young cats, especially those from multicat households, are more commonly affected. Anterior uveitis is the most common ocular manifestation of FIP, although the posterior segment may also be involved. The disease is usually bilateral but not symmetrical. A pyogranulomatous vasculitis allows breakdown of the blood-ocular barrier, and uveitis results. Mild to moderate ocular discomfort, episcleral congestion, hypopyon, aqueous flare, iris oedema and hyperaemia, keratic precipitates and hyphaema may develop (Figure 16.20). As these are all non-specific signs of anterior uveitis, a diagnosis of FIP cannot be made on ocular examination alone. Symptomatic treatment for anterior uveitis may reduce the clinical signs but is not curative.

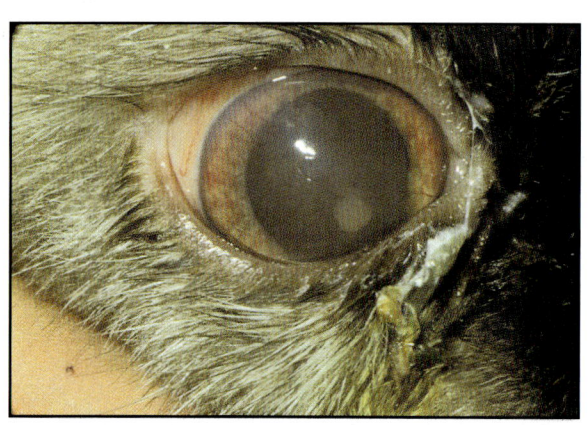

Figure 16.20: Active chronic anterior uveitis in a cat with feline infectious peritonitis, with iris hyperaemia and thickening and corneal oedema. A large keratic precipitate is adherent to the corneal endothelium. A corneal ulcer and superficial neovascularization are also present. The pupil is dilated due to the application of topical atropine.

In the posterior segment, FIP causes a pyogranulomatous chorioretinitis, sometimes with extensive perivascular effusions and vasculitis (Figures 16.21 and 16.22). Retinal haemorrhage and subretinal oedema are non-specific signs of active chorioretinitis. The hyperviscosity syndrome associated with FIP may cause thickened and tortuous retinal blood vessels.

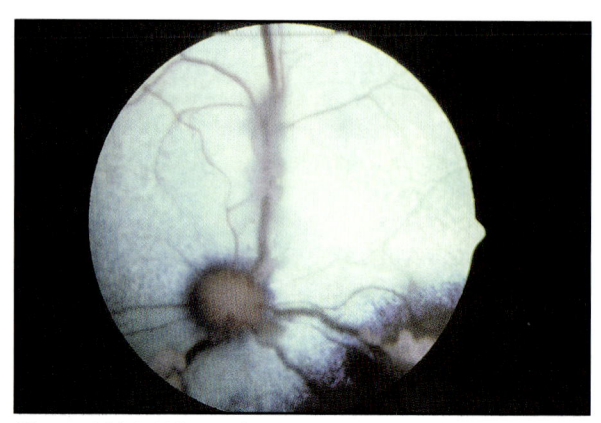

Figure 16.21: Feline infectious peritonitis. Pyogranulomatous perivascular effusions are seen around the superficial retinal venules. (Courtesy of Dr Sheila Crispin.)

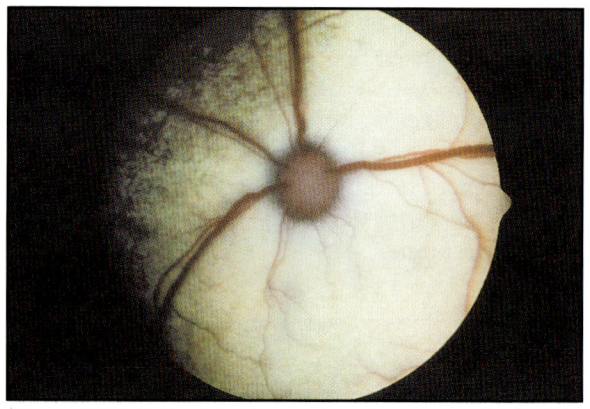

Figure 16.22: Feline infectious peritonitis-associated vasculitis. (Courtesy of Dr Sheila Crispin.)

Feline leukaemia virus: Feline leukaemia virus (FeLV)-induced lymphoma (see Chapter 5) can affect any ocular structure but the anterior segment is its most common ophthalmic target. Lymphoma may present as a focal anterior uveal mass or as an infiltrative lesion. Chronic anterior uveitis usually accompanies the tumour. If neoplastic cells invade the iridocorneal drainage angle or if severe inflammation develops, secondary glaucoma can occur. In some cases posterior segment changes may also develop, including vitreal opacities, neoplastic infiltration of the fundus, retinal haemorrhage, retinal detachment or optic neuritis.

FeLV-induced anaemia and thrombocytopenia may cause pallor of the superficial retinal blood vessels, hyphaema (Figure 16.23) or haemorrhage into the posterior segment. Tumour cell infiltration into the lateral and medial ciliary nerves supplying the

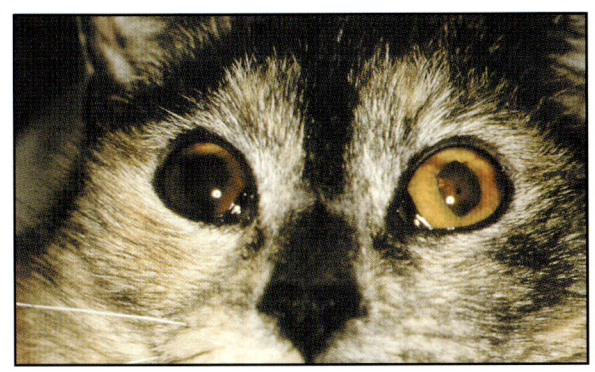

Figure 16.23: Bilateral hyphaema and anterior uveitis in a cat positive for feline leukaemia virus. (Courtesy of Dr Sheila Crispin.)

iris constrictor muscles may cause a static anisocoria (if both are affected) or a hemidilated pupil (if only one is involved).

Feline immunodeficiency virus: Feline immunodeficiency virus (FIV; see Chapter 5) may cause acute, recurrent or chronic anterior uveitis (Figure 16.24). The mechanism may be via immune complex deposition or localization of FIV within the anterior uvea. In late stages of the disease, when immune system suppression begins to develop, secondary ocular infections may occur. This is found commonly in human HIV infections but seems to be less common in the cat. FIV has also been associated with intermediate uveitis (Figure 16.25).

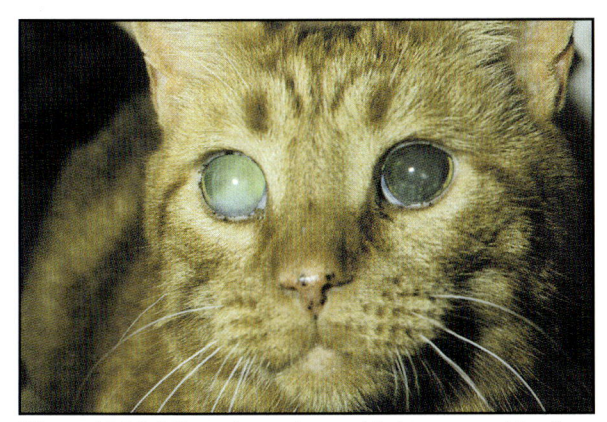

Figure 16.24: Bilateral anterior uveitis in a cat positive for feline immunodeficiency virus. Multiple keratic precipitates are present bilaterally. The pupils are dilated due to the application of topical atropine.

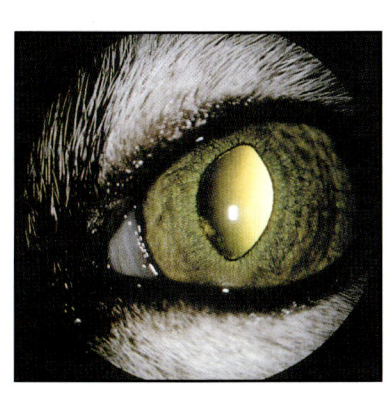

Figure 16.25: Intermediate uveitis (pars planitis) with anterior vitreal inflammatory deposits visible just behind the pupil in a cat positive for feline immunodeficiency virus. (Courtesy of Dr Sheila Crispin.)

Bacterial disease

Penetrating corneal injuries, usually from cat claws, are a common cause of uveitis in the cat, and in such cases intraocular inoculation of bacteria may result (most often *Pasteurella* spp.). Symptomatic treatment for uveitis plus topical antibacterials is usually successful in resolving the condition.

Bartonella henselae, the cause of cat scratch fever in humans, has recently been suggested as a possible cause of feline anterior uveitis, based on the presence of increased aqueous IgG titres to *B. henselae* in an affected cat. Serology for *B. henselae* is not currently available in the UK but may be obtained from some laboratories in the USA.

Protozoal disease

Toxoplasma gondii: Serological studies show that toxoplasmosis is common in the cat, the definitive host of *T. gondii*, but clinical signs are uncommon. If they do occur, many organ systems can be involved, although neurological signs are less common than in the dog.

Ocular infection may cause anterior or intermediate uveitis or chorioretinitis. Anterior uveitis is usually chronic. Active chorioretinitis lesions may appear granulomatous or non-granulomatous, with focal areas of bullous retinal detachment or retinal haemorrhage. Optic neuritis may also occur, and the lesions may be unilateral or bilateral.

Inactive chorioretinal lesions are sometimes identified on routine ophthalmoscopic examination. It is often suspected that these represent previous inflammations due to toxoplasmosis, but since the incidence of anti-*T. gondii* antibodies in the general cat population is high this is difficult to prove. See Chapter 15 for further details on toxoplasmosis.

Mycotic disease

Fungal uveitis occasionally may be encountered in imported cats or in cats with immune suppression. Genera involved include *Cryptococcus*, *Histoplasma* and *Blastomyces*. Well circumscribed granulomatous fundic lesions are the commonest presentation, and the anterior segment is rarely involved (Figures 16.26 and 16.27).

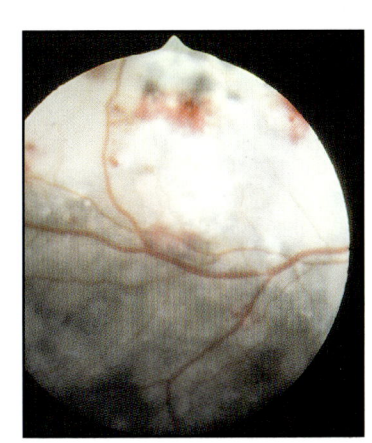

Figure 16.26: Active chorioretinitis in a cat due to cryptococcosis. Subretinal and intraretinal haemorrhages, subretinal oedema and pigment changes within the retinal pigment epithelium are present. (Courtesy of Dr Edward Hall.)

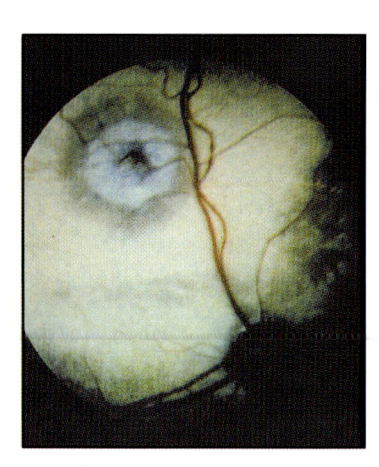

Figure 16.27: Chronic granulomatous fundic lesions in a cat with cryptococcosis. (Courtesy of Dr Sheila Crispin.)

OPTIC NEURITIS

Inflammation of the optic nerve presents as sudden onset blindness, which may be unilateral or bilateral. The pupil is dilated and the pupillary light response absent or sluggish. The ophthalmoscopic appearance depends on whether or not inflammation involves the optic nerve head. If it does, the optic disc appears swollen and hyperaemic and may have areas of haemorrhage. Inflammatory debris in the overlying vitreous may make the optic disc appear out of focus (see Figure 16.16). However, if the optic nerve head is not involved, the fundus appears normal.

Infectious causes of optic neuritis include canine distemper, toxoplasmosis and FIP. Non-infectious causes include local or distant neoplasia. Many cases, however, remain idiopathic.

DRUG DOSAGES

See Appendix 3.

FURTHER READING

Brightman AH, Ogilvie GK and Tompkins M (1991) Ocular disease in FeLV-positive cats: 11 cases (1981-1996). *Journal of the American Animal Hospital Association* **198**, 1049-1051

Collins BK and Moore CP (1999) Diseases and surgery of the canine anterior uvea. In: *Veterinary Ophthalmology, 3rd edn*, ed. KN Gelatt, pp. 755-796. Lippincott Williams and Wilkins, Philadelphia

Crispin SM (1993) The pre-ocular tear film and conditions of the conjunctiva and cornea. In: *Manual of Small Animal Ophthalmology*, ed. SM Petersen-Jones and SM Crispin, pp. 137-171. BSAVA, Cheltenham

Gionfriddo JR (1995) Identifying and treating conjunctivitis in dogs and cats. *Veterinary Medicine* March, 242-253

Gionfriddo JR (1995) The causes, diagnosis, and treatment of uveitis. *Veterinary Medicine* March, 278-284

Glaze MB and Gelatt KN (1999) Feline ophthalmology. In: *Veterinary Ophthalmology, 3rd edn*, ed. KN Gelatt, pp. 997-1052. Lippincott Williams and Wilkins, Philadelphia

Hopper C and Crispin S (1992) Differential diagnosis of uveitis in cats. *In Practice* **14**, 289-297

Lappin MR and Black JC (1999) *Bartonella* spp. infection as a possible cause of uveitis in a cat. *Journal of the American Veterinary Medical Association* **214**, 1205-1207

Martin CL (1999) Ocular manifestations of systemic disease. The dog. In: *Veterinary Ophthalmology, 3rd edn*, ed. KN Gelatt, pp. 1401-1447. Lippincott Williams and Wilkins, Philadelphia

Moore CP, Nasisse MP (1999) Clinical microbiology. In: *Veterinary Ophthalmology, 3rd edn*, ed. KN Gelatt, pp. 259-290. Lippincott Williams and Wilkins, Philadelphia

Stiles J (1999) Ocular manifestations of systemic disease. The cat. In: *Veterinary Ophthalmology, 3rd edn*, ed. KN Gelatt, pp. 1448-1472. Lippincott Williams and Wilkins, Philadelphia

Stiles J (ed.) (2000) *Infectious Disease and the the Eye. Veterinary Clinics of North America* **30**, 971-1167

Wills JM, Howard PE, Gruffyd-Jones TJ and Wathes CE (1988) Prevalence of *Chlamydia psittaci* in different cat populations in Britain. *Journal of Small Animal Practice* **29**, 327-339

Appendices

APPENDIX ONE

Sending Samples by Post

Throughout this Manual reference is made to the submission of samples to diagnostic laboratories. This is usually done via the postal system. However, concerns for the safety of postal workers, laboratory staff and the general public mean that it is essential that all veterinary surgeons send samples in a responsible manner. The following guidance has been prepared for UK veterinary surgeons only and is only valid for sending samples within and to the UK. Other countries have different regulations and local authorities should be contacted for further information.

Royal Mail will accept diagnostic and infectious substances in World Health Organization risk groups 1, 2 and 3 (Figure A1). Substances in risk group 4 and those group 3 items listed in Schedule 9 part 5 of Control of Substances Hazardous to Health, 1994 (COSHH) are prohibited. 'Diagnostic substances' include any animal material, such as faeces, urine, blood and tissues, that is thought unlikely to contain pathogens in groups 2 and 3. These substances may be sent in packaging that meets the guidelines set out in Figure A2.

'Infectious substances' include all substances that are known, or might be reasonably expected, to contain pathogens in groups 2 and 3. The packaging of such samples should follow International Air Transport Authority (IATA) packaging instruction 602, with the sole exception that there is no requirement for 2–3 working days' notice. This packaging instruction specifies, amongst other things, watertight primary and secondary packaging, the latter being able to withstand a defined force (Figure A3). Such packaging has to be obtained from a specialist supplier. It should be marked with 'INFECTIOUS SUBSTANCES' and the name and telephone number of the responsible person. It should also be accompanied by proper documentation, e.g. Shipper's Declaration for Dangerous Goods.

Royal Mail will only accept packages containing diagnostic or infectious substances if posted by a veterinary surgeon or a recognized laboratory or institution. Members of the public should not post infectious or diagnostic samples. It would therefore be inappropriate to ask a client to send a faecal sample from an animal to a veterinary practice or diagnostic laboratory. The client should bring the sample by hand to the practice and the practice should then arrange dispatch to the laboratory.

	Examples
Class 1	Everything that is not Class 2, 3 or 4
Class 2	**Viruses** Feline calicivirus, feline coronavirus, parainfluenza virus 3, contagious pustular dermatitis (orf)
	Bacteria *Actinomyces* spp., *Bacteroides* spp., *Bordetella bronchiseptica*, *Borrelia* spp., *Campylobacter* spp., *Clostridium* spp., *Klebsiella* spp., *Leptospira interrogans*, *Nocardia* spp., *Pasteurella* spp., *Pseudomonas aeruginosa*, some *Salmonella* spp., *Streptococcus* spp.
	Fungi *Aspergillus fumigatus*, *Candida albicans*, *Cryptococcus neoformans*, *Microsporum* spp.
	Parasites *Cryptosporidium* spp., *Giardia intestinalis*, *Leishmania* spp., *Toxocara* spp., *Toxoplasma gondii*
Class 3	**Viruses** Many; although only rabies is likely to be of significance in small animal practice
	Bacteria *Bacillus anthracis*, *Brucella canis*, *Ehrlichia* spp., most *Mycobacterium* spp., some *Salmonella* spp., *Yersinia pestis*
	Fungi *Blastomyces dermatitidis*, *Coccidioides immitis*, *Histoplasma capsulatum*
	Parasites *Echinococcus* spp.
Class 4	**Viruses** No common veterinary examples – group includes Lassa fever, Ebola viruses

Figure A1: Examples of pathogens of veterinary importance grouped according to the World Health Organization risk classification. Group 3 organisms that are listed in Schedule 9 part 5 of Control of Substances Hazardous to Health, 1994 (COSHH) are prohibited by Royal Mail.

1. The specimen is placed in a securely sealed watertight container (e.g. screw-top blood tube). The maximum volume that can be in one container is 50 ml. The use of glass tubes is discouraged.

2. The watertight container is wrapped in sufficient absorbent material to absorb all fluid present in the specimen.

3. The container and absorbent material are sealed in a leak-proof plastic bag. Each container is placed in a separate bag.

4. All the bags are placed in a robust outer container. Such containers include cylindrical light metal containers, strong cardboard boxes with full-depth lids or two-piece polystyrene boxes held together with adhesive tape.

5. The outer container is placed inside a padded envelope that has been clearly labelled with 'PATHOLOGICAL SPECIMEN — FRAGILE. HANDLE WITH CARE' and the sender's name and address (so that Royal Mail can contact the sender in the event of leakage).

Figure A2: Diagnostic samples that might reasonably be thought not to contain infectious organisms from risk groups 2, 3 or 4 may be sent in packaging that meets these guidelines.

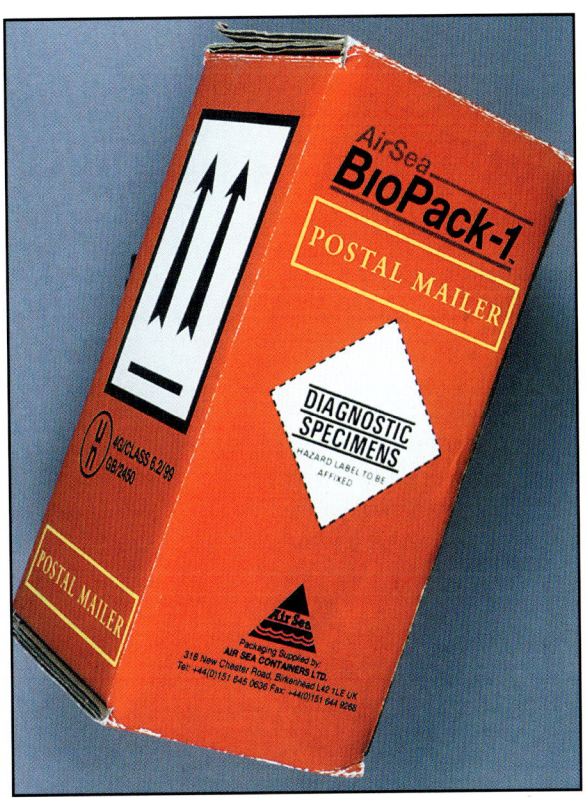

Figure A3: An example of packaging that conforms to IATA packaging instruction 602. Inside the box are polypropylene tubes with plastic closures that act as secondary packaging. The primary packaging (e.g. blood tubes), wrapped in bubble wrap and surrounded with absorbent material, is placed inside. All infectious substances (groups 2 and 3 in Figure A1) should be sent in such packaging.

APPENDIX TWO

Pet Travel Outside the UK and Eire

All information in this Appendix may change and veterinary surgeons are strongly advised to obtain current information on the Pet Travel Scheme from the Ministry of Agriculture, Fisheries and Food.

Post: Ministry of Agriculture, Fisheries and Food, 1a Page Street, London SW1P 4PQ

Tel: +44 (0)207 904 6222

E-mail: quarantine@ahvg.maff.gsi.gov.uk

Internet: http://www.maff.gov.uk/animalh/quarantine

Fax: +44 (0)207 904 6834

PET TRAVEL SCHEME

As an alternative to quarantine, the UK government has introduced the Pet Travel Scheme (PETS). The full PETS will take over from the current pilot scheme in the Spring of 2001. The rules of the pilot scheme are summarized below; any animal not meeting these conditions must go into quarantine as soon as it arrives in the UK.

Species
Applies to cats and dogs only.

Countries, ports and carriers
The PETS is limited to cats and dogs coming into the United Kingdom from certain countries and applies on a limited number of routes, using specified carriers. For the up-to-date list of countries, carriers and routes log on to http://www.maff.gov.uk/animalh/quarantine or http://www.bsava.ac.uk/members.htm .

The current list of countries to which the pilot Pet Travel Scheme applies is shown in the Figure A4.

Microchipping
The animal must be fitted with a permanent number microchip, implanted according to the manufacturer's instructions, so that the microchip number and other details such as the animal's age can be recorded on the rabies vaccination certificate. The microchip should be to ISO standard 11784. If a non-ISO standard microchip is implanted, the owner must

Andorra	Finland	Isle of Man	Portugal (includes Azores and Madeira)
Antigua and Barbuda*	France (includes Martinique*, Guadeloupe*, La Réunion*, French Polynesia*, Wallis and Futura*, New Caledonia* and Mayotte*; excludes French Guyana and St Pierre and Miquelon)	Italy	Republic of Ireland
Ascension Island*		Jamaica*	St Helena*
Australia*		Japan*	St Kitts and Nevis*
Austria		Liechtenstein	St Vincent*
Barbados*		Luxembourg	San Marino
Belgium		Malta	Singapore*
Bermuda*		Mauritius*	Spain (includes Canary Islands; excludes Ceuta and Melilla)
Cayman Islands*		Monaco	
Channel Islands	Germany	Montserrat*	
Cyprus	Gibraltar	Netherlands	Sweden
Denmark	Greece	New Zealand*	Switzerland
Falkland Islands*	Hawaii*	Norway (excludes Svalbard)	Vanuatu*
Fiji*	Iceland		Vatican

Figure A4: *The current list of countries to which the pilot Pet Travel Scheme applies. Other rabies-free islands being considered for the modified version of PETS include: Cape Verde Islands; Cook Islands; Seychelles; St Lucia; and Taiwan.*
* *May have additional conditions and documentary requirements. Contact MAFF for advice.*

be made aware that they may be required to purchase a compatible reader as the authorities may have only ISO standard readers.

The UK legislation recognizes the French system for identifying cats and dogs, whereby the animal is first tattooed with a unique number which is registered on a national database. The animal is then vaccinated against rabies, blood tested and, finally, fitted with a microchip. The owner's copy of the registration document is sent back to the database and returned to the owner with the microchip number on it. Thus dogs and cats that have first been tattooed, in accordance with the rules of the country, and then vaccinated, blood tested and microchipped can qualify for travel to the UK under the PETS. The vet issues an official PETS certificate that shows that they have seen the registration document showing the microchip number.

Pets that are identified solely by tattoo do not meet the rules of the Pet Travel Scheme.

Vaccination

The animal must be vaccinated using an approved inactivated adjuvanted vaccine (and have booster vaccinations at the required intervals) in a qualifying country or in the British Isles. The animal must be at least 3 months old at the time of vaccination and, within the UK, must already be microchipped.

Blood testing

Blood sampling must be carried out by a veterinary surgeon. The optimum time for the blood testing is 30 days after the last vaccination. Vaccine manufacturers have advised that a proportion of vaccinated animals may not show the required 0.5 IU antibody titre on blood testing. If a pet fails to show the required titre, it must be revaccinated and blood tested again.

The blood test must be performed at an accredited laboratory recognized by MAFF. There are currently two in the UK:

- *Veterinary Laboratory Agency:* contact the Rabies Helpline on 01932 357 345 to request the appropriate submission forms and to obtain advice on the correct labelling and means of transmission of the sample
- *BioBest:* Samples should be submitted via your usual clinical pathology laboratory. In case of any questions that the referring laboratory cannot answer, phone 0131 445 6101.

Several other laboratories across the UK are applying for permission to carry out rabies serology. There are also approved laboratories in other European Union countries.

Zoonotic diseases

Treatment for certain parasites carrying potentially serious zoonotic diseases has to be carried out between 24 and 48 hours before returning to the UK, in particular for *Echinococcus multilocularis* (using praziquantel) and ticks (using an acaricide). An official certificate signed by a qualified veterinary surgeon certifying that these treatments have been given should accompany the pet.

Documentation

All pets travelling under the pilot scheme require the following documents:

- Official PETS1 certificate showing that the animal has been identified by its microchip number, has a current rabies vaccination and has had a blood test showing that the vaccine has given satisfactory protection against rabies. The certificate is not valid until 6 months after the date of the blood sample that gave a successful test result
- The French authorities have agreed that a French version of the PETS certificate can be used instead of an export health certificate to accompany dogs and cats travelling to France from the UK. This document is called 'Export of a pet dog or cat to France in accordance with the Pet Travel Scheme' (PETS5). A PETS5 certificate will be issued along with each PETS1 document. Pet owners already in possession of a valid PETS1 certificate will be able to obtain a PETS5 certificate from any Local Veterinary Inspector on production of the original certificate
- Official certificate of treatment against tapeworm (*Echinococcus multilocularis*) and ticks from a veterinary surgeon in the country being visited who has administered the praziquantel
- An official owner declaration form (PETS3 certificate) filled out by the owner.
- Depending on which country is being visited, pet owners may need an export health certificate to show that the animal meets the health requirements of the country (or countries) that it is visiting or travelling through. These requirements may be different from those of the Pet Travel Scheme.

OTHER PRECAUTIONS FOR PETS TRAVELLING ABROAD

Figure A5 (overleaf) lists some infections that pets may be exposed to when travelling abroad and control measures that may be applied.

Infectious agent	Control measures
Leishmania spp. (See Chapter 5)	Avoid taking animals out at dusk when the sandfly vectors are more active. Several products containing synthetic pyrethroids are recommended for use by humans to repel insects such as sandflies; they may provide protection to pets
Dirofilaria immitis (Heartworm) (See Chapter 7)	Administer one of the following within 1 month of exposure to mosquitoes and monthly until the end of the mosquito season. Ivermectin (unlicensed) – low dose 6 µg/kg orally once a month Milbemycin (licensed) – minimum dose 0.5 mg/kg orally once a month Selamectin (licensed) – 6–12 mg/kg once a month
Babesia spp., *Ehrlichia* spp., *Hepatozoon canis*, *Borrelia burgdorferi* (see Chapter 5)	Avoid taking pets into tick areas. Apply a long-acting acaricide prior to travel and possibly during the visit. Suitable acaricides include oral, shampoo or spot-on preparations containing amitraz, fipronil, flumethrin, lufenuron, selamectin and permethrins. The use of collars impregnated with an acaricide may be of some benefit. All pets must be treated with an acaricide 48 hours prior to return to the UK under the Pet Travel Scheme (see above).
Brucella canis	No specific control measures
Angiostrongylus vasorum	Prevent with regular dosing of fenbendazole
Echinococcus multilocularis	Prevent with praziquantel
Spirocerca lupi	No specific control measures
Francisella tularensis	No specific control measures

Figure A5: *Infections that may be encountered when travelling, with some control measures.*

APPENDIX THREE

Drug Dosages

The following table contains the doses of drugs mentioned in the text. Veterinary surgeons unfamiliar with a particular drug should consult the *BSAVA Small Animal Formulary, 3rd edition* or other authoritative source for detailed information on side effects, etc., before prescribing that drug.

Drugs licensed for use in dogs or cats in the UK are in **bold** type.

Drug	Dose	Cautions and Contraindications
Acemannan	2 mg/kg i.p. every 7 days - can also be given slow i.v. or intralesionally	No controlled studies demonstrating efficacy
Aciclovir	Apply every 2-4 hours for 2 days, reducing to every 6 hours thereafter	Less effective than trifluorothymidine in FHV keratitis
Allopurinol	30 mg/kg orally every 24 hours for 30-90 days, then 20 mg/kg orally every 24 hours for 1 week each month	Used with antimonial drugs in leishmaniasis
Amikacin	5-10 mg/kg i.v., i.m. or s.c. every 8 hours or 10-15 mg/kg every 24 hours i.v., i.m. or s.c.	Nephrotoxic/ototoxic when given parenterally Not effective against obligate anaerobes Unpredictable ability to cross blood-brain barrier
Amitraz	**Cats: Use a 0.0125% solution** **Dogs: Demodicosis: Use a 0.05% solution** **Other mites: Use a 0.025% solution**	**Do not use in chihuahuas** **Not licensed for use in cats**
Amoxycillin	7 mg/kg i.m. every 12 hours or 11-22 mg/kg orally every 8-12 hours	Does not cross normal blood-brain barrier Avoid concurrent use of bacteriostatic drugs. Do not mix in same syringe as aminoglycosides Inactivated by β-lactamases (e.g. produced by *Staphylococcus intermedius*) Not usually active against difficult Gram-negative organisms e.g. *Pseudomonas*
Amoxycillin–clavulanate	8.75 mg/kg (combined) i.m. or s.c. every 24 hours or 12.5-25 mg/kg (combined) orally every 8-12 hours	Avoid concurrent use of bacteriostatic drugs. Do not mix in same syringe as aminoglycosides Does not cross normal blood-brain barrier Resistant to β-lactamases Effective against some anaerobes
Amphotericin B	0.025-1 mg/kg diluted in 50-500 ml 5% dextrose (or 40 ml sterile water + 10 ml of 10% Intralipid) by slow i.v. infusion (1-5 hours) every 24-48 hours. Keep animal well hydrated - preloading with intravenous fluids is advisable Maximum dose 4-8 mg/kg is advised by some authors	Nephrotoxic (monitor blood urea nitrogen and creatinine and adjust dose to keep within reference range) Poor blood-brain barrier penetration Synergistic with flucytosine in treatment of cryptococcosis Poor oral absorption Side effects include anaphylactic shock, ventricular fibrillation, non-regenerative anaemia, thrombophlebitis and pyrexia (usually prevented by pretreatment with non-steroidal anti-inflammatory drugs) Lipid-complexed amphotericin is less nephrotoxic but more expensive

Drug	Dose	Cautions and Contraindications
Ampicillin	10–40 mg/kg i.v., i.m., s.c. or orally every 6–8 hours	Does not cross normal blood–brain barrier Avoid concurrent use of bacteriostatic drugs. Do not mix in same syringe as aminoglycosides Inactivated by β-lactamases (e.g. produced by *Staphylococcus intermedius*) Not usually active against difficult Gram-negative organisms e.g. *Pseudomonas* Absorption reduced by food
Aspirin	Cats: 10 mg/kg orally every 48–72 hours Dogs: 10 mg/kg orally every 8–12 hours	Toxic to cats. Do not use more frequently than every 48 hours Suggested for FIP but of no proven benefit Newer non-steroidals are safer antipyretics
Azithromycin	5–10 mg/kg orally every 12–24 hours	Not well studied in small animals May cause vomiting and is acid labile, so best given on an empty stomach
Baquiloprim-sulphonamide *see* **Potentiated sulphonamides**		
Bethanechol	1–5 mg/cat orally every 8 hours 5–25 mg/dog orally every 8 hours	Adverse effects include vomiting and diarrhoea Best given on empty stomach
Bismuth chelate	Animal <30 kg 60 mg orally every 6 hours Animal >30 kg 120 mg orally every 6 hours	Contraindicated if renal disease is present Reduces absorption of tetracyclines
Bromhexine	Cats: 3 mg/cat i.m. every 24 hours; 1 mg/kg orally every 24 hours Dogs: 3–15 mg per dog i.m. every 12 hours or 2–2.5 mg/kg orally every 12 hours	
Buprenorphine	0.006–0.02 mg/kg i.v., i.m. or s.c. every 8 hours or as needed	
Carprofen	2 mg/kg orally every 12 hours for up to 7 days then 2 mg/kg every 24 hours	Not licensed for long-term use in cats
Cefadroxil	Cats: 22 mg/kg orally every 24 hours Dogs: 10–22 mg/kg orally every 12 hours	**May cause pain on injection** **Resistant to some β-lactamases** **Do not mix with aminoglycosides** **Do not use with bacteriostatic drugs**
Cefoxitin	30–40 mg/kg i.v., i.m. or s.c. every 6–8 hours	May cause pain on injection Resistant to some β-lactamases Do not mix with aminoglycosides Do not use with bacteriostatic drugs
Cefuroxime	20–50 mg/kg i.v. every 8 hours	May cause pain on injection Resistant to some β-lactamases Do not mix with aminoglycosides Do not use with bacteriostatic drugs
Cephalexin	10–30 mg/kg i.m., s.c. or orally every 8–12 hours	**May cause pain on injection** **Resistant to some β-lactamases** **Do not mix with aminoglycosides** **Do not use with bacteriostatic drugs**
Cephazolin	20–25 mg/kg i.v. or i.m. every 8 hours	May cause pain on injection Resistant to some β-lactamases Do not mix with aminoglycosides Do not use with bacteriostatic drugs
Chloramphenicol	Cats: 15–30 mg/kg i.v., i.m., s.c. or orally every 12 hours Dogs: 25–60 mg/kg i.v., i.m., s.c. or orally every 8–12 hours Ophthalmic ointment – instil in eye 2–6 times daily	Side effects of systemic use include bone marrow suppression, vomiting and diarrhoea. Cats more likely to show side effects Bacteriostatic at normal doses, 50–100% crosses blood–brain barrier (normal or damaged) Affects plasma levels of many drugs
Chlortetracycline ointment	Three times daily	**Use concurrently with doxycycline in chlamydiophilosis**

Drug	Dose	Cautions and Contraindications
Cholestyramine	1-2 g/dog orally every 12 hours	Constipation may develop
Cimetidine	Cats: 2.5-5 mg/kg i.v., i.m. or orally every 8-12 hours Dogs: 5-10 mg/kg i.v., i.m. or orally every 6-8 hours	May increase plasma levels of many other drugs May effect oral availability of other drugs
Ciprofloxacin	Apply 2 drops to affected eye	
Clarithromycin	5-10 mg/kg i.v. infusion or orally every 12 hours	Little information on use in small animals Avoid use in animals with hepatic disease
Clindamycin	**5.5-11 mg/kg orally every 12 hours**	**Discontinue if diarrhoea develops** **Cross resistance with lincomycin and to a lesser extent erythromycin** **Does not cross normal blood-brain barrier but may cross if barrier damaged** **Upper end of dose range advisable in toxoplasmosis**
Clofazimine	2-12 mg/kg orally every 24 hours for 2-6 months	Adverse effects may include nausea, diarrhoea and renal/hepatic dysfunction
Clotrimazole	Single administration of a 1% solution of clotrimazole solution in a polyethylene glycol base infused into the nasal cavity continuously for 1 hour	See section on aspergillosis (Chapter 6) for technique
Cyclophosphamide	2.2 mg/kg/day orally for 4 consecutive days each week or 8.8 mg/kg orally or 7 mg/kg i.v. once a week	Suggested for FIP but of no proven benefit Myelosuppressive. Haematological monitoring is essential Side effects include haemorrhagic cystitis, vomiting, diarrhoea. Also hepatotoxic and nephrotoxic
Dexamethasone	**0.2-2 mg/kg i.v., i.m., s.c. or orally**	**In bacterial meningitis a high dose may be used once only and only within 12 hours of clinical signs.**
Difloxacin	**5 mg/kg orally every 24 hours**	**Caution in growing animals** **Absorption may be reduced by sucralfate and zinc salts** **No activity against anaerobes** **50-100% crosses blood-brain barrier**
Diphenoxylate	0.05 mg/kg orally every 8 hours	
Doxycycline	**5-10 mg/kg orally every 12 hours**	**Side effects include vomiting and diarrhoea** **Avoid in animals with hepatic disease** **Can cross blood-brain barrier**
Enilconazole	Ringworm: Apply a 0.2% solution to affected areas Nasal aspergillosis: 10 mg/kg instilled into the nasal cavities every 12 hours for 7-10 days	See section on aspergillosis (Chapter 6) for more information on technique. Hepatotoxic if swallowed
Enrofloxacin	**2.5 mg/kg every 12 hours or 5 mg/kg every 24 hours i.m., i.v., s.c. or orally**	**Caution in growing animals** **Absorption may be reduced by sucralfate and zinc salts** **Intravenous route not licensed for veterinary use** **No activity against anaerobes** **50-100% crosses blood-brain barrier**
Epoetin alfa and beta	100 IU/kg s.c. every 8 hours until desired PCV is reached, then once weekly	Prolonged use may induce antibodies and result in lack of efficacy Local and systemic allergic reactions may develop
Erythromycin	10-20 mg/kg orally every 8-12 hours	May cause vomiting and is acid labile, so best given on an empty stomach
Ethambutol	15 mg/kg orally every 24 hours; dose can be reduced from daily to twice weekly for the continuation phase of treatment	Side effects include teratogenicity, vomiting, optic neuritis, CNS signs and thrombocytopenia
Fenbendazole	**20-50 mg/kg orally every 24 hours for 3-7 days or 100 mg/kg orally once in animals older than 6 months**	**Reinfestations may occur** **Therapy may be repeated every 8 weeks if necessary** ***Angiostrongylus* and *Oslerus* require higher end of dose range for 7 days** **Roundworms (e.g. *Toxocara*) and tapeworms require lower end of dose range. Only 60-70% effective against *Dipylidium caninum***

Drug	Dose	Cautions and Contraindications
Fluconazole	Cats: 50 mg/cat every 12 hours i.v. infusion or orally Dogs: 2.5-10 mg/kg every 12 hours orally	Good blood-brain barrier penetration Liver and renal parameters should be monitored monthly (if ALT >250 IU/l discontinue temporarily then reinstate at half previous dose)
Flucytosine	Cats: 25-35 mg/kg every 8 hours i.v. or orally Dogs: 25-50 mg/kg every 6 hours i.v. or orally	Used for cryptococcosis (many other fungal infections are resistant) but drug resistance develops early; therefore do not use as monotherapy Synergistic with amphotericin B but increased risk of nephrotoxicity and is renally excreted Good blood-brain barrier penetration Side effects include diarrhoea, anorexia, vomiting, bone marrow suppression, drug eruptions
Gentamicin	**2-4 mg/kg i.v. (over 30 minutes), i.m. or s.c. every 6-8 hours or 5-10 mg/kg i.v., i.m. or s.c. every 24 hours or 2 mg/kg placed directly into the bladder or (in case of topical preparations) apply every 6-8 hours**	**Nephrotoxic/ototoxic if given parenterally** **No activity against anaerobes** **No activity in abscesses or necrotic tissue** **Also in impregnated beads** **Do not mix with heparin or penicillin in vitro**
Granulocyte colony-stimulating factor (G-CSF)	Cats: 5-25 µg/kg s.c. every 24 hours, for 1-2 weeks) Dogs: 10-100 µg/kg, s.c. every 24 hours, for 1-2 weeks)	Monitor neutrophil count Prolonged use may induce antibodies, resulting in lack of efficacy Local and systemic allergic reactions may develop
Griseofulvin	**15-50 mg/kg orally every 24 hours initially, increasing to 100 mg/kg orally if response is poor**	**Wear gloves when handling** **Contraindicated in pregnancy**
Human pooled immunoglobulin	Dogs: 0.5-1.5 g/kg, i.v. over 6-12 h	Anaphylaxis possible, especially with repeated administration Expensive
Human recombinant interferon alpha 2a	1-30 IU, orally every 24 hours, treat continuously or alternate weeks or 5-25 IU topically (herpetic ulcers) Obtained as 3×10^6 IU - dilute in one litre of saline, aliquot into 1ml volumes, freeze for up to a year. Defrost as required, dilute to required concentration, keep refrigerated for up to a week	If given parenterally at high doses will cause toxicity and induce antibody production Suggested for several feline viruses but efficacy unknown
Idoxuridine	Apply a small amount every 2 hours for 24-48 hours, reducing to every 6 hours thereafter	
Imidacloprid	**Cats: <4 kg 40 mg per cat; >4 kg 80 mg per cat** **Dogs: <4 kg 40 mg per dog; 4-10 kg 100 mg per dog; 10-25 kg 250 mg per dog; >25 kg 500 mg per dog**	**Salivation will be seen if this product is ingested**
Imidocarb	5-6 mg/kg s.c. or i.m. every 2-3 weeks	Adverse reactions include hepatotoxicity, vomiting, swelling and pain at injection site
Isoniazid	10-20 mg/kg orally every 24 hours; maximum 300 mg/day. Doses can be reduced from daily to twice weekly for the continuation phase of treatment	Adverse reactions include vomiting, hepatic damage and seizures (due to Vitamin B6 deficiency)
Itraconazole	5 mg/kg orally every 24 hours	Contraindicated in pregnancy Side effects include anorexia and vasculitis with focal necrotizing dermatitis. Typically resolves after the drug is discontinued Less toxic than ketoconazole Limited blood-brain barrier penetration. Bioavailability improved by administration with food Liver enzymes and haematology should be monitored monthly (if ALT >250 IU/l discontinue temporarily then reinstate at half previous dose)

Drug	Dose	Cautions and Contraindications
Ivermectin	Microfilaricide (dogs): 50 µg/kg orally once Heartworm prophylaxis (dogs): 6-12 µg/kg orally once monthly Heartworm prophylaxis (cats): 24 µg/kg orally once monthly	Definitely not to be used in collie-type dogs or their crosses and its use at this dose is discouraged in all dogs This low dose for heartworm prophylaxis is considered safe in all breeds of dogs and cats
Ketoconazole	5-40 mg/kg orally every 12 hours after meals	Poor blood-brain barrier penetration - itraconazole or fluconazole preferred for CNS infections Side effects are common and include anorexia, hepatotoxicity, depression and vomiting Contraindicated in pregnancy Higher doses are used in nasal or CNS infections
Ketorolac 0.5%	1 drop up to six times daily	
L-Lysine	250-500 mg orally every 24 hours	Preparation must not contain propylene glycol (may be toxic to cats) Used for herpetic ulcers but efficacy unknown
Levamisole	10 mg/kg orally every 24 hours for 7-14 days	Longer courses (30 days) are needed for *Oslerus osleri*
Lithium carbonate	11 mg/kg orally every 12 hours	Toxic to cats May cause nephrotoxicity in dogs
Loperamide	0.04-0.2 mg/kg orally every 8-12 hours	
Lufenuron	**Cats: 30 mg/kg in food once monthly or 40 mg (cats <4.5 kg) or 80 mg (cats >4.5 kg) s.c. every 6 months Dogs: 10 mg/kg in food once monthly**	
Marbofloxacin	**2 mg/kg orally every 24 hours**	**Caution in growing animals Absorption may be reduced by sucralfate and zinc salts No activity against anaerobes 50-100% crosses blood-brain barrier**
Mebendazole	**Ascarids: Animals <2 kg 50 mg orally every 12 hours for 2 days; animals >2 kg 100 mg orally every 12 hours for 2 days Other helminths: Animals <2 kg 50 mg orally every 12 hours for 5 days; animals 2-30 kg 100 mg orally every 12 hours for 5 days; animals >30 kg 200 mg orally every 12 hours for 5 days**	May cause diarrhoea
Meglumine antimonate	100 mg/kg s.c., i.m. or i.v. every 24 hours for 20-40 days	Give i.v. injections slowly Pain and swelling at injection site are common Often give first injection at half the given doseage
Melarsomine	2.5 mg/kg i.m. every 24 hours for 2 days	
Metronidazole	**Cats: 8-10 mg/kg orally every 12 hours Dogs: 15-25 mg/kg orally every 12 hours or 10 mg/kg s.c. or i.v. every 12 hours Doses up to 20 mg/kg i.v. or orally every 12 hours have been recommended for protozoal infections**	**Adverse effects include CNS signs (nystagmus, ataxia and seizures) at high doses Avoid use in liver failure Avoid in pregnant animals Crosses blood-brain barrier Mainly effective against anaerobes**
Milbemycin	0.5 mg/kg orally once for microfilaricide	Use monthly at same dose for prophylaxis May also be useful for demodicosis
Morphine	Cats: 0.1-0.5 mg/kg i.m. or s.c. every 6-8 hours Dogs: 0.25-2 mg/kg i.v. (slow), i.m. or s.c. every 4-6 hours	The greater the pain, the higher the dose that can be used safely Side effects include vomiting and sedation Do not use in pancreatitis
Moxidectin	3 µg/kg orally every month	
Nitrofurantoin	4 mg/kg orally every 8 hours	Do not give to pregnant animals Rapidly concentrated in urinary tract. Therapeutic levels are not obtained in serum

Drug	Dose	Cautions and Contraindications
Nitroscanate	50 mg/kg orally	Do not use in cats Do not break or crush tablets Give with small quantity of food Side effects include vomiting and CNS signs
Omeprazole	0.5–1.5 mg/kg orally every 24 hours	Do not give for more than 2 months
Oxfendazole	10 mg/kg orally every 24 hours for 3 consecutive days	
Oxytetracycline	7–11 mg/kg i.m. or s.c. every 24 hours or 10–20 mg/kg orally every 8 hours Can give i.v. to cats	Side effects include vomiting, anorexia and teeth staining Do not use in young animals Do not use outdated or poorly stored products
Penicillin G	15–25 mg/kg i.v. or i.m. every 4–6 hours	Does not cross blood–brain barrier
Pethidine	Cats: 5–10 mg/kg i.m. or s.c. every 4–6 hours Dogs: 2–10 mg/kg i.m. or s.c. every 3–4 hours	
Phenoxybenzamine	0.25–1 mg/kg orally every 12 hours	Use with extreme caution in animals with pre-existing heart disease
Phenylpropanolamine	1.5 mg/kg orally every 12 hours	May cause behavioural changes
Phosphonylmethoxy-ethyladenine (PMEA)	2.5 mg/kg i.m. every 12 hours	More effective than zidovudine but more toxic
Pimobendan	0.1–0.3 mg/kg orally every 12 hours	Give one hour before feeding
Piperazine	100–200 mg/kg orally every 3 weeks	Use higher dose for hookworm
Potentiated sulphonamides	Trimethoprim/sulphonamide (various) 15 mg/kg orally every 8–12 hours Baquiloprim/sulphadimethoxine: cats: 20–40 mg/kg orally every 24 hours; dogs: 30 mg/kg s.c. every 72 hours or orally every 48 hours	Higher doses for *Pneumocystis carinii* and other protozoal infections Avoid in patients with renal or hepatic disease Side effects include anorexia and blood dyscrasias in cats, immune-mediated blood disorders, immune-mediated polyarthritis; keratoconjunctivitis sicca and dermatological signs in dogs. Suppress thyroid function Do not cross normal blood–brain barrier but may cross if damaged Adequate hydration necessary to prevent renal crystal formation
Praziquantel	3.5–7.5 mg/kg i.m., s.c. or orally once	
Prednisolone	2–4 mg/kg orally every 24 hours (suggested dose for FIP) 1 mg/kg orally every 24 hours (suggested dose for chronic distemper) 1 drop up to six times daily of prednisolone acetate 0.5%	No proven benefit in treating FIP or chronic distemper Dose should be gradually tapered Do not use in uveitis with corneal ulcers
Propionibacterium acnes	Cats: 0.2–0.5 ml i.v. twice weekly for 2 weeks then every 7 days for 20 weeks Dogs: up to 2.0 ml i.v. twice weekly for 2 weeks then every 7 days for 20 weeks	No evidence of efficacy If no improvement after 12 weeks then discontinue Concurrent antibacterial therapy recommended Adverse effects include fever and lethargy
Pyrantel	5 mg/kg orally every 3 months	**Not licensed for cats**
Pyrazinamide	15–40 mg/kg orally every 24 hours; dose can be reduced from daily to twice weekly for the continuation phase of treatment	
Pyrimethamine	1 mg/kg orally every 24 hours for 3 days then 0.5 mg/kg thereafter	Reduce dose by 50% after 3 days Do not use in pregnant animals Folate supplementation advisable as bone marrow suppression possible Usually given with a sulphonamide
Ranitidine	Cats: 2 mg/kg slow i.v. or 3.5 mg/kg orally every 12 hours Dogs: 2 mg/kg slow i.v., s.c. or orally every 12 hours	May affect oral bioavailability of other drugs

Drug	Dose	Cautions and Contraindications
Rifampicin	10-20 mg/kg orally every 12-24 hours; maximum dose 600 mg/day. Dose can be reduced from daily to twice weekly for the continuation phase of treatment	Adverse reactions include hepatotoxicity and CNS disturbances. Some cats show erythema and pruritus Give on an empty stomach Rarely used as monotherapy
Sodium stibogluconate	10-20 mg/kg slow i.v. or i.m. every 24 hours for 20 days	Side effects include pain and swelling at injection site, pancreatitis, haemolytic anaemia and renal dysfunction
Staphylococcus protein A	10 µg/kg i.p. twice weekly for 10 weeks then treat monthly	Anaphylaxis possible Powder needs to be reconstituted and filtered in a sterile fashion
Sucralfate	Cats: 250 mg/cat orally every 8 hours Dogs: 500 mg-2 g/dog orally every 8 hours	Reduce dose in renal disease
Terbinafine	30 mg/kg orally every 24 hours	Also available as a topical preparation
Theophylline	**Cats: 10-20 mg/kg orally every 12-24 hours (sustained release preparation)** **Dogs: 20 mg/kg orally every 8-24 hours**	
Thiacetarsemide	2.2 mg/kg i.v. every 12 hours for 2 days	
Ticarcillin with clavulanate	40-100 mg/kg i.v. or i.m. every 4-6 hours	Do not mix with aminoglycosides in vitro Generally reserved for serious *Pseudomonas* and other difficult Gram-negative infections
Trifluorothymidine	1 drop of 1% solution per eye up to every 4 hours for 5 days	May adversely affect corneal healing so should only be used when a diagnosis of herpetic disease has been confirmed
Trimethoprim-sulphonamide *see* **Potentiated sulphonamides**		
Tylosin	2-10 mg/kg i.m. every 24 hours, 7-11 mg/kg orally every 6-8 hours	May need higher dosages for cryptosporidiosis
Vitamin B1	5-30 mg per cat orally every 24 hours	Suggested for FIP but of no proven benefit
Vitamin C	125 mg per cat orally every 12 hours	Suggested for FIP but of no proven benefit
Zidovudine	5-15 mg/kg orally or s.c. every 12 hours	Monitor for anaemia and signs of hepatotoxicity For oral administration use customised gelatin capsules, for s.c. dilute lyophilate in 5 ml of saline

Index

Entries in **bold** type refer to the main sections for the infectious agents.

Please refer to Appendix 3 for drug dosages.

Abortion 189-90
Abscesses
    cat bite 207
    liver 179-80
    prostatic 193-4
Absidia 150
Accommodation *see* Facilities
Acidophil cell hepatitis 181
Acinetobacter 168
Actinomyces
    cardiovascular system 117
    hepatobiliary system 177
    lymphadenopathy 66, 72
    musculoskeletal system 220
    peritonitis 152
    respiratory tract 112
    skin 207
Adjuvants 46
Adverse effects
    antibacterial drugs 30-2
    antifungal drugs 35
    antiparasitic drugs 38
Aelurostrongylus abstrusus 111
Aeromonas hydrophila 134, 138
Aflatoxins 182
Agar gel immunodiffusion 13
Alaria 134, 148
Alcaligenes 90
Algae
    alimentary tract 150
    eye 261
    hepatotoxicity 182
    skin 216
Alimentary tract 129-50
    algal infection 150
    bacterial infections 131, 132-3, 134-8, 143-4
    defence mechanisms 129
    helminth infections 133, 134, 144-8
    intestine 133-50
    mycotic infections 130, 132, 144, 149-50
    non-infectious diseases 52
    oesophagus 131-2
    oral cavity, pharynx and salivary glands 129-31
    protozoal infections 144, 148-9
    rickettsial infections 144, 150
    stomach 132-3
    viral infections 130-1, 132, 134, 138-44,
    see also individual conditions

Anaemia 73-5
Ancylostoma
    alimentary tract infection 134
    braziliense 146
    caninum
        alimentary tract **145-6**
        anaemia 73, 75
        respiratory tract 112
    ceylanicum 146
    egg size 146
    skin infection 199
Angiostrongylus vasorum
    cardiovascular system **124-5**
    eye 261, 262
    prophylaxis 270
    respiratory tract 111
    zinc sulphate flotation 11
Animal Boarding Establishments Act 1963 51
Anthrax 72
Antibacterial drugs 22-32
    adverse effects 30-2
    bacterial sensitivity testing 23
    combination therapy 23, 25
    dosing regimens 29
    excretion 28-9
    inhibitors of 29
    mode of action 20
    pharmacokinetics 25-9
    physicochemical properties 27
    resistance to 32, 54
    spectrum of activity 23, 24
    see also treatment of individual conditions
Antifungal drugs 33-5
    adverse effects 35
    classification of 33
    mode of action 21
Antiparasitic drugs 34, 36-8
    adverse effects 38
    antiectoparasitic 36-8
    antiendoparasitic 34-6
    mode of action 21, 22
Antiprotozoal drugs 39
Antiviral drugs 32-3
Arthritis, infective 219-24
    bacterial 219-23
    fungal arthritis 224
    musculoskeletal infection 223-4
    mycoplasmal arthritis 224
    protozoal arthritis 224
    rickettsial arthritis 224
    tubercular arthritis 224
    viral arthritis 224
Ascaridiasis 144-5
Aspergillus **94-6**
    alimentary tract 134, 150
    cardiovascular system 119

Aspergillus (continued)
    deflectus 95
    flavipes 95
    fumigatus 8, 14, 95
    musculoskeletal 224, 227
    pancreatitis 182
    respiratory tract 95, 105
    terreus 95
    urinary tract 169
Aujeszky's disease 72, 237

Babesia **75-6**
    anaemia 73
    blood smears 11
    canis 75
    gibsoni 75
    immune-mediated disease 83
    lymphadenopathy 66
Bacillus
    anthracis 72
    piliformis
        alimentary tract 134, **138**
        hepatobiliary system 180
        respiratory tract 90
        urinary tract 168
Bacteraemia 122-4
Bacterial cholangiohepatitis 177
Bacterial endocarditis 120, 122
Bacterial infections
    alimentary tract 131, 132-3, 134-8, 143-4
    cardiovascular system 117-18, 120, 122-3
    eye 254-5, 260, 263
    haemolymphoreticular system 71-2, 74-5
    liver 177-181
    musculoskeletal system 219-23, 224-6, 229
    nervous system
    peritonitis 152, 153
    respiratory tract 105, 107-10
    skin 205-10
    urinary tract 168, 169, 171
Bacterial meningitis 69-70
Bacterial sensitivity testing 23
Bacteriological techniques 5-8
    culture 7-8
    direct identification 5-7
    polymerase chain reaction 8
    serology 8
Bacteroides
    dental disease 131
    drug resistance 24
    hepatobiliary system 177
    musculoskeletal system 220
    neonatal infection 194
    respiratory tract 90, 112
    urinary tract 168
Bartonella 66, **72**
    eye infection 263
Basidiobolius 150
Besnoitia 134, 148
Blastomyces dermatitidis 105, **110**
    eye 263
    lymphadenopathy 66
    musculoskeletal system 224
    urinary tract 169
Blood culture 7, 121, 128
Boarding establishments, vaccination policy 58
    see also Facilities
Bordetella bronchiseptica **99, 102**
    neonatal infection 194
    respiratory tract
        cat flu 100-104

        kennel cough 99-100
        lower 105, 108
Borna disease 245
Borrelia burgdorferi
    cardiovascular system 119
    eye 260
    immune-mediated disease 83
    lymphadenopathy 66
    musculoskeletal system **223-4**
    skin 199, 210
    travel abroad 270
Botulism 132, 248
Bovine herpesvirus-4 169
Brachyspira 138
Breeding establishments 58-9
Bronchoalveolar lavage 11, 92
Brucella
    canis
        eye 260
        immune-mediated disease 83
        lymphadenopathy 66
        musculoskeletal system 227
        reproductive system 187, **189**, 193
        skin 199, 210
    suis 193

Campylobacter
    alimentary tract 136
    coli 136
    jejuni 136
    laridis 136
    upsaliensis 136
Candida
    albicans
        alimentary tract 130, 132
        pancreatitis 182
    alimentary tract **130,** 134, 150
    skin 199, 214
    tropicalis 130
    urinary tract 169
Canine adenovirus
    alimentary tract 134, 140
    eye 254, 260
    hepatobiliary system **180-1**
    immunosuppression 82
    peritonitis 152
    reproductive system 190
    respiratory tract **99,** 105
Canine adenovirus-1 *see* Canine adenovirus
Canine adenovirus-2 *see* Canine adenovirus
Canine calicivirus 134, 143
Canine coronavirus 134, 140-1
Canine distemper virus
    alimentary tract 132, 134, 140
    eye 254, 260
    immunosuppression 82
    musculoskeletal system 224
    nervous system 242-3
    reproductive system 190
    respiratory tract 100, **104-7**
    skin infection 199
    transmission and pathogenesis 107
Canine herpesvirus
    alimentary tract 143
    eye 260
    hepatobiliary system 181
    neonatal infection **194-5**
    renal system 174
    reproductive system 189-90
    respiratory tract 98, 99, 105
Canine influenza virus 100

Canine papilloma virus 66
Canine parainfluenza virus 99, 105
Canine parvovirus type 1 141
Canine parvovirus type 2
    alimentary tract 132, 134, **138–40**
    anaemia 74
    immunosuppression 82
Canine reovirus 99–100
Canine rotavirus 134, 141
Capillaria
    aerophila
        egg size 146
        respiratory tract infection 98, 105
    felis catis 169
    hepatica 182
    plicata 174
    putorii 133
Cardiovascular system 117–28
    bacteraemia and septicaemia 122–4
    endocardial infection 120–2
    intravascular parasites 124–6
    myocardial infection 118–20
    pericardial infection 117–18
    pyrexia of unknown origin 126–7
Caryospora
    alimentary tract 134
    skin 199, 215
Cat bite abscesses 207
Cat flu 100–3
Cat scratch disease 8, 72
CAV-1 *see* Canine adenovirus
CAV-2 *see* Canine adenovirus
CCV *see* Canine coronavirus
Cephalosporium 169
Cervical lymphadenitis 71
Cheyletiella 9, 199, **203**
Chlamydia psittaci var. *felis see Chlamydiophila felis*
Chlamydiophila felis
    alimentary tract 134, 138
    eye 255, **256–7**
    reproductive system 190
    respiratory tract 100, 102, 103
Cholangiohepatitis, bacterial 177
Chorioretinitis 258
Citrobacter 168
Cleaning of animal facilities 57
Clostridium
    alimentary tract 134, 136, 142
    botulinum 132, **248**
    difficile 134, 136
    hepatobiliary system 177
    liver abscess 179, 180
    musculoskeletal system 220, 229
    perfringens
        alimentary tract 134, 136, 137
        musculoskeletal system 229
    piliforme 136
    respiratory tract 90
    skin 207
    tetani 61
        alimentary tract 132
        musculoskeletal system 229
        nervous system **246–8**
Coat brushings 9
Coccidioides immitans
    lymphadenopathy 66
    musculoskeletal system 224
    respiratory tract 105, **110**
Computed tomography
    respiratory tract 91
    septic peritonitis 157
Coniobulus 150

Conjunctivitis 253–7
Corynebacterium
    cardiovascular system 120
    musculoskeletal system 220
    respiratory tract 90, 112
    urinary tract 168
Coxiella burnetti 72
CPV *see* Canine parvovirus type 2
Crenosoma vulpis 105, 111
CRV *see* Canine rotavirus
Cryptococcus neoformans
    cardiovascular system 119
    eye 263, 264
    lymphadenopathy 66
    musculoskeletal system 224, 227
    nervous system 237, 238, **241–2**
    respiratory tract 94–7, 105
    urinary tract 169
Cryptosporidium parvum 134, 148
Ctenocephalides
    canis 199
    felis 199, 200
Culture
    bacterial 7–8
    blood 7–8
    fungi 8
Cyathospirura 132, 133
Cycliospirura felineus 133
Cystic endometrial hyperplasia 187–8
Cytauxzoon felis 73, 75

Dacryocystitis 258
Dark field microscopy 5
Demodex canis 199, **203–5**
    immunosuppression 82
Dental disease 131
Dermacentor reticulates, babesiosis transmission 75
Dermatophilus congolensis 199, 210
Dermatophytosis 210–12
Dioctyphyma renale 174
Dipetalonema reconditum 126
Diphyllobothrium spp. 134, 146
Dipylidium caninum
    alimentary tract 134, 146
    egg size 146
    skin infection 200
Dirofilaria immitis
    blood smears 11
    cardiovascular system **125–6**
    eye infection 261
    immune-mediated disease 83
    respiratory tract 111
Discospondylitis 227–9
Disinfectants 55–6
Dissemination of disease 52–3
Distemper *see* Canine distemper virus
Drug dosages 271–7

ECG *see* Electrocardiography
Echinochasmus perfoliatus 134, 148
Echinococcus 134
    granulosus 147
    multilocularis
        alimentary tract 147
        travel abroad 270
Echocardiography 122, 128
Ectoparasites, laboratory diagnosis 9–10
Ectoparasiticides 36–8
Ehrlichia **86**
    anaemia 73

Ehrlichia (continued)
    blood smears 11
    canis 86
    eye 255, 260
    immune-mediated disease 83, 85-6
    lymphadenopathy 66
    musculoskeletal system 224
    phagocytophilia 86, 255
    platys 260
    travel abroad 72, 270
Eimeria 134, 148
Electrocardiography (ECG)
    endocardial infection 122
    myocardial infection 119-20
    pericardial infection 118
Electron microscopy 3
ELISA *see* Enzyme-linked immunosorbent assay
Embryonic resorption 189-90
Encephalitozoon cuniculi
    renal system 174
    urinary tract 173
Endocardial infections 120-2
Endoparasites, laboratory diagnosis 10-12
Endoparasiticides 34, 36
Endotracheal washing 92
Enteritis *see* Alimentary tract
Enterobacter
    cardiovascular system 123
    faecalis, reproductive tract 194
    respiratory tract 90
    urinary tract 168, 169
Enterococcus
    hepatobiliary system 177, 179
    neonatal infection 194
    urinary tract 168
Enterovirus 134, 143
Entomophoracetes 134
Enzyme-linked immunosorbent assay 16
Epidermophyton floccosum 210
Epididymitis 193
Erysipelothrix 120, 220
Escherichia coli
    alimentary tract 134, 138
    cardiovascular system 120, 123
    hepatobiliary system 177, 179
    musculoskeletal system 220
    neonatal infection 194
    reproductive system 187, 189, 191, 193
    respiratory tract 109, 112
    skin 216
    urinary tract 168, 169
Eugonic fermenter-4 (EF-4) 109
Extrahepatic sepsis 176-7
Eye 251-64
    conjunctivitis and keratitis 253-7
    dacryocystitis 258
    examination 251-3
    optic neuritis 264
    uveitis and retinitis 258-64

Facilities
    cleaning 57
    construction of 53, 55
    isolation 57
    group housing 56
    hygiene 56-8
    management of 56-8
    numbers of animals 56
Fading kittens/puppies 194-5
FCoV *see* Feline coronavirus
FCV *see* Feline calicivirus

FECV *see* Feline enteric coronavirus
Felicola subrostratus 9, 199, 201
Feline astrovirus 134, 143
Feline calicivirus
    alimentary tract 130
    eye 255-6
    immune-mediated disease 83
    musculoskeletal system 224
    respiratory tract **101-2**
    urinary tract 169
Feline coronavirus
    alimentary tract 134, 142
    eradication from catteries 164-5
    hepatobiliary system 181
    immune-mediated disease 83
    lymphadenopathy 73
    peritonitis 152, **158-65**
    renal system 174
    reproductive system 190
    respiratory tract 102
    vaccination 165
    see also Feline infectious peritonitis
Feline cowpox 215
Feline enteric coronavirus 158
Feline herpesvirus-1
    alimentary tract 143
    eye 255-6
    reproductive system 190
    respiratory tract **100-102**
    rhinitis/sinusitis 95
Feline herpesvirus-2 169
Feline immunodeficiency virus **80-83**
    alimentary tract 130
    anaemia 73, 74
    encephalopathy 245-6
    epidemiology 79
    eye 263
    lymphadenopathy 66
    renal infection 174
    tumours 66
Feline infectious peritonitis **158-65**
    anaemia 73
    breed susceptibility 58
    control and prevention 164-5
    eye 262
    fading kittens/puppies 195
    lymphadenopathy 66
    nervous system 238
    respiratory tract 114
    see also Feline coronavirus
Feline leprosy 208-9
Feline leukaemia virus **66-71**
    anaemia 73, 74
    eye 262-3
    immune-mediated disease 83
    immunosuppression 82
    lymphadenopathy 66
    nervous system 238
    peritonitis 152
    renal system 174
    reproductive system 190
    respiratory tract 114
    skin 199
Feline oncornavirus-associated cell membrane antigen (FOCMA) 69
Feline panleucopenia virus *see* Feline parvovirus
Feline parvovirus
    alimentary tract 134, **141-2**
    anaemia 74
    immunosuppression 82
    nervous system 246
    reproductive system 190

Feline poxvirus 107
Feline reovirus 102
Feline rotavirus 134, 142–3
Feline sarcoma virus 199
Feline spongiform encephalopathy 72, 246
Feline staggering disease 245
Feline syncytium-forming virus 169
FeLV *see* Feline leukaemia virus
Filaroides 111
    hirthii 105
    milksii 105
Filobasickiella 224
FIP *see* Feline infectious peritonitis
FIV *see* Feline immunodeficiency virus
Flavobacterium 168
Flea infestation 199, 200–1
Flotation techniques 10–11
Flukes 148
Follicular/pustular smears 9–10
FPV *see* Feline parvovirus
Francisella tularensis 66, 72, 270
Frenkelia 134, 148
Fungal infections
    alimentary tract 130, 132, 144, 149–50
    eye 263
    lower respiratory tract 105, 110
    musculoskeletal system 224, 226–7, 229
    nervous system 241–2
    nose 95–9
    skin 210–14
    urinary tract 169
Fusobacterium
    dental disease 131
    musculoskeletal system 220
    respiratory tract 90, 112
    skin 207

Gastritis 132–3
Gastrointestinal tract *see* Alimentary tract
Genetic susceptibility to disease 58
Genital herpes 191
Giardia intestinalis
    alimentary tract 134, 149
    oocysts 146, 149
Glanders 72
Glycopeptides 20, 24
Gnathostoma 132, 133
Grain mite, egg size 146
Gram stain 6
Granulomas 73
Grooming parlours, vaccination policy 58
Group housing 56

Haemagglutination inhibition 13, 14
Haemobartonella
    canis
        anaemia 75
        blood smears 11
    felis
        acridine orange staining 12
        anaemia 73, **74–5**
        blood smears 11, 12
        transmission 200
Haemophilus felis 90, 94
    respiratory tract 100, 109
    urinary tract 168
Hammondia 134, 148
Harvest mite *see Neotrombicula autumnalis*

Helicobacter
    alimentary tract 132
    felis 132–3
    mustelae 132–3
    pylori 133
Helminth infections 54
    alimentary tract 144–8
    kidney 174
    skin 205
Hepatobiliary system 175–82
    bacterial diseases 177–80
    fungal infections 181, 182
    helminth infections 182
    protozoal diseases 181
    viral diseases 180–1
Hepatozoon canis
    cardiovascular system 119
    musculoskeletal system 229
    travel abroad 270
Herpesvirus *see* Canine herpesvirus, Feline herpesvirus
Heterophyes heterophyes 134, 148
Histoplasma capsulatum
    alimentary tract 134, 150
    eye 263
    lymphadenopathy 66
    respiratory tract 105, 110
    urinary tract 169
Hookworm
    alimentary tract 145–6
    anaemia 75
    skin 205
Host defence mechanisms
    alimentary tract 129
    respiratory tract 89
    skin 197
    urinary tract 167
Hygiene in animal facilities 56–8
Hypoderma 261

Immune-mediated diseases 82–6
Immunoblotting 15–16
Immunochemistry 5
Immunofluorescent antibody assay 14–15
Immunosuppression 75–82
Infective myopathies 229–30
Interspecies spread of disease 52–3
Intestine 133–50
    algal infection 150
    bacterial disease 134–8
    helminth disease 144–8
    mycotic disease 149–50
    protozoal disease 148–9
    rickettsial disease 150
    viral disease 138–44
Investigation of disease outbreaks 59–60
Isolation facilities 57
Isospora 134, 148
    burrowsi 148
    canis 148
        oocysts 146
    felis 148
        oocysts 146, 148
    neorivolta 148
    ohioensis 148
    rivolta 148
Ixodes ricinus, erlichiosis transmission 86

Joint fluid aspirate 122

Kennel cough 99-100
Kennels
    design 55
    vaccination policy 58
Keratitis 253-7
Keratoconjunctivitis sicca 255
Kittening rooms 59
Kittens *see* Neonatal infections
Klebsiella
    musculoskeletal system 220
    neonatal infection 194
    pneumoniae 90
        cardiovascular system 123
        hepatobiliary system 179
    reproductive system 193
    respiratory tract 109, 112, 114
    skin 216
    urinary tract 168, 169
    system 179
Knott's test 11, 12

Laboratory diagnosis 1-17
    bacteriological techniques 5-8
    mycological techniques 8-9
    parasitological techniques 9-12
    samples 1-2
    serological techniques 8, 13-17
    virological techniques 2-5
Larva migrans *see* Toxocara
Latex agglutination 14
Lawsonia intracellularis 134, 138
Leishmania infantum
    anaemia 73
    blood smears 11
    eye 261
    immune-mediated disease **84-6**
    lymphadenopathy 66
    musculoskeletal system 224
    skin infection 214-15
    travel abroad 270
    treatment and prevention 84-5
Leptospira interrogans
    australis 178, 179
    bratislava 177, 178
    canicola 177, 178, 179
        renal system 174
    eye 260
    grippotyphosa 177, 178, 179
    hepatobiliary system 177, 178
    icterohaemorrhagiae 178, 179
        renal system 174
    kirschneri 178
    pomona 177, 178
    renal system 174
    urinary tract 173
Lice infestation 201-2
    laboratory diagnosis 9
Linguatula serrata 94, 98
Linognathus setosus 9, 199, 201
Liver abscessation 179-80
Lower respiratory tract infections (LRTIs) 104-12
Lungworm larvae, sedimentation 11
Lyme disease 223-4
Lymphadenopathy 66, 71-3

Magnetic resonance imaging 91
Malassezia 8, 199
    furfur 216
    globosa 212
    pachydermatis 205, **212-14**, 216
    sympodialis 212, 216

Mange *see individual mites*
Mastitis 190-1
Maternal antibodies 47
Megaoesophagus 132
Meningoencephalitis 69-70, 236
Mesocestoides 134, 146
Metagonimus yokagawi 134, 148
Metorchis conjunctus 182
Metritis 190
Microbial growth inhibition 20
Microbial killing 20
Micrococcus
    respiratory tract 90
    urinary tract 168
Microfilariae, concentration 11
Microsporum 9, 199, **210-11**
    audouinii 210
    canis 8, 9, 210, 211
    equinum 210
    fulvum 210, 211
    gypseum 9, 210, 211
    persicolor 210, 211
Minute virus of canines *see* Canine parvovirus-1
Mites **202-5**
    see also individual mites
Moraxella
    respiratory tract 90
    urinary tract 168
Mucor 134, 150
Multi-animal environments 51-63
    breeding establishments 58-9
    common infectious organisms 52-3, 55
    construction of facilities 53, 55
    disinfection of environments 55-6
    investigation of disease outbreaks 58-9
    management of facilities 56-8
    veterinary practices 59-62
Musculoskeletal diseases 219-30
    discospondylitis 227-9
    infective arthritis 219-24
    infective myopathies 229
    musculoskeletal infection 224-7
    osteomyelitis 224-7
    see also individual conditions
Mycobacterium **108-9**
    alimentary tract infection 134, 137, 149-50
    avium
        respiratory tract 108
        skin 207-8
    bovis
        respiratory tract 108
        skin 207-8
    chelonae 209
    fortuitum 209
    granulomas 66
    lepraemurium 208-9
    lymphadenopathy 73
    microti
        respiratory tract 108
        skin 207-8
    peritonitis 152
    phlei 209
    respiratory tract infection 98, 105, 108-9
    skin infection 199
    smegmatis 209
    tuberculosis
        musculoskeletal system 224
        respiratory tract 108
        skin 207-8
Mycological techniques 8-9, 93
    culture 8-9
    direct identification 8

Mycoplasma **110**
   arthritis 224
   cynos 110
   eye 255, 257
   felis
      respiratory tract 110
      urinary tract 169
   gateae
      respiratory tract 110
      urinary tract 169
   respiratory tract 90, 112
   urinary tract 168
Mycotic infections
   alimentary tract 149-50
   eye 261, 263-4
Myocardial infections 118-20

Nasal infections 94-8
Nasal washing 91
Neisseria
   respiratory tract 90
   urinary tract 168
Neonatal infections 194-5
   septicaemia 194
   streptococcal peritonitis 152
   viral infections 194-5
Neorickettsia
   elokominica 134, 150
   helminthoeca
      alimentary tract 134, 150
      eye 261
Neospora caninum
   cardiovascular system 119
   eye 261
   hepatobiliary system 182
   musculoskeletal system 229
   nervous system **240-1**
   respiratory tract 111
   skin 199, 215
Neotrombicula autumnalis 9, 199, 205
Nervous system 231-49
   altered behaviour 243-6
   cranial or spinal pain 235-6
   diagnosis of infection 231-4
   multifocal signs 236-43
   muscle spasm 246-7
   tetraparesis 248
Neuroborreliosis *see* Borrelia burgdorferi
Nocardia
   asteroides
      cardiovascular system 117
      hepatobilary system 179
      skin 199
   lymphadenopathy 66, 72
   musculoskeletal system 220
   peritonitis 152
   respiratory tract 112
   skin 207, 209
Nosocomial infections 60
   pneumonia 62
   prevention of 61
   veterinary factors in spread of 60-1
Notoedres cati 199

Oesophagitis 132
Oesophagus 131-2
Oestrus ovis 261
Ollulanus tricuspis 132, 133
Opisthorchis felineus 182

Optic neuritis 264
Oral cavity 129-31
Orchitis 193
Oslerus osleri 98, **103-4**, 105
Osteomyelitis 224-7
   bacterial 224-6
   fungal 226-7
   protozoal 227
   viral 227
Otitis 216-17
Otodectes cynotis 10, 199, 205, **217**

Pancreatitis 182-3
Papillomatosis 131
Paragonimus
   egg size 146
   kellicotti 105, 112
Parapneumonic effusion 114
Parasitic gastritis 133
Parasitic infections/infestations
   alimentary tract 133, 134, 144-8, 148-9
   cardiovascular system 124-6
   eye 261-2
   haemolymphoreticular system 75-6, 84-6
   hepatobiliary system 182
   nervous system 239-41
   respiratory tract 98, 103-4, 105, 111-12
   skin 200-5
   urinary tract 174
Parasitological techniques 9-12, 94
   ectoparasites 9-10
   endoparasites 10-12
Pasteurella 52
   cardiovascular system 117
   endocardial infection 120
   eye 263
   multocida 90
   musculoskeletal system 220
   respiratory tract 109, 112
   skin 207
   urinary tract 168, 169
Pediculosis *see* Lice infestation
Pelodera strongyloides 199, 205
Penicillium, respiratory tract **94-6**, 105
Pentatrichomonas hominis 134, 149
Peptostreptococcus anaerobius 131
   musculoskeletal system 220
   respiratory tract 90, 112
   skin 207
Pericardial infections 117-18
Pericardiocentesis 119
Peritonitis 151-66
Pet Travel Scheme (PETS) 268-70
Pharyngitis 131
Phenolic disinfectants 55
Phlebotomus 83
Phycomyces 132
Physaloptera
   canis 133
   praeputialis 133
   rara 133
Plesiomonas shigelloides 134, 138
Plucked hairs, microscopic examination 8
Pneumocystis carinii 105, 111
Pneumonia 62
Pneumonyssoides caninum 94, 98
Polioencephalomyelitis 72
Polymerase chain reaction 3-5, 8
Porphyromonas spp. 207
Posthitis 191
Posting samples 266-7

Preputial discharge 191, 192
Prevention of disease 52
Propionibacterium 90
    acnes 120
Prostatic abscess 193-4
Prostatitis, bacterial 193
Proteus
    cardiovascular system 123
    mirabilis 216
    musculoskeletal system 220
    reproductive system 187, 189, 191, 193
    respiratory tract 90
    skin 199
    urinary tract 168, 169
Prototheca
    alimentary tract 134, 150
    skin 216
    wickhamii 150
    zopfi 150
Protozoal infections 224
    alimentary tract 148-9
    eye 261, 263
    musculoskeletal system 227, 229-30
    respiratory tract 105, 111
    skin 214-15
Pseudomonas 5, 54, 60
    aeruginosa
        cardiovascular system 120, 123
        eye 254, 255
        musculoskeletal system 220
        neonatal infection 194
        reproductive system 187, 189, 191, 193
        respiratory tract 90
        skin 199, 216
        urinary tract 168, 169
    mallei 66, 72
Pseudorabies 72, 237
Pulmonary infection 114
Puppies *see* Neonatal infections
Puppy strangles 71
Pyoderma 206
Pyometra 187-8
Pyothorax 112-14
Pyrexia of unknown origin 126-8
Pythium spp. 134, 150

Q fever 72

Rabies 72, 237, 243-5
Rapid immunomigration assay 16, 17
Red eye 251-2
Renal infections 173-4
    see also Urinary tract infections
Reovirus, alimentary tract 134
    see also Canine reovirus; Feline reovirus
Reproductive tract
    female 185-91
        atrophic vaginitis 187
        cystic endometrial hyperplasia/pyometra 187-8
        herpesvirus 189, 190
        juvenile vaginitis 187
        mastitis 191-2
        metritis 191
        normal bacterial flora 187
        resorption and abortion 189-90
        vaginitis 187
        vulval discharge 186
    male 191-4
        epididymitis 193
        herpesvirus 191

        orchitis 193
        posthitis 191
        preputial discharge 191, 192
        prostatic abscess 193-4
        prostatitis 193
Rescue centres, vaccination policy 58
Respiratory tract diseases 89-115
    aetiology 90
    diagnosis 90-4
    diagnostic tests 93-4
    lower respiratory tract 104-12
        bacterial infections 107-10
        fungal infections 110
        parasitic infections 111-12
        protozoal infections 111
        viral infections 104-7
    nasal infections 94-8
    obtaining diagnostic material 91-2
    pleural and mediastinal infections 112-14
    respiratory tract defence mechanisms 89
    upper respiratory tract 98-104
        parasitic infections 103-4
        respiratory tract infection 99-100, 100-3
    see also individual diseases
Retinitis 258-64
Rhinitis/sinusitis 94, 95
Rhinosporidium seeberi 95, 96
Rhipicephalus sanguineus, babesiosis transmission 75
Rhizopus 150
Rhodococcus 207
    equi
        hepatobiliary infection 177
        necrotizing pyogranulomatous hepatitis 182
        peritonitis 152
Rickettsia
    alimentary tract 150
    conorii 261
    eye 255, 260-1
    musculoskeletal system 224
    rickettsii
        eye 255, 261
        immune-mediated disease **87**
        lymphadenopathy 66
        skin 199, 210
Ringworm *see* Dermatophytosis
Rocky Mountain spotted fever **87**, 210, 224, 261

Salivary glands 129-31
Salmon poisoning disease 150
Salmonella
    alimentary tract 134, **135**, 142
    cardiovascular system 123
    hepatobiliary system 179
    musculoskeletal system 220
    neonatal infection 194
Samples
    laboratory diagnosis 1-2
    sending by post 266-7
    serological testing 13
Sarcocystis 134, 148
Sarcocystis-like coccidia 199
Sarcoptes scabiei 199, **202**
Scabies *see Sarcoptes scabiei*
Sepsis, extrahepatic 176-7
Septic peritonitis 153-8
Septicaemia 122-4
    immunosuppression 82
    neonatal 194
Serological testing
    agar gel immunodiffusion 13
    antibody classes 13

enzyme-linked immunosorbent assay 16
haemagglutination inhibition 13
immunoblotting 15-16
immunofluorescent antibody assays 14-15
latex agglutination 14
paired samples 13
rapid immunomigration assay 16-17
virus neutralizing antibody 13
Serratia marcescens 62
Sialoadenitis 131
Skin infections 197-218
    algal 216-17
    bacterial 205-10
    fungal 210-14
    parasitic 200-5
    protozoal 214-15
    viral 215-16
Skin scrapes 10
Spirocerca lupi 270
Spirometra, alimentary tract 134, 147
Splenitis 183-4
Sporothrix schenkii 199, 214
Sporotrichum, musculoskeletal system 224
Stains
    cytological 5-6
    Gram 6
    haematological 5-6
    Ziehl-Neelsen 6-7
Staphylococcal food poisoning 138
Staphylococcus
    aureus 199
    eye 254, 255
    felis 199
    hepatobiliary system 179
    intermedius
        cardiovascular system 120
        musculoskeletal system 229
        skin 199, 205, 206, 216
    musculoskeletal system 220
    neonatal system 194
    reproductive system 187, 191, 193
    respiratory tract 90
    skin 207
    urinary tract 168, 169
Stomach 132-3
Stomatitis 130
Streptococcus
    canis
        lymphadenopathy 66, 71
        reproductive system 187
        respiratory tract 108
    cardiovascular system 120
    eye 254, 255
    hepatobiliary system 179
    musculoskeletal system 220
    neonatal infection 194
    reproductive system 189, 191, 193
    respiratory tract 90, 108, 112, 114
    skin 207
    urinary tract 168, 169
Strongyloides 134, **147-8**
    felis 148
    planiceps 148
    stercoralis
        alimentary tract 148
        egg size 146
        respiratory tract 112
    tumefaciens 148
Sugar flotation 11
Synovial fluid analysis 221

Taenia
    alimentary tract 134, **147**
    egg size 146
    multiceps 147
    ovis 147
    pisiformis 147
    taeniaeformis 147
Tapeworms 146-7
Tetanus 61, 132, 229, **246-7**
Tetraparesis 248
Thermometers, disinfection of 62
Tick-borne diseases 270
    babesiosis 75-6
    encephalitis 237
    Lyme disease 223-4
    Q fever 72
    Rocky Mountain spotted fever 83, 86, 210, 224, 261
Ticks *see individual species*
Tonsillitis 131
Torovirus 134, 143
Torulopsis 169
Toxascaris leonina
    alimentary tract 134, 144
    egg size 146
Toxocara
    canis **144-5**
        egg size 146
        eye 261
        life cycle 145
        renal system 174
        respiratory tract 105, 111-12
    cati **144-5**
        egg size 146
        life cycle 145
Toxoplasma gondii
    alimentary tract 148
    cardiovascular system 119
    egg size 146
    eye 261, 263
    hepatobiliary system 181
    immunosuppression 82
    musculoskeletal system 229
    nervous system 237, 238, **239-40**
    peritonitis 152
    reproductive system 189, 190
    respiratory tract 105, 111
    skin 199, 215
Transtracheal aspiration 91
Travel
    infections encountered 270
    Pet Travel Scheme 268-70
Trematodes 148
Trichodectes canis 9, 199, 201
Trichophyton 9, 199, **210-11**
    equinum 210
    erinacei 211
    mentagrophytes 9, 210, 211
    rubrum 210
    terrestre 210, 211
    tonsurans 210
    verrucosum 210
Trichosporon 169
Trichuris 134
    campanula 147
    serrata 147
    vulpis
        alimentary tract 147
        egg size 146
Trombiculidiasis *see Neotrombicula autumnalis*
Trypanosoma cruzi 119

Tubercular arthritis 224
Tuberculosis *see* Mycobacterium
Tubulointerstitial disease 173
Tularaemia *see* Francisella tularensis
Tumours 65-73
    feline leukaemia virus 66-71
Tyzzer's disease *see* Bacillus piliformis

Ultrasonography
    cardiovascular system infection 118, 119-20
    liver 176
    nervous system infections 68
    septic peritonitis 157
Ultraviolet fluorescence 8
Uncinaria stenocephala
    alimentary tract 134, 146
    egg size 146
    skin 199
Upper respiratory tract infections (URTIs) 98-104
Ureaplasma 168, 169
Urinary tract infections 167-73
    bacterial 169
    defence mechanisms 167
    reinfection 170
    relapse 170
    routes of infection 167
    superinfection 170
    viral 169
URTI *see* Upper respiratory tract infections
UTI *see* Urinary tract infections
Uveitis 258-64
    anterior 258
    intermediate 258
    ophthalmic examination 251-2
    posterior *see* Chorioretinitis

Vaccination 41-50
    alternatives to 50
    boarding establishments and grooming parlours 58
    breeding establishments and kennels 58
    need for 41
    rescue centres 58
    risks of 48-9
    types of vaccine 42-6
    veterinary practices 58
Vaccines 42-6
    adjuvants 46
    breakdowns 49-50
    chemically inactivated 44
    efficacy 46-8
    genetically engineered subunit 44-5
    genetically modified 44
    lack of efficacy 49
    modified live 43-4
    non-living 44-5
    routes of administration 46
Vaginitis 187
Veterinary practices 60-2
    nosocomial infections 60-1
    specific situations 61-2
    vaccination policy 58
Viral infections
    alimentary tract 130-1, 132, 134, 138-44
    eye 254, 260, 262-3
    haemolymphoreticular 66-71, 74, 80-3
    hepatobiliary system 181-3
    musculoskeletal system 224, 227
    neonatal 194-5
    nervous system 243-7
    peritonitis 158-65
    respiratory tract 104-7
    skin 215-16
    urinary tract 169
Viral stomatitis 130
Virological techniques 2-5, 93
    electron microscopy 3
    haemagglutination 3
    histopathology 5
    immunohistochemistry 5
    isolation 2-3
    polymerase chain reaction 3-5
Virus neutralizing antibody testing 13
Visceral larva migrans 145
Vulval discharge 186, 188

Western blotting *see* Immunoblotting
Whelping rooms 59
    see also Breeding establishments, Facilities
Whipworm *see* Trichuris vulpis

Yersinia
    enterocolitica
        alimentary tract 134, 137
        peritonitis 152
    pestis
        lymphadenopathy 66, 72
        respiratory tract infection **109-10**
    pseudotuberculosis 134, 137

Ziehl-Neelsen stain 6-7
Zinc sulphate flotation 10
Zoonoses
    bartonellosis 72
    chlamydiophilosis 257
    cheyletiellosis 203
    dermatophytosis 210
    leishmaniasis 84
    leptospirosis 179
    mycobacteriosis 108
    plague 109-10
    Q fever 72
    rabies 244-5
    salmonellosis 135
    scabies 202
    toxoplasmosis 239
    tularaemia 72
    visceral larva migrans 145